Oxford Medical Publications

Subcortical Stroke

Subcortical Stroke

Edited by

Geoffrey Donnan
National Stroke Research Institute, Heidelberg West,
Victoria, Australia

Bo Norrving
Department of Neurology, University Hospital, Lund, Sweden

John Bamford
Consultant Neurologist, St James's University Hospital, Leeds, UK

and

Julien Bogousslavsky
Neurology Department, University Hospital, Lausanne, Switzerland

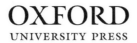

OXFORD
UNIVERSITY PRESS

OXFORD

UNIVERSITY PRESS

Great Clarendon Street, Oxford OX2 6DP

Oxford University Press is a department of the University of Oxford.
It furthers the University's objective of excellence in research, scholarship, and
education by publishing worldwide in

Oxford New York

Auckland Bangkok Buenos Aires Cape Town Chennai
Dar es Salaam Delhi Hong Kong Istanbul Karachi Kolkata
Kuala Lumpur Madrid Melbourne Mexico City Mumbai Nairobi
Sao Paulo Shanghai Taipei Tokyo Toronto

and an associated company in Berlin

Oxford is a registered trade mark of Oxford University Press
in the UK and in certain other countries

Published in the United States
by Oxford University Press Inc., New York

A catalogue record for this title is available for the British Library

Library of Congress Cataloging in Publication Data

Subcortical stroke/edited by Geoffrey Donnan ... [et al.] – 2nd ed.
(Oxford medical publications)
Rev. ed. of: Lacunar and other subcortical infarctions, 1995.
Includes bibliographical references and index.
1. Cerebrovascular disease   2. Cerebral infarction   I. Donnan, G. A. (Geoffrey A.)
II. Lacunar and other subcortical infarctions   III. Series.
[DNLM: 1. Cerebral Infarction. WL 355 S941 2002]
RC388.5 .S87 2002   616.8'1–dc21   2001050040

ISBN 0 19 263157 8 (Hbk.)

10 9 8 7 6 5 4 3 2 1

Typeset by Cepha Imaging Pvt. Ltd.
Printed in Great Britain
on acid-free paper by Biddles Ltd., Guildford & King's Lynn

Preface

Since the first edition of this book in 1995, there have been considerable advances in our understanding of the stroke process, and subcortical stroke has been no exception. The most important of these have been in neuroimaging and therapy. In this new edition, this is reflected by the addition of new chapters and updating of existing ones where appropriate. Chapters in which largely historical matters are addressed have been left unaltered and retained because of their important reference value. Overall, the scope of the book has been broadened, and this is reflected in the title change from 'Lacunar and other subcortical infarctions' to the more inclusive 'Subcortical stroke'.

The classification which we proposed originally for subcortical ischaemic stroke has proven to be surprisingly robust. It has therefore been retained, and many of those involved in the genesis of the classification have been recorded photographically during their deliberations in 1992 at a meeting in Lausanne.

We are also fortunate to have an additional contribution from C. Miller Fisher who continues his active association with the Massachusetts General Hospital in Boston and has an undiminished enthusiasm for this subject in particular.

The current volume is designed to provide an overview and updated reference source for one of the largest subgroups of stroke. We hope the increasingly broad church of stroke investigators and clinicians finds it to be useful.

Geoffrey A. Donnan
Bo Norrving
John M. Bamford
Julien Bogousslavsky

Contents

Part V **Controversies and clinical syndromes**

Part VI **Therapy**

Part VII **Subcortical haemorrhage**

Contributors

P. Amarenco
Service de Neurologie,
Hôpital Lariboisière,
Pierre and Marie Curie University,
Paris,
France.

J. Bamford
Consultant Neurologist
St James's University Hospital,
Leeds,
UK.

C.F. Bladin
Department of Neurosciences,
Box Hill Hospital,
Victoria 3128,
Australia.

P.F. Bladin
Melbourne University,
Austin and Heidelberg Hospitals,
Heidelberg,
Victoria 3084,
Australia.

J. Bogousslavsky
Service de Neurologie,
Centre Hospitalier Universitaire
Vaudois,
Lausanne,
Switzerland.

J. Boiten
Department of Neurology,
St. Anna Hospital,
PO Box 90,
NL-5660 AB Geldrop,
The Netherlands.

M.M. Brown
Institute of Neurology,
University College London,
The National Hospital for Neurology and
Neurosurgery,
Queen Square,
London WC1N 3BG,
UK.

M.G. Bousser
Department of Neurology,
CHU Lariboisière,
2 rue Ambroise Paré,
75010 Paris,
France.

L.R. Caplan
Dana 779,
Neurology Beth Israel Deaconess Medical
Center
330 Brookline Ave
Boston,
Massachusetts 02215,
USA.

H. Chabriat
Department of Neurology,
CHU Lariboisière,
2 rue Ambroise Paré,
75010 Paris,
France.

B.R. Chambers
National Stroke Research Institute,
Austin and Repatriation Medical Centre
Heidelberg West,
Victoria 3081,
Australia.

S.M. Davis
Royal Melbourne Hospital and
University of Melbourne,
Melbourne, Australia.

G.R. de Freitas
Service de Neurologie,
Centre Hospitalier Universitaire
Vaudois, Lausanne,
Switzerland.

G.A. Donnan
Professor of Neurology,
Melbourne University,
Austin and Heidelberg Hospitals,
Heidelberg,
Victoria 3084,
Australia.

A. Elbaz
INSERM Unit 360,
Hôpital de la Salpêtrière,
Paris,
France.

F. Fazekas
Department of Neurology,
Karl-Franzens University,
Auenbruggerplatz 22,
A- 8036 Graz,
Austria.

C.M. Fisher
Neurologist,
Massachusetts General Hospital,
Boston, MA 02114
USA.

J.-J. Hauw
Professor and Head,
Raymond Escourolle Neuropathology
Laboratory,
CHU Pitié Salpêtrière,
47, boulevard de l'Hôpital,
75013 Paris,
France.

S. Hurley
Department of Neurology,
Austin Hospital,
Heidelberg,
Victoria 3084,
Australia.

C.S. Kase
Boston Medical Center,
715 Albany Street, B-605,
Boston, MA 02118,
USA.

L.J. Kappelle
University Department of Neurology,
Rudolf Magnus Institute for
Neuroscience,
University Medical Centre Utrecht,
PO Box 85500,
NL-3508 GA Utrecht,
The Netherlands.

G.A. Lammie
Senior Lecturer in Neuropathology,
Department of Pathology,
University of Wales College of Medicine,
Heath Park,
Cardiff CF14 4XN,
UK.

J. Lodder
Department of Neurology,
University Hospital
PO Box 5800,
NL-6202 AZ Maastricht,
The Netherlands.

C.H. Millikan
Department of Neurology, K-11,
Henry Ford Hospital,
2799 West Grand Boulevard,
Detroit, MI 48202-2689,
USA.

B. Norrving
Department of Neurology,
University Hospital,
S-221 85 Lund,
Sweden.

H.M. O'Malley
Department of Neurology,
Austin Hospital,
Heidelberg,
Victoria 3084,
Australia.

M.W. Parsons
Royal Melbourne Hospital and
University of Melbourne,
Melbourne,
Australia.

L. Quang
Department of Neurology,
Austin Hospital,
Heidelberg, Victoria 3084,
Australia.

G. Roob
Department of Neurology,
Karl-Franzens University,
Auenbruggerplatz 22,
A- 8036 Graz,
Austria.

D. Toni
Department of Neurological Sciences,
University 'La Sapienzà,
Viale dell'Università 30,
00185 Rome,
Italy.

A. Tsiskaridze
Service de Neurologie,
Centre Hospitalier Universitaire
Vaudois,
Lausanne,
Switzerland.

P.-A. Uldry
Service de Neurologie,
Centre Hospitalier Universitaire
Vaudois,
Lausanne,
Switzerland.

J. van Gijn
University Department of Neurology,
Rudolf Magnus Institute for
Neuroscience,
University Medical Centre Utrecht,
PO Box 85500,
NL-3508 GA Utrecht,
The Netherlands.

N.S. Ward
Institute of Neurology,
University College London,
The National Hospital for Neurology and
Neurosurgery,
Queen Square,
London WC1N 3BG,
UK.

S.G. Waxman
Department of Neurology, LCI-707,
Yale University School of Medicine,
PO Box 208018
New Haven, CT 06520-8018,
USA.

C. Weiller
Senior Lecturer,
Neurologische Klinik und
Poliklinik der Universität Essen,
Hufelandstrassse 55,
D-45122 Essen,
Germany.

Part I

History and classification

Chapter 1

The history of lacunes

J.-J. Hauw

La signification d'une découverte ne peut se juger qu'à la lumière de ce qu'étaient nos connaissances, dans ce domaine précis, au moment où elle se produisit. Sa portée ne peut se deviner qu'à la clarté qu'elle jette dans l'intelligence d'une question confuse ou nouvelle. Elle se pressent plus exactement encore à l'impulsion que cette découverte donne à l'analyse de thèmes voisins, différents mais connexes.

The significance of a discovery can only be appreciated in the light of our knowledge, in this precise sphere, at the time of its occurrence. Its impact can be foretold only from the light that it throws on the understanding of a confused or new matter. It is more precisely sensed by the boost given to the analysis of neighbouring, different but closely related, themes.

L. van Bogaert, 1952

Il arrive parfois qu'un point de vue proposé soit rejeté, soit avant d'être intégré, soit après l'avoir été, et qu'il soit cependant repris par la suite, dans un autre contexte, et souvent pour d'autres raisons. La temporalité du précurseur est assez particulière. Il est déplacé, nouveau et novateur au moment de son usage fécond, actuel lorsqu'on l'applique, mais affecté d'un indice culturel de déracinement.

An opinion is sometimes excluded, before or after having been accepted, and is however agreed with later on, in another context, and often for other reasons. The way of locating in time the precursory opinion is somewhat special. It is indeed ill-timed, new and innovating at the time of it's fruitful use, present when it is used, but with a cultural index of deracination.

Judith Schlangers, 1991

The concepts of 'lacune' and 'état criblé' have been debated at length. This fact reflects the difficulties in classifying the acquired small, deep cavities of the human brain and understanding their genesis. It is not my purpose, here, to review every citation of these terms. Such reviews were performed by Poirier and Derouesné (1985) and Besson *et al.* (1992). I will discuss the four critical periods in the development of our present concept of the causes and mechanisms of these lesions, and their authors. The early relevant descriptions of 'lacune', 'état criblé' and a companion lesion, 'atrophie interstitielle du cerveau', relied on macroscopic examination of the brain. They were named by a largely unrecognized neurologist and gerontologist, with expertise in clinico-pathological examination, Max Durand-Fardel (Fig. 1.1). Another milestone in the evolution of thinking was the microscopical description by Pierre Marie, a

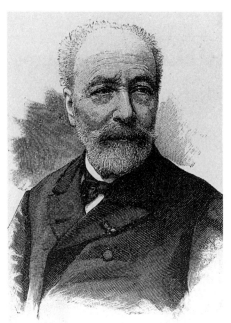

Fig. 1.1 Maxime Durand-Fardel (1816–1899). Courtesy of Institut d'Histoire de la Médecine, Bibliothèque de la Faculte de Médecine de Paris.

Dʳ Mᴀx DURAND-FARDEL

neurologist and neuropathologist. Important contributions to those topics were those of renowned morphologists and scientists, Cécile and Oskar Vogt, and clinicians and anatomists, Charles Foix and Ion T. Niculescu. Ivan Bertrand, a neuropathologist, an influential authority in his time, also contributed to our knowledge. In modern times, the contribution of Charles Miller Fisher, who came back to the clinico-pathological paradigm, and also that of Jacques Poirier and Christian Derouesné, who tried to match the previous descriptions with the modern neuroimaging data, were important.

The precise macroscopic descriptions

Max Durand-Fardel (1816–99) was a medical doctor. In 1835, he won the prestigious title of Interne (Resident) des Hôpitaux de Paris, which allowed the best clinical training. However, although he was a member of numerous medical and scientific societies, and had been nominated 'National Associate Member' of the National Academy of Medicine, he never became 'Médecin des Hôpitaux de Paris' (Physician of University Hospital in Paris) or Professor. He worked for a time as Interne (Resident) and 'Attaché' (Associate) at La Salpêtrière, but the main part of his clinicopathological work was performed at Bicêtre Hospital, where he was also Attaché. His descriptions of diseases in the elderly encompassed neurological and other disorders (Lellouch 1986).

Durand-Fardel coined the terms 'lacune', 'état criblé' and 'atrophie interstitielle du cerveau', in 1842, 1843 and 1854, to describe macroscopically several pathological entities that he separated from other already recognized lesions, such as large infarcts or haemorrhages, and from artefacts such as those induced by putrefaction.

The term lacune, which derives from the Latin 'lacuna', means, in French, an empty space. Although already applied by Dechambre (1838) to the small cavities seen in the core of cerebral infarcts in the course of liquefaction and resorption, it was used in a more modern clinico-pathological concept by Durand-Fardel in 1843. Durand-Fardel described small cavities in the striatum of a patient as 'small lacunes without any change in colour or consistency, from the surface of which it was possible to remove a little cellular tissue containing very small vessels with a thin forceps'. As emphasized by Poirier and Derouesné (1985), he identified these lacunes as healed infarcts, different from small haemorrhages and état criblé.

Etat criblé, which derives from the Latin 'status' and 'cribrare', could be approximately translated from French into 'tissue riddled with holes' or 'sieve-like state' (Haymaker 1969) and meant, in Durand-Fardel's view, 'dilatations of the perivascular space'. It was first described by Durand-Fardel in 1842. In 1854, he wrote:

> When a transverse section of an hemisphere was performed, the white matter appeared riddled with a number of little holes, with sharp edges, usually surrounded by a quite normal white matter, without any alteration in colour or consistency. They were irregularly distributed: sometimes randomly distributed in a somewhat large area, sometimes set up in small clusters, where they were more or less abundant. Their diameter varied: most of them seemed to have been performed with a thin needle that would have been pricked into the cerebral pulp .... a few others would have held a pinhead ... When they were immersed in water, or flooded with current water, a small sectioned vessel was seen getting through each of them, and freely floating. ... These criblures, these holes, which were seen after section of the brain, were thus no more than artificial openings of channels dug into the brain, each of which contained a vessel.

Durand-Fardel suggested that these 'criblures' were caused by vascular congestion:

> It is possible to consider this change, obviously related to the widespread dilatation of vessels, the consequence of repeated blood congestion. The largest vessels that penetrate the brain unremittingly force back the adjacent brain tissue by their dilatation, and lead to the constitution of persisting channels where they feel at ease when emptying after death

> *Durand-Fardel 1842*

Later on, Durand-Fardel clarified this point:

> ... the nervous pulp does not contain, as other parenchymas do, a cellular network, a kind of neutral tissue, where the blood vessels extend and divide, where their volume can be modified without any damage to the tissue that they cross. In the brain, the cellular element and the fibrillary arrangement are so loose that the whole organ appears an homogeneous pulp, without any separation between the vessels lacking themselves part of their sheath and the more delicate and important part of the parenchyma.

> *Durand-Fardel 1854*

He considered that 'état criblé', when evolved and present in the white matter, was a lesion, since it was seen in dementias and chronic delusions. Similar 'criblures' of the white matter were seen in normal ageing. 'However, these 'criblures' were rare, and, above all, they were narrow, being very often slightly distinguishable.' In the same way, in some structures, such as the striatum, 'criblures' were often seen, at any age. In the elderly 'the striatum seemed, in some cases, to have lost more than half its volume: this state, which did not seem to coincide with any specific pathology of the mental functions, was usually associated with an apparent general dilatation of the hemispheric vessels'.

The French 'Atrophie interstitielle du cerveau' translated means 'Interstitial atrophy of the brain'. This disorder was described by Durand-Fardel in 1854:

> An alteration of the cerebral pulp ... seems quite different from the infarct proper, with which it has probably been confused, for we have never as yet found it described. It does not seem due to a change in the consistency of the brain but to a rarefaction of the pulp, by a mere interstitial atrophy, which is preceded by a number of small vacuoles thinly distributed in the cerebral matter, or grouped together. This interstitial atrophy is seen in white and grey matter, more frequently in the former, sometimes as isolated or disseminated pinpoint foci, sometimes as larger hemispheric areas. In the latter case, if a section is performed at the centre of changes, it can be seen that the white matter is rarefied. We do not know any symptom characteristic of this change, which appears to develop usually, if not always, in a latent way. We have given the name of interstitial atrophy to this change for it does not imply any given nature or cause' ...
>
> *Durand-Fardel 1854*

Recognized on macroscopic examination of the brain, interstitial atrophy is tantamount to leuko-araiosis (Hachinski 1987) seen today on neuroimaging (Hauw 1988).

At that time, the matter seemed settled: 'lacunes' (small infarcts) had to be distinguished from 'état criblé' (dilatations of the perivascular space) and from 'atrophie interstitielle du cerveau' (rarefaction of the nervous tissue). However, after Durand-Fardell, the distinction between lacunes and 'criblures' was often lost. Several authors considered lacunes as small haemorrhages, small infarctions or both. In addition, the term lacune was often used to name any small cavity in the brain (for review see Poirier and Derouesné 1985). As an example of the varying and confusing opinions prevalent at the end of the century, Poirier and Derouesné (1985) quoted Brissaud, who wrote the chapter: 'Cerebral softening, Encephalomalacia' in the 'Traité de Médecine' of Charcot, Bouchard and Brissaud (1894). He stated that 'lacunar foci' were cavitated scars of old infarctions due to occlusion of perforating arteries and their branches. However, he did not mention the word 'lacune' in his two lectures on cerebral pseudo-bulbar palsy, and used this word to designate a porencephaly in Lecture No. 24 (Brissaud 1899).

Microscopic description, and the germs of controversies

Pierre Marie (Fig. 1.2) (1853–1940) had a brilliant medical and academic career. He was bom in Paris to a middle-class family. He was the student of C. Bouchard and,

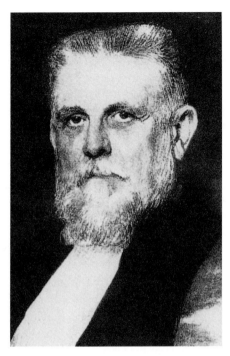

Fig. 1.2 Pierre Marie (1853–1940). From Roussy, *Revue Neurologique* (Paris) 1927, 1, 441–446/c with permission of *Revue Neurologique* and Masson, Paris).

principally, of J.-M. Charcot, of whom he was Interne (Resident), Chef de Clinique (Senior Resident), Head of Laboratory and personal secretary (Guillain 1952). A brilliant clinical neurologist, and a fine observer of pathological preparations, he had little inclination to pursue experimental studies. He was Neurologist at Bicêtre Hospital, and had been named Agrégé (Assistant Professor) of Paris Faculty of Medicine (1899), when he published his famous paper 'Des foyers lacunaires de disintegration et de differents autres états cavitaires du cerveau' (On lacunar foci of disintegration and other cavities of the brain) in *Revue de Médecine* (1901). His macroscopic and histological descriptions were precise, and the conclusions clear— that lacunes are small softenings due to arteriolosclerosis: 'from this description, it can be stated that... the appearance is that of a microscopic infarction' (p. 283). Pierre Marie distinguished lacunes from état criblé, and he largely quoted the description of Durand-Fardel. He insisted upon the distinction between lacunes and cerebral 'porose' (due to putrefaction of the brain). However, there were two ambiguous statements in this description. In the first one (p. 283) he wrote: 'In a general way, it is possible to say that the appearance (of the lacunes) is of a, so to speak, "microscopic softening or hemorrhage" '. Later on (pp. 286–7), he stated:

> ... under the influence of general causes of arteriosclerosis, the vessels that irrigate the brain are deteriorating, the nutrition of the nervous tissue decreases, an atrophy appears, which induces the dilatation of ventricles and perivascular spaces. Progressive vascular lesions induce the rupture or the occlusion of one or a few small branches, and cause one or a few lacunes,

for we know that in the deepest parts of the brain the vessel distribution is terminal, i.e. there is little or no anastomoses, so that any territory the nutritive vessel of which is occluded is unavoidably doomed to necrobiosis.

He noted, in a footnote:

> In a certain number of lacunes, what is striking is that, in the centre of the necrotic focus, one sees permeable vessels of various diameters, with red blood cells filling the lumen. It seems, then, that these vessels should have prevented from necrosis the territory that they cross. On the other hand, in some cases, the dilatation of the perivascular spaces is very marked, and is associated with changes of the adjacent nervous tissue, so it would be possible to wonder whether some lacunes could not be due to a kind of destructive vaginalitis (Pierre Marie meant the progressive destruction of the neighbouring nervous tissue), which would change the contiguous nervous tissue as a kind of progressive corrosion.

Thus, in two different parts of the article, P. Marie suggested that these softenings could be haemorrhagic. It is not clear whether these statements were the result of uncertainties about the pathogenesis of haemorrhagic infarctions, or whether Pierre Marie thought that some lacunes were haemorrhagic in nature. In the footnote, he hypothesized that some of them could be secondary to 'criblures', by the progressive destruction of the neighbouring nervous tissue.

Later on, P. Marie was nominated to the Chair of Pathology in 1907. His assistant was Gustave Roussy, Agrégé of Pathology. Pierre Marie came back to clinical neurology in 1917, when he became, after the death of Jules Dejérine, Chairman of Neurology at Paris (Clinique des Maladies du Système Nerveux) at La Salpêtrière Hospital.

Pierre Marie was a very educated man, who read English and German, which was rare in France at that time. The French–German relationship had been altered by the 1870 war, and the transfer of Alsace and Lorraine provinces from France to Germany. He was highly patriotic, severe, rigid, keeping a strict discipline in his staff, with a strong sense of friendship and charity. He has been described as follows by his student P. Béhague (1952): 'Pierre Marie will leave the memory of a simple and good man, but authoritarian and arrogant, a thought that he could rightly consider as supreme, for it imprinted indelibly on the mind of the men who had the privilege to approach him'.

Different interpretations of Pierre Marie's work

Similar descriptions of lacunes, and the same ambiguities, are found in the works of students and contemporaries of Pierre Marie, such as E. Dupré and A. Devaux (1901) and J. Ferrand (1902). However, it seems clear that two opinions merged progressively. Some authors, such as Cécile and Oskar Vogt, followed the main concept of Pierre Marie: a clear distinction had to be made between lacunes and perivascular dilatations. Other authors, among whom we arbitrarily chose the successors of P. Marie at the head of the Neuropathology Laboratory in La Salpêtrière Hospital, Charles Foix and Ivan Bertrand, emphasized the confusing parts of P. Marie's article. They did not distinguish clearly, and even confused, lacunes and état criblé, which corresponded for them to small infarctions or haemorrhages or perivascular dilatations. They were followed by the majority of neuropathologists until C. Miller Fisher's papers.

The interesting lives of Cécile and Oskar Vogt (Fig. 1.3) have been recorded elsewhere (Haymaker 1951, Kleist 1950, Olszewski 1950, Tommasi 1982, Trelles 1987). Oskar Vogt (1870–1959) was born in Husum, Schleswig (Germany). After his medical studies in Jena, he worked in Zurich (Switzerland). He was the student of Binswanger, and visited Forel and Flechsig. In Paris in 1896–1898, he studied clinical neurology with Pierre Marie, and mainly with Jules Dejérine at La Salpêtrière, and Anatomy with Augusta Dejérine, an American. He met Augustine Marie Cécile Mugnier (1875–1962), a young neurologist from Annecy, Savoie (a new French province, by election) studying with Pierre Marie at the Bicêtre Hospital, whom he married in 1899, against the advice of Pierre Marie, who told her 'to think twice before marrying Oskar Vogt' (Tommasi 1982), but gave them, as a present for the thesis of Cécile, 30 brains from the Bicêtre Hospital, the basis for the famous collection at Neustadt. Oskar Vogt opened, in Berlin, the 'Neurologische Zentralstation',

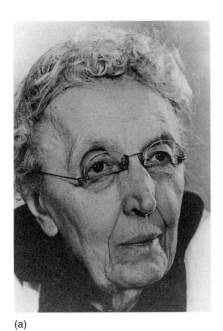 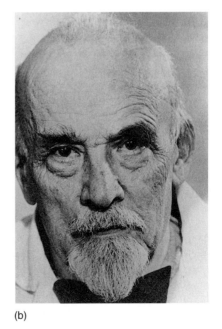

(a)   (b)

Fig. 1.3 (a) Cécile (1875–1962) and (b) Oskar (1870–1959) Vogt. From Tommasi, In: *Conférences lyonnaises d'histoire de la Neurologie et de la Psychiatrie,* (Ed. M. Boucher), Lyon, documentation médicale Oberval, 1982, pp. 191–9, with permission.

which comprised Neuroanatomy and Neuropsychology Departments, and was joined to the Berlin University, as a Neurobiologisches Institute, in 1902. In the same year, he founded, with August Forel, the *'Journal für Psychologie und Neurologie'*, where he published with his wife the masterful paper on the pathology of the striatum in 1920. In this paper, dedicated to Pierre Marie, they called 'status desintegrationis' (disintegration) the pathological states encompassing lacunes (from necrobiosis, infarction or haemorrhage), criblures (dilatations of perivascular spaces of the small vessels), and dysmyelinic state (rarefaction of neurons and myelinated fibres), which could be compared with the 'atrophie interstitielle du cerveau' of Durand-Fardel. In addition, they made a distinction between the precriblures ('status praecribratus') and the criblures ('status cribratus'). The precriblures were isolated, without marked lesions of the nervous tissue, and the criblures were associated with lesions of this tissue.

Charles Foix and Ian T. Niculescu

Charles Foix (Fig. 1.4) (1882–1927) was born in Salies-de-Béarn, in the South of France, from a family of physicians. He studied medicine in Paris. He was Interne 'médaille d'or', a very distinguished qualification among Paris residents that allowed him to spend an additional year of residency in any desired department. He elected to spend it with Pierre Marie, who taught him clinical Neurology at the Bicêtre Hospital. He became head of the Laboratory at Bicêtre Hospital and La Salpêtrière from 1912 to 1919. He served in the First World War as a member of the medical staff on the French front, and then on the East front in Macedonia from 1916 to 1919. When he returned, he was nominated 'Médecin des Hôpitaux', and, later on, 'Agrégé' of the

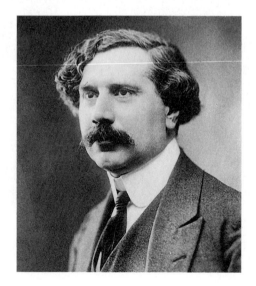

Fig. 1.4 Charles Foix (1882–1927). From Boucher, In: *Conférences Lyonnaises d'histoire de la Neurologie et de la Psychiatrie,* (Ed. M. Boucher), Lyon, documentation médicale Oberval, 1982, 201–8 with permission.

Faculty of Medicine of Paris, with the support of Henri Claude. After practising in a number of hospitals, he settled down in Bicêtre Hospital for 2 years, then went on to Ivry Hospital, where he developed a school of neurology based upon clinico-pathological correlations which could be considered as competition to that in La Salpêtrière. He was a sensitive and charming person, with a good sense of humour. A poet, and a humanist, he had been deeply impressed by the misfortunes of the French soldiers in the East campaign (Boucher 1982, Roussy 1927).

Ian T. Niculescu (1895–1957) was born in Focsani in Moldavia (Romania). He studied medicine in Bucharest with Gheorghe Marinescu, who taught him neurology, histology, and pathology of the nervous system. Following the tradition of Victor Babes in the Institut Pasteur, he came to Paris in 1922, with his wife Maria (Fig. 1.5), a young neurologist who had conducted her medical studies in Paris, to work with Pierre Marie and Joseph Babinski at La Salpêtrière. He went on to the Bicêtre Hospital, where he worked mainly with Charles Foix, and then to Ivry Hospital, until May 1924, when he returned to Romania. In Bucharest, he taught histology as Assistant until 1937, when he took the Chair of Histology. He was thus essentially more a histologist, although he became 'Medic Primar Neurolog' (First-Class Neurologist) at Central Hospital of Bucharest in 1929. (Niculescu 1992, Petrescu 1978). He was an enthusiastic teacher, and a great humanist, who later went through difficult periods of time with great dignity. He had a great admiration for Charles Foix.

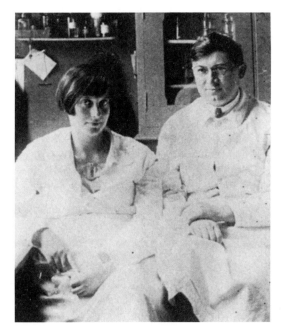

Fig. 1.5 Maria and Ian Niculescu (1895–1957). From S.I. Niculescu: *Ian T. Niculescu maestri, prieteni, contemporani,* 1992, Bucarest, Eminescu.

Although refering to Pierre Marie, these authors used the classification of Cécile and Oskar Vogt, with a quite different meaning. They distinguished small infarcts (which they called 'microscopic', even if they could be seen with the naked eye), small haemorrhages, and lacunes of disintegration, which were the genuine lacunes (and that they considered as the evolved stage of 'état criblé'). These were classified into four groups:

(1) perivascular disintegration, only seen after histological examination of sections stained for myelin, which was the initial lesion;

(2) the 'precriblate' state: this appeared later on;

(3) the criblate state;

(4) 'lacunes' of Pierre Marie.

Charles Foix and Ian T. Niculescu considered, for a time, that the precriblate state was identical to the status desintegrationis of Cécile and Oskar Vogt (Foix 1923, Foix and Nicolesco 1923); however, it could be better compared to 'status precribratus' of these authors (Nicolesco 1959). Their description of this lesion is similar to that of the 'atrophie interstitielle du cerveau' of Durand-Fardel, although they stated that it was seen especially in the basal ganglia:

> this is . . . a sort of rarefaction that can be compared to that of a tissue the roof of that has been worn out, and that would have acquired a kind of lucency; this can be guessed on macroscopic examination of the unfixed brain, and is very well seen with the naked eye on sections stained with any myelin method.
>
> *Foix and Nicolescu 1923*

The 'lacunes of Pierre Marie', had a constant finding of 'vaginalite destructive', in other words the lesions of progressive destruction of the neighbouring nervous tissue. They stated:

> . . . we will use the term lacunes only for lacunes of disintegration proper . . . . Lacunes of disintegration, as described by Pierre Marie, are a frequent change in the elderly'. However, all cavities that look like lacunes are not, far from it, lacunes of disintegration. As a matter of fact, lacune-looking lesions can have three main origins: disintegration proper; microscopic softenings; punctiform haemorrhages . . . . Lacunes of disintegration . . . . are nearly specific for basal ganglia, and far more frequent in the putamen. Any lacune-looking lesion of some volume seen in another region, must be suspected to be a microscopic softening.
>
> *Foix and Nicolescu 1923*

Charles Foix and Niculescu distinguished lacunes from the small infarctions for the following reasons:

> in contrast to microscopic softenings, compound granular cells were rare or absent (in lacunes); this is an important difference for compound granular cells are seen for a long time in microscopic softenings, probably because the pathological process is ongoing.

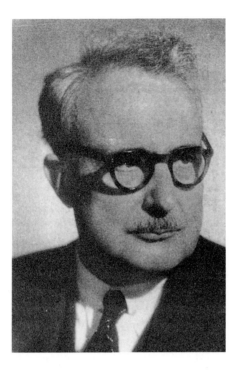

Fig. 1.6 Ivan Bertrand (1893–1965). From Alajouanine, *Presse Med* 1966, 74, 1093–5, with permission.

In the same way, the central vessel of these small lesions appeared permeable, as noted by P. Marie.

Foix and Nicolescu 1923

Ivan Bertrand (Fig. 1.6) (1893–1965) was bom in Oran (Algeria). After his medical studies in Algiers, where he specialized in histology, he moved to Paris. He worked in the pathology laboratory of the Faculty of Medicine, where he was a student of Gustave Roussy and of Pierre Marie. Ivan Bertrand followed Pierre Marie when he left the Chair of Pathology for the famous Clinique des Maladies du Système Nerveux, in 1917. He succeeded Charles Foix as the Chair of Neuropathology in La Salpêtrière Hospital, working with Pierre Marie, and, when he retired, with his successors, Georges Guillain, Théophile Alajouanine, and Paul Castaigne. He retired in 1964. Far from being only a clinical neuropathologist, Ivan Bertrand was interested in physiology, especially electroencephalography. In his book on 'The Processes of Disintegration of the Nervous Tissue' (Bertrand 1923), he clearly grouped together 'état lacunaire' (seen mainly in the basal ganglia) and 'état criblé' (seen in the white matter) as small infarctions to be distinguished from lacunes.

The modern period

Charles Miller Fisher, following meticulous clinico-pathological observations (1965, l969, 1982), confirmed the descriptions of Durand-Fardel that lacunes were small, deep infarcts. Fisher showed that they were caused by occlusion of small perforating arteries of the brain and that they could induce a variety of clinical signs and symptoms. These lacunes, he wrote, were the consequence, in most cases, of an occlusion of small arteries by arteriolosclerosis induced by high blood pressure. Fisher performed pathological observations of serial sections of the small arteries whose occlusion had led to a lacune. He described the segmental disorganization of the vessel wall as 'lipohyalinosis' (a mixed lesion combining fibrosis, hyalinosis, fibrinoid necrosis, and endothelial proliferation of the vessel wall of arterioles, and atherosclerosis of small arteries) that induced the vessel occlusion. The small size of the infarcts and their location in restricted areas allowed their identification and their precise localization on clinical grounds. Fisher principally emphasized the frequency of lacunar hemiplegia already described by Foix and co-workers under the names 'petits ramollissements en chapelets' (string of small softenings [of the pons]) (Foix and Hillemand 1926), or 'ramollissements sylviens profonds partiels' (partial softenings of the deep territory of the sylvian artery) (Foix and Levy 1927). He then described pure sensory stroke (Fisher 1965b) and the dysarthria–clumsy hand syndrome (Fisher 1967b). This was in contrast to the previous neurological symptoms and signs attributed to lacunes, which had mainly concerned multiple lacunes. Their consequences had been described as 'pseudo-bulbar palsy', lacunar gait (marche à petits pas), and eventually spasmodic paraplegia and dementia. The clear concepts brought by C.M. Fisher helped the clinical recognition of occlusions of small perforating arteries.

Several neuropathologists adopted this restrictive and clear definition (Miller 1983; Mohr 1982), which was used in the Neuropathology Laboratory of La Salpêtrière (Gautier 1976; Escourolle and Poirier 1977). However, there is still no real consensus on the meaning of 'état lacunaire' and 'état criblé', as demonstrated by the discussion following the paper of P.O. Yates (1975). describing how J.-C. Gautier and R. Escourolle showed three slides to C. Miller Fisher and P.O. Yates, who gave different interpretations.

Jacques Poirier and Christian Derouesné, however, proposed a return to the macroscopic definition of the term lacune being a small cavity in the brain. This could easily match neuroimaging data. Since this may be confusing, they suggested a clinico-pathological classification. This led first to the division of lacunes into three types: type I (small infarction), type II (small haemorrhage), type III (perivascular dilatation), with four subgroups: IIIa: small criblures; IIIb: large criblures (associated with neuronal loss and astrogliosis of the adjacent nervous tissue); IIIc: isolated giant criblures of the lenticular nucleus; IIId: expansive lacunes (Poirier and Derousné 1984).

History undoubtedly provides enlightening perspectives. These selected examples of varying opinions on the classification and the mechanism of the acquired small deep cavities of the human brain suggest that some of the controversies may come either from misinterpretations of texts, or, perhaps from the intrusion of non-scientific reasons into descriptions and interpretations. The clinico-pathological, or only pathological point of view, of the different authors might also explain some discrepancies. However, most differences are likely to be due to simpler reasons:

(1) the mere description of these lesions is not complete today—the thorough observations of C.M. Fisher on small deep infarcts have no counterparts for the other types of small cavities;

(2) as a consequence, with the exception of these infarctions, and of small haemorrhages, the mechanism of other lesions (lumped together under the name of 'état criblé') remains largely hypothetical.

Neuropathology of the cerebral arterial system is not very fashionable at present. The work needed for better understanding of all types of lacunes has to be undertaken, as it was for small deep infarcts. The advent of modern radiological methods might provoke such a challenge.

Acknowledgements

The help of Mrs V. Leroux-Hugon (Bibliothèque Charcot, La Salpêtrière) and L. François (Service de Documentation et Archives, Assistance Publique des Hôpitaux de Paris) is gratefully acknowledged. The comments by Prs and Drs S. Duckett, C. Duyckaerts, C. Hausser-Hauw, J.-C. Gautier and M. Serdaru were appreciated.

Chapter 2

Commentary on subcortical strokes

C.M. Fisher

Introduction

This chapter is in response to an invitation from the Editors to comment in general on the current lacunar infarct scene. Since the other chapters cover every facet of the subject, the broad-ranging assignment has been interpreted as an invitation to record recent personal experiences and review old precepts.

Concerning high blood pressure

High blood pressure is by far the most important cause of vascular disease of the brain, the heart, the legs, etc. If the blood pressure were kept at 120/80 mmHg, almost all serious vascular disease would be prevented. All preventive efforts should be directed to the control of the blood pressure (BP). Stroke neurologists must be knowledgeable about the practical aspects of the subject.

The central importance of high BP as the cause of lacunar infarcts was evident from early on. (Incidentally, the term high BP is preferred personally to hypertension as having more impact for patients.) The systolic BP is determined more accurately and therefore is more reliable. Measurement of the diastolic BP is much less reliable because of falsely high readings (Spence *et al.* 1978). Experts disagree on which Korotkoff sound to use as the end point. All complications of high BP correlate better with the systolic BP than with the diastolic (Gubner 1962). Systolic BP by itself with a normal diastolic pressure is a risk factor for stroke and coronary heart disease (SHEP Study 1991). Major life insurance companies now require only systolic BP measurements in determining underwriting risks; the present writer discontinued routine measurement of the diastolic BP some 25 years ago (Fisher 1985).

An important matter concerns the circumstances in which the BP is measured—at the doctor's office, clinic, emergency department, in hospital, at home, at a community health centre, etc. How long should the patient rest before the BP is measured? Preferably, it should be taken when the patient first arrives and, if indicated, again at the end of the visit. How many measurements, under what circumstances, and made by whom constitute a baseline? Is the patient seated or lying? Measurement of postural changes may be relevant. Is the cuff wide enough? A reliable judgement that the BP is the same in the two arms can be made by comparing the radial pulses. Taking the BP in the two arms is usually unnecessary.

Preferably, patients should take their own pressures at home. After exercise, the BP may remain elevated for an unduly long period. Exercise may benefit the heart but at the same time potentiate any tendency to cerebral atheroma. Left ventricular hypertrophy and A/V nicking of the retinal arteries should be noted. Achieving a reliable representative determination of the BP may not be easy.

The possible effect of bed rest after admission to the hospital is illustrated in the following anecdote. During the 1940s, the most promising treatment of high BP was a rice diet. A formal trial of the diet was carried out at the Rockefeller Institute in New York City. To qualify for enrolment, the BP had to be at least 230/130 mmHg. A clinical fellow, a member of the medical staff, related that it was 'amazing' how many of these severe hypertensives became normotensive after 2 or 3 days at rest in hospital without treatment. The conclusion is, first, normal BP in the hospital does not necessarily reflect the level in everyday life and, secondly, high BP persisting while the patient is in the hospital may pose a particular threat. While on the subject of hospitalization, it should be mentioned that many resident physicians literally never take a patient's BP, relying on nurses' readings. Stroke neurologists should remain engaged.

Concerning the matter of what constitutes normal BP, an editorial in the *Lancet* indicated that there is a consensus that BP higher than 140 mmHg systolic requires antihypertensive drug therapy (Alderman 2000). The present writer agrees. Clinical judgement is necessary, however. For example, systolic BP of 150 mmHg in patients over the age of 80 could be excepted. By the same token, a BP of 140 mmHg in a patient who has had a haemorrhage associated with congophilic angiopathy can be reduced to 120 mmHg or lower.

High BP is a risk factor for stroke and coronary artery disease mainly because it promotes a vascular deposit of atherosclerosis in the form of cholesterol plaques. Certainly, abnormal blood lipids play a role and must be treated. However, control of high BP is crucial. Some 40 years ago in a post-mortem pathological study of the small cerebral arteries, the plan was to compare four groups of cases: cases with atherosclerosis of the cerebral arteries, with and without clinical hypertension; and cases with no atherosclerosis of the cerebral arteries, again with and without clinical hypertension. Three of the four categories were readily filled by appropriate cases, but no cases qualified for the group atherosclerosis of the cerebral arteries with clinically normal BP (C.M. Fisher and R.D. Adams unpublished data). In other words, when the BP was normal, atherosclerosis of the intracranial cerebral arteries did not occur. No high BP—no cerebral atherosclerosis. This dictum has proved reliable over the years. It is likely that the rule also holds good for symptomatic atherosclerosis of the cervical internal carotid and vertebral arteries.

There is an important mechanical or physical factor in the deposition of atheroma in the cerebral arteries. First, as just stated, without high BP, atherosclerosis does not involve the intracranial arteries. When atheromoa does occur, it is deposited chiefly at bifurcations, branchings, and curves, sites where special physical forces are operative.

The junction of the two vertebral arteries to form the basilar artery is especially predisposed to the deposition of atheroma. When one vertebral artery is large and the other small, atheroma is deposited selectively on the wall of the basilar artery just distal to the small vertebral artery. Atherosclerotic deposition in the superficial arteries over the cerebellum is indicative of high BP and of a special proclivity to atheroma. Deposition of atheroma in the penetrating arteries arising from the middle cerebral, anterior cerebral, posterior cerebral, and basilar arteries requires the presence of high BP. Hence the strong relationship of hypertension to lacunar infarcts and lacunar strokes.

There has been no mention so far of the role of high BP in hypertensive cerebral haemorrhage, bleeding in congophilic angiopathy, ruptured saccular aneurysm, and the formation of dolioectasia of the basilar artery.

There should be zero tolerance for high BP. Some years ago, in closing a lecture to internists, the challenging statement was made "if a patient of yours has a stroke, it is your fault". Although clearly overstated, as an axiom it has considerable merit. The statement is well remembered by the audience.

According to colleagues in cardiology, there has not been a study of the effect of cardiac rate on systemic vascular disease. If systolic high BP is a crucial factor, it is reasonable to expect that the number of systolic thrusts an artery is subjected to per minute or hour could affect the damaging physical forces. At 55 beats per minute, there would be 79 200 beats per day; at 70 beats per minute, there would be 100 800 beats per day, an increase of 20 per cent. A study of the matter should be feasible. Healthy individuals over the age of 80 not infrequently have a pulse of 50–60 beats per minute, sometimes under the influence of β-blockers.

The mechanism by which an atherosclerotic plaque precipitates a stroke has not been studied methodically in the cerebral arteries. In the case of the coronary arteries, it has been demonstrated that a haemorrhage occurs into a coronary artery plaque, narrowing the arterial lumen further, then rupturing into the lumen and causing a local intravascular thrombosis. This is obviously a relevant matter in lacunar strokes, particularly when anticoagulant therapy is used. In a study of 20 cases of lacunar infarction, the infarct and its artery of supply were studied in their entirety in serial sections, 8 μm thick. There was no evidence that haemorrhage into a plaque played any part in the occlusive process. Usually, the blockage was due to a fatty plaque causing severe arterial narrowing resulting in thrombosis distally. In 47 cases of symptomatic carotid occlusion, the surgically removed carotid endarterectomy plaques were fixed in their entirety and sectioned in unbroken serial sections of 8 μm thickness (Fisher and Ojemann 1986). In no case was there evidence of haemorrhage into a plaque at the site of greatest stenosis. When occlusion was complete, a mural thrombus appeared immediately distal to the site of greatest stenosis. In these two studies, the occlusion appeared to have been precipitated by crucial arterial stenosis by atheroma.

In several autopsied cases of recent basilar artery thrombosis secondary to severe atherosclerotic narrowing of the arterial lumen, inspection of the site of occlusion carefully sectioned with a razor blade followed by microscopic studies failed to reveal haemorrhage into the plaque as the mechanism of occlusion.

The absence of haemorrhage into plaques is consistent with the clinical picture in cerebral thrombosis which often presents with recurrent transient ischaemic attacks (TIAs) as a prodrome to the stroke. This is true in lacunar infarction as well as in occlusion of the carotid, basilar, vertebral, middle cerebral, anterior cerebral, and posterior cerebral arteries. There may be two or a hundred TIAs. Haemorrhage into a plaque followed by occlusion of the affected artery would be inconsistent with the well-established rule that TIAs reflect tight arterial stenosis. Also against the idea of haemorrhage into a plaque is failure of anticoagulants to precipitate a stroke, presumably due to haemorrhage into an atherosclerotic plaque. One might speculate that haemorrhage into a plaque in coronary artery disease may be the result of movement of the cardiac wall during systole. The mechanism of occlusion in cerebral arteries appears to differ from that in coronary arteries.

A recent lacunar stroke with pathological study

Recently, at the weekly Massachusetts General Hospital Neuropathological Conference, the case presentation was that of a 88-year-old woman who had been living independently when she was found in bed one day with right-sided weakness and slurred speech. She was immediately admitted to an outside hospital. The blood pressure was 170 mmHg. There was moderate right facial weakness and a pronator drift of the right arm. The legs were equally strong. A computed tomography (CT) scan of the head was normal. The patient's difficulty swallowing was severe enough to require the services of a consultant. She was confused. On the fifth day of the stroke, she was transferred to a Rehabilitation Hospital where examination disclosed dysarthria, right facial weakness, drooling, choking on liquids, and slight slowness of finger movements on the right. She was mentally clear.

On day 18 of her stroke, she developed venous thrombosis of the right leg complicated by pulmonary embolism. Heparin therapy resulted in thrombocytopenia (32 000) within 24 h, with widespread bleeding. Pulmonary complications resulted in death on day 23.

Neuropathological examination, with the brain cut in coronal sections, revealed a recent pale lacunar infarct involving the left putamen and extending upwards to involve the posterior limb of the internal capsule in a segment about 1 cm wide with its anteriol border exactly at the genu. The infarct, after crossing the internal capsule, extended upwards to involve the body of the caudate nucleus, 5 cm posterior to the head of the caudate.

Why present such a mundane case? Recent lacunar infarcts rarely come to neuropathological examination, and then only as the result of intercurrent illness, since by themselves they pose little threat. The present writer was the only one present at the conference who had ever previously seen a recent infarct of the internal capsule, pathologically. CT and magnetic resonance imaging (MRI) have replaced pathological study. Yet the anatomical specimen provides quite a different dimension of experience. Imaging in the horizontal plane precludes an adequate three-dimensional reconstruction.

The motor deficit involved mainly the face and swallowing. The localization of the infarct to the anterior 1 cm of the posterior limb of the internal capsule was plainly seen as a 23-day softening which was sharply delimited. Sparing of the right leg with minimal involvement of the right arm and hand were clearly understood. The severity of the dysarthria and the presence of choking were unusual with a unilateral lesion. On carefully examining the internal capsule on the right side, a region of old non-cavitated ischaemic damage was found in almost the mirror position of the infarct on the left side. The severity of the bulbar involvement reflected old damage on the opposite side.

When the recent infarct was seen to extend to involve the body of the caudate nucleus, it was suggested that this could explain the patient's mental confusion. This view ran counter to personal experience, and further details of the patient's confused state were sought. It was learned that the patient's mind was clear during the first 3 days in hospital, whereupon she rather abruptly became agitated, anxious, and disoriented, yelling that everyone was trying to kill her. Forty-eight hours later, she had returned to normal. The confused state had not come on at the time of the stroke but with a delay of 3 days and associated with agitation. The possibility of a withdrawal reaction existed, and enquiry revealed that the patient was a social drinker who took one or two ounces of whisky each evening. It is likely that the patient's delirium was a withdrawal reaction. It is not rare that abstinence delirium occurs in persons who use only one or two ounces of liquor each evening. More pertinent here is that the incorrect suggestion that a lesion of the caudate was responsible was rectified.

The case illustrates a somewhat unexpected phenomenon, namely the absence of aphasia with lacunar capsular lesions. When the cortex of the left hemisphere is damaged, the corticobulbar fibres often carry the pattern of motor aphasia. Yet ischaemic damage to corticobulbar fibres in the capsule seems never to assume a pattern that gives rise to the slightest element of aphasic utterance.

The reader may note in this account a certain enthusiasm for the neuropathological approach. That perception is correct, for this writer, whose work was grounded in clinico-pathological correlation, regrets the almost complete disappearance of the method from the current scene. He would claim that never has he failed to be instructed by the neuropathological examination of the brain. There is no adequate substitution for seeing the actual tissue. Neuropathological studies help to prevent unwarranted speculation. In not a single lacunar infarct has the underlying vascular pathology been investigated methodically in the past 25 years. The nature of the blockage of an artery of Percheron has never been studied. The contribution of diabetes mellitus to small artery disease of the brain should be investigated. The white matter lesions, more common with high BP, should be studied more methodically.

A case of ataxic hemiparesis with pathological laughing

Unusual events associated with lacunar strokes are still appearing on the scene. A 54-year-old man while on vacation developed an unsteady gait, drooping of the left side of the face, drooling from the left side of the mouth, and choking on fluids. He could not hold a fork or a dish in the left hand. When he ran his left hand through his hair, the fingers tingled as if asleep. His left hand tended to fall off the steering wheel of his car. For the first 3 days, he laughed excessively and uncontrollably even when discussing serious affairs. The laughter was described as guffawing. His friends attributed his behaviour to an excess of alcohol, while the patient claimed to have taken little. On day 3 of the stroke, for 15 min he saw vertical 'squiggling worms' about 2–5 cm long, moving from above down in front of both eyes, possibly more on the left side. They were dull rather than bright and interfered with vision although they were not blinding. There was no associated headache or diplopia.

When examined on day 7 of his stroke, he thought he was much improved. The BP was 160/100 mmHg. His mind was clear. The ocular movements were intact without nystagmus. There was slight dysarthria. The left eyebrow was 1 mm lower and the left corner of the mouth was 2 mm lower than on the right side. Strength in the left limbs was about normal except for definite weakness of adduction and abduction of the fingers. He could go up on the toes of each foot. The tendon reflexes were slightly brisker on the left and there was a left Babinski sign. Sensation was normal, including number writing on the left palm.

On the finger–nose test on the left there was dysmetria of 1 cm amplitude with one oscillation in transit. Tapping with the left index fingertip on the thumb was markedly dysmetric. On the left heel–knee–tibia test, the heel slid off the shin. Shin tapping with the left heel showed gross dysmetria. On the Romberg test, there was a 4 cm sway. The patient was unable to balance on the left foot with the eyes closed.

MRI showed a 1 cm T_2 hyperintensity in the right mid-pontine base.

It is well known that pathological laughter is associated with intra- and extra-axial lesions in the posterior cranial fossa, especially with tumours. The present case illustrates a short-lived episode related to a right unilateral infarct of the pons. The basilar artery was fully patent. The history seemed reliable, although the symptoms were dismissed by the patient's associates. Further experience is needed. The patient reported tingling of the left fingertips on running his fingers through his hair. This is attributed to minimal involvement of the medial lemniscus. The visual disturbance was not accounted for.

Pathological laughter is a dramatic neurological event. Its occurrence unassociated with pathological crying has been related to unilateral and bilateral strokes (Ceccaldi et al. 1994). The present case would be the first one associated with a unilateral basis pontis infarct. Often the lesions responsible for pathological laughter are complex, involving more than one system. Demonstration that a pontine lacunar infarct can be causative may be important when considering the underlying mechanism.

The subject is of more than passing interest, since the expression of emotion is involved. The James–Lange theory holds that the sensation associated with the outward expression of emotion constitutes the affect, i.e. we laugh, and the sensation of laughter constitutes the emotion of happiness, amusement, etc. Yet subjects with pathological laughter usually disclaim associated mirth, amusement, or humour, contradicting the James–Lange theory. The nature of the trigger that sets off spells of laughter has not been identified. The patient cannot deliberately bring on a spell via their thoughts or even by relating humorous stories. The stimulus comes from outside the person. Moreover, the patient cannot control the outburst. One might speculate that impulses arising in the cerebral hemispheres normally descending in the pyramidal systems prevent laughter, except when a certain emotion prevails. A partial interruption of the pyramidal tracts, even as low as the pons, in some individuals, sets the stage for non-emotional social situations to trigger a well-organized laughter mechanism existing in the brainstem from early life. Smiling occurs in infants aged 2 or 3 weeks. Bilateral partial motor lesions more frequently permit the laughter phenomenon, whereas it has not been reported in the locked in syndrome. Because of their limited size and sharp demarcation, lacunar lesions are particularly suited for clinico-anatomical studies of the most fundamental matters.

The case is also of interest with regard to motor activity in general. Laughing normally is involuntary, automatic. In pathological laughter, laughing is doubly automatic, if that were possible. The activity is inappropriate, unnatural, imposed on the person, foreign. It is an 'alien phenomenon', alien laughter.

Aprosody with a lacunar infarct in the anterior limb of the right internal capsule

An intelligent vivacious 68-year-old woman rather abruptly began to act depressed. After 3 or 4 days she was persuaded by her friends to see a physician. The patient disclaimed depression and did not understand what her friends found wrong with her. On examination, she conveyed the impression of severe depression. Her face was expressionless, glum. She was fully cooperative and her answers were given in a matter-of-fact, flat monotone with minimal if any inflection or change in rhythm or pitch. There was no gesturing with the hands or shoulders. The neurological examination was within normal limits. The lack of animation bore a superficial resemblance to abulia, but responsiveness was intact. The BP was 170/110 mmHg. CT showed as the only abnormality a rectangular region of decreased density in the anterior limb of the right internal capsule without involvement of the head of the caudate nucleus.

Attempts at getting her to speak with inflection and lilt produced only minor changes. She did not smile even when presented with humorous material. She could interpret the various emotional facial expressions of her examiners. She insisted that she was in no way depressed. When it was explained to her, she understood that she had aprosodic speech, but seemed to have little or no insight into what the deficit consisted of. Consequently, she did not agree with advice that she should interrupt her office work temporarily as this involved meeting the public.

The case illustrates a remarkable interruption of the apparatus for efferent emotional expression particularly in the domain of speech (Ross 1985). It is an example of a discrete strategically located lacunar infarct creating a lesion that rivals a surgeon's skill. For the stroke neurologist, Nature's secrets are revealed in Her experiments.

The personal account of a pure motor hemiplegic stroke

When Professor Alf Brodal, the distinguished Norwegian neuroanatomist, suffered a severe left pure motor hemiplegia at the age of 62, he turned his personal misfortune to the gain of others by making detailed self-observations with the special perceptiveness that only a neuroscientist could bring to the task. His personal account of the nuances of neurological deficit and recovery in stroke and their pathophysiologic significance is must-reading for the stroke neurologist (Brodal 1973). (i) When other minor or transient manifestations are added to a purely motor deficit, it is customary to speak of 'pure motor hemiplegia plus'. In this regard, Professor Brodal addresses the transient occurrence of dizziness and nystagmus at the onset of his stroke, suggesting a contribution from cortical vestibular neurons. (ii) Next he describes the exhausting mental effort required in attempting voluntary innervation of muscles unwilling to contract. (iii) There follows a discussion of the value of passive movement in retraining. (iv) The question of a muscle sense and a patient's appreciation or feeling of spasticity is discussed. (v) Professor Brodal then undertakes a keen analysis of the physiology of movement in the early stage of recovery. (vi) Although the paralysis involved the left side, face, arm, and leg, there was an unexplained but definite change in hand-writing (right hand). This raised the question of whether the control of the motor units of the hand is strictly unilateral. This is unlikely, but also contributing was a disturbance of uncrossed cerebellar connections. (vii) Although cranial nerve nuclei receive a bilateral innervation, the marked dysarthria was attributed to failure of the bilateral supply to support the exquisitely fine movements of speech adequately. Dysarthria occurs after left as well as right pyramidal lesions. Impairment of swallowing is explained similarly. Two months after the stroke, there was an inability to shout, indicative of impairment of respiratory control.

Regarding higher mental function, Professor Brodal became much more easily tired than previously, from mental work. There was a marked reduction in the power of concentration. It was difficult to follow the arguments in scientific papers. These changes are attributed to the loss of unrecognized higher functions, normally residing in the non-dominant hemisphere. A role for depression was disclaimed.

The author's view that no area of the brain can be spared or dispensed with was supported by the painful awareness that in recovery, even in a purely motor stroke, the patient was 'not as he was'. The specificity of the morphological organization of the nervous system and the multiplicity of connections led him to conclude that for optimal function we need the whole brain. The apparent harmlessness of minor strokes is questioned.

In discussing the process of recovery, Professor Brodal refers to the earliest suggestions that there exists a process called neuronal plasticity.

The author's self-observations are valid even though his assumption that there was only a single capsular lesion may be incorrect. The stroke occurred before the introduction of CT. Also there was a history of a pure sensory stroke 1 year before

The present writer is greatly indebted to the Editors for this opportunity to share his recent experiences and ruminations.

Chapter 3

Classification of subcortical infarcts

G.A. Donnan, B. Norrving, J.M. Bamford, and
J. Bogousslavsky

Background

Controversy has surrounded the categorization of infarcts in the subcortex for many years and, in particular, the relevance of the concept of lacunar infarction. If anything, the introduction of sophisticated imaging techniques such as computed tomography (CT) and magnetic resonance imaging (MRI) has intensified the debate because the original classification was essentially a clinical one based on limited clinico-pathological correlations; latterly, the more recent and frequent clinico-radiological correlations have exposed the frailty of this classification. Specifically, it has been shown that a number of different pathologies may express identical clinical syndromes, the best example of which is the myriad of reported pathologies causing pure motor hemiplegia. The burgeoning number of publications in this area suggests that there is a real need to develop a structure for their classification and terminology. This may enable patients with common clinical, radiological, and perhaps pathological features to be grouped more precisely to allow the study of pathogenesis, prognosis, and, hopefully, treatment. The genesis of the proposed classification came from a meeting on 'Lacunar and Other Subcortical Infarctions' held in Lausanne, Switzerland in 1992. The major participants are shown in Fig. 3.1.

Before presenting the classification, it must be made clear what needs are to be satisfied when proposing a classification of stroke subtypes. Specifically, what type of classification is of the most use to the most people?

Types of classification

Broadly, stroke classification may be clinical, clinico-radiological, or clinico-pathological (WHO Task Force on Stroke and Other Cerebrovascular Disorders 1989, National Institute of Neurological Disorders and Stroke 1990). In the acute phase, classification of cerebral infarction syndromes must, by necessity, be mainly clinical, given that CT is unable to give reliable information concerning infarct topography for the first few days after the event. Since MRI is not yet routinely available in many countries and its role is still undergoing evaluation, it is more difficult to include in a standard stroke management algorithm. For most clinicians,

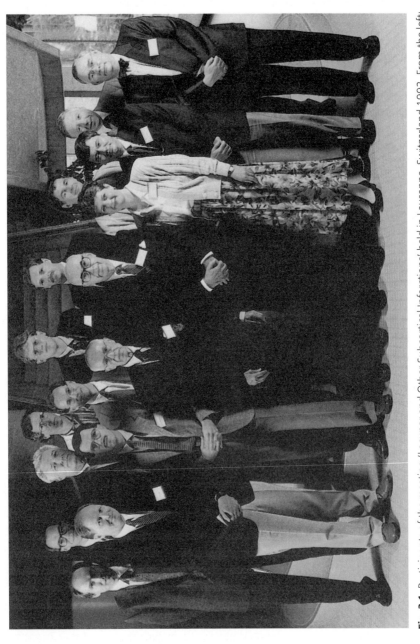

Fig. 3.1 Participants of the meeting 'Lacunar and Other Subcortical Infarctions' held in Lausanne, Switzerland 1992. From the left: J.M. Bamford, C. Weiler, G.A. Donnan, F. Regli, J. Bogousslavsky, C.P. Warlow, B. Norrving, C.H. Millikan, J. Boiten (rear), B.R. Chambers (rear), C.M. Fisher, C.M. Helgason, M. Hommel, J.J. Hauw, L.R. Caplan, J.P. Mohr.

therefore, only a clinical classification of ischaemic stroke subtypes is possible during this early period and may be the only practical one to adopt for patient entry into acute trials of therapy. For example, in the Australian Streptokinase Trial (ASK) where trial entry is restricted to ischaemic stroke occurring within the preceding 4 h (with CT scan used to exclude haemorrhage), patients are classified as hemispheric, subcortical, or brainstem, depending on the presence or absence of cortical or brainstem signs (Donnan et al. 1993). In the Oxfordshire Community Stroke Project, the clinical classification of partial anterior cerebral infarcts (PACIs) total anterior cerebral infarction (TACI), lacunar infarcts (LACIs), and posterior cerebral infarcts (POCIs) was used (Bamford et al. 1991). This is practical classification for clinical trial entry in that each clinical pattern has an expected outcome based on epidemiological studies. However, the distinction of subcortical infarct types requires a more refined approach and greater certainty of diagnosis. Hence the concept of when the diagnosis is made (within the first few days or later) becomes important, because with increasing time from the stroke and introduction of other diagnostic modalities, the degree of certainty of diagnosis increases.

For example, it is well recognized that the clinical expression of the lacunar syndrome of pure motor hemiplegia may result from either a single penetrator territory infarct, a restricted striatocapsular infarct (with no cortical signs), or a restricted infarct in the territory of the anterior choroidal artery (again without cortical signs). While the latter two radiological correlates of a lacunar syndrome probably are uncommon, their recognition is important because their pathogenesis is quite different from that of single penetrator territory infarction. Striatocapsular infarcts are most frequently the result of emboli from the heart or carotid vessels (Bladin and Berkovic 1984, Donnan et al. 1991), the mechanism of anterior choroidal artery territory and thalamic infarcts are varied and poorly understood (Helgason et al. 1986, Bougousslavsky et al. 1988a), whereas single penetrator territory infarcts are generally considered to be due to in situ vessel disease (Bamford and Warlow 1988). Hence the confirmation of the involvement of a single penetrator on CT scan (or MRI) may increase the certainty of diagnosis of a true lacunar infarct and its underlying mechanism of development. A further degree of certainty concerning the mechanism of infarction may be achieved by the use of other investigative techniques such as ultrasonography (carotid and cardiac). Because of these issues, it was felt that the classification should be a clinico-radiological one.

In order to make the classification robust enough to allow expansion in future years to include infarct patterns not yet described (with related clinical features) and also to account for the obvious fact that ischaemic stroke syndromes must relate to arterial territories, the classification has been based on arterial anatomy; this applied to sections of the brain supplied by named arteries and the borderzones between them (Bogousslavsky 1992). Notes have been provided to enable this chapter to act as a ready reference to the usual or more commonly seen clinical expression of the radiological features. In no way should it be regarded as an exhaustive list of the complete range of clinical expressions of each infarct type, but is designed to help house officers, physicians, radiologists, and others to refer quickly to the commonly expected clinico-radiological associations they may have under consideration.

A final word needs to be said about 'lacunar syndromes'. As stated in a review (Bogousslavsky 1992), the sensitivity and specificity of the clinical syndrome need to be established. If the term is to be retained, it should be restricted to a clinical situation where the mechanism of infarction involves transient or permanent occlusion of a single penetrating artery with a high degree of probability. A clinico-radiological definition may be the most precise one, and, given the increasing availability of MRI (Hommel *et al.* 1990), ultimately realistic. The use of the term 'lacune' as a purely radiological phenomenon, as is currently practised by many of our radiological colleagues, should be actively discouraged since, in many instances, it undoubtedly leads less aware clinicians down an inappropriate management pathway. In general, radiological descriptions of infarct patterns need to be couched in neutral pathophysiological terms so that the clinician is left to draw his or her own conclusions concerning the mechanism of infarction based on recognized clinico-radiological association and other information. It is hoped that this chaper will facilitate this process.

Subcortical cerebral infarction: classification and terminology

This classification is divided into two sections. Section A is a broad framework which has the potential to accommodate later clinical and radiological descriptions as they are developed. Currently well-described clinical syndromes are marked with an asterisk and are discussed in more detail in Section B.

Section A: Classification based on arterial territory

A. Infarcts in the territories of deep perforators

1. Middle cerebral artery

    (a) Presumed single perforator involvement (lacunar infarct)*

    (b) Multiple perforator involvement

    (i) Striatocapsular*

    (ii) Extended large subcortical*

2. Anterior choroidal artery

    (a) Presumed single perforator (lacunar infarct)*

    (b) Multiple perforators*

Section A: Classification based on arterial territory (*continued*)

  3. Anterior cerebral artery

    (a) Presumed single perforator (lacunar infarct)*

    (b) Multiple perforators

  4. Posterior communicating artery

  5. Posterior cerebral artery

B. Infarcts in the territories of superficial perforators*
   [White matter medullary branches from the superficial pial (cerebral) arteries]

C. Borderzone infarcts between A and B

    (a) Confluent (total)*

    (b) Non-confluent (partial)*

D. Other infarcts including combinations of A, B, and C and the concept of leukoariosis*

E. Unclassified infarcts

Section B: Notes on specific syndromes*

1. Presumed single perforator artery territory infarcts (lacunar infarcts)

(1) *Location:* commonly internal capsule, striatum, or thalamus.

(2) *Mechanism:* small vessel disease, the precise nature of which remains uncertain since few cases have been studied pathologically. Described phenomena include lipohyalinosis secondary to the effects of hypertension, *in situ* atheroma either at the mouth or along the length of the penetrating vessel. Emboli from large vessels or heart thought to be uncommon, but frequency is uncertain.

(3) *Clinical features:* there are five recognized classical (lacunar) syndromes:

    (a) pure motor hemiparesis;

    (b) sensorimotor stroke;

    (c) pure sensory stroke;

    (d) dysarthria clumsy hand syndrome;

    (e) ataxic hemiparesis. Face, arm, and leg involvement are characteristic for (a), (b), and (c). The most important clinical feature is the absence of cognitive symptoms or signs (except in the case of thalamic infarcts). Other clinical presentations have been described but are less specific for single perforator territory infarction *per se.*

(4) *CT/MRI appearance:* small circular or oval changes <1.5 cm diameter (approximately). In a substantial proportion of cases, CT may be negative which may suggest the presence of a brainstem lacunar infarct.

2. Striatocapsular infarcts

(1) *Location:* caudate, anterior of limb of internal capsule, putamen.

(2) *Mechanism:* middle cerebral artery origin occlusion due to embolus (cardiac or internal carotid artery origin), middle cerebral artery pathology (atheroma, arteritis, dissection), other mechanisms uncertain.

(3) *Clinical features:* hemiparesis with neuropsychological dysfunction, arm weakness greater than face or leg. Occasionally cortical signs may be minimum or absent.

(4) *Subtypes:*

   (a) caudate head;

   (b) caudatocapsular;

   (c) putamental;

   (d) putamenocapsular.

(5) *CT/MRI appearance:* comma-shaped changes in the striatum.

3. Internal borderzone infarcts (subcortical junctional infarcts)

(1) *Location:* paraventricular region, high internal capsule.

(2) *Mechanism:* distal middle cerebral artery occlusion (beyond perforating vessels and before bifurcation), severe extracranial carotid occlusive disease. Anterior and posterior subtypes may be due to occlusion of superior or inferior divisional branches of the middle cerebral artery, but this remains to be proven.

(3) *Clinical features:* usually varying degrees of hemiparesis with hemisphere-specific neuropsychological dysfunction.

(4) *Subtypes:*

   (a) Confluent internal borderzone infarct:

      (i) anterior

      (ii) posterior

      (iii) total

    (b) Partial internal borderzone infarct (non-confluent):

       (i) anterior

       (ii) posterior

       (iii) total

(5) *CT appearance:* confluent or non-confluent hypodensity in periventricular region.

4. Anterior choroidal arterial territory infarcts

(1) *Location:* low internal capsule, medial globus pallidus.

(2) *Mechanism:* uncertain. Perhaps *in situ* disease of vessel (smaller infarcts), or embolism (larger infarcts).

(3) *Clinical features:* hemiparesis, hemianaesthesia, hemianopia, or a combination of these. Neuropsychological dysfunction may be a feature of larger infarcts.

(4) *CT/MRI appearance:* changes of oval shape in low internal capsule encompassing the territory of more than a single perforator territory.

5. Thalamic infarcts

(1) *Location:* thalamic regions.

(2) *Mechanism: in situ* disease of small vessel or mouth of parent artery, cardioembolism (paramedian territory), other causes are rare.

(3) *Subtypes (dependent on arterial territory):* tuberothalamic, posterior thalamo-subthalamic paramedian, thalamogeniculate pedicle, posterior choroidal.

(4) *Clinical features:* a variety of syndromes with moderate motor and sensory signs, memory impairment, dysphasia if the left thalmus involved, neglect if right involved. Additional distinguishing features include: confusion, behavioural changes, and eye movement disorders (posterior thalamo-subthalamic paramedian artery); contralateral ataxia (thalamogeniculate pedical). Posterior choroidal artery infarcts may produce an isolated homonymous horizontal sectoranopia.

(5) *MRI appearance:* small circular or oval-shaped changes in the thalamus.

6. White matter medullary infarcts

(1) *Location:* centrum semiovale, external/extreme capsule (territory of the medullary penetrators from the pial middle cerebral artery system).

Section B: Notes on specific syndromes* (*continued*)

(2) *Mechanism:* uncertain, but most probably larger infarcts due to embolism (heart to artery, or artery to artery) and smaller infarcts due to *in situ* small vessel disease.

(3) *Clinical features:* small infarcts may cause a partial hemiparesis including single limb involvement. Larger infarcts have similar clinical expressions to pial middle cerebral artery territory infarcts.

(4) *CT/MRI appearance:* circular/oval shape in the centrum semiovale/external extreme capsular region.

7. Extended large subcortical infarcts

(1) *Location:* hemispheric white matter/internal capsule/basal ganglia.

(2) *Mechanism:* large vessel disease (internal carotid and/or middle cerebral artery occlusion).

(3) *Clinical features:* same as large middle cerebral artery territory infarct with dense hemiplegia and neuropsychology dysfunction appropriate to the affected hemisphere.

(4) *CT/MRI appearance:* extended involvement of hemispheric white matter and basal ganglia with cortical sparing.

8. Leukoariosis

(1) *Location:* periventricular region (lateral ventricles) and centrum semiovale.

(2) *Mechanism:* uncertain. Hypertensive mechanisms may be involved.

(3) *Clinical features:* presumed cognitive decline or asymptomatic.

(4) *CT/MRI appearance:* involvement of periventricular and central core of hemispheric white matter.

Part II

Pathology and neurochemistry of subcortical strokes

Chapter 4

Pathology of lacunar infarction

G.A. Lammie

Introduction

Autopsy is often expected to reveal the precise nature, extent, and underlying cause of a disease, resolving the diagnostic uncertainties so common during life. However, autopsy conclusions may be limited by, amongst other things, a lack of clinical information (e.g. a history of atrial fibrillation), the fleeting nature of some pathologies (such as lysed thromboemboli), the possibility of sampling errors (small lesions in large organs, as well as in inaccessible lesions such as small or intra-osseous vessels), even on occasion an embarrassment of pathological riches (multiple potential sources of emboli), and, importantly, the difficulty of inferring mechanism from morphology. A pathological diagnosis may be, therefore, as subjective and inferential as the clinical, and cause is often best couched in terms of probabilities.

Nevertheless, pathological studies have been pivotal to our current understanding of lacunar infarction. In this chapter, I review this contribution, clarify the limitations inherent in a traditional autopsy-based approach, and suggest possible avenues of future pathological research.

Pathology of the brain lesion

The low case fatality rate of lacunar infarction (Bamford *et al.* 1987) means that most autopsy lesions are old, healed cavities, by definition small in size and located deep within the brain. The imprecision of the terms 'small' and 'deep', and the variety of causes of a brain cavity have generated semantic arguments about the definition and usefulness of the term 'lacune'. It is important, therefore, that the pathologist should carefully document the number of lesions, their size, location, and microscopic appearance, qualifying any use of the term 'lacune'. In 1984, Poirier and Derouesne provided a neuropathological classification of 'lacunes' which remains useful: Type I lacunes are irregular cavities, containing variable amounts of degenerate brain parenchyma, lipid-laden macrophages, and blood vessels, surrounded by a rim of gliotic, sometimes rarefied brain (Fig. 4.1a). The histological features of developing and healed lesions are comparable with those seen in large vessel and cortical infarcts. This observation, together with the demonstration in some cases of an occluded feeding artery, underlies the assumption that these cavities represent old, small

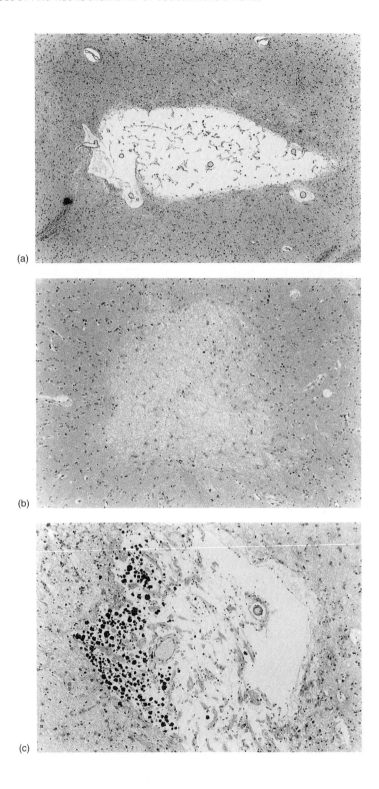

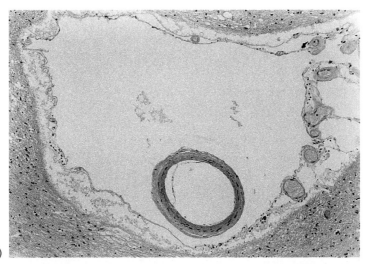

(d)

Fig. 4.1 Pathological types of lacune. (a) A small, old type I lacune containing fragments of gliovascular tissue, occasional macrophages, and blood vessels. (b) An incomplete lacunar infarct (so-called type Ib lacune), comprising a well-defined focus of rarefaction, gliosis, and hypocellularity. The lesion is devoid of neurons and oligodendroglia, but is not cavitated. (c) An irregular cavity containing numerous haemosiderin-laden macrophages (left), as well as tissue debris and blood vessels. This is more likely to represent an old haemorrhagic infarct than an old, deep-seated microhaemorrhage (type II lacune). (d) A modestly diltaed perivascular space (type III lacune) with a lining layer of flattened epithelial-like cells. There is no evidence of previous tissue destruction within the cavity, which contains a histologically normal vessel.

infarcts. This type of lacune is, numerically and clinically, the most significant, and has been reported in 6–11 per cent of selected autopsy brain series (Fisher 1965*a*, Tuszynski *et al.* 1989).

A variant type I lacune has been described (Lammie *et al.* 1998), which is characterized by loss of only selectively vulnerable cellular elements, falling short of coagulative pan-necrosis with cavitation. This so-called 'incomplete' lacunar infarct (Fig. 4.1b) mirrors its fully cavitated counterpart in size, shape, and distribution, suggesting a common underlying cause (i.e. arterial obstruction), but perhaps of shorter duration and/or lesser severity (Lassen 1982). There has been suggestion that these lesions are caused by the effects of oedema ('oedema-related gliosis') rather than being primarily ischaemic in origin (Ma and Olsson 1993, 1997). Whilst not denying the possible importance of oedema-mediated tissue damage in any brain infarct, the available evidence suggests that type I lacunes should be regarded as infarcts, either 'complete' or 'incomplete' (Lammie 1998).

Type II lacunes are similar in size and distribution to type I, but are distinguished by the presence of numerous haemosiderin-laden macrophages (Fig. 4.1c). That these represent old, small haemorrhages (Poirier and Derouesnse 1984) and are therefore distinct from type I lesions is perhaps questionable. Many, perhaps the majority, of cerebral infarcts of any size have at least some haemorrhagic component microscopically, and it seems likely that many blood-stained cavities are old, haemorrhagic microinfarcts. Perivascular red cell extravasation and haemosiderin deposits, often associated with dilated perivascular spaces but not necessarily with brain cavitation, are also common in aged brains. Overall, although incidental acute microhaemorrhages are occasionally found in deep grey nuclei at autopsy, as a pathologically verified cause of a lacunar syndrome they must be considered a rarity.

Type III lacunes are dilatations of the perivascular (Virchow–Robin) space, rounded and regular in profile, surrounded by a single layer of epithelial-like cells and by compressed or mildly gliotic brain, often with corpora amylacea (Fig. 4.1d). They usually contain one or more segments of a normal artery. Four variants of dilated perivascular space have been described, based on their number and volume (Poirier and Derouesne 1984). Their cause has been ascribed variously to arterial wall permeability or interstitial fluid drainage disorders (Benhaiem-Sigaux *et al.* 1987, Derouesne *et al.* 1987, Pollock *et al.* 1997), to cerebral atrophy (Van Swieten *et al.* 1991), to mechanical stress from pulsating arterioles (Hughes 1965), as well as to perivascular inflammatory (Marie 1901) or other unspecified 'lytic' agents (Moore 1954). The clinical significance of type III lacunes is apparently restricted to their radiological distinction from small infarcts, and to rare documented examples of 'expanding' lacunes which behave as space-occupying lesions (Poirier 1983, Benhaiem-Sigaux *et al.* 1987, Derouesne *et al.* 1987).

In summary, small, deep brain cavities may have more than one pathological substrate. The most significant clinically are infarcts, pathological investigation into the cause of which is now discussed.

Pathology of the vessel lesion

From the vantage point of the 21st century, it is difficult to overestimate the importance of C.M. Fisher's clinico-pathological studies of lacunes, which he began in the middle of the 20th century (Fisher 1965*a*). By meticulous serial section autopsy reconstructions of the vascular supply to a total of 68 lacunar infarcts in 18 brains, he demonstrated that the majority appeared to be caused by two types of arterial pathology, namely intracranial atherosclerosis and so-called 'segmental arterial disorganization' or 'lipohyalinosis' (Fisher 1969, 1977, 1978*a*, 1979, Fisher and Caplan 1971, Fisher and Tapia 1987). This body of work remains the cornerstone of our current understanding of lacunar infarct pathogenesis (Fisher 1982, 1991). Much of the controversy his research generated relates to terminological semantics and to flawed interpretation of, and unwarranted extrapolation from, his observations, very often by those with little or no neuropathological experience. Certainly, there have been no convincing pathological data since which seriously challenge his conclusions and, although the relative importance of atherosclerosis and 'lipohyalinosis' in the present era of controlled hypertension may have changed, they remain the chief suspects. They form the pathological basis of the so-called 'lacunar hypothesis', which subsequently has received widespread, if not universal, clinical and epidemiological support.

Atherosclerosis

In Fisher's series, intracranial atherosclerosis affecting arteries 200–800 μm in diameter caused larger (5 mm or more in diameter), more often symptomatic, lacunar infarcts than did lipohyalinosis. He identified stenotic or occlusive plaques, either in the proximal portion of the relevant perforating artery ('microatheroma'), at its origin ('junctional atheroma'), or in the parent artery itself ('mural atheroma') (Fisher 1991). Although limited by the inevitably small number of cases, there was suggestion that certain anatomic sites are particularly prone to develop atheroma-related lacunes, for example pontine branches of the basilar artery (Fisher and Caplan 1971, Fisher 1977). The mechanism of infarction he showed was related either to occlusive thrombus complicating a plaque or to severely stenotic, non-occlusive plaque, in the latter case presumably mediated by post-stenosis hypoperfusion (Pullicino 1993).

Subsequent clinical studies have to some extent reinforced the idea that intracranial large vessel atheroma may obstruct the mouth of deep perforators (Bogousslavsky *et al.* 1991*a*), but much remains to be learned of the relationship between atherosclerosis and lacunar infarction. In particular, researchers have been slow to apply the coronary paradigm of the unstable atherosclerotic plaque (Davies 2000) to cervicocranial atheroma. Although it has been shown that coronary-type rupture of unstable plaque is the usual cause of fatal carotid sinus thrombosis (Lammie *et al.* 1999), the relevance of intra- and extracranial atherosclerotic plaque instability to lacunar infarction is unknown. Perhaps the relatively low frequency of large vessel atheromatous sources of emboli in lacunar stroke patients compared with those with cortical infarcts (Lodder *et al.* 1990) reflects in part an inability to detect during life mildly stenotic, yet potentially embolic, unstable large vessel atheroma. This and related subjects require pathological, as well as correlative pathological–radiological, study.

'Complex' small vessel disease (Lipohyalinosis)

The other vascular lesion of pathologically proven relevance to lacune formation is a destructive small vessel (40–200 μm diameter) lesion characterized in the acute phase by fibrinoid necrosis and, in the more commonly observed healed phase, by loss of normal wall architecture, collagenous sclerosis, and mural foam cells (Fig. 4.2a). This lesion, for which Fisher coined the descriptive term 'lipohyalinosis', causes smaller (3–7 mm diameter), less often symptomatic, infarcts than those caused by atherosclerosis, particularly in the striatocapsule and thalamus (Fisher 1969, 1978*a*).

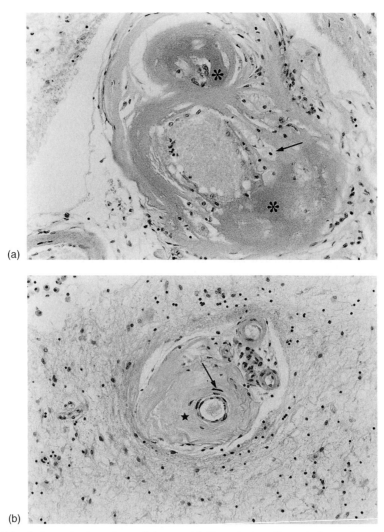

Fig. 4.2 Intrinsic cerebral small vessel disease. (a) 'Complex' small vessel disease (or 'lipohyalinosis'), showing an asymmetric, disorganized arterial wall with fibrinoid material (*) and mural foam cells (arrow). (b) 'Simple' small vessel disease (hyaline arteriolosclerosis), showing concentric hyaline vessel wall thickening (star), with a few residual smooth muscle cell nuclei (arrow).

The same, or a similar, lesion is thought to underlie the majority of 'hypertensive-type' primary intracerebral haemorrhages (Feigin and Prose 1959, Masuda *et al.* 1983, Rosenblum 1993), although how the same vessel lesion causes both infarction and haemorrhage is unclear. Although perhaps less prevalent today in the era of controlled hypertension (Masuda *et al.* 1983, Fisher 1991, Lammie *et al.* 1997), such lesions are still seen at autopsy in relation to lacunar infarcts. What remain uncertain are the proportion of symptomatic lacunar infarcts that nowadays are due to this lesion, the nature of its relationship with hypertension, and the underlying (molecular) mechanism.

'Simple' small vessel disease (arteriolosclerosis)

The term 'lipohyalinosis' is misused consistently to describe almost any small cerebral vessel pathology. It is distinct from, and should not be confused with, the concentric hyaline wall thickening (hyaline arteriolosclerosis) that is seen to some degree in the large majority of aged brains, particularly from individuals who were hypertensive or diabetic (Fig. 4.2b). The terms 'simple' and 'complex' cerebral small vessel disease have the merits of simplicity and descriptive accuracy, and are perhaps less likely to be confused in the future.

By whatever name, arteriolosclerosis or simple small vessel disease, with concomitant structural vascular remodelling (Baumbach and Heistad 1989), appears to encroach on the vessel lumen and is therefore often invoked as a cause of brain ischaemia. It is a consistent feature of brains with diffuse white matter disease or leukoaraiosis (Furuta *et al.* 1991), an association which is usually assumed to be causal. Certainly the arteriolosclerotic vessel is unlikely to be an effective autoregulatory organ, but it is also possible that the association reflects merely a common insult, such as abnormal vessel permeability, which may result in both white matter rarefaction and concentric small vessel thickening (Lammie *et al.* 1997). Similarly, whilst the severity of simple small vessel disease does appear to correlate with the presence and number of lacunes (Dozono *et al.* 1991), there currently is no direct evidence that this form of small vessel pathology is their cause. Finally, the relationship between simple and complex small vessel disease is unclear; for example, does simple small vessel disease precede or predispose to complex?

Miscellaneous small vessel pathologies

Whilst atherosclerosis and complex small vessel disease are the most important pathologically verified vessel lesions causing lacunar infarcts, it is perhaps unsurprising that a variety of other mechanisms and pathologies have also been invoked. There are reports linking small, deep infarcts with miscellaneous infections (due to secondary endarteritis and direct or immune-mediated vasculitis), with cardiogenic and artery-to-artery embolism, with thrombosis in, or compression by, both micro- and saccular aneurysms, with vasculitis (infective, primary, or due to collagen vascular disease), with arterial dissection, and with *in situ* thrombosis due to a range of hypercoaguable states (reviewed in Pullicino 1993). Such mechanisms can be verified pathologically to at least some degree, whereas other proposed mechanisms, such as vasospasm, turbulent carotid siphon flow, and oedema, cannot. However, with the possible exception of embolism, these miscellaneous causes are unlikely to be responsible for more than a small minority of symptomatic lacunes.

With specific regard to embolism, it is clear that small emboli from a variety of cardiac and arterial sources can, and on occasion do, enter perforating vessels and cause small, deep infarcts (Blackwood *et al.* 1969, Amarenco *et al.* 1992), perhaps more often in the centrum ovale than in the deep grey nuclei (Lammie and Wardlaw 1999). Often, but not necessarily always, such embolic small, deep infarcts are associated with multiple cortical infarcts. Although clinical studies suggest that cardiac and carotid embolism are unlikely causes of lacunar infarction, adequate autopsy-based study into the potential contribution of embolism to lacunar infarction is lacking. It should be emphasized, however, that the pathologist often can only infer, rarely prove, an embolic cause, for example if small vessel studies are normal or if small vessel thrombus is found in the absence of underlying thrombogenic vessel wall pathology or a documented clotting tendency.

Limitations of an autopsy-based approach

Failure to advance our understanding of the pathogenesis of lacunes significantly since Fisher's observations at least partly reflects the complexity of the problem— lacunes are a heterogeneous entity, not only in terms of number, size, and anatomic location, but also pathogenetically. In addition, for the pathologist, there are limitations inherent in a traditional autopsy-based approach. The low case fatality of lacunar infarction (Bamford *et al.* 1987) means that very few acute vessel lesions come under the microscope; most are of long standing, and may therefore represent as much a response to injury as its cause. In the rare instance of a fresh lesion coming to autopsy, the technical difficulties in tracing the lesion's blood supply are considerable, perhaps currently unfundable in a prospective study of adequate size. Meanwhile, novel approaches to visualizing cerebral small vessels in autopsy brains have been few (Challa *et al.* 1990) and have had limited application. Finally, and perhaps most importantly, the classical descriptions of 'lipohyalinosis' have not shed light on the underlying mechanism of vessel wall damage. This research, therefore, has not translated into rational treatment or prevention, aside from the treatment of its associated risk factors, in particular hypertension.

The future role of pathology in lacune research

In the light of this, has pathology a role in the future of lacune research? Certainly, there is a need to apply modern concepts of atherosclerosis biology to the cervicocranial arteries, in order to reassess the embolic, low flow and thrombotic potential of intra- and extracranial atherosclerotic plaques, both stable and unstable. There will also be a need for pathological verification of emerging cerebrovascular imaging modalities, as well as for continued pathological validation of stroke subtyping in clinically defined stroke cohorts.

It is, however, the experimental pathologist who has, for the first time, access to tools with which to explore the molecular genetic pathogenesis of complex small vessel disease, and its relationship to stroke. For example, the pathological hallmark of the acute causal small vessel lesion in lacunar stroke, namely fibrinoid necrosis, represents a potentially important 'intermediate phenotype'. If, as seems likely, small vessel stroke reflects a combination of both genetic and environmental risk factors, such intermediate phenotypes, being influenced by a smaller number of genes than stroke itself, have the potential to improve the power of genetic linkage and association studies, as well as to provide insight into underlying mechanisms (Boerwinkle *et al.* 1999). Experimental identification of genes conferring susceptibility to develop small vessel fibrinoid necrosis will focus and rationalize genetic polymorphism association studies in human stroke cohorts.

Fibrinoid necrosis—pathophysiology and genetic susceptibility

Fibrinoid necrosis has long been recognized as the histological hallmark of malignant or accelerated hypertension, both naturally occurring and experimentally induced (Gustaffson 1997). *In vivo* observation of vessels, including pial arterioles, during experimental hypertension (Byrom 1954, Mackenzie *et al.* 1976) has shown that fibrinoid necrosis is preceded by alternating segments of vessel constriction and dilatation. This appears to be followed by excessive endothelial permeability and tunica media necrosis, specifically in dilated vessel segments (Gustafsson 1997). Although high blood pressure *per se* may induce fibrinoid necrosis (Hill 1970), most cerebral lesions today appear not to occur in the context of accelerated hypertension, and there is therefore increasing interest in the role of underlying hypertension-associated endothelial dysfunction and neurohumoral mechanisms. For example, components of the renin–angiotensin system may mediate small vessel lesions via local vasoconstrictor and other vasculotoxic effects, rather than as a direct consequence of raised blood pressure. Whatever the precise underlying mechanism(s), the evidence is that fibrinoid necrosis may reflect, at least in part, pathological vasoconstriction and/or vasorelaxation. Our own unpublished observations suggest that diabetic cerebral vessels are particularly prone to develop fibrinoid necrosis, and that this may be linked to a reduced endothelial nitric oxide-induced vasodilator tone. A clinical corollary of this putative link between fibrinoid necrosis and abnormal vessel tone is that cerebrovascular reactivity, which reflects the dilatory capacity of cerebral arterioles, is impaired in patients with hypertension and diabetes mellitus, and may be an independent risk factor for lacunar infarction (Molina *et al.* 1999).

If fibrinoid necrosis is a function of disordered cerebrovascular reactivity, then this may reflect not only the structural and functional effects on small cerebral vessels of ageing, hypertension, diabetes, and other risk factors, but also an inherent or genetic susceptibility. This might explain why some patients suffer cortical and others lacunar stroke in the face of broadly similar risk factor profiles. Recent insights into the genetic basis of established animal models of stroke are potentially important in this regard. For example, in the stroke-prone spontaneously hypertensive rat (SHRSP), chromosomal regions have been identified which may harbour blood pressure-independent predisposing genetic factors (Rubattu *et al.* 1996), and stroke may associate and co-segregate with impaired endothelium-dependent vasorelaxation (Volpe *et al.* 1996). The SHRSP does suffer cerebral microinfarcts and haemorrhages as well as fibrinoid small vessel lesions (Yamori *et al.* 1976, Fredriksson *et al.* 1985, 1988) and, despite having blood pressure levels not often seen in modern clinical practice, may yet prove a useful model of human small vessel stroke. Conversely, in rats transgenic for liver-expressed prorenin, classical 'hypertensive' end-organ damage, including fibrinoid necrosis, is observed without a rise in blood pressure (Veniant *et al.* 1996). In this model, it has been speculated that the vessel lesions may be mediated by excessive vasoconstriction, perhaps via locally generated angiotensin II.

These and other animal models, using fibrinoid necrosis as a small vessel stroke intermediate phenotype, clearly have potential to uncover candidate genes in the human disease. It is intriguing, therefore, that from provisional genetic polymorphism data, genes implicated in these animal models and encoding potential mediators of small vessel tone are being linked to lacunar stroke. Thus, specific polymorphisms of the angiotension-converting enzyme and endothelial nitric oxide synthase (eNOS) genes appear to associate with lacunar stroke (see Chapter 8). Perhaps fibrinoid necrosis and small vessel stroke are manifestations of an evolving and dynamic interplay between abnormalities of vessel wall structure and function. These abnormalities may be partly inherited and partly acquired, the latter as a result of ageing and chronic diseases such as hypertension and diabetes mellitus.

Summary

Clinico-pathological study has formed the basis of our current understanding of lacunar infarction. Although pathogenetically heterogeneous, current evidence suggests that two distinct vasculopathies underlie the majority of clinically relevant lesions, namely atherosclerosis and what may usefully be termed complex small vessel disease (or 'lipohyalinosis'). The relative importance of these two pathologies, and of other putative causes less amenable to pathological study, in particular embolism, remains unclear. The relationship between atherosclerosis and lacunar infarction requires more detailed traditional pathology study, whilst the aetiopathogenesis of complex small vessel disease may yield to the experimental pathologist using genetically defined animal models.

Chapter 5

Leukoaraiosis

N.S. Ward and M.M. Brown

Introduction

Leukoaraiosis is a term coined by Hachinski *et al.* (1987) from the Greek roots 'leuko' (white) and 'araiosis' (rarefied) to describe the radiological appearances of patchy or diffuse abnormalities in the deep white matter, which appear as low attenuation on computed tomography (CT) or high intensity signals on T_2-weighted magnetic resonance imaging (MRI) sequences. The abnormalities are seen characteristically in the periventricular regions, especially around the horns of the lateral ventricles, and in the centrum semiovale. A multitude of other terms have been used by radiologists to describe these appearances, some of which imply pathogenesis (Table 5.1). The suggestion of Hachinski *et al.* was that 'leukoaraiosis' could provide a purely descriptive term appropriate for both CT and MRI that should be used in place of these other labels without implying pathogenesis or aetiology. The invention of the term has served to focus attention on the enigma of the pathogenesis and clinical correlates of this common radiological finding. Hachinski's ultimate hope was that leukoaraiosis would be replaced by more accurate terminology when 'labelling is replaced by understanding'.

Most observers would agree on the presence of severe leukoaraiosis on CT or MRI (Fig. 5.1), but the definition of leukoaraiosis was deliberately vague and allows the inclusion of almost any periventricular white matter abnormality short of infarction. Infarcts can usually be distinguished from leukoaraiosis by the fact that they are well demarcated, wedge-shaped and may have cortical extensions. Infarcts follow a specific vascular territory, may involve the internal capsule, basal ganglia, or thalamus, and are often associated with enlargement of the ipsilateral ventricle or sulcus, whereas leukoaraiosis is associated with more diffuse enlargement of the ventricles. However, the appearances of infarction merge into those of a patchy area of leukoaraiosis, and different machines, settings, and sequences of CT or MRI may be more, or less, sensitive to the presence of leukoaraiosis, which is in any case a purely visual interpretation. Early studies included almost any MRI signal change around the ventricles within the definition of leukoaraiosis. However, it is now recognized that hyperintense foci (stripes) seen around the rim of the lateral ventricles and small T_2 bright hyperintense foci at the angle of the ventricular horns (CAPS) are a normal phenomenon in elderly patients (Kertesz *et al.* 1988, Leifer *et al.* 1990, Van Swieten *et al.* 1991),

Table 5.1 Synonymous nomenclature of radiological deep white matter lesions culled from the literature

Binswanger's disease (BD)

Diffuse white matter disease

Leukoaraiosis

Patchy white matter lesions

Periventricular arteriosclerotic leuko-encephalopathy

Periventricular leukomalacia

Periventricular lucency (PVL)

Periventricular white matter lesions

Progressive subcortical vascular encephalopathy

Stripes, caps, and unidentified bright objects (UBOs)

Subacute arteriosclerotic encephalopathy

Subcortical arteriosclerotic encephalopathy (SAE)

White matter low attenuation (WMLA)

White matter signal hyperintensities (WMSHs)

Small vessel disease

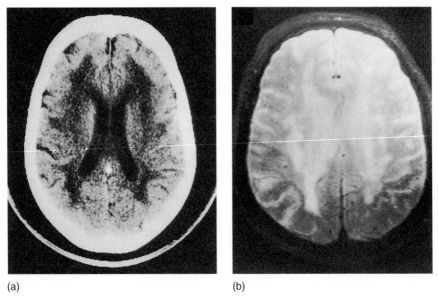

(a)   (b)

Fig. 5.1 Typical appearances of leukoaraiosis on CT (a) and MRI (b) scans at the level of the lateral ventricles.

Table 5.2 Differential diagnosis of leukoaraiosis

Atherosclerotic small vessel ischaemia

Granulomatous angiitis and other vasculitides

CADASIL

Multiple sclerosis

Acute disseminated encephalomyelitis

Post-traumatic demyelination

Obstructive and communicating hydrocephalus

Progressive multifocal leukoencephalopathy

Lymphoma

Tumour oedema

Congenital leukodystrophy

Gangliosidosis

Mucopolysaccharidosis

HIV encephalopathy

whereas thick irregular periventricular signal change can be regarded as pathological. Many scales for rating CT or MRI white matter changes are in operation, although none are ideal (Scheltens *et al.* 1998).

The radiological findings of diffuse changes in the white matter, taken on their own, can be indicative of a very wide variety of pathological process affecting the white matter (Table 5.2). In children and in younger adults, the differential diagnosis includes metabolic disorders, such as leukodystrophy. These disorders usually produce diffuse changes throughout the white matter, rather than the more patchy abnormalities seen in leukoaraiosis resulting from vascular disease. Another important non-vascular cause of patchy periventricular lucencies is multiple sclerosis. Here the radiological distinction may be difficult, if not impossible. The age of the patient is a guide, but is not reliable. The association with other vascular lesions, particularly lacunes in grey matter, may help to point to vascular aetiology rather than multiple sclerosis. The characteristic distribution of the lesion in multiple sclerosis around the ventricular horns may also help and may be distinguishable by the appearance of T_1-weighted spin-echo sequences (Uhlenbrock and Sehlen 1989). Magnetic resonance spectroscopy may also be useful in distinguishing these white matter diseases (Confort-Gouny *et al.* 1993). If other causes of white matter disease can be excluded, leukoaraiosis is usually attributed to cerebrovascular disease. Any form of vascular disease involving the blood supply of the deep white matter, including cerebral autosomal dominant arteriopathy with subcortical infarcts and leukoncephalopathy (CADASIL; see Chapter 9) and vasculitis, may result in leukoaraiosis, but in most cases the underlying pathology is likely to be subcortical arteriosclerosis. The evidence supporting this assumption is reviewed in the remainder of this chapter.

Incidence

Before the advent of CT scanning, subcortical arteriosclerotic encephalopathy (Binswanger's disease) was thought to be an extremely rare condition. Soon after the introduction of CT, it was realized that periventricular lucencies were a relatively common finding and it was suggested that the combination with dementia was diagnostic of subcortical arteriosclerotic encephalopathy (Loizou *et al.* 1981). As CT became more widely available and the definition improved, it soon became clear that identical appearances could be found in non-demented patients with cerebrovascular disease, in apparently normal elderly subjects, and also in demented patients with Alzheimer's disease. In one study, 9 per cent of 105 normal elderly volunteers (aged 59–91 years) were found to have leukoaraiosis on CT (Steingart *et al.* 1987). In another study, leukoaraiosis was found in as many as 22 per cent of 37 neurologically normal volunteers (Kobari *et al.* 1990a). Irrespective of cognitive state, leukoaraiosis becomes increasingly common with increasing age. In unselected series, it is rare below the age of 60, but in a selected CT study in Japan, Goto *et al.* (1981) reported white matter lesions in 5 per cent of nearly 5000 scans. The prevalence increased by 10 per cent in each successive decade after the age of 60.

MRI is much more sensitive to white matter changes than CT. In one study, incidental MRI lesions (areas of increased signal intensity on T_2-weighted images that could not be explained directly by the patient's clinical diagnosis or CT scan) were found in 22 per cent of patients under the age of 40, 57 per cent of patients aged 41–60, and in 90 per cent of patients over the age of 60 years (Awad *et al.* 1987). In this study, obvious areas of T_2 abnormality corresponding to the type of diffuse abnormalities typically seen on CT were not encountered in any patient younger than 40 years of age, but were present in 10 per cent of patients aged between 41 and 60 years and in 30 per cent of patients over the age of 60 years. The presence and severity of these incidental lesions correlated significantly with age and with risk factors for cerebrovascular disease. This was not a study of normal subjects, and the incidence of abnormalities detected by MRI may be less in the normal population. However, Van Swieten *et al.* (1991) performed post-mortem MRI on the brains of 40 consecutive patients over the age of 60 years who came to autopsy and had died from causes other than brain disease, and found moderate or severe periventricular lesions in 10 per cent of the patients aged between 60 and 69 years, and in 50 per cent between the ages of 80 and 89. It can therefore be concluded that leukoaraiosis is a common radiological finding particularly in the elderly. Its pathological significance is less clear.

Risk factors

A number of studies have documented a clear association of CT-evident leukoaraiosis with vascular risk factors. In the study of Inzitari *et al.* (1987), a history of hypertension was present in two-thirds of demented patients with leukoaraiosis compared with half that number in patients without leukoaraiosis, although there was no difference in mean diastolic blood pressure between subjects with and without leukoaraiosis. However, hypotension, orthostatic hypotension, and labile hypertension have also been found to be significantly associated with the presence of leukoaraiosis on CT (McQuinn and O'Leary 1985, Raiha et al. 1993, Tarvonen-Schroder et al. 1996). The possible significance of these findings in relation to the aetiology of leukoaraiosis is discussed below. A history of stroke was four times more frequent in patients with leukoaraiosis, occurring in 25 per cent of those with leukoaraiosis compared with 2 per cent of those without leukoaraiosis. Other studies have confirmed this association of leukoaraiosis with hypertension and stroke (Gupta et al. 1988, Hijdra et al. 1990). Similarly, both discrete and diffuse deep white matter abnormalities on MRI scan are also associated with vascular risk factors (Awad et al. 1986a, 1987).

Clinical features

Dementia

Although leukoaraiosis is found in apparently normal subjects, numerous studies document a stronger association with dementia. For example, Inzitari et al. (1987) found leukoaraiosis on CT of 35 per cent of 140 patients with dementia. Significantly, leukoaraiosis was found in all patients who were classified on other grounds as having multi-infarct dementia, and 38 per cent of patients in whom the dementia was attributed to a combination of vascular disease and Alzheimer's disease (mixed dementia). However, leukoaraiosis was also found in 33 per cent of those with dementia of Alzheimer type. In another large series of 233 demented patients, Erkinjuntti (1987a) reported leukoaraiosis on CT in 72 per cent of patients with multi-infarct dementia and 19 per cent of patients with Alzheimer's disease. In at least a fifth of cases of dementia attributed to vascular disease, leukoaraiosis is found on CT without evidence of cortical infarction (Erkinjuntti 1987b). These findings suggest that subcortical white matter ischaemia may be a more important cause of vascular dementia than multiple cortical infarcts.

There is also some evidence that the finding of leukoaraiosis may be associated with intellectual decline short of frank dementia. In the study of Steingart et al. (1987) of 105 normal elderly volunteers recruited to a dementia study, nine patients were found to have leukoaraiosis and had a significantly lower mean psychometric score than the 96 controls without leukoaraiosis. The difference remained significant even after adjusting for the possible confounding effects of age, sex, education, or asymptomatic cerebral infarction detected on CT. In this series, leukoaraiosis was also found to be significantly associated with abnormalities of gait and primitive reflexes, including extensor plantar responses, rooting, and palmomental responses, suggesting that even in apparently normal individuals leukoaraiosis is a marker of subclinical pathology.

The pattern of cognitive abnormalities found in patients with CT-evident leukoaraiosis shows the features characteristic of subcortical dementia such as slowing of information processing and impaired attention (Junque et al. 1990,

Kertesz *et al.* 1990). This is consistent with the suggestion that leukoaraiosis contributes to dementia and is not merely a coincidental sequel to dementing disease processes in the cortex. As well as dementia, leukoaraiosis has been linked with other psychiatric manifestations, including depression, apathy, disinhibitive behaviour, paranoia, and emotional lability, which may imply disruption of frontal connections (Summergrad and Peterson 1988). It is not clear whether these psychiatric manifestations can occur without intellectual impairment.

The relationship between leukoaraiosis detected by MRI and intellectual decline is less clear, probably because MRI detects much milder lesions. Several reports have demonstrated that leukoaraiosis is evident on CT only in those cases which show severe lesions on MRI (Awad *et al.* 1987, Lechner *et al.* 1988). Awad *et al.* (1986*a*) found no association between subcortical areas of increased signal intensity and dementia in 240 consecutive MRI scans, but this may be because they included single and remote isolated incidental lesions and only a small number of demented patients. Kobari *et al.* (1990*b*) showed that remote subcortical white matter lesions observed on T_2-weighted MRI showed no correlations with cognitive impairment and suggested that these represent clinically silent, tiny infarcts of white matter in otherwise normal brains. In studies where only moderate or severe periventricular white matter lesions are included, a clearer association between the presence of diffuse white matter abnormalities detected by MRI and dementia emerges (Brant-Zawadzki *et al.* 1985, Kinkel *et al.* 1985, Tanaka *et al.* 1989, Junque *et al.* 1990, Kertesz *et al.* 1990). In patients with MRI-detected leukoaraiosis, the severity of intellectual decline correlates both with the size of the lateral ventricles (Tanaka *et al.* 1989, Pujol *et al.* 1991) and with the degree of callosal atrophy (Yamauchi *et al.* 2000), presumably reflecting the severity of associated white matter tissue loss.

In conclusion, in contrast to CT, the majority of small subcortical lesions seen in the white matter on MRI are not associated with clinical findings, but they may be an early indicator of vascular disease that may progress to more extensive leukoaraiosis and dementia. It is probably only a matter of degree and distribution of white matter damage that distinguishes the patient with normal intellect from the patient with frank dementia.

Other clinical features

The clinical features of patients with pure leukoaraiosis determined by CT were compared with an age-matched control group without such CT findings. Dementia was found to be the strongest association, but other clinical features included gait disorder, urinary incontinence, personality changes, night-time confusion, and difficulty with activities of daily living. Focal signs were not found to be more common in either group, but have been reported in groups of patients with pathologically confirmed subcortical arteriosclerotic encephalopathy (see below) and stroke-like episodes (Tarvonen-Schroder *et al.* 1996).

Clinico-pathological correlates of leukoaraiosis

Diffuse atrophy of the deep white matter associated with dementia and severe arteriosclerosis was first delineated by Otto Binswanger in 1893 (Blass *et al.* 1991). Binswanger himself distinguished the condition from arteriosclerotic brain degeneration with involvement of the cortex, which we would now refer to as multi-infarct dementia. Curiously, in Binswanger's cases, the atrophy spared the frontal white matter, which does not correspond with our present-day observations of leukoaraiosis. To avoid the imprecision, it is preferable to refer to the pathological changes attributed to Binswanger's disease as subcortical arteriosclerotic encephalopathy, and to reserve the eponym for patients with full-blown syndrome of progressive dementia associated with the characteristic clinical features and radiological findings described in this chapter. Prior to CT, the condition was considered extremely rare and the clinical features associated with the characteristic pathology were not clearly described until Caplan and Schoene's paper in 1978, in which five patients with pathologically confirmed subcortical arteriosclerotic encephalopathy, and six patients with similar clinical findings, were studied retrospectively. The majority of their 11 patients had had persistent hypertension and a history of acute stroke-like episodes. In addition, there was typically fluctuation in the clinical picture, with the subacute accumulation of focal neurological symptoms and signs over weeks to months, associated with a long plateau periods and the development of dementia of varying degrees. The dementia had features characteristic of subcortical involvement, particularly abulia, bradyphrenia, and poor concentration. There were also prominent pyramidal signs and pseudobulbar palsy. The pathology was characterized by diffuse regions of white matter loss with gliosis, hydrocephalus, and severe thickening of the small penetrating arterioles. Babikian and Ropper's (1987) review of the literature revealed 46 pathologically confirmed cases, and found similar features. The typical pathological findings in subcortical arteriosclerotic encephalopathy are illustrated in Fig. 5.2.

Fredriksson *et al.* (1992) studied 14 cases of pure subcortical arteriosclerotic encephalopathy selected from their autopsy files, and again emphasized the history of chronic hypertension, and invariably progressive fluctuating mental changes (forgetfulness, abulia, emotional lability, and impaired cognitive function). A history of multiple lacunar strokes, particularly pure motor stroke, was common, and these occurred on average every fourth year. Dementia characterized by agitation and confusional episodes occurred in the later stages in the majority. The clinical signs were those of decreased mobility resulting from a small-stepped gait (13/14 cases), pseudobulbar palsy, and urinary incontinence. Rigidity (occasionally cogwheel in type) and impaired ocular movement were found in half the patients. Histologically, the deep white matter changes in these cases were characterized by lacunar infarcts surrounded by large areas of incomplete infarction, oedema, and gliosis associated with demyelination and pallor on myelin staining (Brun *et al.* 1992).

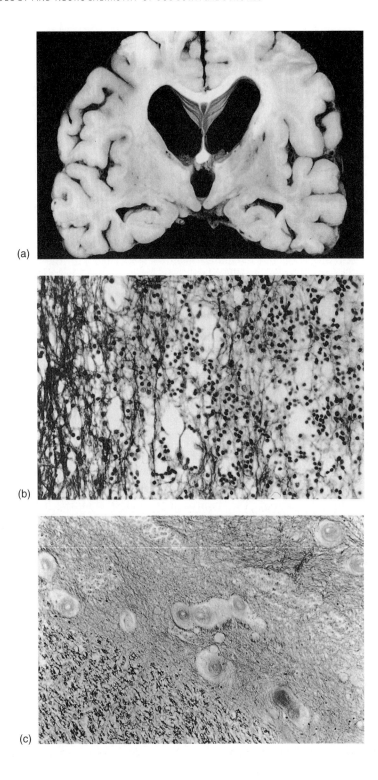

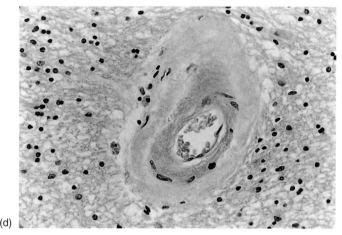

(d)

Fig. 5.2 Pathological findings in subcortical arteriosclerotic encephalopathy. (a) Gross macroscopic appearance showing thinning and discoloration of the white matter, lacunar infarcts, and ventricular enlargement. (b) High power microscopic appearance of the deep white matter stained for myelin showing patchy demyelination. (c) Low power microscopic appearance of the deep white matter showing hyalinization and thickening of the penetrating arterioles, with perivascular gliosis and demyelination. (d) High power microscopic appearance of a penetrating arteriole showing marked hyalinisation and thickening of the vessel wall.

Electron microscopy studies suggest that the majority of this pallor is due to loss of whole nerve fibres and only partly due to thinning of the myelin sheaths of the remaining nerve fibres (Yamanouchi *et al.* 1989). Brun *et al.* (1992) have now clearly described the vascular abnormalities associated with subcortical arteriosclerotic encephalopathy. The large arteries at the base of the brain and the convexity of the brain were affected by atherosclerosis, while the penetrating arteries were affected by two types of microangiopathy. In type I, fibrotic wall thickening (small vessel arteriosclerosis) occurred in all brain regions, but was severe only in the deep penetrators to periventricular white matter where highly fibrillary connective tissue (fibrohyalinosis) caused arteriolar narrowing. In type II microangiopathy, focal wall necrosis with eosinophilic fibrin strands, erythrocytes, and siderophages in the vessel and surrounding perivascular region (fibrinoid necrosis) was found in the shorter highly branched penetrating arterioles of cortex and deep grey matter nuclei. These changes were associated with small infarcts, microaneurysms, and fibrotic or thrombotic vessel occlusion, but spared the deep white matter.

The next question to consider is whether the changes of leukoaraiosis detected radiologically in elderly patients are the result of the same pathological processes and underlying microscopic vascular changes invariably present in the arterioles supplying the white matter in subacute arteriosclerotic encephalopathy. The clinical features associated with leukoaraiosis are certainly similar to those associated with subcortical arteriosclerotic encephalopathy and, on the whole, pathological studies correlating radiology with neuropathology have confirmed that leukoaraiosis usually results from similar pathological changes. Lotz *et al.* (1986) reported that the autopsy findings in 18 out of 20 patients in whom deep white matter radiolucent areas had been identified on CT confirmed a diagnosis of subcortical arteriosclerotic encephalopathy. In these patients, a triad of demyelination, loss of axons, and fibrous thickening of the walls of small arteries was found in the affected areas of the white matter. One case was found to have metastatic carcinoma, the abnormalities on CT being attributed to oedema, and one case had obstructive hydrocephalus, emphasizing that the differential diagnosis of white matter low attenuation includes other well-recognized pathology. Hypertension was present in 17 of the cases, but dementia was only documented in seven, which supports the suggestion that CT findings of leukoaraiosis in apparently normal elderly patients also represent the results of small vessel disease, although in this study the patients were not examined prospectively. Other studies of the pathology underlying subcortical lesions on CT have been reported in which the patients have been selected by pre-existing motor and cognitive deficits (Goto *et al.* 1981, Kinkel *et al.* 1985). The pathological findings in these patients include sharply delineated areas of necrosis, diffuse demyelination, small infarcts, and dilation of the ventricular system associated with thickening of small vessels.

The explanation for many of the focal white matter lesions seen on MRI is less certain. Studies in which patients have not been selected specifically for the presence of motor and cognitive deficits reveal a broad spectrum of possible pathological processes underlying these lesions. Kirkpatrick and Hayman (1987) examined at post-mortem, without radiology, 15 clinically healthy subjects aged between 52 and 72 years, and found unsuspected small white matter lesions in 12 patients. In eight of these, the lesions were due to perivascular demyelination, particularly in the centrum semiovale, associated with sclerotic tortuous arterioles. They distinguished these lesions from subcortical arteriosclerotic encephalopathy by the absence of tissue necrosis, small size, and relatively limited extent. Other unsuspected lesions found included small arteriovenous malformations, diverticulum of the lateral ventricle extending into the white matter, and an isolated central white matter infarct. They suggested that all these lesions could provide the basis of leukoaraiosis seen on MRI in healthy elderly patients. A number of authors have carried out pathological studies on brains in which MRI has been performed on the formalin-fixed brain specimens after death. Braffman *et al.* (1988) examined 23 elderly brains. Fifteen hyperintense white matter foci were found in seven brains. Six of the lesions were pathologically the result of infarction, two were small foci of gliosis, and two were plaques of demyelination. One brain cyst and a congenital diverticulum of the lateral ventricle were found, but these could be distinguished by different MRI sequences. Awad *et al.* (1986*b*) performed post-mortem MRI on the brains of seven consecutive elderly patients dying of neurological causes, and an eighth patient who underwent MRI in life, 11 days before death. Many of the lesions on MRI could be attributed to dilated perivascular spaces. Vascular ectasia and arteriosclerosis were found more frequently in MRI-positive areas and, in addition, there were patchy zones of gliosis associated with pallor on myelin stains. Only one area of true infarction was noted. The MRI signal did not appear to differentiate between milder forms of histological changes in which there were only enlarged perivascular spaces and vascular ectasia, and more severe forms in which there were myelinated fibre loss and gliosis. Marshall *et al.* (1988) reported similar findings.

The definitive study of post-mortem MRI was carried out by Van Swieten *et al.* (1991) on the brains of 40 patients over the age of 60 years who had died from causes other than brain disease. Eleven patients with moderate or severe lesions of the white matter on MRI were examined pathologically and contrasted with eight normal patients. The presence of periventricular lesions on MRI correlated well with the severity of demyelination and astrocytic gliosis in the white matter. Demyelination was always associated with an increased ratio between the wall thickness and the external diameter of the small arterioles (up to 150 μm). A variable degree of axonal loss was present in the white matter of all the brains with demyelination. Dilated perivascular spaces were also found, but their presence correlated less well with the demyelination and arteriosclerosis. The findings confirm that extensive demyelination and gliosis secondary to arteriosclerosis is the major cause of periventricular leukoaraiosis detected by MRI and that arteriosclerosis is the primary arteriological factor.

Association with lacunes

Not long after Binswanger delineated the association of dementia with white matter atrophy, Pierre Marie (1901) described the pathological features of the lacunar state (état lacunaire) in which multiple subcortical lacunes were also associated with dementia as well as bilateral corticospinal and corticobulbar signs (pseudobulbar palsy). The existence of these two separate causes of vascular dementia remains disputed a century later. Fisher (1982) has doubted the existence of a clinical syndrome attributed to the lacunar state on the grounds that multiple lacunes are found frequently at post-mortem without a history of dementia, while the clinical picture of the lacunar state may be present with only a few lacunes present at post-mortem. On the other hand, Roman (1987) has suggested that Binswanger's disease and lacunar dementia are the same disease because of the similarities of the clinical features. This fudges the issue of whether diffuse white matter damage or discrete areas of focal infarction, or both, are necessary for the development of cognitive impairment.

The understanding of ischaemia of the white matter has not been helped by semantic confusion and the differences of interpretation concerning the pathology of lacunes (Poirier and Derouesne, 1985). Since Fisher introduced the concept of a clinical syndrome associated with lacunar infarction, lacunes have been considered by clinicians mainly as the result of small deep infarcts caused by occlusion of perforating vessels. However, the term has also been used to describe the dilation of the perivascular space surrounding small perforating vessels. These lacunes contain a patent blood vessel and are particularly common in the hemispheric white matter of elderly patients. It is this type of lacune which, when multiple, constitutes the cribriform state ('état criblé' or 'status cribrosus') (Fig. 5.3). These perivascular lacunes may appear to compress surrounding tissues and on occasions may appear to destroy the adjacent brain.

Pathological studies have shown there is a very close association between the presence of lacunes and more diffuse white matter changes of subcortical arteriosclerotic encephalopathy. In Babikian and Ropper's review (1987), 93 per cent of pathologically proven cases of subcortical arteriosclerotic encephalopathy were associated with lacunar infarcts. Del Ser *et al.* (1990), in a careful clinical pathological study of 28 cases of dementia with only vascular lesions on histological examination, also showed that there was a significant relationship between deep lacunar infarcts, deep white matter demyelination, and cognitive decline. In the clinico-pathological study of Brun *et al.* (1992) of 14 cases of 'pure' subcortical arteriosclerotic encephalopathy, multiple lacunes were found in all cases in the centrum semiovale, the striatum, the thalamus, the internal capsule, and, to a lesser extent, infratentorially. In this study, an average of 11 lacunes were present in each case, and widening of the perivascular tissue spaces (i.e. the cribriform state) was also seen in the same areas, but to a lesser extent. The majority of lacunes occurred in the same sites as the other histological changes characteristic of subcortical arteriosclerotic encephalopathy. On the other hand, Van Swieten *et al.* (1991) found a lacunar infarct in only two out of six brains with severe periventricular lesions, demyelination, and arteriosclerosis, which compared with five out of the seven brains with normal white matter. This suggests that leukoaraiosis is not associated invariably with lacunes, at least in the absence of clinical neurological disease. In this study, there was a closer association of leukoaraiosis with dilated perivascular spaces, which were found in six out of seven brain specimens with severe demyelination, and in two out of four brains with moderate demyelination, but in only one brain specimen with normal white matter.

It seems likely that the association of leukoaraiosis and subcortical arteriosclerotic encephalopathy with lacunar infarcts and dilated perivascular spaces reflects a shared pathophysiology, namely arteriosclerosis of the penetrating arterioles. The distinction may be that in leukoaraiosis the brunt of the disease is borne by small arterioles below 150 μm in size, whereas lacunar infarcts are caused by occlusion of larger penetrating arterioles between 400 μm and 1 mm in diameter, and that pure subcortical arteriosclerotic encephalopathy and the lacunar state are two ends of a spectrum of small vessel disease.

It remains uncertain whether either diffuse white matter changes or multiple lacunes are sufficient to cause dementia by themselves, or whether a combination of these pathologies is necessary for dementia to occur. However, the study by Wolfe *et al.* (1990) has confirmed that multiple lacunar infarcts are associated with cognitive

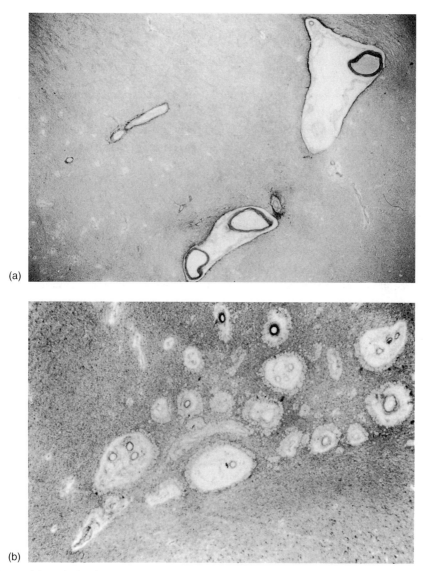

(a)

(b)

Fig. 5.3 (a) Marked enlargement of perivascular spaces in the deep white matter associated with diffuse demyelination. (b) Low power microscopic appearance of the deep white matter showing the cribriform state secondary to perivascular dilation of the penetrating arterioles.

impairment, especially frontal lobe deficits, but this paper did not establish whether leukoaraiosis was associated with the multiple lacunar infarcts or not. It is well recognized that very small areas of infarction in the paramedian thalamic region may result in dementia (Katz *et al.* 1987) and so it seems reasonable to conclude that the pathogenesis of subcortical dementia associated with small vessel disease is complex and depends to a variable degree on the site and number of lacunar infarcts and the presence of more diffuse ischaemic white matter lesions. Where insidious mental changes, gait disturbance, and pseudobulbar palsy are present, these may be the result of the more diffuse white matter ischaemia. However, since three-quarters of all lacunes are found in traditionally 'silent' areas, it remains possible that the gradual accumulation of such lacunar infarcts can be responsible for progressive dementia or gait disturbance. Where focal signs or stroke-like episodes occur in patients with leukoaraiosis, it is likely that these result from lacunar infarction rather than the more diffuse changes.

Pathophysiology of leukoaraiosis

Association with vascular factors

The association of leukoaraiosis with the clinical and pathological findings of subcortical arteriosclerotic encephalopathy and a history of hypertension suggests that arteriosclerosis of the penetrating arteries supplying the deep white matter is fundamental to the mechanism of the white matter changes. The changes have been interpreted as those of partial ischaemia without infarction, which is consistent with haemodynamic ischaemia rather than occlusion of arterioles secondary to thrombo-embolism. A number of mechanisms have been proposed to explain the white matter abnormalities. One suggestion is that arteriosclerosis results in increased arteriolar wall permeability, vasogenic oedema, and secondary chronic hypoxia (Benhaiem-Sigaux et al. 1987). However, it seems more plausible that arteriosclerotic vessels will be less permeable and that the perivascular dilation results from impairment of local nutrition in the capillary-free zone surrounding the arterioles (Kirkpatrick and Hayman 1987). This could account for a degree of perivascular demyelination, but would be unlikely to account for the more widespread white matter changes seen on CT or at pathological examination in classical cases of subcortical arteriosclerotic encephalopathy. One further possibility is that perivascular dilation results simply from mechanical stress caused by movement of tortuous hypertensive vessels and is unrelated to the process of demyelination.

A striking feature of leukoaraiosis and subcortical arteriosclerotic encephalopathy is that the white matter changes spare the subcortical u-fibres. This is consistent with the pathology being confined to the terminal supply of the penetrating arterioles. The periventricular regions and white matter of the centrum semiovale are supplied by the very long penetrating arteries travelling from the pial vessels on the surface of the cortex, while the centrum semiovale is also supplied from the surface of the cortex around its periphery by penetrating vessels. De Reuck (1971) has described this anatomy in detail. It can be seen from the beautiful microinjection specimens of Salaman (1973) (Fig. 5.4) that the deep white matter areas most affected by leukoaraiosis are those least well supplied by penetrating arterioles and, in addition, they are at the end of the territory of these vessels where the perfusion pressure

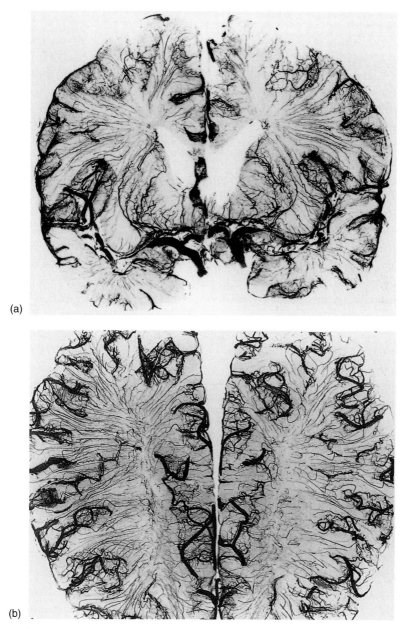

(a)

(b)

Fig. 5.4 Microinjection radiological plates showing the centripetal arteriolar blood supply of the periventricular regions (a) in a coronal slice at the level of the frontal horns, and (b) in an axial slice at the level of the centrum semiovale (from Salamon 1973).

will be lowest. These areas are therefore likely to be particularly vulnerable to borderzone ischaemia and hypotensive episodes (Moody *et al.* 1990). In addition, the density of capillaries is less in the white matter than in grey matter, and this is reflected by a volumetric blood flow in white matter which is normally about one-fifth of that of the cortex. This may make axons of neurons in white matter more vulnerable to diffuse ischaemia than the cortex. It is also possible that there are differences in metabolism between grey and white matter which make the latter more vulnerable to ischaemia.

There is considerable evidence confirming that vascular dementia of Binswanger's type may be associated with haemodynamic factors. For example, Sulkava and Erkinjuntti (1987) reported six cases in which dementia of acute onset occurred in clear temporal association with cardiac arrhythmias or hypotension, judged at the time insufficient to require resuscitation. All the patients were elderly, and hypo-volaemia secondary to diuretic therapy may have contributed. All the patients were found to have white matter leukoaraiosis and not the more usual cortical borderzone infarction attributed to hypotension. In another CT study, 10 out of 11 patients with confluent white matter lucencies had disordered blood pressure regulation, including labile hypertension with wide fluctuations of systolic pressure in three patients, and symptomatic orthostatic hypotension in another three (McQuinn and O'Leary 1987). Tarvonen-Schröder *et al.* (1996) found that systolic blood pressure less than 130 mmHg and orthostatic hypotension were more common in subjects with leukoaraiosis on CT, compared with those with normal CT scans. The severity of CT changes correlated with blood pressure instability, although not with dementia, which was not found in all patients. In some cases of subcortical arteriosclerotic encephalopathy, systemic factors, including metabolic disturbance, congestive cardiac failure, and respiratory hypoxia, appear to have interacted with small vessel disease to cause the selective damage of white matter (Garcia-Albea *et al.* 1987).

A large longitudinal study over 15 years of 382 elderly patients in Sweden showed that high blood pressure at screening was associated with the development of both leukoaraiosis and dementia, but also that blood pressure declined before dementia onset and was then similar to or lower than that in non-demented subjects (Skoog *et al.* 1996). To what extent the decline in blood pressure before dementia onset was the cause or the consequence of vascular brain damage was uncertain. However, in a more detailed study by Fredriksson *et al.* (1992), 14 cases of post-mortem-confirmed subcortical arteriosclerotic encephalopathy were described with clinical information from repeated examinations over a long pre-morbid observation time of up to 18 years. All the patients with onset before 68 years of age had a history of hypertension, but in the symptomatic phase of the disease serial measurements of blood pressure showed that the systolic pressure was highly variable. In eight out of 10 cases, antihypertensive treatment was stopped 2 or 3 years after the onset of symptoms because of declining blood pressure measurements associated with rapidly progressive neurological symptoms. These studies strongly suggest that relative hypotension accelerates the course of the disease.

Interestingly, leukoaraiosis is not generally associated with severe carotid artery disease but, in the presence of lacunar infarcts, internal carotid artery occlusion was associated with leukoaraiosis (Streifler *et al.* 1995). The absence of leukoaraiosis in subjects with internal carotid artery occlusion without lacunar infarcts suggests that any impairment of blood flow in the affected hemisphere does not cause white matter damage unless there is associated pre-existing small vessel arteriosclerosis (Yamauchi *et al.* 1999).

Cerebral blood flow (CBF) studies have confirmed that impairment of white matter CBF is associated with leukoaraiosis. Kobari *et al.* (1990*b*), using the stable xenon-enhanced CT method, showed a reduction of the CBF in frontal white matter and also in basal ganglia and cortex. The severity of leukoaraiosis correlated well with the reduction in regional CBF in the cortex, but not in the white matter, but this may reflect technical difficulties in measuring the very low flow values found in the white matter of patients with leukoaraiosis.

In our own studies, we measured white matter CBF using stable xenon-enhanced CT in 10 patients with leukoaraiosis before and after administration of a cerebral vasodilator, acetazolomide (Brown *et al.* 1990). The measurements demonstrated that leukoaraiosis is accompanied by markedly impaired vasodilatory capacity in the deep white matter with relatively preserved cortical vasodilatory capacity (see Fig. 5.5). Isaka *et al.* (1994) also reported impaired vasodilatory capacity in patients with leukoaraiosis. These findings support the hypothesis that the radiological changes are the result of haemodynamic ischaemia.

Patients with leukoaraiosis may therefore be particularly vulnerable to mild falls in blood pressure, which may not cause any symptoms or signs, but may damage the white matter. Whether leukoaraiosis results from constant gradual ischaemia in such patients, or from single or multiple episodes of unrecognized hypotension, such as might occur during the night, remains to be determined.

Association with hydrocephalus

Hydrocephalus was noted by Binswanger in his original descriptions, and has been a constant feature of the gross microscopic appearances of patients with subcortical arteriosclerotic encephalopathy. For example, widening of the ventricles was reported in 93 per cent of cases reviewed by Babikian and Ropper (1987), although it was only found in 78 per cent of the series of Brun *et al.* (1992). A number of studies have confirmed an association between radiological leukoaraiosis and hydrocephalus (Tanaka *et al.* 1989, Pujol *et al.* 1991). It is usually assumed that the widening of the ventricles reflects periventricular tissue loss 'ex vacuo'. However, the features of subcortical arteriosclerotic encephalopathy are very similar to those of 'normal' pressure hydrocephalus and, since ventricular enlargement is found in

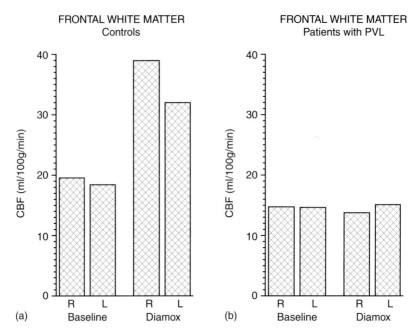

Fig. 5.5 Mean cerebral blood flow (CBF) in the frontal white matter measured by the stable xenon method in (a) 10 control subjects and (b) 12 patients with leukoaraiosis (PVL) on CT in the right (R) or left (L) hemisphere. CBF was measured under baseline conditions and then repeated after an intravenous injection of a cerebral vasodilator, acetazolamide (Diamox). CBF approximately doubled in the frontal white matter of control subjects ($P < 0.01$) (a), but there was no increase in CBF at all in the patients with leukoaraiosis (b).

both conditions, they may be indistinguishable clinically (Gallassi *et al.* 1991). A number of cases have been described in which normal pressure hydrocephalus with moderate response to shunting has been associated with the finding at post-mortem of florid hypertensive vascular disease with lacunar infarcts in the periventricular white matter (Earnest *et al.* 1974, Koto *et al.* 1977). It was suggested that hypertensive vascular disease had, in these cases, been the initiating factor in developing normal pressure hydrocephalus. Kimura *et al.* (1992) measured CBF by xenon CT in seven patients in whom normal pressure hydrocephalus had developed after subarachnoid haemorrhage, before and after shunting. Widespread reductions in CBF were seen in the cortex, subcortical white matter, and thalamus before shunting. After shunting, clinical improvement correlated significantly with normalization of CBF in subcortical white matter, raising the possibility that hydrocephalus plays a role in the pathogenesis of subcortical white matter lesions by inducing relative hypo-perfusion. It remains uncertain whether this association represents true cause and effect, or simply diagnostic confusion between the syndromes of normal pressure hydrocephalus and subcortical arteriosclerotic encephalopathy.

Association with Alzheimer's disease

A number of studies have documented an association between radiological leukoaraiosis and Alzheimer's disease. A significant percentage of patients with Alzheimer's disease are diagnosed as having mixed dementia with features of both Alzheimer's disease and cerebrovascular disease but, even when patients with pure Alzheimer's disease are considered, as many as 30 per cent of patients are found to have leukoaraiosis (George *et al.* 1986, Steingert *et al.* 1987, Kertesz *et al.* 1990). The aetiology of leukoaraiosis in Alzheimer's disease remains uncertain, but Brun and Englund's (1986) histopathological study strongly suggests that white matter changes in Alzheimer's disease are the result of a pathology similar to subcortical arteriosclerotic encephalopathy. Sixty per cent of patients dying of Alzheimer's disease showed white matter abnormalities consisting of areas of incomplete infarction, characterized by partial loss of myelin associated with fibrohyaline sclerosis and thickening of the local arterial and capillary walls. Scheltens *et al.* (1995) reported similar findings, which can be distinguished from subcortical arteriosclerotic encephalopathy by the absence of hypertensive small vessel changes. There was no relationship between the white matter abnormalities and the degree of involvement of the overlying grey matter, making it unlikely that the changes were simply the result of degeneration secondary to cortical neuronal loss. Moreover, the white matter changes were associated with the signs of cardiovascular disease and, in many cases, a history of hypotension, or a terminal blood pressure which was low relative to previously documented hypertension, suggesting that the white matter changes could be the result of hypoperfusion. Similar neuropathological findings were found in a study of 10 patients with Alzheimer's disease who had had pre-mortem CT scans, but the severity of the post-mortem changes did not correlate with the ante-mortem findings of leukoaraiosis on CT (Rezek *et al.* 1987). This may well be because there was a long interval between CT and death. It has been suggested that hypoperfusion of the deep white matter in Alzheimer's disease may be due to associated cerebral amyloid angiography of the meningocortical segments of the long perforating arterials (Gray *et al.* 1985). These authors studied 12 patients with diffuse haemorrhagic cerebral amyloid angiopathy and found subcortical arteriosclerotic encephalopathy in eight, four of whom also had Alzheimer's disease. These findings have not been confirmed. The aetiology of leukoaraiosis in Alzheimer's disease remains an intriguing enigma.

Prognosis

There is increasing evidence that the finding of leukoaraiosis has significant clinical implications. Those with leukoaraiosis carry a poorer prognosis in terms of death, stroke, and myocardial infarction (Inzitari *et al.* 1995, 1997). In addition, the presence of leukoaraiosis in post-stroke patients significantly increases the incidence of dementia (van Kooten *et al.* 1997), and the incidence of intracranial haemorrhage in those patients anticoagulated after their stroke (Gorter *et al.* 1997). It is not yet clear whether this last effect is related to increasing age and hypertension (Inzitari *et al.* 1990).

Conclusions

This chapter has sought to establish that the radiological appearances of leukoaraiosis and the pathological findings of subcortical arteriosclerotic encephalopathy are closely related, and in most cases reflect haemodynamic ischaemia of the white matter secondary to arteriosclerotic thickening of the penetrating arteries supplying the white matter. The clinical accompaniments of leukoaraiosis range from apparently normal findings to severe dementia characteristic of Binswanger's disease. There is a close association between leukoaraiosis and lacunar infarcts, and it is likely that the clinical features depend both on the severity and on the location of associated lacunar infarcts and ischaemic white matter changes. The exact anatomical and pathological substrate necessary for dementia to be associated with leukoaraiosis remains uncertain. Further careful clinico-pathological studies and a better understanding of the pathophysiological behaviour of the small vessels of the brain are needed. The enigma remains of the occasional patient who has very marked radiological changes in the periventricular white matter but who appears clinically normal. From the point of view of management, it is clear that careful control of hypertension while avoiding hypotension, especially in the elderly patient with long-standing arterial disease, is essential to prevent the development or deterioration in dementia. It is also now becoming clearer that the presence of leukoaraiosis even in asymptomatic individuals has significant clinical implications which cannot be ignored.

Chapter 6

Molecular mechanisms of subcortical versus cortical infarction

S.G. Waxman

Introduction

Based on differences in their cellular organization, it might be expected that different molecular mechanisms would trigger secondary cell death in white matter of the central nervous system (CNS) as opposed to grey matter. Axons and associated myelin sheaths, oligodendrocytes, and astrocytes constitute the major cellular constituents of white matter tracts. Synaptic transmission does not occur in white matter, and pre- and postsynaptic specializations are not present. Grey matter, on the other hand, is where synaptic transmission occurs; neuronal cell bodies and dendrites are present in the grey matter, and are impinged upon by synaptic terminals so that there is a high density of pre- and postsynaptic specializations. These synaptic specializations provide a substrate for excitotoxic cell injury within grey matter.

   As might be expected, in the absence of synapses, excitotoxic mechanisms play a smaller role, if any, in causing irreversible dysfunction in white matter. Consistent with this prediction, exposure to even high concentrations of the excitatory neurotransmitters glutamate or aspartate (10 mM, applied for extended periods in the absence of Mg^{2+} and in the presence of 0.1 mM glycine) does not produce dysfunction in the rat optic nerve, a representative white matter tract (Ransom et $al.$ 1990). Nevertheless, Ca^{2+}-mediated cell death does occur in white matter where it can be triggered by anoxic/ischaemia (Stys et $al.$ 1990, Waxman et $al.$ 1991), and the underlying molecular routes for Ca^{2+} influx (Stys et $al.$ 1992a, Fern et $al.$ 1995) as well as some regulatory mechanisms that modulate Ca^{2+} influx (Fern et $al.$ 1994, 1995) are beginning to be understood. The molecular mechanisms that underlie anoxia/ischaemia-triggered Ca^{2+} influx into white matter axons, and the modulatory mechanisms that regulate this Ca^{2+} influx, suggest neuroprotective approaches which may limit irreversible dysfunction in subcortical stroke, which has a predilection for white matter. This chapter will review our current understanding of the molecular pathophysiology of anoxic/ischaemic injury of white matter.

Slow Na$^+$ channels, the Na$^+$–Ca^{2+} exchanger, and anoxic/ischaemic injury of white matter

The critical role of Ca^{2+} influx from the extracellular milieu into the intracellular compartment of axons in anoxic white matter has been demonstrated in experiments (Stys *et al.* 1990) using the rat optic nerve model (Davis and Ransom 1987). This model, together with quantitative analysis of the compound action potential (CAP) (Stys *et al.* 1991), permits an estimation of functional *integrity* of a white matter tract, i.e. it provides a measure of the proportion of white matter axons that are capable of generating and conducting action potentials after various insults. Using this model, Stys *et al.* (1990) showed that during a 60 min period of total anoxia, the development of irreversible dysfunction of white matter is critically dependent on the presence of extracellular Ca^{2+} (Fig. 6.1). If the optic nerve is perfused with 2 mM Ca^{2+} (a concentration similar to that within the

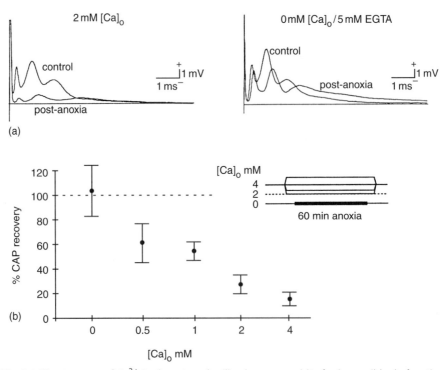

Fig. 6.1 The presence of Ca^{2+} in the external milieu is a prerequisite for irreversible dysfunction of the optic nerve by a 60 min anoxic challenge. (a) Optic nerve CAPs before and after 60 min of anoxia in normal (2 mM) Ca^{2+}, and in zero-Ca^{2+} bathing solution. Note the significantly enhanced CAP recovery when Ca^{2+} is absent. (b) The degree of CAP recovery after 60 min of anoxia is dependent on the concentration of extracellular Ca^{2+} [Ca]$_o$. The percentage recovery of the CAP is a monotonic function of [Ca]$_o$ in the domain between 0 and 4 mM. Modified from Stys *et al.* (1990).

extracellular space of the normal CNS) during a 60 min anoxic insult, only about 30 per cent of the axons recover the ability to conduct axon potentials as measured by the area under the CAP. However, if Ca^{2+} is removed from the external solution that bathes the nerve and ethleneglycobis(β-aminoethyl)ether tetaacetic acid (EGTA) is added to buffer residual Ca^{2+}, 100 per cent of optic nerve axons recover the ability to conduct action potentials after a 60 min anoxic insult (Stys et al. 1990). These results show that anoxia-induced irreversible dysfunction of this white matter tract is critically dependent on the presence of extracellular Ca^{2+}, suggesting that Ca^{2+} influx into an intracellular compartment mediates cell death. Ultrastructural studies have demonstrated that this intracellular compartment lies within axons. After 60 min of anoxia, axons within the optic nerve display dissolution of the cytoskeleton with nearly total loss of microtubules in many axons (Waxman et al. 1992), similar to pathological changes that have been reported in myelinated axons following exposure to the Ca^{2+} ionophore A23187 (Schlaepfer 1977) and after incubation in elevated Ca^{2+} (Schlaepfer and Bunge 1973). Exposure of the anoxic optic nerve to zero-Ca^{2+} perfusate during the anoxic period protects the axonal cytoskeleton from damage (Waxman et al. 1993). These experiments demonstrate that axons constitute an important target for Ca^{2+} influx in anoxic white matter.

A major route for Ca^{2+} influx in anoxic CNS white matter involves the Na^+–Ca^{2+} exchanger (Stys et al. 1992a). This antiporter molecule, which operates with a stoichiometry of 3:1, normally extrudes one Ca^{2+} ion as it carries three Na^+ ions down their concentration gradient, from the extracellular milieu where its concentration is high into the intracellular compartment where it is low (Blaustein and Santiago 1977, Rasgado-Flores and Blaustein 1987). If the cell membrane is depolarized and/or the intracellular Na^+ concentration is increased so that the transmembrane gradient is collapsed or reversed, the Na^+–Ca^{2+} exchanger can operate in a reverse (calcium influx) mode, importing Ca^{2+} to the intracellular compartment (Baker et al. 1969, Cerveto et al. 1989).

The influx route for Ca^{2+} in the anoxic optic nerve involves the reverse mode of the Na^+ and Ca^{2+} exchanger, which is triggered by depolarization and Na^+ influx via persistent Na^+ channels. Sucrose gap studies in the optic nerve have demonstrated the presence of a non-inactivating tetrodotoxin (TTX)-sensitive Na^+ conductance (Stys et al. 1993). This non-inactivating Na^+ conductance is active close to resting potential, and persists after depolarization that is sufficient to abolish classical transient Na^+ currents (Fig. 6.2). Anoxia produces elevated extracellular K^+, and resultant depolarization in CNS white matter (Ransom et al. 1992). This activates the non-inactivating Na^{2+} conductance, permitting a persistent influx of Na^+ which collapses the transmembrane gradient for this ion (Stys et al. 1992a, 1993). The increase in intracellular Na^+, coupled with depolarization, triggers reverse operation of the Na^+–Ca^{2+} exchanger which carries damaging levels of Ca^{2+} into the cytoplasm (Stys et al. 1992a).

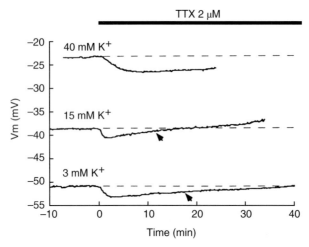

Fig. 6.2 A persistent Na$^+$ conductance is present in optic nerve and is active at resting potential. These gap recordings show d.c. potentials (which represent an attenuated mean of resting potentials in multiple axons). Application of the Na$^+$ channel blocker tetrodotoxin (TTX, 2 mM) results in a hyperpolarizing shift in the d.c. potentials, indicating that an Na$^+$ conductance contributes to resting potential. The hyperpolarizing shift is present at rest (3 mM K$^+$ in extracellular solution) and in optic nerves depolarized by exposure to elevated (15 mM and 40 mM) extracellular K$^+$ From Stys *et al.* (1993).

The functional importance of this mechanism of Ca^{2+} influx in anoxic white matter is suggested by several types of experiments. As shown in Fig. 6.3a and b, there is nearly total functional recovery of the optic nerve after 60 min of anoxia when Na$^+$ influx is blocked by removal of Na$^+$ from the extracellular milieu or by exposure to TTX, a neurotoxin which blocks Na$^+$ channels. Consistent with a role for persistent Na$^+$ channels in this cascade, experiments in which the optic nerve was exposed to TTX at various times during a 60 min anoxic challenge (Fig. 6.3c) indicate that Na$^+$ influx continues throughout the anoxic period. As seen in Fig. 6.4, approximately 70 per cent recovery of the CAP occurs when the optic nerve is subjected to anoxia in the presence of inhibitors of the Na$^+$–Ca^{2+} exchanger such as benzamil and bepridil; these results, together with experiments in which the transmembrane Na$^+$ gradient was changed, show that reverse Na$^+$–Ca^{2+} exchange carries Ca^{2+} into the axonal intracellular compartmenting anoxia (Stys *et al.* 1992a). Ultrastructural evidence for the coupling of Na$^+$ influx and damaging Ca^{2+} influx is provided by experiments which show that damage to the axonal cytoskeleton is prevented almost entirely by exposure of white matter to TTX during a 60 min anoxic challenge (Waxman *et al.* 1994). Electron probe microanalysis (LoPachin and Stys 1995, Stys and LoPachin 1998) has confirmed the presence of elevated intracellular Na$^+$ levels in anoxic white matter axons, and has shown that as axoplasmic Na$^+$ increases, there is a parallel elevation in calcium content, providing additional evidence for reverse

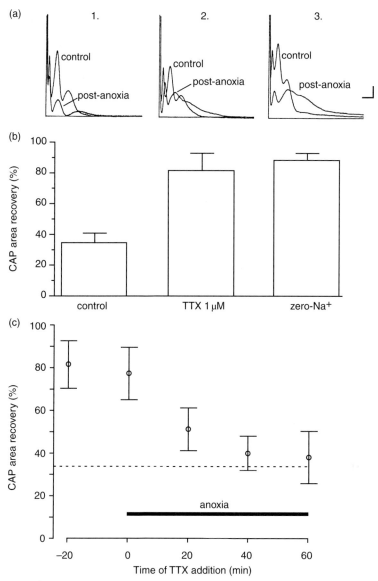

Fig. 6.3 The Na^+ channel blocker tetrodotoxin (TTX) and perfusion in zero-Na^+ solution both protect the optic nerve from a 60 min anoxic challenge. (a) Representative CAPs before and after a 60 min anoxic challenge in normal solution (1), with the addition of 1 mM TTX (2), and with perfusion in zero-Na^+ solution (3) throughout the anoxic period. (b) Exposure to 1 μM TTX or zero-Na^+ solution significantly improves CAP recovery (to $81.5 \pm 11\%$, $P < 0.0001$; and $88.0 \pm 5\%$, $P < 0.0001$, respectively) compared with controls ($36.7 \pm 7\%$). (c) Effects of 1 μM TTX, applied at various times during a 60 min anoxic challenge. CAP recovery decreases gradually as introduction of TTX is delayed with respect to onset of anoxia, suggesting that Na^+ influx begins soon after the onset of anoxia and continues throughout the 60 min anoxic period. Modified from Stys et al. (1992a).

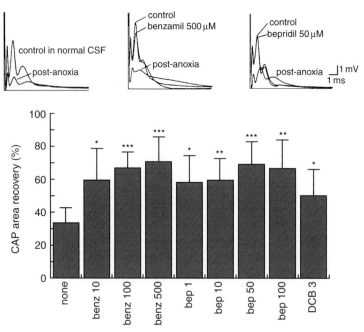

Fig. 6.4 Blockers of the Na^+–Ca^{2+} exchanger are neuroprotective in the anoxic optic nerve. Benzamil (benz), bepridil (bep), or dichlorobenzamil (DCB) were applied 60 min before the start of a 60 min anoxic challenge and continued until 15 min after reoxygenation, when normal solution was resumed. Post-anoxic activity was measured 60 min after reoxygenation. Benzamil significantly improves recovery of the CAP area in a dose-dependent manner over a concentration range of 10–500 mM. Bepridil (1–100 mM) and dichlorobenzamil (3 mM) also significantly improve recovery. Benzamil has no effect on the pre-anoxic response at 10 and 100 mM and reduces CAP area modestly to 61.1 ± 20 per cent of control at 500 mM in a reversible manner. Bepridil and dichlorobenzamil have no effect on pre-anoxic responses at the concentrations shown. $*P < 0.01$; $**P < 0.001$; $***P < 0.0001$; $n = 7$–10 for each drug and concentration. Modified from Stys et al. (1992a).

Na^+–Ca^{2+} exchange. The Na^+ channel/Na^+–Ca^{2+} exchanges cascade is illustrated diagramatically in Fig. 6.5.

Ca^{2+} channels as a parallel route for axonal injury in white matter

In addition to persistent Na^+ channels and the Na^+–Ca^{2+} exchanger which provide a major route for Ca^{2+} influx in anoxic white matter, L-type and N-type Ca^{2+} channels appear to provide a parallel pathway for influx of Ca^{2+} into the intracellular compartment of optic nerve axons when they have been injured (Fern et al. 1995b). Although the subcellular distribution and function of Ca^{2+} channels in white matter axons are not yet clear, there is evidence which suggest that Ca^{2+} channels are

EXTRACELLULAR

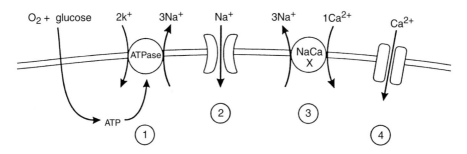

INTRACELLULAR

Fig. 6.5 Pathophysiological events leading to axonal injury in anoxic/ischaemic white matter. Anoxia/ischaemia leads to depletion of ATP with resultant run-down of ATPase activity (1) and depolarization. Persistent Na^+ channels (2) provide a route for sustained Na^+ influx, collapsing the transmembrane Na^+ gradient. Depolarization and the collapsed Na^+ gradient both favour reverse Na^+–Ca^{2+} exchange (3) which results in influx of Ca^{2+} into the intracellular compartment. Voltage-gated Ca^{2+} channels (4) provide a parallel route for Ca^{2+} entry into the intracellular compartment.

expressed in optic nerve axons (Lev-Ram and Grinvald 1987) and optic nerve glia (Barres *et al.* 1989, 1990). Pharmacological blockage of L-type Ca^{2+} channels provides significant protection of the rat optic nerve from anoxic injury; simultaneous block of L-type and N-type Ca^{2+} channels provides even greater protection (Fern *et al.* 1995*b*). Fern *et al.* (1995*b*) suggested the presence of three types of pharmacologically distinct Ca^{2+} channels in CNS white matter, two of which are involved in anoxic injury. Imaizumi *et al.* (1999) extended this type of analysis to spinal cord white matter and showed, in a dorsal column preparation, that L-, N-, and possibly R-type calcium channels permit damaging Ca^{2+} influx into anoxic white matter axons.

Autoregulation as a modulator of Ca^{2+}-mediated injury in white matter

The two injury pathways discussed above, reverse Na^+–Ca^{2+} exchange triggered by Na^+ entry and Ca^{2+} influx via Ca^{2+} channels, may be subject to modulation by endogenous neuroactive molecules. As shown in Figs 6.6 and 6.7, irreversible dysfunction in anoxic axons of optic nerve can be modulated by neurotransmitters and neuromodulators including γ-aminobutyric acid (GABA) and adenosine (Fern *et al.* 1994, 1995*a*). A number of lines of evidence indicate that extracellular concentrations of GABA (Shimada *et al.* 1993) and adenosine (Van Wylen *et al.* 1986,

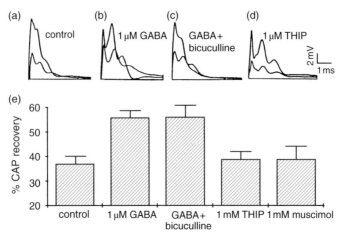

Fig. 6.6 GABA is neuroprotective, acting via GABA-B receptors, in the anoxic optic nerve. (a–d) Superimposed pre- and post-anoxic CAPs taken under control conditions (a) and in the presence of various agents applied prior to anoxia (b–d). The larger of each CAP pair is the pre-anoxic recording and the smaller CAP is the post-anoxic recovery. (a) Under control conditions, the mean post-anoxic CAP recovery after anoxia was 36.5 ± 2.9 per cent ($n = 10$). (b) GABA (1 μM) significantly increased recovery to 55.7 ± 2.5 per cent ($n = 16$, $P < 0.002$). (c) The selective GABA-A antagonist bicuculline (100 μM), added with GABA, did not attenuate the protective effect of 1 μM GABA. (d) The selective GABA-A agonist THIP had no protective effect against anoxia. (e) Data summary showing that mean recovery in 1 μM GABA + bicuculline was 56.1 ± 4.4 per cent ($n = 12$), recovery in 1 μM THIP was 38.5 ± 2.9 per cent ($n = 8$), and recovery in 1 mM muscimol (a selective GABA-A agonist) was 38.6 ± 4.8 per cent ($n = 7$). From Fern *et al.* (1995a).

Hagberg *et al.* 1987, Meghji *et al.* 1989, Ballarin *et al.* 1991) in the CNS increase during anoxia or ischaemia. Fern *et al.* (1994, 1995a) have demonstrated that in response to anoxia, GABA and adenosine are released into the extracellular compartment from endogenous stores within white matter. These two substances can act alone or synergistically, at nanomolar concentrations, by binding to GABA-B and adenosine receptors which activate G-protein and protein kinase C, as part of an autoprotective feedback loop that limits the development of irreversible dysfunction in the anoxic optic nerve (Fig. 6.8). Although 'downstream' events in this autoprotective pathway are not yet understood, they could involve modulation of Na^+ conductance, Na^+–Ca^{2+} exchange, or voltage-gated Ca^{2+} channels; there is, for example, evidence for protein kinase C-mediated down-regulation of Na^+ channels (Li *et al.* 1993, Numann *et al.* 1994) and of the Na^+–Ca^{2+} exchanger (Mene *et al.* 1991).

Potential therapeutic approaches

In principle, delineation of the molecular mechanisms outlined above might be expected to provide a basis for the development of new therapeutic strategies for

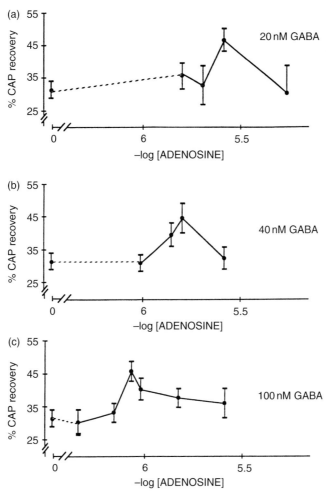

Fig. 6.7 Adenosine is neuroprotective in the anoxic optic nerve. Moreover, adenosine acts synergistically with GABA. Graphs show the neuroprotective effect of adenosine (% CAP recovery after 60 min of anoxia) at various adenosine concentrations. Low concentrations of GABA alter the adenosine dose–response relationship. (a–c) Protective effect of various adenosine concentrations applied in the presence of 20, 40, or 100 nM GABA, respectively. Note that the concentration of adenosine that produced maximum protection was shifted to the left at higher GABA concentrations ($n = 4$–16). From Fern et al. (1994).

subcortical stroke. Although more needs to be learned, the available data proved a substrate for discussion of a number of potential clinical approaches:

Alteration of extracellular ion concentrations

As might be predicted from the molecular mechanisms described above, nearly complete neuroprotection of anoxic white matter (optic nerve; 60 min of anoxia) can

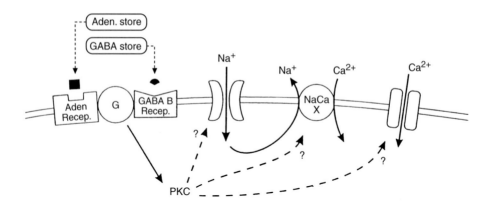

Fig. 6.8 The autoprotective feedback loop in white matter. Anoxia/ischaemia triggers release of adenosine and GABA from endogenous stores. Activation of adenosine receptors and GABA-B receptors activates an intracellular cascade involving a G-protein and protein kinase C (PKC) which decreases susceptibility to anoxia. PKC may limit Ca^{2+} influx by modulating Na^+ channels, the Na^+–Ca^{2+} exchanger, and/or voltage-gated Ca^{2+} channels.

be achieved by removal of Ca^{2+} (Stys *et al.* 1990) or Na^+ (Stys *et al.* 1992*a*) from the extracellular milieu for the *total* period of anoxia. However, because transmembrane ion gradients shift during anoxia/ischaemia (see, for example, Ransom and Philbin 1992, Ransom *et al.* 1992), removal of Na^+ from the extracellular milieu for only the latter part of the anoxic period can worsen the functional outcome; Na^+ influx into the intracellular compartment during early phases of anoxia (prior to removal of extracellular Na^+) followed by subsequent lowering of extracellular Na^+ levels can produce a reverse transmembrane Na^+–Ca^{2+} exchange (Stys *et al.* 1992*a*). Manipulation of extracellular ionic concentrations does not appear to be clinically applicable.

Na^+ channel blockade

The Na^+ channel-blocking drugs TTX and saxitoxin (STX) can provide substantial protection from anoxic injury of CNS white matter (Stys *et al.* 1992*a*). There is at least 81.5 per cent recovery of optic nerve CAP area after a 60 min anoxic insult if the optic nerve is exposed to 1 µM TTX throughout the anoxic period (this may represent an underestimate, since TTX is not completely removed from the perfusate following the anoxic period and will tend to attenuate the CAP). Lower concentrations of TTX result in progressively less recovery in a dose-dependent manner. STX is also neuroprotective although not to the same extent as TXX (58.2% recovery at 1 µM).

The neuroprotective effects of TTX in the optic nerve model have been demonstrated at the ultrastructural level, with preservation of the axonal cytoskeleton even after 60 min of anoxia if optic nerves are exposed to 1 µM TTX (Waxman *et al.* 1994). TTX is also neuroprotective in the anoxic dorsal columns (Imaizumi *et al.* 1997).

Interestingly, block of action potential electrogenesis with TTX is not a prerequisite for protection of white matter from anoxia. TTX at 10 nM does not produce significant conduction block in the optic nerve, but nevertheless is neuroprotective (56.4% recovery of CAP; Stys *et al.* 1992*b*). It has been demonstrated that neurons express multiple, molecularly distinct Na^+ channels (Black *et al.* 1996, Dib-Hajj *et al.* 1998) which display different sensitivities to TTX (see Caffrey *et al.* 1992, Elliott and Elliott 1993, Cummins and Waxman 1997, Cummins *et al.* 1999). The molecular identity of the channel(s) responsible for the neuroprotective effect of TTX in the anoxic optic nerve and spinal cord are not known. Neither TTX nor STX can be used safely in the clinical domain, but their efficacy as neuroprotective agents for white matter under experimental conditions shows that specific blockade of voltage-dependent Na^+ channels can be neuroprotective in white matter.

Tertiary anaesthetics

These tertiary amine drugs reversibly block both Na^+ and (to a lesser extent) K^+ channels (Narahashi *et al.* 1967, Strichartz 1973, Strichartz 1976, Cahalan 1978, Stole 1988). Stys *et al.* (1992*b*) demonstrated that lidocaine and procaine can both significantly improve post-anoxic recovery of the optic nerve CAP (1 mM lidocaine provides 88.5% recovery, and 1 mM procaine provides 93.8% recovery). As with TTX, neuroprotection of smaller degree was provided by concentrations of tertiary anaesthetic that did not block normal conduction (Fig. 6.9). For example, 0.1 mM lidocaine reduced the control CAP area, under normoxic conditions, only slightly (to 92% of control values) but was significantly protective against a 1 h anoxic challenge (CAP area recovered to 74.1% of control). Procaine (0.1 mM) did not reduce the area of the normoxic CAP, but still significantly protected the optic nerve from anoxic injury (72.4% CAP recovery). Whether this phenomenon is due to a threshold effect, whereby non-specific blockage of a proportion of Na^+ channels provides neuroprotection without compromising axonal conduction because of its high safety factor, or to specific blockade of a particular channel subtype is not known.

Quarternary anaesthetics

Because of the participation of non-inactivating Na^+ channels in anoxic injury of white matter (Stys *et al.* 1992*a*, 1993), Stys *et al.* (1992*b*) suggested that quaternary anaesthetics, which bind preferentially to open Na^+ channels (Wang *et al.* 1987, Khodorov 1991), might provide neuroprotective ions in anoxic/ischaemia white matter). As shown in Fig. 6.9, QX-314 and QX-222 have neuroprotective effects in the anoxic optic nerve at concentrations that do not affect action potential conduction

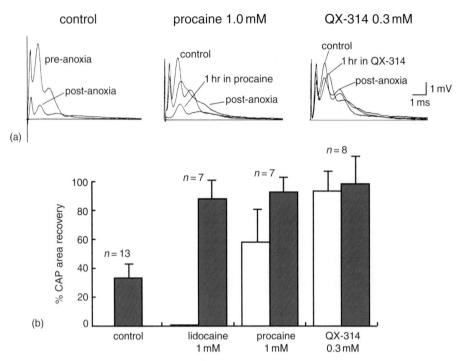

Fig. 6.9 Tertiary and quaternary anaesthetics are neuroprotective in the anoxic optic nerve. CAPs and graphs of CAP area show CAP recovery after 60 min of anoxia. Top: representative CAPs from optic nerves showing the effects of local anaesthetics on excitability and on recovery from anoxia. Responses are shown in normal CSF before anoxia after 60 min of exposure to drug (procaine and QX-314), and after 60 min of anoxia. Procaine improves outcome from anoxia but strongly depresses the CAP. QX-314 allows complete recovery of the CAP area after anoxia and had only a small effect on the CAP at the protective concentration. Bottom: open bars represent the area under the CAP 60 min after perfusion with drug and before the onset of anoxia. Stippled bars show recovery of the CAP area after 60 min of anoxia and 1–3 h of wash in normal solution. 'Control' represents recovery in normal solution with no drug added. Lidocaine, procaine, and QX-314 significantly improve outcome, but highly protective concentrations of tertiary anaesthetics depress the CAP far more than do quaternary anaesthetics at equally protective concentrations. Lidocaine abolished measurable excitability at 1 mM ($P < 0.00001$, compared with control). At 0.3 mM, QX-314 had a minimal effect on the pre-anoxic CAP area, yet resulted in virtually complete recovery of the CAP after anoxia ($P < 0.00001$, compared with control). Modified from Stys et al. (1992b).

(Stys *et al.* 1992*b*). QX-314 was most effective at 0.3 mM where it reduced the normoxic CAP only minimally (94.4% of control) but provided full recovery (99.6%) of the CAP after 60 min of anoxia.

QX-222 provides optimal neuroprotection at 3 mM (CAP recovery to 81.4% of control) without detectable reduction in the area of the normoxic CAP (Stys *et al.* 1992*b*).

The dissociation of the conduction-blocking and neuroprotective effects of tertiary and quaternary anaesthetic agents may be due in part to their non-selective ion channel-blocking properties, i.e. their block of K^+, as well at Na^+ conductance. Since action potential electrogenesis depends on the ratio of Na^+ to K^+ conductance (Jack et al. 1983, Sontheimer and Waxman 1992), it would be expected that concomitant, partial block of both conductances would tend to preserve action potential conduction. Moreover, the preferential block of open channels (Wang et al. 1987, Khodorov 1991) or of non-inactivating channels (Stafstrom et al. 1985) by quaternary compounds might permit these molecules to act selectively at Na^+ channels that remain open during periods of anoxia/ischaemia, thus providing neuroprotection without compromising electrogenic activity in unaffected CNS regions.

Antiepileptic drugs

The antiepileptic drugs phenytoin and carbamazepine are known to block Na^+ channels and appear to provide a degree of neuroprotection in anoxic white matter (Fern et al. 1993). Phenytoin at $1\,\mu M$ has a significant neuroprotective effect in the anoxic optic nerve (57.8% recovery after 60 min of anoxia) (Fern et al. 1993). These neuroprotective effects were observed at concentrations somewhat below the normal therapeutic free plasma and cerebrospinal fluid (CSF) concentration range ($4–8\,\mu M$) (Goodman and Gilman 1987, Levy et al. 1989) and below the concentrations that are normally required for a block of Na^+ channels ($5–500\,\mu M$) (Catterall 1981, Matsuki et al. 1984, Willow et al. 1984, Schwartz and Grigat 1989, Backus et al. 1991). Carbamazepine is also neuroprotective in the anoxic optic nerve model (Fern et al. 1993). Carbamazepine at $10\,\mu M$ increased CAP recovery after 60 min of anoxia to 59.2 per cent. A neuroprotective effect for carbamazepine could be detected in the anoxic optic nerve even at very low concentrations; $50\,nM$ carbamazepine increased post-anoxic recovery of the CAP to 44.3 per cent (Fern et al. 1993). As with phenytoin, neuroprotective effects of carbamazepine have been observed at concentrations below those that have been reported to be required for Na^+ channel block in model systems (Schauf et al. 1974, Catterall 1981, Willow et al. 1984, 1985, Schwarz and Grigat 1989, Wakamori et al. 1989, Backus et al. 1991). It is possible that the neuroprotective efficacy of phenytoin and carbamazepine may reflect the voltage-dependent manner in which these drugs block Na^+ channels (Willow et al. 1985, Schwarz and Grigat 1989).

Antiarrhythmic agents

Antiarrhythmic drugs appear to act via use-dependent block of Na^+ channels (Ragsdale et al. 1991). Stys (1995) studied arrhythmic agents as possible neuroprotective drugs for white matter, using a 60 min anoxic challenge in the optic nerve model. In this study, tocainide (1 mM) provided substantial neuroprotection ($\sim78\%$ CAP recovery) while having minimal effects on the normoxic action potential. Prajmaline (10 and $30\,\mu M$) had a neuroprotective effect with recovery of the CAP of 76–82 per cent, with only a small reduction in normoxic conduction. Ajmaline (100 μM) was also neuroprotective, yielding CAP recovery to approximately 79 per cent of control values, while having only a small effect on the normoxic CAP. Disopyramide was neuroprotective at doses of 30–300 μM, with optimal protection (68% CAP recovery) at 100 μM, a dose where the normoxic CAP is reduced by only a small amount, to 90 per cent. Bupivacaine is neuroprotective but tended to produce depression of normoxic conduction. Procainamide did not provide neuroprotection (Stys 1995). Stys and Lesiuk (1996) found that mexiletine (10 μM–1 mM) was significantly neuroprotective in the anoxic optic nerve model, with CAP recovery improved to 52.9 per cent at 100 μM. They also observed neuroprotection in an *in vivo* model of white matter ischaemia (Stys and Lesiuk 1996).

Calcium channel blockers

Fern *et al.* (1995*b*) observed that the L-type calcium channel antagonists verapamil (90 μM and 50 μM) and nifedepine (2.5 μM) provide significant neuroprotection in the anoxic optic nerve (CAP recovery 51.3, 65.6, and 54.3%, respectively; Fern *et al.* 1995*b*). Simultaneous block of L- and N-type calcium channels via co-application of 50 μM diltiazem and 1 μM ω-conotoxin (CgTx GVIA) results in greater neuroprotection (CAP recovery 73.6%) than diltiazem alone, although ω-conotoxin CgTx GVIA alone did not provide significant protection.

Neuroprotection of anoxic white matter by diltiazem and verapamil is dose dependent with a plateau of approximately 50 μM. In contrast, nifedepine showed maximal protection at 2.5 μM, with a lower degree of protection at higher concentrations (Fern *et al.* 1995*b*). A lack of neuroprotective effect at higher nifedepine concentrations may be due to a blocking effect on the actions of adenosine (O'Regan *et al.* 1990, 1991) and GABA (O'Regan *et al.* 1992); as discussed above, both of these molecules participate in an autoregulatory loop (Fern *et al.* 1994, 1995*a*) which tends to protect white matter from anoxic injury.

Blockade of $Na^+–Ca^{2+}$ exchange

Stys *et al.* (1992*a*) demonstrated neuroprotective effects of three drugs that block the $Na^2–Ca^{2+}$ exchanger, bepridil (Kaczorowski *et al.* 1989) and two derivatives of amiloride, benzamil and dichlorobenzamil (Kleyman and Cragoe 1988), in the anoxic optic nerve model (Stys *et al.* 1992*a*). The neuroprotective effect of benzamil is dose dependent (71% recovery of the CAP at 500 μM with smaller degrees of protection at lower doses). Bepridil shows optimal neuroprotection at 50 μM (69% CAP recovery). Bepridil and benzamil also block voltage-gated calcium channels (Galizzi *et al.* 1986, Kleyman and Cragoe 1988, Garcia *et al.* 1990). In addition, benzamil expresses inhibitory effects on Na^+ channels (Kleyman and Cragoe 1988); 500 μM benzamil reduces CAP area in the normoxic optic nerve to 61 per cent of control values (Stys *et al.* 1992*a*). Although the neuroprotective effects of benzamil and bepridil may, in part, reflect the latter activities, a significant part of the neuroprotective action of these drugs in anoxic white matter appears to be due to block of reverse Na^+-Ca^{2+} exchange.

GABA and adensosine

As shown by Fern *et al.* (1994; 1995*a*), the anoxic injury cascade in CNS white matter is subject to modulation via an autoprotective mechanism which involves GABA (which acts via GABA-B receptors) and adenosine (which acts via adenosine receptors). GABA and adenosine appear to act synergistically, via convergent actions of adenosine receptors and GABA-B receptors, on a common G-protein which activates protein kinase C (Fig. 6.8). Co-administration of nanomolar concentrations of GABA shifts the concentration dependence of the protective effects of adenosine to lower concentrations, and vice versa (Fig. 6.7).

GABA has its maximal neuroprotective effect at a concentration of 1 μM (56% recovery of the optic nerve CAP after 60 min of anoxia), with a smaller degree of protection at lower or higher concentrations. Baclofen, a GABA-B agonist, has a similar effect, with maximal protection at 1 μM. The protective effect of GABA requires 30 min of exposure prior to onset of anoxia, and appears to require exposure to GABA throughout the anoxic period (Fern *et al.* 1995*a*). The available evidence suggests that GABA is released from endogenous stores within white matter during anoxia. Nipecotic acid, which inhibits GABA uptake and can enhance release of GABA from endogenous stores (Brown and Marsh 1978, Sakatani *et al.* 1992), has a neuroprotective effect in the anoxic optic nerve (Fern *et al.* 1995*a*).

Like GABA, adenosine has a neuroprotective effect in white matter, with a maximal effect at a concentration 2.5 μM (Fern *et al.* 1994). As with GABA, adenosine's neuroprotective effects require tens of minutes to develop, and reach maximal levels only after 60 min of pre-exposure to adenosine. The dose–response curve for the protective effects of adenosine is shifted to lower concentrations as GABA levels increase. In the presence of 20 nM GABA, maximal protection is found at 2.5 μM adenosine, while in the presence of 100 nM GABA, adenosine's protective effect is greatest at 900 nM (Fig. 6.7). Drugs that block adenosine re-uptake can increase extracellular adenosine levels (Jacobson *et al.* 1992, Rudolphi *et al.* 1992). The adenosine uptake inhibitor propentofylline, which passes the blood–brain barrier (DeLeo *et al.* 1988, DeLeo and Kreutzberg 1988, Andine *et al.* 1990, Jacobson *et al.* 1992), is neuroprotective in the anoxic optic nerve; 1 mM propentofylline increases the degree of CAP recovery (to 48%) (Fern *et al.* 1994).

Other drugs

A neuroprotective effect has been observed for diazepam in the anoxic optic nerve (69.2% CAP recovery at a concentration of 1 μM, and 76% recovery at 10 μM; Fern *et al.* 1993), at concentrations higher than those used clinically (20–40 nM; Goodman and Gilman 1987, Levy *et al.* 1989). Neuroprotection is, however, produced by concentrations below those required to block Na^+ channels (5–500 µM) (Backus *et al.* 1991). The mechanism of action for this neuroprotective activity is not understood.

Hypothermia

Stys *et al.* (1992*c*) demonstrated that mild hypothermia is neuroprotective in white matter. Lowering of temperature by 2.5 °C (i.e. from 37 to 34.5 °C) during the period of anoxia provided significant neuroprotection in the optic nerve model (CAP recovery 64.6%). Reduction of temperature to 32 °C during a 60 min anoxic insult is even more neuroprotective (CAP recovery 100.5%) (Stys *et al.* 1992*c*). Lowering of temperature during the anoxic insult appears to be required for neuroprotection. Hypothermia immediately following anoxia at 37 °C does not have a neuroprotective effect. We do not yet understand the mechanisms underlying the protective effect of hypothermia in anoxic white matter. The rate of oxygen consumption is decreased by 6–8 per cent/ °C (compared with the rate at 37 °C) by hypothermia in both grey and white matter (Nishizaki *et al.* 1988). One possibility (Stys *et al.* 1992*c*) is that hypothermia may affect the rate of calcium transport by the Na^+-Ca^{2+} exchanger in anoxic white matter.

Glutamate and glial cell damage in white matter

Although axons do not appear to be a target of excitotoxic (glutamate-triggered) injury in anoxic white matter, recent evidence (Li *et al.* 1999) suggests that reverse Na^+-dependent glutamate transport may result in increased glutamate levels that injure white matter oligodendrocytes and/or myelin. α-Amino-3-hydroxy-5-methyl-4-isoxazole proprionic acid (AMPA) and kainate receptors are expressed by oligodendrocytes and white matter at densities sufficient to support glutamate-mediated injury (Matute *et al.* 1997, MacDonald *et al.* 1998). Li *et al.* (1999) found that the broad-spectrum glutamate antagonist kynurenic acid (1 mM) and the selective AMPA antagonist GYK 152466 (30 µM) are neuroprotective in the anoxic spinal cord. Their study suggests that, even in the absence of synaptic specializations or membrane rupture, anoxia triggers reverse Na^+-dependent glutamate transport from an intracellular pool (possibly within axons) into the extracellular compartment. Their immunohistochemical results provide additional evidence suggesting that glutamate injures oligodendrocytes and/or myelin sheaths within white matter.

Overview and prospects

As outlined above, a complex ensemble of molecules contributes to the development of anoxic/ischaemic injury within white matter of the CNS. White matter axons are susceptible to the effects of abnormal influxes of calcium that travel through several routes, including reverse Na^+-Ca^{2+} exchange triggered by persistent Na^+ channels, and by a parallel pathway involving Ca^{2+} channels. In addition, oligodendrocytes and/or myelin sheaths appear to be susceptible to glutamate-triggered injury, resulting from reverse Na^+-dependent glutamate transport. Some of the steps involved in these destructive events appear to be subject to modification by neurotransmitters such as GABA and by neuromodulators such as adenosine.

Subcortical stroke is a frequent event and represents a major medical challenge. Moreover, even the more common large hemispheric strokes (e.g. infarctions in the middle of the cerebral territory) often include white matter, as well as grey matter, within their region of injury. Thus, there is a pressing need for the development of therapies which will prevent, or at least limit, irreversible damage that occurs as a consequence of anoxia/ischaemia in white matter. The complexity of the network of molecular mechanisms that contributes to anoxic/ischaemic injury of white matter presents a challenge to those who wish to understand its pathophysiology. At the same time, it represents multiple targets for therapeutic intervention. Hopefully, as we understand the molecular pathophysiology of calcium-mediated injury of white matter in greater detail, it will be possible to harness some of these molecular mechanisms so that they can be used therapeutically.

Acknowledgements

Supported in part by grants from the Medical Research Service and the Rehabilitation Research Service, Department of Veterans Affairs, the National Multiple Sclerosis Society, the Paralyzed Veterans of America, and the Eastern Paralyzed Veterans Association.

Part III

Risk factors and genetic aspects

Chapter 7

Risk factors for lacunar infarction

J. Boiten and J. Lodder

Introduction

Stroke has an enormous impact on public health as a leading cause of death and permanent disability. Identifying and modifying risk factors for stroke may reduce mortality and morbidity. Many studies have revealed various risk factors for stroke. Stroke is a heterogeneous group of disorders, and the question is whether the ischaemic stroke subgroups such as lacunar infarcts are associated with distinct risk factor profiles. Unfortunately, ischaemic stroke subtypes were not distinguished in many studies.

Lacunar infarcts have a unique pathophysiological mechanism. Most of them are caused by local obstruction of a small perforating artery due to small vessel disease (SVD) (Fisher 1965a, 1969, 1979). However, the vascular risk factor profile is not unique, because territorial infarcts (which have a distinct pathogenesis) have a similar risk factor profile, even with regard to hypertension. What determines whether (mainly) small or (mainly) large vessels, or both become affected in the presence of similar risk factors still remains unclarified. Possibly, genetic susceptibility determines which subtype of stroke occurs in the presence of a similar atherogenic milieu. There are several arguments that favour a genetic susceptibility in ischaemic stroke: familial aggregation of stroke (Kiely et al. 1993), higher concordance rates for stroke in homozygotic than in dizygotic twins (Brass et al. 1992), and the existence of several mendelian and mitochondrial diseases, which may cause ischaemic stroke, and in particular cerebral SVD (Alberts 1991, Rastenyte et al. 1998). Furthermore, angiotensin-converting enzyme (ACE) I/D polymorphism has been described as a risk factor for lacunar stroke (Markus et al. 1995). The genetic aspects of lacunar infarction are described extensively in Chapter 8.

The known risk factors account only for part of the risk of lacunar stroke. Several lacunar stroke patients do not have one of the known risk factors. Therefore, additional risk factors should be looked for and investigated in the future. For instance, Lammie et al. (1997) found in an autopsy study that many lacunar stroke cases lacking classic risk factors had other factors known to enhance small vessel permeability.

The unmodifiable risk factors for lacunar stroke include age, gender, and, probably, heredity (genetic susceptibility) and ethnicity (Table 7.1). Detecting these

Table 7.1 Risk factors for lacunar infarctions

Unmodifiable risk factors	Possible (less well documented) risk factors
Age	Hypercholesterolaemia
Gender	Alcohol consumption
Heredity	Elevated hematocrit
Ethnicity	Oral contraceptives
Modifiable risk factors	Elevated fibrinogen
Hypertension	Hyperhomocysteinaemia
Diabetes	Physical inactivity
Cigarette smoking	Obesity
Ischaemic heart disease	and others
TIA	

unmodifiable risk factors is important to identify persons who are at higher risk for lacunar infarcts and in whom risk factors should be treated vigorously.

Modifiable risk factors for lacunar stroke include hypertension, diabetes mellitus, cigarette smoking, ischaemic heart disease, and transient ischaemic attack (TIA). Other possible (less well documented) risk factors for lacunar stroke are hypercholesterolaemia, hyperhomocysteinaemia, alcohol consumption, use of oral contraceptives, physical inactivity, obesity, elevated haematocrit, elevated fibrinogen, etc.

There are many studies on lacunar infarction, but only a few well-designed studies investigated risk factors for lacunar infarction. There are three case–control studies, which determined the relative risks for lacunar infarction of several vascular risk factors (Table 7.2) (Gandolfo *et al.* 1988, You *et al.* 1995, Boiten *et al.* 1996). One case–control study used hospital controls and made no adjustment for confounding variables (Gandolfo *et al.* 1988). The other two studies used community controls and performed a multivariate logistic regression analysis to adjust for confounding variables (You *et al.* 1995, Boiten *et al.* 1996). The risk of lacunar stroke was significantly increased by hypertension, diabetes, and cigarette smoking. TIA also increased the risk of lacunar infarction, but was investigated in only one study. History of ischaemic heart disease (or ischaemic ECG abnormality) was a risk factor for lacunar infarction (Gandolfo *et al.* 1988, Boiten *et al.* 1996), but heart disease in general was not (You *et al.* 1995).

Established risk factors for lacunar infarction

Age and sex

Age is the most important risk factor for stroke. For each 10 years after age 55, the stroke rate more than doubles for both men and women (Wolf *et al.* 1992*b*, Brown *et al.* 1996, Sacco *et al.* 1997). As for stroke in general, age is also an important risk

Table 7.2 Risks for lacunar infarction from case–control studies

Risk factor	Cases n (%)	Controls n (%)	OR/RR[a]	95% CI
Hypertension				
Gandolfo et al. (1988)	70 (65)	63 (29)	4.7	2.9–7.6
You et al. (1995)	140 (69)	66 (33)	8.9	4.2–18.8
Boiten et al. (1996)	138 (48)	159 (18)	4.5	3.3–6.1
Diabetes				
Gandolfo et al. (1988)	23 (21)	24 (11)	2.0	1.1–3.5
You et al. (1995)	36 (18)	13 (6)	2.3	1.0–5.5
Boiten et al. (1996)	58 (20)	72 (8)	3.6	2.3–5.5
Cigarette smoking				
Gandolfo et al. (1988)	59 (55)	86 (40)	2.3	1.3–4.3
You et al. (1995)	91 (45)	41 (20)	6.6	2.9–14.8
TIA				
Gandolfo et al. (1988)	37 (34)	6 (3)	35.0	14.2–86.5
Heart disease				
Gandolfo et al. (1988)[b]	31 (29)	19 (9)	4.3	2.3–8.0
You et al. (1995)	51 (25)	34 (17)	1.0	0.5–1.9
Boiten et al. (1996)[b]	61 (21)	69 (8)	2.6	1.7–3.8
Hypercholesterolaemia				
Gandolfo et al. (1988)	48 (44)	81 (38)	1.3	0.8–2.2
You et al. (1995)	42 (22)	43 (22)	0.9	0.5–1.8

[a] Relative risk (RR) was estimated by means of the Mantel–Haensczel matched chi-square method for multiple controls (Gandolfo et al. 1988). Odds ratio (OR) was estimated by multivariate logistic regression analysis (You et al. 1995, Boiten et al. 1996). CI = confidence interval.
[b] Ischaemic heart disease [clinical (Boiten et al. 1996) or on ECG (Gandolfo et al. 1988)].

factor for lacunar infarction. The incidence of lacunar infarction increases with age (Bamford et al. 1987, Sacco et al. 1991, Norrving and Staaf 1991). The mean age of the patients suffering from lacunar infarction ranged widely from 58 to 72 years in various studies (Gross et al. 1984, Bamford et al. 1987, Foulkes et al. 1988, Gandolfo et al. 1988, Norrving and Cronqvist 1989, Ghika et al. 1989, Anzalone and Landi 1989, Arboix et al. 1990a, Boiten and Lodder 1991a, Norrving and Staaf 1991, Sacco et al. 1991).

In most studies, men are more often affected than women (Donnan et al. 1982, Gandolfo et al. 1988, Anzalone and Landi 1989, Ghika et al. 1989, Norrving and Cronqvist 1989, Arboix et al. 1990a, Boiten and Lodder 1991a, Norrving and Staaf 1991). Incidence rates of lacunar infarction were higher for men, independently of age (Norrving and Staaf 1991, Sacco et al. 1991).

Hypertension

Hypertension is the most important modifiable risk factor for stroke, with age-adjusted relative risks of about 3 (Wolf et al. 1992a). The risk of stroke increases with blood pressure level (MacMahon *et al.* 1990). Clinical trials showed that hypertension treatment reduces stroke incidence (Collins *et al.* 1990).

The importance of hypertension as a specific risk factor for lacunar infarction is controversial. The controversy originates from the different frequencies of hypertension in both clinical and pathological studies. In 1965, Fisher described a pathological study in 1042 consecutive adults of whom 114 (11%) had one or more lacunes. All but three of Fisher's 114 patients had documented hypertension. Consequently, Fisher (1965*a*) concluded that lacunar infarcts are directly related to hypertension. More recently, he continued to find an association between hypertension and lacunar infarcts in 80–90 per cent of cases (Fisher 1982, 1991).

In another autopsy study of 2859 patients, 169 (6%) had lacunar infarctions (Tuszynski *et al.* 1989). Hypertension was the most common risk factor for lacunar infarcts, being found in 64 per cent of the patients. The value of risk factor data from this study is limited because data were obtained retrospectively by chart review. As indicated above, the frequency of hypertension in the pathological series of Fisher (1965*a*) was much higher, namely about 97 per cent. This difference may be explained by differences in the definition of hypertension. Fisher (1965*a*, 1982, 1991) defined hypertension as a blood pressure of greater than 140/90 mmHg, whereas Tuszynski *et al.* (1989) defined it as greater than 160/95 mmHg. Another autopsy study of 1086 cases, of which 532 (49%) had one or more lacunes, showed that hypertensive (>160/95 mmHg) and borderline hypertensive (>140/90 and <160/95 mmHg) patients had more lacunes than normotensive patients, whereas diastolic hypertension was more strongly related to the number of lacunes than systolic hypertension (Dozono *et al.* 1991).

Besides pathological studies, there are many clinical studies providing data on hypertension in lacunar infarction. Table 7.3 shows the frequency of hypertension in lacunar infarction. It was noted how hypertension was defined, when indicated. In these clinical studies, between 44 and 75 per cent of patients with lacunar infarcts had hypertension. Differences in the definitions of hypertension may, in part, explain differences in the frequency of hypertension between these studies. Some authors did not indicate at all how hypertension was defined and/or the timing of the recording (Mohr *et al.* 1978, Nelson *et al.* 1980, Pullicino *et al.* 1980, Foulkes *et al.* 1988, Tegeler *et al.* 1991). The lowest frequency of hypertension (44%) was found in a population-based study (Lodder *et al.* 1990). In this study, pre-stroke measurements were also available. The higher prevalence of hypertension in the hospital-based studies might result from the fact that blood pressure measurements in the post-stroke period were used, which in some cases probably did not reflect pre-stroke blood pressure levels reliably. Some studies also did not indicate how many blood pressure recordings on separate occasions in a patient were used because using single blood pressure measurements to define hypertension might lead to overdiagnosis. Most studies defined hypertension as blood pressure recordings of more than 160/90 mmHg (pre- and post-stroke, or only post-stroke) and known hypertension with treatment

Table 7.3 The frequency of hypertension in clinical studies of lacunar infarction

Reference	Definition[a]	Lacunar infarct			Non-lacunar infarct			OR[b]	95% CI
		Total *n*	*n*	%	Total *n*	*n*	%		
Mohr et al. (1978)	?	131	–	75	–	–	–	–	–
Nelson et al. (1980)	?	37	27	73	–	–	–	–	–
Pullicino et al. (1980)	?	42	24	57	122	52	43	1.80	0.88–3.65
Donnan et al. (1982)	b, d	69	50	72	–	–	–	–	–
Loeb et al. (1986)	a	154	116	75	111	66	59	2.08	1.22–3.53
Foulkes et al. (1988)	?	337	–	75	–	–	–	–	–
Gandolfo et al. (1988)	b, c, (a)	108	70	65	–	–	–	–	–
Anzalone and Landi (1989)	b, c	88	57	65	–	–	–	–	–
Ghika et al. (1989)	a	100	59	59	–	–	–	–	–
Norrving and Cronqvist (1989)	b, c	61	32	53	61	27	44	1.39	0.68–2.83
Arboix et al. (1990a)	a	227	164	72	–	–	–	–	–
Lodder et al. (1990)	c	102	45	44	202	95	47	0.89	0.55–1.43
Boiten and Lodder (1991a)	b, c	103	51	50	94	35	37	1.65	0.94–2.91
Norrving and Staaf (1991)	b, c	180	94	52	–	–	–	–	–
Tegeler et al. (1991)	?	55	33	60	54	30	56	1.20	0.56–2.57
Mast et al. (1995)	b	184	134	73	453	290	64	1.54	1.04–2.29
You et al. (1995)	b	203	140	69	–	–	–	–	–
Boiten et al. (1996)	b, c	287	138	48	582	260	45	1.24	0.93–1.65

[a] Definition of hypertension: a $\geq$ 160/95 mmHg; b = clinical treatment; c $\geq$ 160/90 mmHg; d = diastolic >95 mmHg.

[b] OR = odds ratio; CI = confidence interval.

(Anzalone and Landi 1989, Norrving and Cronqvist 1989, Boiten and Lodder 1991*a*, Norrving and Staaf 1991, Boiten *et al.* 1996). The frequency of hypertension in these studies was quite similar, ranging from 48 to 65 per cent. Besides differences in definitions of hypertension, differences in study methods (e.g. definition of lacunar infarction) may also partly explain the different frequency of hypertension.

The case–control studies show that the risk of lacunar infarction is increased 5- to 9-fold by hypertension (Table 7.2), demonstrating that hypertension is a very important risk factor for lacunar infarction. However, a lot of lacunar infarct patients do not have hypertension. Several clinical studies, except one (Mast *et al.* 1995), showed that the frequency of hypertension did not differ between lacunar and non-lacunar infarct patients (Table 7.3).

Hypertension is therefore associated with both large vessel atherosclerosis and SVD. Patients with hypertension therefore seem no more likely to develop lacunar than non-lacunar infarction. Obviously, hypertension is an important but not a unique risk factor in lacunar infarction.

Diabetes mellitus

Diabetes mellitus is also a major risk factor for stroke in general. The association of stroke and diabetes is independent of other vascular risk factors, which are often present in diabetic patients (obesity, hypertension, hypercholesterolaemia). The relative risk of stroke is increased independently 2- to 3-fold in patients with diabetes (Sacco *et al.* 1997). Diabetes can cause a small vessel arteriolopathy, especially in the retina and kidney, and might therefore also be a risk factor for cerebral SVD causing lacunar infarction.

Fisher (1965*a*) found diabetes mellitus in only 11 per cent of his pathological cases. The number of lacunar infarcts was approximately the same in diabetic as in non-diabetic persons. This led him to conclude that cerebral SVD is usually not related to diabetes mellitus. However, in the autopsy study of Tuszynski *et al.* (1989), 34 per cent of the cases had diabetes mellitus although a definintion of diabetes was not provided.

Case–control studies show an independent relative risk of lacunar infarction in diabetic patients of from 2 to 3.6 (Gandolfo *et al.* 1988, You *et al.* 1995, Boiten *et al.* 1996) (Table 7.2), which is similar to the risk of ischaemic stroke in general. In Table 7.4, the frequency of diabetes mellitus in lacunar infarction in various clinical studies is shown. Again, it is worth mentioning that many of these studied did not provide a definition of diabetes. The frequency of diabetes ranged from 2 to 37 per cent. All clinical studies showed that the frequency of diabetes mellitus did not differ between patients with lacunar and those with non-lacunar infarction (Table 7.4). These studies demonstrate that diabetes mellitus is as important a risk factor for lacunar infarction as it is for cerebral infarction in general, but that it is not a unique risk factor for cerebral SVD causing lacunar infarction.

Diabetes mellitus is commonly associated with other risk factors, most frequently hypertension (Dyken 1991, Sacco *et al.* 1997). Weisberg (1988) reported from prelimininary data that diabetes mellitus combined with hypertension might be a major risk factor for lacunar infarction. Others reported the association of hypertension and diabetes mellitus in about 20 per cent of the lacunar infarct patients (Arboix *et al.* 1990*a*). In two other studies, 15 and 23 per cent of the lacunar infarct patients had diabetes mellitus associated with hypertension, which, however, did not differ significantly from the frequency in non-lacunar infarction (10 and 17%) (Boiten and Lodder 1991*a*, Mast *et al.* 1995).

Cigarette smoking

Cigarette smoking is an independent risk factor for stroke, specifically brain infarction (Wolf *et al.* 1988, Shinton and Beevers 1989). A meta-analysis (32 separate studies) showed that the (pooled) relative risk of cigarette smoking for cerebral infarction was 1.92 (Shinton and Beevers 1989). There is a dose–response relationship between the number of cigarettes and risk of stroke (Wolf *et al.* 1988, Shinton and Beevers 1989).

Table 7.4 The frequency of diabetes mellitus in clinical studies of lacunar infarction

Reference	Definition[a]	Lacunar infarct			Non-lacunar infarct			OR[b]	95% CI
		Total n	n	%	Total n	n	%		
Mohr et al. (1978)	?	131	–	29	–	–	–	–	–
Nelson et al. (1980)	?	37	3	8	–	–	–	–	–
Pullicino et al. (1980)	?	42	–	2	122	–	6	0.40	0.05–3.36
Donnan et al. (1982)	?	69	6	9	–	–	–	–	–
Loeb et al. (1986)	?	154	–	25	111	–	25	1.01	0.57–1.76
Foulkes et al. (1988)	?	337	–	27	–	–	–	–	–
Gandolfo et al. (1988)	a, d	108	23	21	–	–	–	–	–
Anzalone and Landi (1989)	a, e	88	17	19	–	–	–	–	–
Ghika et al. (1989)	b	100	37	37	–	–	–	–	–
Norrving and Cronqvist (1989)	?	61	5	8	61	6	10	0.82	0.24–2.84
Arboix et al. (1990a)	c	227	64	28	–	–	–	–	–
Lodder et al. (1990)	?	102	13	13	202	19	9	1.41	0.66–2.98
Boiten and Lodder (1991a)	a, b	103	28	27	94	25	26	1.03	0.55–1.93
Norrving and Staaf (1991)	a	180	28	16	–	–	–	–	–
Tegeler et al. (1991)	?	55	19	35	54	16	30	1.25	0.56–2.81
Mast et al. (1995)	a	184	53	29	453	96	21	1.44	0.96–2.17
You et al. (1995)	a	203	36	18	–	–	–	–	–
Boiten et al. (1996)	a, b	287	58	20	582	120	21	1.10	0.77–1.58

[a] Definition of diabetes mellitus: a = treated with diet or medication, or both; b = two or more fasting serum glucose levels ≥ 6 mmol/l; c = abnormal fasting glucose level and/or glucose tolerance test; d = two glucose levels ≥ 110 mg%; e = fasting glucose level ≥ 140 mg%.
[b] OR = odds ratio; CI = confidence interval.

In two case–control studies, smoking increased the risk of lacunar infarction 2.3 and 6.6 times (Gandolfo et al. 1988, You et al. 1995) (Table 7.2). In these studies, definition of smoking differed (especially differentiating between current and ex-smokers) as well as controlling for confounding variables, which may have caused the different relative risks.

Of the lacunar stroke patients, 28–68 per cent smoked cigarettes (Table 7.5). The frequency of smoking was similar in patients with lacunar infarction to that in those with non-lacunar infarction [68 versus 69%; odds ratio (OR) 0.94; 95% confidence interval (CI) 0.57–1.58] (Lodder et al. 1990), indicating that smoking is a non-specific risk factor for lacunar infarction.

Heart disease

Heart disease in general, including ischaemic or coronary heart disease, is a risk factor for stroke (Dyken 1991, Norris and Hachinski 1991, Sacco et al. 1997), and the major

Table 7.5 Frequency of other risk factors in clinical studies of lacunar infarction

Reference	No. of patients	Ischaemic heart disease		Previous TIA		Smoking	
		n	%	*n*	%	*n*	%
Mohr et al. (1978)	131	–	–	–	23	–	–
Loeb et al. (1986)	154	25	16	52	34[c]	–	–
Foulkes et al. (1988)	337	–	20[a]	–	13	–	–
Gandolfo et al. (1988)	108	31	29[d]	37	34	59	55
Anzalone and Landi (1989)	88	–	–	20	23	30	34
Ghika et al. (1989)	100	–	–	–	–	33	33
Norrving and Cronqvist (1989)	61	–	8[a]	15	25	–	51
Arboix et al. (1990a)	227	58	26[b]	40	18	–	–
Lodder et al. (1990)	102	40	39	18	18	69	68
Boiten and Lodder (1991a)	103	27	26	–	–	–	–
Norrving and Staaf (1991)	180	31	17[a]	29	16	51	28
Tegeler et al. (1991)	55	–	–	4	7	21	38
You et al. (1995)	203	51	25[e]	–	–	91	45
Boiten et al. (1996)	287	61	21	–	–	–	–

[a] Sum of patients (percentage) with myocardial infarction and patients (percentage) with angina.
[b] Heart disease also including dysrhythmia.
[c] RIA, reversible ischaemic attack.
[d] Ischaemic ECG abnormalities.
[e] Heart disease in general.

cause of death among stroke survivors (Dyken 1991). In the case–control studies, heart disease in general was not a risk factor for lacunar infarction (You *et al.* 1995, Table 7.2), whereas ischaemic heart disease increased the risk of lacunar infarction 2.6–4.3 times (Gandolfo *et al.* 1988, Boiten *et al.* 1996). These findings support the view that embaligenic heart disease is an unlikely cause of lacunar infarction. Of lacunar infarct patients, 8–47 per cent have a history of ischaemic heart disease (Table 7.5). The frequency of coronary heart disease did not differ between patients with lacunar and non-lacunar infarction in some studies (Lodder *et al.* 1990, Boiten and Lodder 1991a). However, in another study, lacunar infarct patients had ischaemic heart disease significantly less often than non-lacunar infarct patients (OR 0.63, 95% CI 0.45–0.88) (Boiten *et al.* 1996).

Transient ischaemic attacks

It is questionable whether one should consider TIAs as a risk factor or just another form of stroke (Dyken 1991). TIAs can, however, identify patients with a high risk of stroke, and could therefore be considered as a risk factor (Dyken 1991, Sacco *et al.* 1997). Even after adjustment for other vascular risk factors, TIAs are an independent risk factor for stroke (Howard *et al.* 1994, Sacco *et al.* 1997). In clinical studies, between 7 and 34 per cent of the lacunar stroke patients experienced previous TIAs (Table 7.5). Compared with control subjects, lacunar infarct patients had a previous TIA significantly more often (34 versus 3%), which gave a relative risk of 35 (Table 7.2; Gandolfo *et al.* 1988). The frequency of previous TIA did not differ significantly between patients with lacunar and those with non-lacunar infarction (18 versus 18%; Lodder *et al.* 1990). Therefore, previous TIA could be considered as a risk factor for lacunar infarction as it is for ischaemic stroke in general.

Possible risk factors for lacunar infarction

Many less well documented risk factors for stroke have been described (Sacco *et al.* 1997). For some of these risk factors, data are available for lacunar infarction.

Hypercholesterolaemia

There is a discussion as to whether hypercholesterolaemia is a risk factor for stroke. On the one hand, epidemiological studies failed to show an association between stroke and cholesterol (Prospective Studies Collaboration 1995) but, on the other hand, lowering of plasma cholesterol reduces stroke risk in patients who have not yet had a stroke (Hebert *et al.* 1997). There are no trials of cholesterol lowering in stroke patients.

Case–control studies show that hypercholesterolaemia is not a risk factor for lacunar infarction (Gandolfo *et al.* 1988, You *et al.* 1995) (Table 7.2). In 16–44 per cent of lacunar stroke patients, hyperlipidaemia was present (Gandolfo *et al.* 1988, Anzalone and Landi 1989, Ghika *et al.* 1989, Norrving and Cronqvist 1989, You *et al.* 1995).

Alcohol consumption

Many studies suggest a J-shaped association between customary alcohol consumption and ischaemic stroke (Camargo 1989). Heavy drinking increases the risk, whereas light to moderate drinking probably decreases risk. Recently, it was reported from a prospective cohort study (Physicians' Health Study) that light to moderate alcohol consumption reduced the risk of ischaemic stroke in men (Berger *et al.* 1999).

In a case–control study, alcohol consumption did not increase the risk of lacunar stroke (You *et al.* 1995). Alcohol consumption by a subject was defined as ever having drunk alcohol in his or her lifetime. In this study, 75 per cent of lacunar infarct patients and 71 per cent of controls had consumed alcohol by this defintition.

Other possible risk factors

In the case–control studies, high haematocrit and use of oral contraceptives were not risk factors for lacunar infarction (Gandolfo *et al.* 1988, You *et al.* 1995). Individuals who undertook regular physical exercise were at lower risk of lacunar infarction (12 versus 27%, OR 0.3, 95% CI 0.1–0.7) (You *et al.* 1995).

A nested case–control study within the British Regional Heart Study cohort showed a strong independent association between homocysteine concentration and risk of stroke (Perry *et al.* 1995). Other studies also showed that hyperhomocysteinaemia is associated with an increased stroke risk (Sacco *et al.* 1997, Hankey 1999). However, there are no data available yet on ischaemic stroke subtypes such as lacunar infarction. Obviously, these possible risk factors warrant further investigation in lacunar infarct patients.

Two lacunar infarct subtypes?

Recently, we hypothesized that single and multiple lacunar infarcts constitute two distinct lacunar infarct entities with a distinct risk factor profile and a distinct type of underlying SVD (Boiten 1991, Boiten *et al.* 1993). We developed our hypothesis on the basis of the discrepancy in the rate of hypertension between the pathological studies by Fisher and clinical studies. Fisher found that almost all his lacunar cases had hypertension (Fisher 1965*a*), whereas clinical studies showed that many lacunar infarct patients do not have hypertension (see above). Almost all the lacunar cases of Fisher had multiple lacunar infarcts, whereas in clinical studies most patients have a single lacunar infarct. Probably, single and multiple lacunar infarcts constitute distinct entities. Subsequently, others also investigated the risk factor profile of single and multiple lacunar infarcts (Mast *et al.* 1995, Mochizuki *et al.* 1997, Spolveri *et al.* 1998). Table 7.6 shows the frequency of hypertension and diabetes mellitus in the two lacunar infarct subtypes. Two studies did not use logistic regression models to investigate the independent association of the risk factor with multiple lacunar infarcts (Mochizuki *et al.* 1997, Spolveri *et al.* 1998). Patients with multiple lacunar infarcts more often had hypertension and diabetes than those with a single

Table 7.6 Risk factors for single and multiple lacunar infarcts

Risk factor	Single lacunar infarct			Multiple lacunar infarct			OR[a]	95% CI
	Total *n*	*n*	%	Total *n*	*n*	%		
Hypertension								
Boiten *et al.* (1993)	79	34	43	21	15	71	2.64	0.79–8.90
Mast *et al.* (1995)	144	101	70	40	33	82	2.54	1.07–6.03
Mochizuki *et al.* (1997)[b]	15	13	86	10	9	90		
Spolveri *et al.* (1998)[b]	39	19	49	35	24	69		
Diabetes								
Boiten *et al.* (1993)	79	21	27	21	6	29	1.35	0.36–5.13
Mast *et al.* (1995)	144	37	26	40	16	40	2.26	1.13–4.52
Mochizuki *et al.* (1997)[b]	15	2	13	10	5	50		
Spolveri *et al.* (1998)[b]	39	7	18	35	8	23		

[a] OR = odds ratio; CI = confidence interval.
[b] These studies did not use logistic regression models to investigate the independent association of the risk factor with multiple lacunar infarcts.

lacunar infarct. The association of multiple lacunar infarcts with hypertension is more convincing than the association with diabetes. These studies support the hypothesis of two distinct lacunar infarct entities, of which multiple lacunar infarcts are more strongly associated with hypertension and probably also with diabetes.

There is also a pathogenetic basis for the existence of two distinct lacunar infarct entities. Fisher (1965a, 1969, 1979) described two types of SVD. In most of his patients, he found lipohyalinosis (or arteriolosclerosis), affecting the smaller penetrating arteries. These patients had multiple, usually clinically asymptomatic, lacunar infarcts, whereas almost all of them had hypertension. Fisher related this type of SVD particularly to hypertension. Furthermore, he described another type of SVD, causing larger and usually symptomatic lacunar infarcts. This second type of SVD is characterized by microatheromata, which occlude the larger penetrating arteries. These small atheromata are probably similar to the large vessel atheromata, except for their size.

We hypothesized that clinically, patients with multiple lacunar infarcts probably suffer from lipohyalinosis, whereas patients with a single lacunar infarct suffer from microatheromatosis. The similarity of small vessel atheromata and large vessel atheromata explains that the vascular ('atherogenic') risk factor profile is similar in lacunar stroke patients (with a single lacunar infarct) and non-cardioembolic, territorial stroke patients.

Conclusions

The risk factor profile of lacunar infarction constitutes, besides age and gender, hypertension, diabetes, cigarette smoking, previous TIA, and probably ischaemic heart disease. These vascular risk factors are not specific for lacunar infarction. Of the two lacunar infarct subtypes, that with multiple lacunar infarcts is more strongly related to hypertension and probably also to diabetes. Several lacunar stroke patients do not have any of these classic risk factors, and therefore searching for new risk factors is an important endeavour.

An as yet unresolved question is what determines whether mainly smaller (as in lacunar infarcts) or mainly larger (as in non-lacunar infarcts) vessels will become affected in the presence of the same atherogenic milieu. Probably, genetic susceptibility determines the type of stroke which evolves.

Chapter 8

Genetic susceptibility and lacunar stroke

A. Elbaz and P. Amarenco

Introduction

Understanding the genetic basis of lacunar stroke (LacS) may help understand the aetiology and pathogenesis of this particular ischaemic stroke (IS) subtype (ISType); this, in turn, may have consequences in terms of treatment or prevention.

Two main questions are to be answered. First, does genetic susceptibility play a role in the aetiology of LacS? In other words, does LacS aggregate in families and, if so, do genetic factors account for part of this aggregation, or is it only the consequence of the familial aggregation of other cardiovascular risk factors? Secondly, if genetic susceptibility does play a role in the aetiology of LacS, which specific genetic factors increase its risk? What is the importance of their attributable risk? Do they interact with environmental risk factors?

As we will discuss below, family studies in the context of stroke are difficult and, to our knowledge, no study has investigated specifically the familial aggregation/ segregation of LacS. A limited number of studies have investigated the role of candidate genes in the aetiology of LacS as part of larger studies on IS, but our knowledge on the genetic susceptibility of LacS is still very limited. In this review, we will first discuss methodological issues concerning genetic studies on IS (including LacS), and then summarize the results of recent genetic studies in this field. We will not address the issue of IS in the context of monogenic (mendelian, mitochondrial) diseases.

Genetic studies on lacunar stroke: methodological considerations

The investigator aiming to study the genetic basis of IS, including that of LacS, has to consider several particularities which have important implications for study design.

Aetiological heterogeneity

The main difficulty of genetic studies on IS is related to the aetiological heterogeneity underlying this disease. Under a simplistic model, genes may play a role in IS at least at two different levels: (1) they may increase the risk of the underlying cause of IS (see below) or (2) they may increase the risk of a complication of the underlying disease (e.g. thrombus formation) (Elbaz and Amarenco 1999).

(1) If genetic susceptibility does play a role at this level, the genes involved, or at least the strength of their effect, may differ according to ISTypes (atherothrombotic, lacunar, cardioembolic, dissections, etc). Although ISTypes share several environmental risk factors, there is some evidence that in the case of IS recurrence, the recurrent and the first event belong more frequently to the same subtype (Samuelsson *et al.* 1996*a*, Yamamoto and Bogousslavsky 1998). This observation is compatible with different genetic factors involved in different ISTypes. Many studies have investigated the role of specific candidate genes in IS without distinguishing LacS from other ISTypes; based on the results of such studies, it is not possible to draw conclusions about the relationship between genes and LacS, unless we hypothesize that the role of genes is independent of ISTypes. We do not believe, however, that such a hypothesis is warranted for many candidate genes at the present time.

(2) Alternatively, genes that are involved in the final stages of IS aetiology (e.g. thrombosis) may increase the risk of IS independently of its underlying cause. Still, being able to assess whether a given gene is a risk factor for IS, whatever the subtype is, is interesting and important by itself.

Hence, classifications of patients into homogeneous groups from an aetiological perspective are an important issue in genetics studies of IS. How *pure* LacS (i.e. due to small vessel disease) can be distinguished from other ISTypes is thus a central problem—which is beyond the scope of this chapter. We will just point out that it is far from being an easy task because pathological confirmation can only be obtained in exceptional instances; besides, some lacunes may be due to large vessel or heart disease. A way of dealing with this problem may be to exclude from genetic studies of LacS those patients who have a clinical/radiological diagnosis of LacS, as well as another potential IS cause (e.g. atrial fibrillation, carotid stenosis). In addition, some authors have suggested that the risk factors of multiple asymptomatic lacunes and a single symptomatic lacune may not be the same (Boiten *et al.* 1993), whereas other authors do not believe this is likely (Longstreth *et al.* 1998).

Finally, lacunes usually account for approximately 20 per cent of the total number of IS, and this should be taken into account when evaluating the power of a given study to detect an association between a polymorphism and LacS.

Intermediate phenotypes

When studying IS risk factors, one should keep in mind that what we could call *intermediate phenotypes* (e.g. lipohyalinosis in LacS, carotid stenosis in atherothrombotic strokes, atrial fibrillation in cardioembolic strokes) are involved in the mechanism of the disease. Concerning LacS, the intermediate phenotype cannot be measured readily and we can only detect those subjects who have already suffered a

LacS. Surrogates for the intermediate phenotype would be helpful, because their risk factors, and in particular their genetic determinants, can be studied. Could white matter hyperintensities (WMHs) represent such a surrogate? The pathogenesis of WMHs and their relationship to LacS or lipohyalinosis are still not well understood, but it is likely that ongoing studies will help to clarify these issues.

Incidence and study designs

The incidence of IS rises sharply with increasing age. It is less frequent than myocardial infarction and occurs at a mean older age; estimates of LacS incidence are available (Bamford *et al.* 1987, Sacco *et al.* 1991, Petty *et al.* 1999). Large cohorts have to be followed for long periods of time in order to ascertain a sufficient number of IS: for instance, in the Physician's Health Study (PHS), 22 071 men had to be followed for 12 years in order to ascertain 348 strokes (ischaemic and haemorrhagic) (Zee *et al.* 1999). As a consequence, if we are interested in specific ISTypes (e.g. lacunes), very large cohorts are needed. It is often difficult in such cohorts to classify strokes according to their aetiology. Besides, classifications of events and diagnoses are likely to change over time because of changes in diagnostic procedures and an increasing number of investigations available. Case–control studies are therefore likely to be a more feasible and less expensive approach. Besides, compared with other risk factors, genetic risk factors have the advantage of not being prone to recall bias, of not being modified by the disease, and of being less prone to measurement errors. Still, the limitations of case–control studies in this context must be recognized (see below).

Family studies

Family studies may represent a first step in order to elucidate the genetic component of a disease. However, this is a difficult approach for IS. First, such studies are highly sensitive to the reliability of the information obtained for relatives. In IS, such information is often difficult to collect (for instance in parents who are most often deceased at the time of the study); when available, discrimination between IS and haemorrhages is problematic or impossible in many cases. Distinguishing the different ISTypes in relatives is even more difficult. Second, several IS risk factors have a genetic component and are characterized by a certain degree of familial aggregation; this may be a source of confounding.

Although studies on the familial aggregation of stroke have been reported (Brass *et al.* 1992, Kiely *et al.* 1993, Graffagnino *et al.* 1994, Wannamethee *et al.* 1996, Jousilahti *et al.* 1997, Kubota *et al.* 1997, Liao *et al.* 1997, Nicolaou *et al.* 2000)—some of them suggesting that there may be a familial component—there are no studies to our knowledge that have specifically investigated the familial aggregation and recurrence risks of LacS.

Association studies

Most of the data available to date on genetic susceptibility of LacS come from case–control studies that compared distributions of genotypic/allelic frequencies of candidate genes in cases and controls (association studies). Population stratification, survival bias, and asymptomatic LacS among controls may represent limitations of these studies.

In the first case, when cases and controls differ in ethnic background, bias can occur if the allelic frequencies differ across ethnic groups, and if there are differences in incidence rates according to ethnicity. To overcome this problem, investigators have suggested the possibility of matching cases and controls on ethnicity (Khoury and Yang 1998); however, the feasibility of this strategy has not been well evaluated, and the methods needed to assess ethnicity are not well defined. Family-based studies (e.g. transmission disequilibrium test) have been proposed as a solution (Spielman and Ewens 1996). However, this is not likely to be a feasible design in the context of IS, because most of the parents are dead at the time of the study; sibship-based methods have been elaborated, but they have limited power and require large numbers of subjects (Spielman and Ewens 1998, Schaid and Rowland 1998).

Incidence-prevalence bias may arise if prevalent cases are included in the study and if survival is related to the gene under investigation. If cases are included early after the event, this is not likely to be a major issue, because early IS case fatality rates are rather low, especially in LacS in which they are close to the null (Bamford *et al.* 1987, 1991, Sacco *et al.* 1991, Peltonen *et al.* 1998, Petty *et al.* 2000). Conversely, ascertainment of prevalent cases may bias the results. This is also important when patients with LacS are compared with cases with other stroke ISTypes, because survival after stroke varies across ISTypes.

There is evidence that the prevalence of asymptomatic LacS increases with age and that it is quite important among old subjects (Longstreth *et al.* 1998, Bryan *et al.* 1999). It is therefore likely that a proportion of controls included in case–control studies of IS actually had asymptomatic lacunes, which would remain undiagnosed, unless a brain magnetic resonance imaging (MRI) or computed tomography (CT) scan was also performed in controls. This is a source of further difficulties in the design of such studies.

Published studies usually have relied on comparisons between cases and controls. If we hypothesize that a particular candidate gene is associated with a given ISType, another way of analysing the data would be to compare cases with cases according to ISTypes; we view this strategy as a complementary one. When doing so, analyses should take into account that there may be several differences between ISTypes (e.g. in age or sex). Again, such analyses are meaningful (in terms of power) only if a sufficient number of subjects have been included for each subtype.

Finally, association studies have relied on a candidate gene approach. The choice of the candidate genes to be studied usually is based on pathophysiological considerations, and until now it has been dictated largely by the results of similar studies in the context of myocardial infarction. It is likely that a better understanding of the anatomical basis and pathogenesis of LacS would help to guide researchers towards genes more specifically involved in LacS. Besides, there have been major advances in molecular techniques, and it will soon be possible to start considering genome-wide association studies (Boerwinkle *et al.* 1999).

Lacunar stroke: association studies

In the last 5 years, there have been many reports of association studies in the context of IS (Elbaz and Amarenco 1999). Some of them have, in addition, examined the relationship between candidate genes and IS according to ISTypes. It should be emphasized, however, that many were not designed primarily to study the relationship between candidate genes and ISTypes, due to the small sample sizes involved. Table 8.1 summarizes the results of several studies which investigated different candidate genes in LacS. When possible, we present their findings for LacS, for controls, as well as for another ISType. The methods used in these studies to (i) select patients (i.e. prevalent or incident cases), (ii) select controls (population-based, hospital-based, relatives, undefined), (iii) classify IS events into ISTypes, and (iv) analyse the data (matched or unmatched, uni- or multivariate analyses) are highly variable from one study to another; this is a major source of difficulties when trying to compare the results of these studies. Significant results are indicated, and three examples will be discussed briefly.

Angiotensin-converting enzyme (ACE)

The ACE I/D polymorphism has been widely investigated in relation to several phenotypes (e.g. coronary artery disease, hypertension, cardiomyopathy, intima-media thickness) with varying results (for a review of the role of ACE, see Villard and Soubrier 1996). It is also the gene which has been investigated most often in IS, but studies on their relationship have yielded conflicting results. A meta-analysis found a modest but significant association between the DD genotype and IS (Sharma 1998). However, in a study nested in the PHS cohort, no association between the ACE I/D polymorphism and stroke was found (Zee *et al.* 1999). Markus *et al.* (1995) reported no overall association between this polymorphism and IS, but they observed an association between the DD genotype and LacS ($n = 18$). Similar findings were observed in the GÉNIC study: there was no association of IS with the I/D polymorphism overall, but an association was found among men with LacS (manuscript in preparation). Other studies did not confirm an association between the ACE I/D polymorphism and LacS (Table 8.1). In particular, no relationship was found in the largest of these studies (Ueda *et al.* 1995). In this study, patients were classified into ISTypes using a clinical classification; it is not certain whether or not this may have introduced some misclassification.

Table 8.1 Candidate genes and lacunar stroke

	Lacunar cases n (%)	Cases with other IS subtypes n (%)	Controls 1 C_1 n (%)	Controls 2 C_2 n (%)
ACE I/D				
Doi et al. (1997)	n = 123	n = 34	n = 271	
		Cortical infarcts		
II	51 (41.0)	13 (38.0)	115 (42.0)	
ID	53 (43.0)	14 (41.0)	126 (46.0)	
DD	19 (15.0)	7 (21.0)	30 (11.0)	
Catto et al. (1996)[§]	n = 130	n = 242	n = 215	
		TACI/PACI		
II	32 (24.6)	68 (28.1)	50 (23.2)	
ID	61 (46.9)	109 (45.0)	102 (47.4)	
DD	37 (28.5)	65 (26.9)	63 (29.3)	
Markus et al. (1995)	n = 18	n = 242	n = 137	
		Large vessel		
II	2 (11.1)	10 (23.3)	36 (26.3)	
ID	5 (27.8)	21 (48.8)	71 (51.8)	
DD	11 (61.1)[†]	12 (23.3)	30 (21.9)	
Ueda et al. (1995)[§]	n = 163	n = 253	n = 188	
		TACI/PACI		
II	41 (25.0)	66 (26.0)	41 (22.0)	
ID	91 (56.0)	139 (55.0)	105 (56.0)	
DD	31 (19.0)	48 (19.0)	42 (22.0)	
Notsu et al. (1999)	n = 74	n = 101	n = 213	n = 174
		SBI		
II	32 (43.0)	33 (33.0)	86 (41.0)	67 (39.0)
ID	34 (46.0)	56 (55.0)	92 (44.0)	77 (44.0)
DD	8 (11.0)	12 (12.0)	31 (15.0)	30 (17.0)
ecNOS Glu298Asp, Markus et al. (1998)	n = 75	n = 105	n = 236	
		Large vessel		
GG	32 (42.7)	38 (36.2)	96 (40.7)	
GT	33 (44.0)	52 (49.5)	104 (44.1)	
TT	10 (13.3)	15 (14.3)	36 (15.3)	
Glu298Asp, Elbaz et al. (2000b)	n = 95	n = 106	n = 95*	
		Large vessel		
GG	47 (49.5)	49 (46.2)	32 (33.7)	
GT	34 (35.8)	41 (38.7)	46 (48.4)	
TT	14 (14.7)[†]	16 (15.1)	17 (17.9)	

(continued)

Table 8.1 (continued) Candidate genes and lacunar stroke

	Lacunar cases n (%)	Cases with other IS subtypes n (%)	Controls 1 C$_1$ n (%)	Controls 2 C$_2$ n (%)
27 bp intron 4, Yahashi *et al.* (1998)	*n* = 58	*n* = 18	*n* = 91	
		Large vessel		
bb	43 (74.1)	14 (77.8)	67 (73.6)	
ab	14 (24.1)	4 (22.2)	24 (26.4)	
aa	1 (1.7)	–	–	
Factor XIII Val34Leu Catto *et al.* (1998)[§]	*n* = 176	*n* = 353	*n* = 434	
		TACI/PACI		
Val/Val + Val/Leu	99 (56.3)	184 (52.1)	254 (58.3)	
Leu/Leu	77 (43.8)	169 (47.8)	182 (41.7)	
Elbaz *et al.* (2000a)	*n* = 94	*n* = 105	*n* = 94*	
		Large vessel		
Val/Val	58 (61.7)	66 (62.9)	37 (39.4)	
Val/Leu	29 (30.8)	29 (27.6)	49 (52.1)	
Leu/Leu	7 (7.5)[†]	10 (9.5)	8 (8.5)	
Factor VII R353Q Nishiuma *et al.* (1997)	*n* = 118[‡]	–	*n* = 83 Hypertensives	*n* = 97 Non-hypertensives
RR	76 (92.0)		106 (90.0)	86 (89.0)
RQ + QQ	7 (8.0)		12 (10.0)	11 (11.0)
MTHFR C677T Markus *et al.* (1997)	*n* = 75	*n* = 116	*n* = 161	
		Large vessel		
CC	33 (44.0)	55 (47.4)	76 (47.2)	
CT	35 (46.7)	50 (43.1)	63 (39.1)	
TT	7 (9.3)	11 (9.5)	22 (13.7)	
Notsu *et al.* (1999)	*n* = 74	*n* = 108	*n* = 209	*n* = 92
		SBI		
CC	23 (31.0)	44 (41.0)	86 (41.0)	39 (43.0)
CT	33 (45.0)	53 (49.0)	92 (44.0)	39 (43.0)
TT	18 (24.0)	11 (10.0)	31 (15.0)	14 (15.0)
Markus *et al.* (1997)[§]	*n* = 72	*n* = 139	*n* = 173	
		TACI/PACI		
CC	25 (35.0)	72 (51.8)	81 (46.0)	
CT	41 (57.0)	53 (38.1)	76 (43.0)	
TT	6 (8.0)	14 (10.0)	16 (9.0)	

(continued)

Table 8.1 (continued) Candidate genes and lacunar stroke

	Lacunar cases n (%)	Cases with other IS subtypes n (%)	Controls 1 C_1 n (%)	Controls 2 C_2 n (%)
Glycoprotein IIb HPA-3				
Carter et al. (1999)	n = ?	n = ?	n = 423	
		Large vessel		
aa	(36.1)	(41.4)	187 (44.2)	
ab	(53.3)	(46.0)	183 (43.3)	
bb	(10.7)	(12.6)	53 (12.5)	
ApoE				
Kessler et al. (1997)	n = 34	n = 70	n = 225	
		Large vessel		
22	2 (5.9)	–	1 (0.4)	
23	4 (11.8)	6 (8.6)	24 (10.7)	
33	18 (52.9)	39 (55.7)	149 (66.2)	
24	–	4 (5.7)	6 (2.7)	
34	8 (23.5)	20 (28.6)[†]	43 (19.1)	
β-Fibrinogen G455A				
Kessler et al. (1997)	n = 34	n = 66	n = 218	
		Large vessel		
GG	20 (58.8)	35 (53.0)	109 (50.0)	
GA	14 (41.2)	25 (37.9)	102 (46.8)	
AA	–	6 (9.1)[†]	7 (3.2)	
Nishiuma et al. (1998)	n = 66 Hypertensives	n = 19 AICLA	n = 85 Hypertensives	n = 84 Non-hypertensives
GG	50 (76.0)	12 (63.0)	71 (84.0)	74 (88.0)
GA + AA	16 (24.0) [†]versus C_2	7 (37.0) [†]versus $C_{1,2}$	14 (16.0)	10 (12.0)
Apo(a) size polymorphism				
Notsu et al. (1999)	n = 70	n = 144	n = 194	
		SBI		
Alleles I–IV –	42 (60.0)	88 (61.1)	137 (70.6)	
+	28 (40.0)[†]	56 (38.9)[†]	57 (29.3)	

*Controls individually matched to lacunar cases.

[†]$P < 0.05$ for the comparison between cases and controls.

[‡]Sixty-four patients with overt LacS and 54 hypertensives patients with silent brain infarction (SBI) on MRI.

[§]Patients classified into ISTypes according to the Oxfordshire Community Stroke Project Classification (Bamford et al. 1991).

Endothelial nitric oxide synthase

Nitric oxide (NO) synthesized from L-arginine by the endothelial constitutive nitric oxide synthase (ecNOS) is constantly released from arterial and arteriolar endothelium. NO plays a key role in the relaxation of vascular smooth muscle cells

(VSMCs); it reduces VSMC proliferation, adhesion of platelets and leukocytes, endothelial permeability, and extracellular matrix collagen synthesis. Conversely, an excess of NO may be harmful because of its oxidative role. In animal models, ecNOS inhibition accelerates atherosclerosis (Cayatte *et al.* 1994), while L-arginine administration prevents it. In humans with atherosclerosis, abnormalities in the endothelial NO pathway have been shown. A genetic contribution of ecNOS to plasma NO metabolite levels has been demonstrated (Wang *et al.* 1997, Adachi and Wang 1998). Several polymorphisms have been identified in the ecNOS gene, in particular a polymorphism located in exon 7 which modifies its coding sequence (Glu298Asp) (Shimasaki *et al.* 1998). Although enhanced vascular responsiveness recently has been shown to be associated with the Asp allele of this polymorphism—subjects carrying this allele may have a lower production of NO—this finding does not strictly prove the functionality of the polymorphism (Philip *et al.* 1999).

In the GÉNIC study, the frequency of the GG genotype was significantly higher in cases compared with controls, and this genotype was associated with a modest increase in the risk of IS [odds ratio (OR) 1.49, 95% confidence interval (CI) 1.13–1.96] (Elbaz *et al.* 2000*b*). After stratification on ISTypes, its frequency was significantly higher in cases than in controls only among LacS (OR 2.00, 95% CI 1.05–3.80); this difference remained significant after adjustment for other risk factors. In all other ISTypes, the ORs associated with the GG genotype were greater than 1, but not significantly; after adjustment for other risk factors, the association was considerably attenuated in the atherothrombotic stroke group (OR 1.01; 95% CI 0.49–2.06). There was also evidence in favour of a synergistic interaction between the GG genotype and low-density lipoprotein (LDL) cholesterol level in determining the risk of LacS. As already hypothesized by others in the context of myocardial infarction (Adachi and Wang 1998), this association may be explained by the oxidative role of NO. NO reacts with superoxide to generate a powerful oxidant, peroxynitrite, which is known to be highly cytotoxic. In addition, peroxynitrite increases lipid oxidation and oxidized LDL plays a central role in the oxidative theory of atherosclerosis. Although these findings need to be replicated in another sample due the small sample sizes involved, the relationships between NO, LDL, and LacS deserve further investigation.

Markus *et al.* (1998) were the first to report a study on the relationship between this polymorphism and IS, and they did not find any association between them. However, the frequency of the GG genotype (*nn* in their study) was higher in 75 LacS cases (42.7%) than in other ISTypes (*n* = 286, 33.2%; *P* = 0.13). In another study by MacLeod *et al.* (1999), the G allele was also more frequent in cases (69.7%) than in controls (65.0%), but this difference was only significant at the *P* = 0.08 level and no analyses according to ISTypes were performed. Finally, no association between a 27 bp polymorphism in intron 4 of the ecNOS gene and LacS was found in a Japanese study (Yahashi *et al.* 1998).

Factor XIII

Factor XIII (FXIII) is a transglutaminase consisting of two catalytic A-subunits and two carrier protein B-subunits. When activated by thrombin, FXIIIa catalyses the formation of covalent ε-(γ-glutamyl)-lysyl bounds between fibrin monomers, thus stabilizing the fibrin clot and increasing its resistance to fibrinolysis. FXIIIa is also implicated in the cross-linking of several other proteins, such as α-2 antiplasmin, fibronectin, and collagen. Mutations of the FXIII A-subunit have been related to FXIII deficiency, a rare autosomal recessive disorder characterized by a tendency for spontaneous bleeding (including intracranial haemorrhages at a young age) and impaired wound healing.

A common $G \rightarrow T$ polymorphism, leading to a valine (Val) to leucine (Leu) substitution three amino acids from the thrombin activation site, has been described in exon 2 of the FXIII A-subunit gene (Mikkola *et al.* 1994). The frequency of the Leu allele has been shown to be lower in subjects with myocardial infarction or deep venous thrombosis than in controls (Kohler *et al.* 1998b, 1999, Catto *et al.* 1999, Franco *et al.* 1999, Wartiovaara *et al.* 1999). Because the mutant allele is associated with a higher activity of the enzyme, this protective effect is not well understood. It has been hypothesized that increased rates of FXIII activation could lead to ineffective cross-linking, or that the kinetics of the cross-linking reactions may be disrupted due to the effects of FXIIIa on other proteins (Kohler *et al.* 1998a).

Catto *et al.* (1998) investigated the relationship between stroke and the Val34Leu polymorphism; they found that the mutant allele was more frequent in cases with haemorrhagic stroke (54.8%) than in controls (41.7%), while no significant difference was observed between cases with IS (46.5%) and controls, or between cases with LacS and controls. However, the frequency of the Leu allele in the control group was lower than in other studies carried out by the same team in the same country (Kohler *et al.* 1998b, 1999, Catto *et al.* 1999). In the GÉNIC study, the frequency of carriers of the Leu allele was significantly lower in cases compared with controls (OR = 0.53, 95% CI = 0.40–0.70) (Elbaz *et al.* 2000a). After stratification on ISType, no heterogeneity of this association was observed. The ORs associated with the Leu allele were lower than 1 in all ISTypes; the strongest and most significant association was observed among LacS, and carrying this allele was associated with an important risk reduction in LacS risk (OR = 0.32, 95% CI = 0.16–0.65). Adjustment for other risk factors did not modify these results. Thus, these findings suggest that being a carrier of the Leu allele is protective for both arterial and venous disease. It is also interesting to note that the negative association between the polymorphism and IS was observed for all ISTypes (although with different strengths of association) and that the frequency of the Leu allele was very similar in the different ISTypes. This is in agreement with the role of FXIIIa as a stabilizer of the fibrin clot, which can be hypothesized to be a mechanism in common for IS of different causes.

Genetic determinants of white matter hyperintensities

The cause of WMHs is certainly complex and not yet well understood, but it is believed that ischaemic factors are involved (Pantoni and Garcia 1997). Carmelli *et al.* (1998) reported a twin study on environmental and genetic determinants of WMHs. They found that the heritability of WMHs volume was 71 per cent and that proband concordance rates for large amounts of WMHs were 61 per cent in monozygotic versus 38 per cent in dizygotic pairs, compared with a prevalence of 15 per cent in the entire sample. These results are in favour of a genetic component for WMHs.

There have been few reports on the relationship between WMHs and genes. In a study from Austria in which MRI was performed in 280 subjects (50–75 years old) randomly selected from an official residents register, it was found that carrying the $\varepsilon2/\varepsilon3$ genotype for the apolipoprotein E (ApoE) polymorphism was associated with microangiopathy-related cerebral damage (including WMHs and LacS; OR = 3.00, 95% CI = 1.35–6.69) (Schmidt *et al.* 1997). In a report from the Cardiovascular Health Study on the relationship between ApoE, MRI abnormalities, and cognitive function in 3469 participants (≥65 years) recruited from Medicare files, it was mentioned that no relationship between the ApoE $\varepsilon4$ allele and infarcts ≥3 mm, the number of infarcts, sulci width, ventricle size, or white matter changes was found (Kuller *et al.* 1998).

Studies in animals

In view of the complexity of genetic studies on IS in humans, studies in animals are an interesting approach, and they have brought important contributions. Although some of these results may not have direct implications for LacS, they highlight the interest of animal studies (homogeneity of genetic background, control of the environment). Rubattu *et al.* (1996) performed a genome-wide screen in F_2 rats obtained by mating SHR (spontaneously hypertensive stroke-resistant rats) and SHRSP (stroke-prone spontaneously hypertensive rats), with latency to stroke as the phenotype of interest. They identified three major blood pressure-independent QTLs (quantitative trait loci), that accounted for 28 per cent of the phenotypic variance; one of them (STR2) co-localized with the loci of atrial and natriuretic factors. Interestingly, positive associations between the G1837A (intron 2, $OR_A = 1.64$, 95% CI = 1.01–2.65) and G664A (exon 1, $OR_A = 2.00$, 95% CI = 1.17–3.19) polymorphisms in the gene encoding atrial natriuretic peptide and stroke ($n = 348$) in humans were found in a case–control study nested in the PHS (Rubattu *et al.* 1999). Both ischaemic and haemorrhagic strokes were included in the study, but analyses restricted to 281 ischaemic strokes yielded similar results.

Jeffs *et al.* (1997) performed a genome-wide scan in F_2 rats obtained by mating SHRSP and WKY rats in order to identify genetic factors determining large brain infarcts after occlusion of the middle cerebral artery (MCA). They identified a blood pressure-independent QTL on chromosome 5, which accounted for 67 per cent of the phenotypic variance of the infarct size; this QTL co-localized with the loci of atrial and natriuretic factors. Using MRI, it has also been demonstrated that ischaemic sensitivity in the SHRSP rats was inherited as a dominant trait and was independent of blood pressure after MCA occlusion (Gratton *et al.* 1998).

Conclusions

Our knowledge of the genetic factors underlying LacS remains limited; there have been a few isolated positive results—which remain to be replicated—while others have been negative. It is likely that increasing development of genetic markers and molecular techniques will allow us to gain insight into the genetic factors involved in IS. This will help to improve our knowledge of IS risk factors, and may have therapeutic implications. Furthermore, if gene–environment interactions are implicated, this may also help to prevent a proportion of events, for instance by reducing the environmental exposure in those genetically susceptible.

Because IS in humans is such an aetiologically complex disease, a key issue concerns the genetic factors underlying the different ISTypes. This implies that (i) efforts should be made in order to define and study homogeneous groups of patients, and (ii) large samples of patients are needed. In order to succeed, the creation of networks of collaborating researchers using similar methodologies should be promoted. Efforts should also be directed towards investigation of genetic factors involved in intermediate phenotypes such as WMHs.

Although we are entering an era in which genome-wide association studies are considered, we also believe that a better understanding of the pathogenesis and the anatomical basis of LacS would greatly contribute to guide researchers towards genes specifically involved in LacS.

The implementation of alternative study designs (e.g. sib-pair, family-based studies) should be discussed. As illustrated by the identification of mutations in the *Notch3* gene responsible for cerebral autosomal dominant arteriopathy with subcortical infarcts and leukoencephalopathy (CADASIL), identification of large pedigrees in which IS segregates as a monogenic trait should be helpful. In addition, genetic studies in animal models of IS are important tools and will certainly have a decisive role in the next years.

Acknowledgements

We wish to thank the many persons who have contributed to the GÉNIC study.

Chapter 9

Cerebral autosomal dominant arteriopathy with subcortical infarcts and leukoencephalopathy

H. Chabriat, and M.G. Bousser

Introduction

CADASIL (cerebral .autosomal dominant arteriopathy with subcortical infarcts and leukoencephalopathy) (Tournier-Lasserve *et al.* 1993) is a systemic small artery disease which was identified during the past decade, using clinical, magnetic resonance imaging (MRI), pathological, and genetic tools (Tournier-Lasserve *et al.* 1993). The disease is due to mutations of the Notch3 gene on chromosome 19 (Joutel *et al.* 1996). The identification of the CADASIL gene was crucial to determine precisely the different aspects of the clinical phenotype and to understand better the natural history of this new cause of dementia of both subcortical type and pure vascular origin. This was also an essential step to obtain a genetic test which is now used routinely to confirm the diagnosis of the disease.

History

In 1955, Van Bogaert reported two sisters belonging to a family originating from Belgium with a 'subcortical encephalopathy of Binswanger's type of rapid course' with onset during mid-adulthood (Van Bogaert 1955). Their clinical presentation included dementia, gait disturbances, pseudobulbar palsy, seizures, and focal neurological deficits. Two other sisters had died aged 36 and 43 years after a progressive dementia. Their father had a stroke at age 51 and died after a myocardial infarct. Pathological examination revealed widespread areas of white matter rarefaction in the brain associated with multiple small infarcts mainly located in the white matter and basal ganglia.

In 1977, Sourander and Walinder, proposed a hereditary origin for the disease. They called it 'hereditary multi-infarct dementia', a familial condition observed in a Swedish pedigree and characterized by dementia associated with pseudobulbar palsy occurring 10–15 years after recurrent stroke-like episodes (Sourander and Walinder 1977). Age of onset was between 29 and 38 years; age at death varied from 30 to 53 years. The authors reported brain lesions in three cases, identical to those observed by

Van Bogaert also caused by a small vessel disease in the brain. The wall of the small arteries was thickened, causing a reduction of their lumen. Atherosclerosis of basal arteries was found only in one family member. In the pedigree, the condition followed an autosomal dominant pattern of transmission.

Up to 1993, several families with a similar presentation had been reported using numerous eponyms. We also reported a large family originating from the western part of France in a region called 'Loire-Atlantique' first as 'recurrent strokes in a family with diffuse white-matter and muscular lipidosis—a new mitochondrial cytopathy?' (Bousser *et al.* 1988), secondly as 'Autosomal dominant syndrome with stroke-like episodes and leukoencephalopathy' (Tournier-Lasserve *et al.* 1991) and later as 'Autosomal dominant leukoencephalopathy and subcortical ischemic strokes' (Baudrimont *et al.* 1993). Because of the confusion caused by all these different names, in 1993 we proposed the acronym CADASIL to designate this disease and to highlight its main characteristics (Tournier-Lasserve *et al.* 1993). In 1993, when the gene was mapped on chromosome 19, the term CADASIL was adopted. The identification of the Notch3 gene in 1996 was a crucial step to investigate the pathophysiology of the disease which is essential to open up rapidly therapeutic avenues.

Clinical phenotype

After the gene mapping was conducted in 1993, the study of families with proven linkage to the CADASIL locus improved the understanding of the natural history and the determination of the complete clinical spectrum of the disease.

CADASIL is a disease of mid-adulthood. The mean age at onset of symptoms is 37 years (Desmond *et al.* 1999). However, it varies from 4 to 68 years in different reports mainly because migraine was sometimes considered to be the initial symptom of the disease. The age of onset of ischaemic events can also differ widely among individuals even within a given family. Elsewhere, it has been reported that age of onset does not differ significantly according to gender (Chabriat *et al.* 1995c, Vahedi *et al.* 1996, Dichgans *et al.* 1998). When considering the two most frequent symptoms of the disease, stroke and/or dementia, the mean age at onset does not differ between different generations. The duration of the disease varies between 10 and 30 years. Mean age at death is about 65 years, but it varies from 30 to 80 years in the reported affected pedigrees.

The earliest clinical manifestations of CADASIL are attacks of migraine with aura (International Headache Society 1988). Despite their frequency, which is four times that of the general population (Chabriat *et al.* 1995c, Dichgans *et al.* 1998), these manifestations are inconstant and are observed in 20–30 per cent of symptomatic subjects. They occur at a mean age of 28 ± 11 years (Desmond *et al.* 1999). The first attacks occasionally occur before the age of 20 years and before the appearance of MRI signal abnormalities (Hutchinson *et al.* 1995, Verin *et al.* 1995). They were not present in the first reports of affected families which focused only on the oldest subjects who had a severe clinical impairment (Sourander and Walinder 1977). Their frequency can vary greatly among the affected pedigrees (Vahedi *et al.* 1996). No subject suffering from migraine with aura was reported in the family studied by Sabbadini *et al.* 1995). Conversely, in 40 per cent of families, more than 60 per cent of symptomatic subjects had a history of migraine with aura (Chabriat *et al.* 1995*b*, Verin *et al.* 1995). Within some families, migraine with aura is the most important clinical aspect of the phenotype. Thus, in one French family, six of the seven symptomatic members had a pure history of migraine with aura (Chabriat *et al.* 1995*b*). The frequency of migraine attacks can also vary greatly among affected subjects, from one attack in their life time to several attacks per month (Chabriat *et al.* 1995*b*). As usually observed in migraine with aura, the most frequent neurological, symptoms associated with headache are visual and/or sensory. However, the frequency of attacks with basilar, hemiplegic, or prolonged aura, according to IHS diagnosis criteria, is noticeably high (International Headache Society 1988, Chabriat *et al.* 1995*b*, Verin *et al.* 1995). A few patients have been reported with severe attacks including unusual symptoms such as confusion, fever, meningitis, or coma (Chabriat *et al.* 1995*b*), reported only exceptionally in migraine with aura (Fitzimons and Wolfenten 1991, Frequin *et al.* 1991).

Stroke is the most frequent clinical manifestation of the disease. About two-thirds of symptomatic subjects have had transient ischaemic attacks or a completed stroke (Desmond *et al.* 1999). These events occur at a mean age of 41 ± 9 years (extreme limits from 20 to 65 years) (Chabriat *et al.* 1995*c*, Dichgans *et al.* 1998, Desmond *et al.* 1999). Two-thirds of them are classical lacunar syndromes: pure motor stroke, ataxic hemiparesis, pure sensory stroke, and sensory motor stroke. Other focal neurological deficits of abrupt onset are observed: less frequently dysarthria either isolated or associated with motor or sensory deficit, monoparesis, paresthesiae on one limb, isolated ataxia, non-fluent aphasia, and hemianopia (Chabriat *et al.* 1995*c*), these latter deficits can also be secondary to lacunar infarcts. The ischaemic manifestations are isolated in 40 per cent of cases, particularly at the onset of the disease. Most frequently, they are associated with migraine with aura, mood disturbances, or dementia (Chabriat *et al.* 1996). We are aware of only two patients over 60 years of age with a large artery cortical infarct associated with lacunar lesions. The onset of the neurological deficit can be progressive over several hours. Some neurological deficits occur suddenly and are associated with headache. When they are transient, they can mimic attacks of migraine with aura. Ischaemic events usually occur in the absence of vascular risk factors. However, they are also observed in some patients with one or several vascular risk factors, most frequently in tobacco users and/or hypertensive subjects. The influence of such factors on the clinical and/or MRI phenotype remains unknown (Chabriat *et al.* 1996).

About 20 per cent of CADASIL patients have a history of severe episodes of mood disturbances. Again, their frequency is widely variable between families (Chabriat *et al.* 1995*a, b*) Most patients have severe depression of the melancholic type, sometimes alternating with typical manic episodes (Chabriat *et al.* 1995*b*, Verin *et al.* 1995, Dichgans *et al.* 1998). The diagnosis of bipolar mood disorder is sometimes considered before an MRI examination (American Psychiatric Association 1987). Thus, differential diagnosis with a psychiatric disease can be difficult, particularly when such mood disturbances are the initial symptom and are isolated. The late onset of recurrent depressive episodes or of bipolar disorders, their poor response to treatment, their association with a cognitive impairment, and even the sole presence of a family history of stroke, migraine with aura, or dementia should lead to MRI being performed. The association of any of these symptoms with white matter signal abnormalities at MRI is suggestive of CADASIL and should prompt investigations to confirm this diagnosis. The exact causes of mood disturbances in CADASIL remain undetermined. The location of ischaemic lesions in basal ganglia and/or in frontal white matter may play a key role in their occurrence (Aylward *et al.* 1994, Bhatia and Mansden 1994).

Dementia is the second most common clinical manifestation of CADASIL. It is reported in one-third of symptomatic patients. The location of cerebral lesions explains the 'subcortical' aspect of the cognitive deficit. The neuropsychological deficit with a progressive or stepwise course is mainly responsible for attention deficit, apathy, and memory impairment (Davous and Fallet-Bianco 1991, Chabriat *et al.* 1995*c*, Davous and Bequet 1995). Aphasia, apraxia or agnosia are rare or observed only at the end stages of the disease (Davous and Fallet-Bianco 1991, Salvi *et al.* 1992). The cognitive deficit is often subtle, particularly at the onset of the disease, and can only be detected using a battery of neuropsychological testing. Some tests can even detect cognitive alterations before the age of 35 years. In our experience, the Wisconsin or Trail Making tests are the most sensitive examinations to detect a recent cognitive alteration (Taillia *et al.* 1998). The cognitive deficit can occur either suddenly or stepwise, but it can also occur progressively in the total absence of ischaemic events, mimicking a degenerative dementia (Chabriat *et al.* 1995*c*, Verin *et al.* 1995). The frequency and severity of the cognitive decline are variable in different members of a given family. The exact determinants of this variability are currently being investigated. The variable location and the severity of cerebral tissue damage might play a key role. In a positron emission tomography (PET) study of two affected brothers, one demented and the other asymptomatic, a severe cortical metabolic depression was found in the demented subject who only had infarcts within the basal ganglia and thalamus. Furthermore, we recently observed that the severity of white matter microstructural damage is strongly related to the clinical status in CADASIL (Chabriat *et al.* 1999*b*). This is in agreement with the correlations observed between the clinical status and the load of T_1 lesions within the white matter (Dichgans *et al.* 1999). Therefore, the degree of tissue destruction or neuronal loss is important for the cognitive status of CADASIL patients. When dementia is present, at a mean age of 60 years, it is observed in the absence of any other clinical manifestations in only 10 per cent of cases. Most often, other clinical manifestations of the disease have already occurred (migraine with aura, stroke). Dementia is always associated with pyramidal signs, pseudobulbar palsy, gait difficulties, and/or urinary incontinence (Bousser and Toutnier-Lasserve 1994a). The cognitive and functional decline is progressive. The patient becomes bedridden and often dies after pulmonary complications of swallowing difficulties. Baudrimont *et al.* (1993) reported one CADASIL patient who died after the occurrence of a deep cerebral haematoma. Dementia is present in 90 per cent of cases and death occurs at a mean age of 65 years with a wide range from 30 to 77 years.

Other neurological manifestations have been occasionally reported for CADASIL. Focal or generalized seizures have been observed in 6–10 per cent of cases (Chabriat *et al.* 1995c, Dichgans *et al.* 1998). Deafness of acute or rapid onset has been observed in several cases (Tournier-Lasserve *et al.* 1991). The lack of cranial nerve palsy, spinal cord disease, and symptoms of muscular origin is noteworthy in CADASIL. The cause of the radiculopathy reported in one case by Ragno *et al.* (1995) has not been determined.

Neuroimaging

MRI is essential for diagnosis of CADASIL. It is always abnormal in symptomatic subjects (Tournier-Lasserve *et al.* 1993, Bousser and Tournier-Lasserve, 1994b, Chabriat *et al.* 1995c). In addition, the signal abnormalities can be detected during a pre-symptomatic period of variable duration. MRI signal abnormalities are observed as early as 20 years of age. After age 35, all subjects with the affected gene have an abnormal MRI (Chabriat *et al.* 1995c, Joutel *et al.* 1996). The frequency of asymptomatic subjects with abnormal MRI decreases progressively with ageing among gene carriers, and becomes very low after 60 years.

MRI on T_1-weighted images shows punctiform or nodular hyposignals in basal ganglia and white matter (Fig. 9.1). T_2-weighted images show hypersignals in the same regions often associated with widespread areas of increased signal in the white matter (Bousser *et al.* 1994b, Skehan *et al.* 1995). The severity of the signal abnormalities is variable. These lesions increase dramatically with age in affected patients. In subjects aged under 40 years, T_2 hypersignals are usually punctate or nodular with a symmetrical distribution, and predominate in periventricular areas and in the centrum semiovale (Fig. 9.2) Later in life, white matter lesions are diffuse and can involve all of the white matter including the u-fibres under the cortex. The scores evaluating the severity of the lesions based on a semi-quantitative rating scale significantly increase with age not only in white matter but also in basal ganglia and brainstem. The frontal and occipital periventricular lesions are constant when MRI is abnormal. The frequency of signal abnormalities in the external capsule (two-thirds of cases) and in the anterior part of the temporal lobes (40%) is noteworthy (Bousser *et al.* 1994b, Skehan *et al.* 1995, Chabriat *et al.* 1996). Brainstem lesions are observed mainly in the pons (Chabriat *et al.* 1999a). The medulla is usually spared. Cortical or

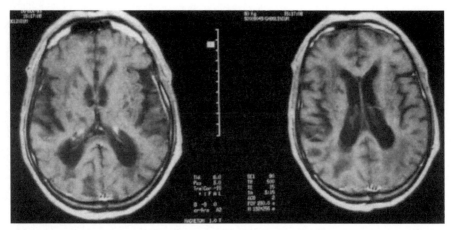

Fig. 9.1 T_1-weighted images in one CADASIL patient with dementia and a long history of recurrent stroke events showing multiple hyposignals in the white matter and basal ganglia.

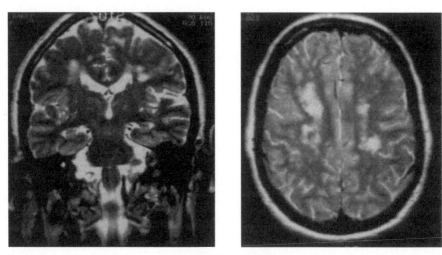

Fig. 9.2 T_2-weighted MRI in one asymptomatic subject showing white matter signal abnormalities located in the centrum semiovale predominating in the periventricular lesions.

cerebellar lesions are exceptional. They have been observed in only two cases aged over 60 years. A CT scan can reveal the white matter and basal ganglia lesions but is much less sensitive than MRI (Chabriat *et al.* 1997).

New MRI methods have been recently used to understand better the pathophysiology of CADASIL. With measures of the mean diffusivity of water and its anisotropy in the brain (Chabriat *et al.* 1999*b*), we demonstrated the crucial role of microstructural white matter alterations in the clinical status of CADASIL. More recently, we performed MRI perfusion showing a severe reduction of cerebral blood flow and blood volume within the abnormal white matter of CADASIL patients. With acetazolamide challenge, a reduction in vasoreactivity was observed at the same level. The results suggest that the reduction of the arteriolar lumen and/or the loss of the vessel compliance might play a role in the tissue loss observed in this disease (Chabriat *et al.* 2000).

Cerebral angiography obtained in 14 patients belonging to seven affected families was normal except in one case with a detectable narrowing of small arteries (Chabriat *et al.* 1995c). Weller *et al.* (1996) reported a worsening of the neurological status in two CADASIL patients after angiography, which was found to be normal with a possible vasospasm in one. One subject had a severe headache, vomiting, confusion, somnolence, and a grand mal seizure that resolved within several hours. Dichgans and Petersen (1997) later confirmed the high frequency of neurological complications after angiography in CADASIL patients. Ultrasound studies and echocardiography are usually normal. Cerebrospinal fluid examination is usually normal, but oligoclonal bands with pleiocytosis have been reported (Chabriat *et al.* 1997). Recently, an isolated increase in complement factor B was detected in three CADASIL patients (Unlu *et al.* 2000). Electromyogram examination is essentially normal. A monoclonal immunoglobulin was detected in the serum of two cases of our first family, but not in the other affected pedigrees (Tournier-Lasserve *et al.* 1991).

Pathology

Macroscopic examination of the brain shows a diffuse myelin pallor and rarefaction of the hemispheric white matter sparing the u-fibres (Gutierrez-Molina *et al.* 1994, Ruchoux *et al.* 1995). Lesions predominate in the periventricular areas and centrum semiovale. They are associated with lacunar infarcts located in the white matter and basal ganglia (lentiform nucleus, thalamus, caudate) (Gutierrez-Molina *et al.* l994, Ruchoux *et al.* 1995). The most severe hemispheric lesions are the most profound (Davous and Fallet-Blanco 1991, Baudrimont *et al.* 1993, Ruchoux *et al.* 1995). In the brainstem, the lesions are more marked in the pons and are similar to the pontine rarefaction of myelin of ischaemic origin described by Pullicino *et al.* (1995). The macroscopic study of the cortex is essentially normal, but a case has been reported recently in a woman with diffuse brain lesions, including microlacunar infarcts (diameter < 200 μ) within the cortex, mainly in layer 6 adjacent to the white matter (Ruchoux *et al.* 1995). No territorial or borderzone infarct has been reported so far at post-mortem. Intracerebral haemorrhage has been occasionally reported (Baudrimont *et al.* 1993).

Microscopic investigations show that the wall of cerebral and leptomeningeal arterioles is thickened, with a significant reduction of the lumen (Baudrimont *et al.* 1993). Such abnormalities can also be detected by leptomeningeal biopsy (Lammie *et al.* 1995). Some inconstant features are similar to those reported in patients with hypertensive encephalopathy (Zhang *et al.* 1994), duplication and splitting of internal elastic lamina, adventitial hyalinosis and fibrosis, and hypertrophy of the media.

However, a distinctive feature is the presence of a granular material within the media extending into the adventitia (Davous and Fallet-Blanco 1991, Estes *et al.* 1991, Baudrimont *et al.* 1993, Gray *et al.* 1994*b*, Gutierrez-Molina *et al.* 1994, Zhang *et al.* 1994, Lammie *et al.* 1995, Ragno *et al.* 1995, Ruchoux *et al.* 1995, Sabbadini *et al.* 1995, Schroder *et al.* 1995, Malandrim *et al.* 1997). The periodic acid–schiff (PAS) positive staining suggested the presence of glycoproteins; staining for amyloid subtance and elastin is negative (Baudrimont *et al.* 1993, Ruchoux *et al.* 1995, Ruchoux and Maurage, 1997). Immunohistochemistry does not support the presence of immunoglobulins. In contrast, the endothelium of the vessels is usually spared. Sometimes it is not detectable and is replaced by collagen fibres (Zhang *et al.* 1994). On electron microscopy, the smooth muscle cells appear swollen and often degenerated, some of them with multiple nuclei. There was a granular, electron-dense, osmiophilic material within the media (Gutierrez-Molina *et al.* 1994). This material consists of granules of about 10–15 nm diameter (Zhang *et al.* 1994). It is localized close to the cell membrane of the smooth muscle cells where it appears very dense. The smooth muscle cells are separated by large amounts of the unidentified material. In a single case, these vascular abnormalities were found associated with typical lesions of Alzheimer's disease (Gray *et al.* 1994*a*).

Ruchoux *et al.* (1994, 1995) made the crucial observation that the vascular abnormalities observed in the brain were also detectable in other organs. The granular and osmiophilic material surrounding the smooth muscle cells as seen with electron microscopy is also present in the media of arteries located in the spleen, liver, kidneys, muscle, and skin, and also in the wall of carotid and aortic arteries (Ruchoux *et al.* 1994, 1995). These vascular lesions can also be detected by nerve biopsy (Schroder *et al.* 1995). The presence of this material in the skin vessels now allows the diagnosis of CADASIL to be confirmed during life using punch skin biopsies (Furby *et al.* 1998), although the sensitivity and specificity of this method have not yet been completely established (Ruchoux *et al.* 1994, 1995, Sabbadini *et al.* 1995).

Genetics

The study of the first and very large French family allowed confirmation of the autosomal dominant pattern of transmission and mapping of affected gene on chromosome 19 in 1993 (Tournier-Lasserve *et al.* 1993). A crucial step for this mapping was the use of neuroimaging data for the genetic linkage analysis. Joutel *et al.*, 3 years later, identified different mutations within the *Notch3* gene as the cause of the disease. (Joutel *et al.* 1996). They reported a sporadic mutation of the *Notch3* gene (Joutel *et al.* 2000*b*). The frequency of *de novo* mutation remains to be investigated, particularly in patients with clinical features of the disease but without a positive familial history.

The *Notch3* gene was unknown in humans. Mutations of homologous genes, *Notch1* and *Jagged1*, located on chromosomes 9 and 20, are implicated respectively in a T-cell acute lymphoblastic leukaemia/lymphoma and in a developmental disorder, the Alagille syndrome (Joutel and Tourmier-Lasserve, 1998). The *Notch3* gene encodes a 2321 amino acid protein, with an extracellular domain containing 34 epidermal growth factor (EGF)-like repeats and three Lin repeats associated with an intracellular and a transmembrane domain. Stereotyped missense mutations, within EGF-like repeats, only located in the extracellular domain of the Notch3 protein, are observed in CADASIL patients. This extracellular domain is thought to interact with structurally similar ligands, also containing EGF repeats, such as the Delta and Serrate proteins. However, today, the actual ligands of the Notch3 receptor remain unknown. The mutations observed in CADASIL lead to an uneven number of cysteine residue which may alter the function of the Notch3 receptor. Dichgans *et al.* (2000) recently showed, using a three-dimensional model of the protein, that the presence of unpaired cysteine residue might cause an abnormal folding of the protein. The recent contribution of Joutel *et al.* (2000*a*) provides important insights into the role of this protein in the pathophysiology of CADASIL. These authors first demonstrated that in normal tissues the Notch3 protein is expressed exclusively in vascular smooth muscle cells. They also showed that the protein usually undergoes a proteolytic cleavage leading to two fragments: one extracellular and one intracellular. In CADASIL patients, the extracellular fragment accumulates dramatically at the cytoplasmic membrane of smooth muscle cells within vessels. This accumulation is found near to but not within the characteristic granular osmiophilic material seen by electron microscopy. An abnormal clearance of the Notch3 ectodomain from the smooth cell surface is presumed to cause this accumulation (Joutel *et al.* 2000*a*). These results finally emphasize that the vascular smooth muscle cell is playing a key role in the pathophysiology of CADASIL.

The genetic testing of CADASIL is also now available. The detection of the most frequent mutations of the *Notch3* gene (within exons 3 and 4) is easily performed routinely. For the other mutations, in the absence of an already known target (known mutation within the family), genetic testing is hampered by the numerous exons requiring analysis. Diagnostic testing with immunostaining using anti-Notch3 antibodies might be easier than electron microscopy and genetic analysis (Joutel *et al.* 2000*a*).

Conclusion

CADASIL is a systemic genetic disease of vascular smooth muscle cells. The recent developments in genetic and pathological research suggest that the accumulation of the ectodomain of the Notch3 protein is associated with the severe ultrastructural alterations of the arteriolar wall observed in this disease. Other data suggest that the arteriolar wall changes may result in cerebral hypoperfusion causing 'chronic ischaemia' and leading to the progressive accumulation of tissue lesions. These lesions predominate in the most vulnerable cerebral areas possibly, because of the particular angioarchitecture of the brain. Finally, both the variable severity of the tissue destruction within the white matter and basal ganglia and their different locations might be the main sources of the important variability of the clinical severity which can be observed in a given family.

The research performed on CADASIL is not only crucial to determine the best target for future prevention of the disease, but is also important to understand better the pathophysiology of small artery diseases. We think that CADASIL should be considered as a unique model to investigate the determinants of vascular dementia, the clinical correlates of ischaemic white matter lesions, and the natural history of tissue damage associated with small artery diseases. Furthermore, the identification of the *Notch3* gene will be helpful in the group of cerebral vascular disorders associated with leukoaraiosis.

Part IV

Investigating subcortical stroke

Chapter 10

MRI and other neuroimaging modalities for subcortical stroke

S.M. Davis and M.W. Parsons

Introduction

The widespread introduction of computed tomographic (CT) imaging in the 1970s allowed non-invasive diagnosis of lacunar infarcts, previously identified as clinical syndromes and confirmed only via autopsy studies (Fisher 1965a, Caplan 1980, Nelson *et al.* 1980). However, it was evident that CT scanning was frequently insensitive, particularly with acute infarcts. By the late 1980s, magnetic resonance imaging (MRI) had become widely available and this modality allowed more sensitive detection of lacunar infarcts, particularly those in the brainstem (Arboix *et al.* 1990a, Hommel *et al.* 1980). However, as with CT scanning, the diagnostic sensitivity with MRI was greater when it was performed a few days after stroke onset, rather than at the hyperacute stage (Table 10.1).

With the advent of these neuroimaging techniques, the lacunar hypothesis originally developed by Fisher (1965a) could be systematically evaluated *in vivo* (Table 10.2). Studies were performed to test the first part of the hypothesis that the five lacunar syndromes (pure motor hemiparesis, pure sensory syndrome, sensori-motor syndrome, ataxic-hemiparesis, and dysarthria–clumsy hand syndrome) were associated with radiological evidence of lacunar infarcts. To test the second part of the hypothesis, namely that lacunar syndromes were due to small vessel vasculopathy, rather than embolism from proximal sources, studies were performed using brain imaging, cardiac investigation with echocardiography, and large vessel investigation with duplex Doppler and digital subtraction angiography (Bamford and Warlow 1988, Gan *et al.* 1997).

The more recent advent of echoplanar MRI has provided new insights into acute brain ischaemia (Warach *et al.* 1995, Barber *et al.* 1998a, Davis *et al.* 2000). These techniques have enabled rapid, non-invasive measurement of impaired diffusion of water in the infarct core (diffusion-weighted imaging, DWI) as well as rapid, non-invasive measurement of regions of hypoperfusion (perfusion imaging, PWI). In general, the DWI lesion represents the non-viable ischaemic core, or tissue destined for infarction. Recent studies have shown that DWI is the diagnostic modality of choice for cerebral infarction (Barber *et al.* 1998a, Davis *et al.* 2000,

Table 10.1 Comparison of conventional neuroimaging modalities for subcortical infarcts: CT, contrast CT, MRI, and gadolinium-enhanced MRI

	Advantages	Disadvantages
CT	Widely available Inexpensive Sensitive for haemorrhage	Poor sensitivity for acute lacunar infarction
MRI	Improved sensitivity for acute infarction versus CT	Less widely available Possibly less sensitive for acute haemorrhage
MRI with gadolinium	More sensitive for acute infarction versus CT or MRI	Longer procedure Slight risk of hypersensitivity Cost of gadolinium

Table 10.2 Testing the lacunar hypothesis with neuroimaging

	Clinical lacunar syndromes = small, deep infarcts	Small, deep infarction = small vessel disease
CT	High positive predictive value (87%) of clinical syndrome for detecting small, deep infarct. Hemorrhage may mimic clinical lacunar syndrome	Moderate positive predictive value (75%) of small, deep infarct on CT for presumed lacunar mechanism with no evidence of a proximal, embolic source
MRI	Positive predictive value of 81% for finding a *relevant* infarct	69% with small, deep infarct have a presumed lacunar mechanism
DWI	Positive predictive value approaches 100% for detection of small, deep infarcts if a clinical lacunar syndrome is present	New evidence that 16–50% of patients with small, deep infarcts have DWI patterns suggesting a non-lacunar pathology

Parsons *et al.* 2000), and the diagnostic accuracy of DWI for acute subcortical infarction exceeds 90 per cent (Singer *et al.* 1998). Furthermore, studies with DWI, PWI, and magnetic resonance spectroscopy (MRS) have started to provide new insights into the pathogenesis of lacunar infarction, as well as allowing more sensitive and specific diagnosis (Table 10.3).

Subcortical infarction includes a large variety of infarct types, including lacunar, striatocapsular, internal watershed, anterior and posterior choroidal artery, and brainstem infarcts. This review has focused on the imaging of patients with classical lacunar syndromes.

CT scanning in subcortical infarction

Fisher pioneered the demonstration of the small vessel, arterial lesions underlying lacunar infarcts and definition of the lacunar syndromes in the 1960s (Fisher 1965*a*, 1967, 1969, Fisher and Cole 1965, Fisher and Curry 1965). The term 'lacunar infarct' came into use, whereby both the pathological features and underlying aetiology

Table 10.3 Newer MR techniques for subcortical infarction

	Advantages	Disadvantages
DWI	Images ischaemic core More sensitive for acute lesions than conventional imaging Allows distinction of acute versus old lunar infarcts Rapid scan time	Relatively limited availability Possibly less sensitive than CT for acute haemorrhage
PWI	Assessment of brain perfusion Complementary information to DWI May indicate potential for reperfusion therapy	Limited data in subcortical infarction Invasive
MRA	Assessment of vessel patency	Limited data in subcortical infarction
MRS	Measurement of brain metabolism Improves prediction of stroke outcome	Limited data in subcortical infarction

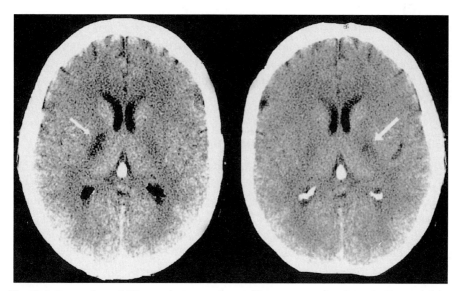

Fig. 10.1 Comparison of CT scans in two patients with pure motor hemiparesis. The patient on the right has a typical small vessel infarct in the internal capsule. CT of the patient on the left shows a larger striatocapsular infarction, suggesting a proximal embolic pathogenesis.

(typically small vessel disease, rather than embolism) were inferred from the clinical syndromes. With the introduction of CT scanning, radiological confirmation of lacunar syndromes became possible (Fig. 10.1). Hence, Nelson *et al.* (1980) studied 37 patients with a clinical lacunar syndrome, based on Fisher's earlier descriptions. The majority of these had pure motor hemiplegia. The CT scans were performed at variable times after stroke onset. In this series, small, deep 'lacunar' infarcts (usually < 1.5 cm in diameter as initially described by Fisher) were shown in approximately 50 per cent of patients. The investigators also found that a significant proportion of patients (six of 37) had 'large superficial infarcts'. This group had a lower incidence of hypertension, and they therefore suggested that the clinical diagnosis of lacunar syndrome did not necessarily predict a small, deep infarct. Furthermore, they found that large vessel, carotid disease was not uncommon and considered that a search for carotid embolism via angiography remained appropriate. Weisberg (1979) found 10 patients with lacunes on CT in a series of 33 patients with pure motor hemiplegia.

Donnan and colleagues (1982) performed a systematic study using serial CT scanning in patients with clinical lacunar syndromes. They studied 75 patients with clinical features of lacunar infarcts and found that 69 per cent had evidence of capsular infarction, as the only region concordant with the clinical syndrome. In 31 per cent of patients, no lesion was seen on CT and there was no evidence of cortical infarction. They identified partial lacunar syndromes in about one-third of cases, including isolated monoparesis and dysarthria. This study also showed that the sensitivity of scanning improved with time, although most CT changes were evident within 10 days. In patients with frequent lacunar transient ischaemic attacks (TIAs), termed the 'capsular warning syndrome' (Donnan et al. 1982), there was an increased likelihood of CT confirmation of infarction. Interestingly, a negative scan did not suggest a better stroke prognosis.

Conventional magnetic resonance imaging

In the 1980s, brain MRI was shown to be superior to CT in the diagnosis of cerebral infarction, particularly in relation to small, deep infarcts and posterior fossa ischaemia (Fig. 10.2). (Davis et al. 1989). Brown et al. (1988) studied 22 patients with lacunar TIAs or infarcts with MRI and CT. They concluded that MRI was significantly superior to CT scanning, lacunar infarcts being evident as focal areas of decreased signal intensity on T_1-weighted imaging, with increased signal intensity on T_2-weighted imaging. They showed that T_2-weighted imaging was the superior technique for detection of acute rather than chronic lesions.

Rothrock and colleagues (1987) analysed 31 patients with presumed lacunar stroke and found that MRI detected small, deep lesions relevant to the symptoms in 74 per cent of cases. They also concluded that MRI was diagnostically superior to brain CT in the acute setting and that MRI helped distinguish acute from chronic ischaemic lesions.

Other studies confirmed these findings. Hommel et al. (1990) studied 100 patients hospitalized with a lacunar infarct. Of these, 79 had one of the five classical lacunar syndromes, while 21 per cent had less typical lacunar presentations. They found that 89 per cent of patients had demonstration of a lacunar infarct compatible with the signs and symptoms. However, in 16 per cent of patients, at least two lacunar-type

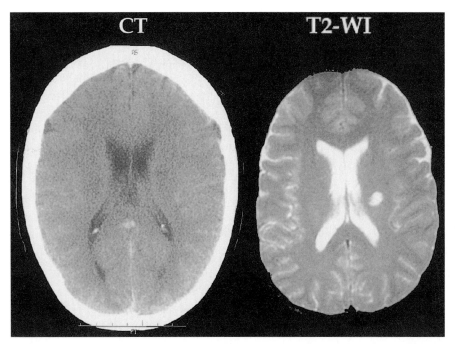

Fig. 10.2 CT at 48 h after onset of right pure motor hemiparesis does not reveal a definite abnormality. Concurrent T$_2$-weighted imaging clearly identifies the infarct.

lesions could have explained the signs and symptoms. There was a good correlation between the presence of lacunar infarction and classical lacunar syndromes. Nonetheless, in 5 per cent of their patients, the lacunar syndrome was actually found to be due to a deep intracerebral haemorrhage, and 3 per cent had a large artery occlusion. Various studies showed that MRI was particularly sensitive in the diagnosis of brainstem lacunes, obviating the problem of bone artefacts (Davis *et al.* 1989, Hommel *et al.* 1990). These latter authors found pontine lacunes in 30 per cent of those patients with classical lacunar syndromes.

Arboix and colleagues (1990*a*) studied 227 patients with lacunar infarcts, of whom a subset had both MRI and CT. They found that MRI was clearly superior, particularly for lacunes in either the pons or internal capsule. The diagnostic sensitivity was increased from 44 per cent with CT, to 78% with MRI in their series, confirming earlier reports (Arboix *et al.* 1990*a*). As in other series of lacunar infarcts, they emphasized the benign natural history, including the relative lack of mortality and low percentage of medical complications. More recently, Stapf *et al.* (2000) also showed that classical lacunar syndromes were highly predictive for small, deep infarcts on MRI. They therefore questioned the cost-efficacy of MRI in this setting, provided that a CT scan had been performed to exclude non-ischaemic pathology.

One of the problems with conventional MRI is the common finding of multiple lacunar lesions and the inherent difficulty in deciding which infarct is responsible for the presenting syndrome. Various investigators have emphasized that lacunes are often multiple and asymptomatic (Arboix *et al.* 1990*a*, Roman 1996).

The benign prognosis of lacunar infarcts was emphasized by a number of investigators. For example, Samuelsson *et al.* (1996*b*) assessed functional outcome in 81 consecutive patients with a first-ever stroke, who had clinical and MRI findings compatible with lacunar infarction. Only 6 per cent of patients died during follow-up. In this group, 21 per cent of patients had recurrent strokes over 3 years, mainly recurrent, lacunar infarcts. Functional outcome was usually favourable. The severity of motor impairment and white matter disease were both strong predictors of a poor functional outcome (Samuelsson *et al.* 1996*b*).

Gadolinium contrast enhancement with MRI in lacunar infarction

Regli *et al.* (1993), in a prospective case series, evaluated the use of gadolinium-DTPA, contrast-enhanced MRI, prior to acquisition of T_1-weighted images. Precise clinico-topographic correlation was significantly improved after gadolinium-DTPA administration, with demonstration of lesional enhancement (Fig. 10.3). However, they found that 23 per cent of the patients showed no enhancement within 7 days of acute infarction.

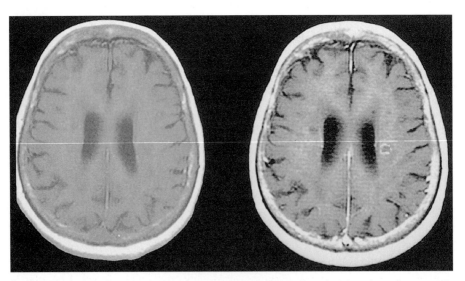

Fig. 10.3 Comparison of T_1-weighted scans before and after the administration of contrast 7 days after lacunar stroke. The pre-contrast scan (left) shows subtle deep white matter hypodensities bilaterally, but the age of the lesions is not clear. The post-contrast scan (right) shows a small region of reduced signal in the left internal capsule surrounded by contrast enhancement, indicating recent infarction.

Neuroimaging with CT and MRI and validation of the lacunar hypothesis

Bamford and Warlow (1988) reviewed the two parts of the lacunar hypothesis, namely that there were a small number of distinct clinical syndromes specifically associated with small, deep infarcts or lacunes and that, secondly, these generally were due to small vessel arteriopathy rather than embolism. These authors emphasized the need for further patho-radiological correlations and pointed out that small, deep infarcts on CT and MRI did not necessarily correlate with pathological lacunes. Furthermore, they emphasized the insensitivity of CT scanning for the diagnosis of posterior fossa lacunes. They indicated that the lacunar syndromes could be due to small, deep haemorrhages and that the distinction could not be made reliably on clinical criteria. They considered that partial lacunar syndromes (e.g. monoparesis rather than symmetrical motor weakness in 'pure motor hemiplegia') were reasonably validated lacunar patterns. Notwithstanding these reservations, they concluded that the classical lacunar syndromes would generally predict the finding of small, deep infarcts on neuroimaging, with the caveat that haemorrhages could mimic lacunar syndromes perfectly.

Concerning the second part of the lacunar hypothesis, namely the relationship between a qualitatively distinct small vessel arteriopathy and a lacunar infarction, they found that the evidence was less clear. Indirect evidence suggested that extracranial large vessel disease and cardioembolic sources were less frequent in patients with lacunar infarcts, but various studies still showed that a significant minority of patients with small, deep infarcts had ipsilateral carotid stenosis (Landau 1989).

Concurrently, a number of investigators consistently have challenged these lacunar hypotheses. For example, Millikan and Futrell (1990) argued that the 'lacunar hypothesis' was a fallacy, because small cerebral infarcts were not caused solely by a combination of hypertension and small vessel disease. They indicated that photochemical damage to the carotid artery of rats could produce microemboli to the brain, resulting in cavitary lesions resembling human lacunar infarcts. They concluded that lacunar infarcts were simply small strokes, which had been investigated using standard protocols to exclude a proximal embolic source.

Gan et al. (1997) more recently tested the lacunar hypothesis using a cohort of 591 patients with cerebral infarction, of whom 225 had lacunar syndromes. Pure motor hemiplegia was the most common type. They found that lacunar syndromes had an overall positive predictive value of 87 per cent for detecting radiological lacunes (CT or MRI), particularly in those with pure sensory stroke and ataxic hemiparesis. This was one of the first studies to test the second part of the lacunar hypothesis. In patients with lacunar syndromes and radiological correlation of a pertinent small, deep infarct, there was a positive predictive value of final diagnosis of a lacunar mechanism in 75 per cent of cases. However, nearly 25 per cent of the patients with a lacunar syndrome confirmed on imaging had non-lacunar mechanisms for infarction, namely large vessel disease, cardioembolism, or a cryptogenic source. Hence, they concluded that non-invasive neurovascular and cardiac evaluations were still warranted, even in patients with classical lacunar syndromes.

Other series using MRI confirmed these findings. Staaf *et al.* (1998) studied 32 patients with sensorimotor stroke, finding a relevant infarct in 81 per cent of patients. They found that small vessel disease was the most likely cause in 69 per cent, but 31 per cent had either a potential cardioembolic or large vessel source, or infarcts incompatible with perforating artery disease. Similarly, Gorman and colleagues (1998) evaluated 45 cases with ataxic hemiparesis and found that this syndrome generally predicted a small, deep infarct, either in the pons or in the internal capsule. In those where there was complete evaluation, the majority could be attributed to small vessel disease, but a minority were likely to be due to embolism from proximal arteries or a cardiac source.

Lacunar infarcts are found commonly on MRI in elderly individuals being investigated for other pathologies. Longstreth *et al.* (1998) studied the risk factors and functional consequences of lacunar infarcts in elderly people. In the cardiovascular health study, a longitudinal study of people aged 65 years and over, 3660 participants had brain MRI. Lacunes were defined as subcortical infarcts 0.3–2.0 cm in diameter. In 23 per cent of subjects, they found one or more lacunes. These were generally single (66%) and silent (89%), without any history of TIA or stroke. They found that lacunes defined by MRI were common in older people and associated with factors likely to promote or reflect small vessel disease, with independent predictive factors including age, diastolic blood pressure, creatinine, and pack-years of smoking.

Recent advances in MRI: DWI, PWI, and MR spectroscopy

The advent of echoplanar MRI in the 1990s enabled rapid and non-invasive assessment of the ischaemic infarct core (DWI) and cerebral perfusion (PWI). DWI measures alterations in the diffusion of water molecules. Hyperintense DWI lesions are evident as early as 3 min after the onset of ischaemic injury and reflect a reduction in the apparent coefficient of water (ADC). This is due to disruption of high energy metabolism, leading to failure of ion pumps and resulting in cytotoxic oedema. These regions generally progress to frank infarction, although early reversibility has been shown in animal models (Minematsu *et al.* 1992) and more recently in human infarcts (Kidwell *et al.* 2000).

In the first 6 h after ischaemic stroke, DWI has an extraordinarily high sensitivity and specificity (Lovblad *et al.* 1998, Barber *et al.* 1999*a*). Hence, DWI usually enables the detection of acute infarcts within the first few hours of onset, at a time when CT and conventional MRI are relatively insensitive, particularly for small, deep lesions (Fig. 10.4). Furthermore, DWI is helpful in ageing a lesion, given that the hyperintense signal typically lasts 7–10 days.

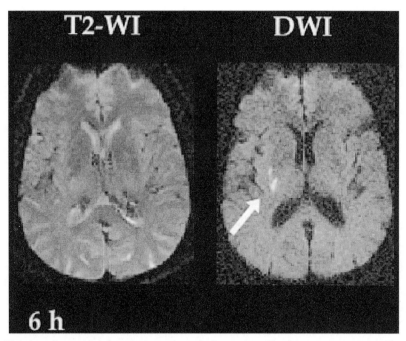

Fig. 10.4 A patient with left pure sensory stroke imaged at 6 h after symptom onset. The T$_2$-weighted image is normal. DWI clearly identifies an acute area of infarction in the posterior limb of the right internal capsule.

Studies using DWI have shown that this technique allows sensitive and accurate diagnosis of lacunar infarction, and the ability to discriminate between acute and old lesions. Singer *et al.* (1998) studied 39 patients with a clinical diagnosis of acute subcortical infarction, 7 h to 4 days after onset, using both DWI and conventional MRI. They found a very high accuracy of 95 per cent with DWI and noted that in 10 per cent of cases, the acute infarction was not detected on conventional MRI. As in other studies, conventional MRI showed both the acute lesion and multiple other lesions. In contrast, delineation of the acute lesion with DWI was possible in all cases of multiple lacunes, corresponding to the acute clinical symptomatology (Fig. 10.5). Similarly, Noguchi *et al.* (1998) used DWI to study 35 patients with lacunar infarcts. They were also able to identify acute small infarcts and to separate these from chronic infarcts, based on the DWI signal and ADC ratios. In three patients, small hyperacute brainstem infarcts (within 6 h of onset) were seen only with DWI and, in five patients, fresh small infarcts adjacent to multiple old infarcts could only be distinguished with DWI. Other reports have shown the superiority of DWI over conventional MRI for the diagnosis of clinically relevant, small, penetrating artery infarcts (Oliveira-Filho *et al.* 2000). In one study, conventional MRI including FLAIR imaging failed to identify the relevant infarct in almost one-quarter of cases (Lindgren *et al.* 2000).

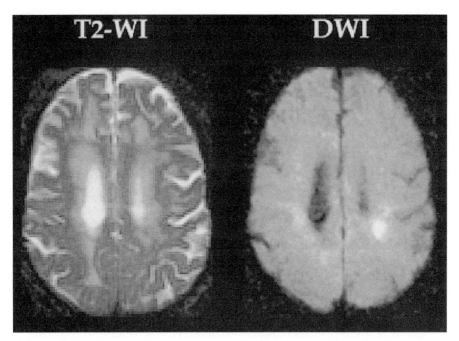

Fig. 10.5 A patient with acute right sensorimotor stroke with MRI 3 days after symptom onset. T$_2$-weighted imaging shows extensive deep white matter ischaemic change; however, the acute lesion is not delineated. DWI identifies the acute infarct responsible for the patient's symptomatology.

Newer MRI techniques may eventually contribute to a modification of the lacunar hypothesis. There is accumulating evidence that acute DWI identifies a subset of patients presenting with typical lacunar syndromes who have a pattern of ischaemic lesions suggesting an embolic pathogenesis. A recent study used DWI to determine whether clinical lacunar syndromes predicted lacunar infarcts (Lindgren *et al.* 2000). Twenty-three patients with clinical lacunar syndromes had DWI within 3 days of onset. In most cases, acute lacunar syndromes correlated with small subcortical infarcts compatible with single-penetrator occlusion. However, a small number had cortical involvement.

Several other reports have confirmed that multiple acute lesions are evident on DWI in some patients presenting with classical lacunar syndromes, implying that a proportion of cases may well be due to embolism (Ay *et al.* 1999*a*, Gerraty *et al.* 2000, Lindgren *et al.* 2000)(Fig. 10.6). In a study of 62 patients with classical lacunar syndromes studied with DWI within 3 days, 16 per cent had multiple regions of increased signal intensity. The index lesion could be identified in the hemisphere or brainstem, while these 'subsidiary infarcts' usually occurred in leptomeningeal artery territories and were more often associated with an embolic stroke source (Ay *et al.* 1999*a*). Our group recently found that in 16 patients with clinical presentations

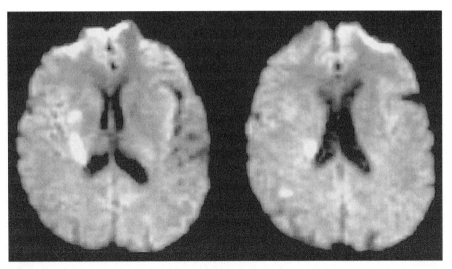

Fig. 10.6 DWI at 10 h after onset of lacunar infarct with sensorimotor stroke. There are discrete lesions in the internal capsule, caudate nucleus, and parietal cortex, indicating a proximal source of embolism, rather than a single small vessel lesion.

of subcortical infarcts, 10 had some evidence to suggest an embolic aetiology (Gerraty *et al.* 2000). This was indicated by a pattern of multiple, acute lesions in more than one single small vessel territory.

DWI may also provide insights into the pathophysiology of lacunar syndromes. A study of the mechanism of capsular warning syndrome indicated that DWI could show ischaemic lesions in the basal ganglia, adjacent to motor pathways (Norrving 1999). They suggested that the episodes could suggest transient metabolic dysfunction in motor tracts adjacent to ischaemic lesions. Schonewille *et al.* (1999) used DWI to study 43 patients presenting acutely with classical lacunar syndromes. They confirmed that lacunar syndromes can be caused by heterogeneous lesions, including deep ischaemic infarcts, but also superficial infarction and haemorrhage. Furthermore, lesions in the same location can give rise to a variety of clinical lacunar syndromes.

Bolus-tracking PWI makes use of the signal loss that occurs during the dynamic tracking of the first part of an intravenous paramagnetic contrast agent (Kucharczyk *et al.* 1993). A signal intensity–time curve is obtained from whole-brain T_2-weighted perfusion scans, performed every second following the intravenous injection of gadolinium. Different haemodynamic measurements can be obtained, such as relative cerebral blood volume (rCBV), relative cerebral blood flow (rCBF), and mean transit time (MTT). Although PWI has been used mainly to study cortical stroke, it shows promise in providing further insights into subcortical infarction. In our series of patients presenting with lacunar syndromes studied with both acute PWI and DWI, some had perfusion lesions suggesting that *in situ* small vessel disease was not the source of infarction (Gerraty *et al.* 2001)(Fig. 10.7).

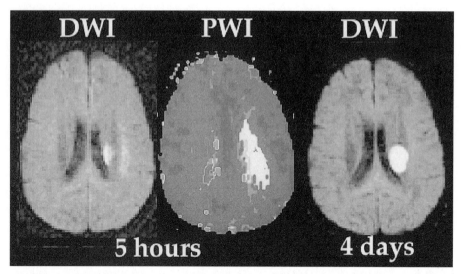

Fig. 10.7 DWI at 5 h after onset of pure motor hemiparesis shows a small infarct in the internal capsule which, in isolation, suggests lacunar infarction. However, concurrent PWI shows a larger lesion indicating hypoperfusion in the internal carotid 'watershed' region, implying non-lacunar pathology. Follow-up DWI at 4 days shows expansion of the lesion. The size of this infarct is larger than that typically seen with small vessel disease.

A further application of acute PWI and DWI in subcortical infarction is the potential to guide acute stroke therapy, such as thrombolysis. There is increasing evidence that the area of acute PWI–DWI mismatch represents the ischaemic penumbra, and thus may identify tissue potentially salvageable with rapid reperfusion (Barber *et al.* 1998*b*). Whilst studies have concentrated on cortical stroke, patients with subcortical infarction may have PWI–DWI mismatch (Fig. 10.7), and therefore may benefit from thrombolytic therapy. The NINDS trial showed that patients with lacunar infarction did in fact benefit from intravenous tissue plasminogen activator (Natioanl Institute of Neurological Disorders and Stroke 1995). PWI combined with DWI may help determine whether all patients with lacunar infarction, or only the subset with PWI–DWI mismatch, benefit from thrombolysis.

In addition, MRI can allow concurrent determination of extracranial and intracranial vascular patency via magnetic resonance angiography (MRA), performed at the same time as the PWI studies. The current resolution of MRA does not allow visualization of small penetrating arteries. However, MRA may identify more proximal sources of embolism, which can result in subcortical infarction and present as a clinical lacunar syndrome.

Magnetic resonance spectroscopy (^{1}H MRS) provides information about alterations in brain biochemistry in acute infarction (Graham *et al.* 1995, Pereira *et al.* 1999, Parsons *et al.* 2000). We found that ^{1}H MRS was particularly useful in identifying patients with subcortical infarction who were likely to have a poorer prognosis than

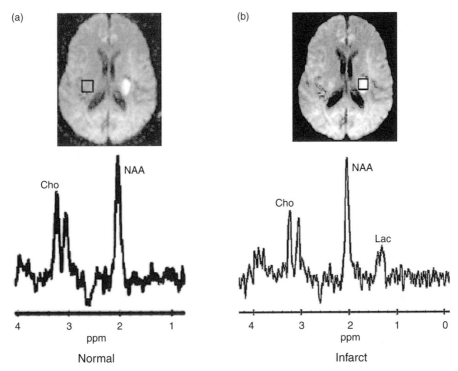

Fig. 10.8 MRS of an acute capsular infarct showing the presence of lactate in the infarct core (a). This contrasts with a normal spectrum in the contralateral internal capsule (b). Despite a small infarct, this patient had a poorer than expected prognosis, based on infarct size alone. The presence of acute lactate in subcortical infarcts may herald infarct expansion and worse functional outcome.

on the basis of DWI infarct size alone (Parsons *et al.* 2000). The presence of a high lactate level despite relatively small acute infarct size predicted subsequent infarct expansion and poorer functional outcome (Fig. 10.8). Reduced *N*-acetylaspartate (NAA) has been shown in subcortical ischaemic stroke (Lai *et al.* 1995). Kang *et al.* (2000) found changes in cortical NAA levels in patients with large subcortical infarcts and clinical evidence of cortical dysfunction, but not in patients with isolated subcortical syndromes. We found that reductions in lesional NAA, particularly at the subacute stage, were associated with a worse clinical outcome (Parsons *et al.* 2000).

Conclusions

The development of neuroimaging techniques has allowed improved diagnosis of clinical lacunar syndromes. Furthermore, they have enabled closer exploration of the lacunar hypothesis. CT scanning has provided many insights into subcortical infarction. However, CT is insensitive for acute diagnosis. Whilst conventional MRI is superior to CT in the diagnosis of acute lesions, it is still relatively insensitive. DWI is the most exciting new development in the investigation of acute subcortical stroke. DWI allows very early identification of acute lesions. In addition, it has allowed a more rigorous assessment of the lacunar hypothesis by identifying a subset of patients presenting with classical lacunar syndromes who may have a proximal embolic pathogenesis. Other new MRI techniques such as PWI, MRS, and MRA have not been studied as extensively as DWI, but offer the potential to improve diagnosis and prediction of prognosis, as well as aid in guiding acute therapy for subcortical stroke.

There remains a small element of doubt as to the sensitivity of DWI in identifying acute haemorrhage, which may mimic classical lacunar syndromes. If future research clarifies this concern, it is now widely predicted that DWI will replace CT as the imaging modality of choice for acute stroke.

Chapter 11

Carotid angiography in patients with subcortical ischaemia

L.J. Kappelle and J. van Gijn

Introduction

Since direct puncture of the carotid artery and injection of sodium iodide was introduced by Moniz in 1927 (Moniz 1940), angiographic techniques have been replaced by much safer procedures. Nowadays, intra-arterial digital subtraction angiography (IDSA), performed via the femoral artery, is the most informative method to visualize the cervico-cranial vasculature. Unfortunately, this procedure is associated with a 1 per cent overall incidence of neurological deficit and a 0.5 per cent incidence of persistent neurological deficit or death (Grzyska *et al.* 1990, Hankey *et al.* 1990, Heiserman *et al.* 1994, Derdeyn *et al.* 1995). During the last years, magnetic resonance angiography (MRA) and spiral computed tomography (CT) angiography have been introduced (Marks 1996, Neumann Haeflin *et al.* 2000). These methods are safe and, therefore, are being used more and more for visualization of the arteries in the neck and the intracranial arteries (Magarelli *et al.* 1998). To date, there are no studies comparing ISDA with MRA or spiral CT angiography in patients with subcortical infarcts.

Angiography of the extracranial vessels is indicated only if the results will influence therapeutic management or give information about prognosis. Carotid endarterectomy (CEA) is indicated in patients with transient or minor cerebral ischaemia in the territory of the internal carotid artery (ICA) who have an extracranial stenosis of this artery of more than 70 per cent of the original lumen (Barnett *et al.* 1998, ECST Group 1998). Consequently, the major reason for performing carotid angiography (CA) in patients with subcortical ischaemia is to identify those patients who might benefit from CEA.

Both the European and the North American CEA trials included patients with ischaemia in the striatum, internal capsule, corona radiata, and centrum semiovale, because the blood supply to these area originates from the ICA. Infarcts in the thalamus are not usually an indication for CEA, because the thalamus is supplied mainly by the posterior circulation (Damasio 1983, Bogousslavsky *et al.* 1988*a*). The chief arteries in the territory of the ICA that supply the deep regions of the brain are the anterior choroidal artery (AChA), the medial and lateral lenticulostriate arteries, and the recurrent artery of Heubner (Damasio 1983). In the European study, the small number of lacunar infarcts did not allow conclusions about the efficacy of CEA in patients with these infarcts and severe ICA stenosis (Boiten *et al.* 1996). The NASCET investigators defined a probable lacunar infarct as a lesion with a diameter of less than 1 cm (Inzitari *et al.* 2000). They found a non-significant benefit of CEA [relative risk reduction of CEA 53%, 95% confidence interval (CI) –100 to 81%] in patients with a symptomatic lacunar infarct and an ICA stenosis of more than 70 per cent (Inzitari *et al.* 2000).

Important causes of subcortical ischaemia other than atherosclerosis that can be diagnosed by CA are dissection of the ICA (Levine *et al.* 1988), moyamoya disease (Bruno *et al.* 1988), and saccular aneurysm (Fisher *et al.* 1988). Neurocysticercosis, syphilis, and other forms of vasculitis have also been reported (Mohr 1986, Del Brutto 1992, Cantu *et al.* 1998, Dawson and Starkebaum 1999, Padovan *et al.* 1999). CA may be needed for the diagnosis of these rare causes and for exclusion of more common causes.

Subcortical ischaemia can be divided into different subtypes according to the cause. The pathogenesis of these different forms of subcortical ischaemia is discussed in previous chapters and may serve as a guideline for the decision as to whether CA with a view to CEA should be performed. In this chapter, studies of CA in various anatomically defined categories of subcortical ischaemia will be reviewed.

Lacunar infarcts

Lacunar infarction is caused by an occlusion of a small perforating vessel in the deep area of the brain or the brainstem. This occlusion can be the result of a localized vasculopathy or can be caused by (micro)embolization. Which of these two possible mechanisms should be considered the most important cause is a matter of debate (Millikan and Futrell 1990, Van Damme *et al.* 1991, Bogousslavsky 1992, Horowitz *et al.* 1992, Hupperts *et al.* 1997*a*). This dilemma cannot be resolved by autopsy studies because embolic material usually disappears within hours or days after stroke. Furthermore, small strokes are only rarely lethal, and enlightenment from autopsy material can hardly be anticipated.

ICA stenosis is found in 20–25 per cent of patients with lacunar infarcts (Zeumer *et al.* 1981, Gorsselink *et al.* 1984, Loeb *et al.* 1986, Kappelle *et al.* 1988, Thajeb 1993, Boiten *et al.* 1996, Inzitari *et al.* 2000). However, ICA lesions may well be a general marker of atherosclerosis rather than a specific factor contributing to lacunar infarction (Stein *et al.* 1962, Faris *et al.* 1963, Junquist *et al.* 1991, Ricci *et al.* 1991). In both the ECST and the NASCET studies, lacunar infarcts were uncommon and were more likely to be associated with a milder degree of ICA stenosis (Boiten *et al.* 1996, Inzitari *et al.* 2000). In NASCET, no relationship to plaque irregularity and ulceration was observed (Inzitari *et al.* 2000).

The low incidence of severe carotid lesions in patients with lacunar infarcts and their uncertain relationship to actual infarction has led several investigators to advise against CA (Olsen *et al.* 1985, Caplan and Stein 1986, Kappelle *et al.* 1988, Norrving and Cronqvist 1989, Boiten and Lodder 1991*a*, Chamorro *et al.* 1991, Fisher 1991, Tegeler *et al.* 1991, Donnan 1992). Others suggested that emboli from extracranial sources are common causes of occlusion of small penetrating arteries (Ghika *et al.* 1989, Orgogozo and Bogousslavsky 1989, Millikan and Futrell 1990, Cacciatore and Russo 1991, Laloux and Brucher 1991, Horowitz *et al.* 1992, Mendez and Estanol 1993). In a primate model, emboli were far less likely to reach small perforating arteries than surface arteries; only 6 per cent of sephacryl spheres with a mean diameter of 68 µm blocked deeply localized perforators (Macdonald *et al.* 1995). Consequently, embolism was considered a relatively unlikely cause of lacunar infarcts (Macdonald *et al.* 1995).

If ipsilateral ICA stenosis was more common than contralateral ICA stenosis, this would support a causative role for the carotid lesion. Only few studies allow us to study this in patients with lacunar infarcts (Norrving and Cronquist 1989, Boiten and Lodder 1991*a*, Tegeler *et al.* 1991, Boiten *et al.* 1996, Mead *et al.* 1998). Although the total number of patients in these series is small, ipsilateral carotid disease was somewhat more common than contralateral carotid disease. Only in the cohort of the European Carotid Surgery Trial did this difference reach statistically significance (Boiten *et al.* 1996). These findings support the notion that carotid disease can be important in the pathogenesis of lacunar infarcts rather than simply an associated condition (Mead *et al.* 1999).

The occurrence of lacunar infarcts secondary to local obstruction of the orifice of deep penetrating arteries by intracranial large vessel disease may be underestimated (Caplan 1989, Bogousslavsky *et al.* 1991*a*, Thajeb 1993, Lyrer *et al.* 1997, Adachi *et al.* 2000). In the Lausanne Stroke Registry, 320 of the 1800 patients had lacunar infarcts; in 26 of them no obvious cause was detected (Bogousslavsky *et al.* 1991*a*). Angiography was performed in 16 of these 26 patients, resulting in 10 intracranial stenoses of the parent large artery (Bogousslavsky *et al.* 1991*a*). Tan and Halsey (1990) propose that lacunar infarcts may occur with stenosis of the middle cerebral artery (MCA), when this results in a reduced perfusion pressure rather than in occlusion of a lenticulostriate artery, but this has not been confirmed so far. Intracranial arterial dolichoectasia may also cause occlusion of deep penetrating arteries. Among 387 residents of Rochester who had brain CT or magnetic resonance imaging (MRI) for first cerebral infarction, 12 (3.1%) had dolichoectasia (Ince *et al.* 1998). Patients with dolichoectasia were more likely to have had a stroke fitting a clinical and radiographic pattern of lacunar infarction than those without (Ince *et al.* 1998).

Striatocapsular infarcts

Striatocapsular infarcts are typically comma-shaped infarcts involving the putamen, the anterior limb of the internal capsule, and the caudate nucleus (Nicolai *et al.* 1996). The affected areas of striatocapsular infarcts correspond to the territories of the

Table 11.1 Results of carotid angiography in patients with clinical and CT scan evidence of striatocapsular infarction

Series of patients with striatocapsular infarct	No. of patients	No. of carotid angiograms	Carotid angiography: no. of patients with	
			Intracranial abnormalities	Extracranial abnormalities
Bladin and Berkovic (1984)	11	7	5[a]	1
Caplan et al. (1990)[b]	18	7	0	2
Levine et al. (1988)	24	24	13	9
Weiller et al. (1990)	29	29	9	15
Donnan et al. (1991)	50	27	12	3
Thajeb (1993)	5	5	3	2
Nakano et al. (1995)	5	5	3	2

[a] One carotid artery was studied post-mortem.
[b] Only caudate infarcts.

lenticulostriate arteries. Occlusion of the orifices of the lenticulostriate arteries at the level of the proximal part of the MCA is the main cause of these relatively large subcortical infarcts. Stenosis or occlusion of the extracranial ICA, documented by CA, has also been described (Table 11.1). In these patients, the carotid lesion may be the source of embolism. Levine *et al.* (1988) performed CA in a series of 24 patients with striatocapsular infarcts; only two of these were normal, and ICA abnormalities were found in 17 patients. In five patients, occlusion of the MCA was caused by emboli from the heart. In the study of Weiller *et al.* (1990), all 29 patients with striatocapsular infarcts underwent CA. The result was normal in 13 of the 29 patients; in eight of these 13 patients, a source of embolism in the heart was present. Combined abnormalities of the ICA and MCA were found in eight patients (Weiller *et al.* 1990). Nicolai *et al.* (1996) found 56 large striatocapsular infarcts among 1053 patients with a first-ever supratentorial infarct. Angiography, performed in 24 of these 56 patients, identified occlusion of the common carotid artery in five and of the ICA in two other patients. Stenosis of a large intracranial or extracranial artery was found in 15 patients; the remaining two patients had no abnormalities of the extracranial or intracranial vessels (Nicolai *et al.* 1996). Other series included small numbers of patients (Table 11.1), or selected only patients with occlusion of the ICA or MCA (Takagi and Shinohara 1981, Adams *et al.* 1983, Araki *et al.* 1983, Ringelstein *et al.* 1983, Bogousslavsky and Regli 1984*a*, Caplan *et al.* 1985, Saioto *et al.* 1987, Bozzao *et al.* 1989, Caplan 1989, Waterston *et al.* 1990, Thajeb 1993, Croisille *et al.* 1994, Lyrer *et al.* 1997, Nishida *et al.* 2000).

Anterior choroidal infarcts

Isolated infarcts in the entire territory of the AChA are usually associated with occlusion of this artery itself, but with normal findings of the extracranial ICA

Table 11.2 Results of investigations of the internal carotid artery in patients with anterior choroidal artery infarctions

Series of patients with infarction in the territory of the AChA	No. of patients	No. of carotid angiograms	Patients with extracranial abnormalities of the ICA
Mason et al. (1983)	4	1	0
Decroix et al. (1986)[a]	16	13	8
Helgason et al. (1986)	5	2	1
Paroni Sterbini et al. (1987)	28	27	3
Bruno et al. (1989)[b]	31	31	4
Mohr et al. (1991)	11	8	1
Leys et al. (1994)	16	15	4

[a] Results of Doppler examination.
[b] Twelve patients had only duplex ultrasound examination.

(Decroix et al. 1986, Helgason et al. 1986, Paroni Sterbini et al. 1987, Bruno et al. 1989, Fisher et al. 1989, Weiller et al. 1990, Mohr et al. 1991, Mayer et al. 1992) (Table 11.2). This differs from the situation with, for instance, infarction in the territory of the posterior inferior cerebellar artery, in which the occlusion usually affects the parent vessel, in that case the vertebral artery (Fisher et al. 1961).

Hupperts et al. (1994) compared angiographic findings of patients with AChA infarcts with those of patients with lacunar infarcts or with superficial infarcts. They found that significant carotid stenosis was found more often with AChA infarcts than with lacunar infarcts located outside the area of the AChA [adjusted odds ratio (OR) 8.9; 95% CI 1.4–55] (Hupperts et al. 1994). ICA stenosis appeared less frequent in patients with AChA infarcts than in those with superficial infarcts (OR 0.33, 95% CI 0.15–0.74) (Hupperts et al. 1994). Takahashi et al. (1994) studied 12 patients with an infarct in the territory of the AChA and angiographic evidence of obstruction of this artery. Complete occlusion of the AChA at its origin was found in seven, stenosis in three, and the ICA was occluded without filling of the AChA in the remaining two patients (Takahashi et al. 1994).

Little is known about intracranial vascular abnormalities in patients with AChA infarcts; Bruno et al. (1989) described one siphon stenosis among 17 angiograms. Only one other case of narrowing of the petrous portion of the carotid artery of unspecified severity has been described (Helgason et al. 1988). Occlusion of the AChA can be compensated for the collateral supply to the AChA territory from branches of the posterior cerebral, posterior communicating, and middle cerebral arteries, which may become visible with CA (Helgason et al. 1988, Mohr et al. 1991).

In the end, the pathogenesis of AChA infarcts remains a matter of debate. Some maintain that AChA infarcts usually result from intrinsic small vessel disease, and that the diagnostic and therapeutic management of these patients should be the same as that of patients with lacunar infarcts (Masson *et al.* 1983, Helgason *et al.* 1986, Bruno *et al.* 1989), but others attribute these to large vessel disease and argue that the usually extensive collateral supply is probably the main cause of the restricted size of the AChA infarct (Fisher *et al.* 1989, Mayer *et al.* 1992, Leys *et al.* 1994). Possible sources of embolism from the heart are found in 10–25 per cent (Decroix *et al.* 1986, Paroni Sterbini *et al.* 1987, Bruno *et al.* 1989, Mohr *et al.* 1991, Hupperts *et al.* 1994, Leys *et al.* 1994).

Internal borderzone infarcts

Hypoperfusion of the subcortical region, together with insufficient blood supply by collaterals, may result in 'internal borderzone infarctions' (IBIs), occurring between the deep territories of the anterior and middle cerebral artery or between the superficial and deep territories of the MCA. Consequently, IBIs are usually associated with occlusion or severe stenosis of the ICA (Wodarz 1980, Ringelstein *et al.* 1983, Bogousslavsky and Regli 1986*a*, Bladin and Chambers 1993, Hupperts *et al.* 1997*a*, Gandolfo *et al.* 1998, Del Sette *et al.* 2000) or of the MCA (Bozzao *et al.* 1989, Angeloni *et al.* 1990). IBIs usually involve parts of the basal ganglia, the internal capsule, the corona radiata, and the centrum semiovale.

Bogousslavsky and Regli (1986*a*) described nine patients with IBI; in seven patients, severe stenosis of the ICA was found, and in two the result of CA was normal. In another study, eight patients with IBI were found among 107 patients with ICA occlusion (Ringelstein *et al.* 1983). In a group of 18 patients with IBI, 12 had severe carotid disease (Bladin and Chambers 1993). Hennerici *et al.* (1998) mentioned that IBI occurred significantly more often in patients with carotid obstructive disease than in patients with atrial fibrillation (36% versus 16%). A comparison between patients with isolated IBI and with other types of cerebral infarcts demonstrated an independent causal role of carotid stenosis or occlusion (Gandolfo *et al.* 1998). Among 1253 patients participating in NASCET, 108 had an IBI; 81 of these patients showed an ICA stenosis of more than 50 per cent (Del Sette *et al.* 2000). Patients with IBI were about twice (relative risk: 1.9; 95% CI 1.4–2.6) more likely to have greater than 70 per cent ICA stenosis than patients with lacunar infarcts (Del Sette *et al.* 2000).

In a study of 36 patients with MCA occlusion who were studied within 6 h of the ictus, seven patients with IBI were found (Bozzao *et al.* 1989). One patient showed MCA occlusion just distal to the origin of the lenticulostriate arteries, three patients had MCA occlusion distal to the origin of pial branches to the temporal lobe, and three showed occlusion of pial MCA branches (Bozzao *et al.* 1989).

Conclusion

CA or other non-invasive techniques should be considered in order to visualize severe lesions of the extracranial part of the ICA in patients who may benefit from CEA.

In patients with large subcortical infarcts caused by embolism or by haemodynamic factors, examination of the ICA is particularly indicated, whereas in patients with small, deep infarcts this is probably less rewarding. CA may be useful also for the diagnosis of rare causes of subcortical ischaemia.

Acknowledgements

The author thanks C.J.M. Frijns, MD for useful comments on earlier versions of this chapter.

Chapter 12

Electroencephalography in patients with small, deep infarcts

L.J. Kappelle and A.C. van Huffelen

Introduction

When Fisher (1965a) revitalized the concept of the small deep ('lacunar') infarction in the 1960s, there were no brain imaging techniques to confirm this diagnosis during life. Since lesions were limited to subcortical structures and spared the cortex, specific clinical features in conjunction with a normal electroencephalogram (EEG) were obligatory for the diagnosis (Fisher and Curry 1965, Caplan and Young 1972, Caplan 1976, Haferkamp 1977).

After the introduction of X-ray computed tomography (CT) and later magnetic resonance imaging (MRI), EEG was no longer mandatory in the evaluation of patients with (possible) small, deep infarcts. Consequently, the EEG was increasingly disregarded in the clinical series of small, deep infarcts that were published during the last 20 years. However, little attention was paid to newer and more objective methods of investigation that became available in the EEG laboratories. Particularly, the development of refined quantitative analysis of the EEG (qEEG) has increased the likelihood of detecting the subtle abnormalities that are characteristic of small lesions in the subcortical structures.

Electroencephalographic data

In contrast to cortical and large subcortical infarcts, the EEG in patients with small, deep infarcts rarely shows focal or more diffuse slow activity. However, rather subtle changes in the physiological patterns such as the alpha and the mu rhythm are characteristic. EEG abnormalities that might be detected on visual assessment in this context are frequency decrease of the alpha rhythm on the side of the lesion, and diminished reactivity to eyes opening (alpha blocking). In addition, frequency decrease and enhancement of the mu rhythm, as well as decreased reactivity of the mu rhythm to hand movements, may be found on the side of the infarction (Fig. 12.1) (Pfurtscheller et al. 1981, van Huffelen et al. 1984). In recent years, qEEG techniques that can be used to detect minor abnormalities in patients with small ischaemic lesions that escape the EEG interpreter on visual assessment have been applied (Sainio et al. 1983, van Huffelen et al. 1984, Jonkman et al. 1986, Jackel et al. 1987,

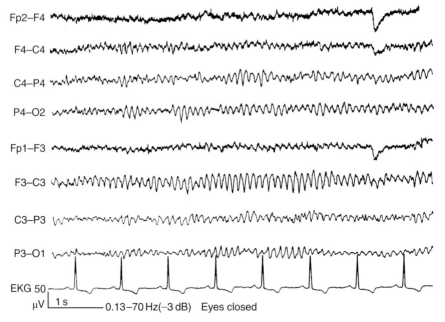

Fp2–F4

F4–C4

C4–P4

P4–O2

Fp1–F3

F3–C3

C3–P3

P3–O1

EKG 50
μV ⌊ 1 s ⌋ ———— 0.13–70 Hz(–3 dB)   Eyes closed

Fig. 12.1 EEG recording of a 66-year-old woman 3 days after the onset of a right-sided pure motor hemiparesis. The CT scan showed a small, deep infarct in the left corona radiata. An abundant mu rhythm in the left central region (C3) is visible.

Nuwer *et al.* 1987*a,b*, Jackel and Harner 1989, Kappelle *et al.* 1990). Brain mapping can help to give a quick impression of such abnormalities in the qEEG (Nuwer *et al.* 1987*b*, Jackel and Harner 1989). For the assessment of small, deep lesions, qEEG should include symmetrical derivations with special attention to the central (mu rhythm) and the posterior (alpha rhythm) regions. Different approaches have been followed, all departing from power spectral analysis using the Fast Fourier Transform (Tolonen 1984).

Several authors have used broad-band power data, which reflect the abundance as well as the amplitude of the different activities (delta, theta, alpha, beta). This technique is valuable for an objective evaluation of cortical infarcts (Nagata *et al.* 1984), but in the spontaneous EEG it may be inappropriate to demonstrate the subtle abnormalities in alpha and mu rhythm parameters that are present in small deep infarcts (Kappelle *et al.* 1990). A more sophisticated and rewarding use of the broad-band parameters can be made by studying asymmetries in both the abundance and the reactivity of the alpha and mu rhythms (Pfurtscheller *et al.* 1981, van Huffelen *et al.* 1984).

Alpha band parameters may indicate asymmetry (enhancement on the side of the lesion) as well as decreased blocking in patients with apparently normal EEG on visual assessment (van Huffelen *et al.* 1984). However, the most prominent changes in the EEG and qEEG of patients with small, deep infarcts are found in the mu rhythm

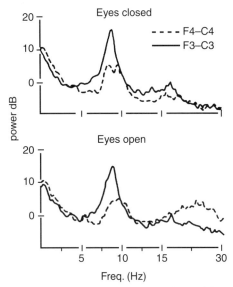

Fig. 12.2 Power spectrum of the F3–C3 and F4–C4 derivations of the same EEG as in Fig. 12.1, showing the asymmetry of the mu rhythm in eyes open as well as eyes closed condition. On the left side (F3–C3), solid line), the power of the mu rhythm is much larger than that on the right side (F4–C4, dotted line). Note the preponderance of the lower mu frequencies.

(Figs 12.1 and 12.2). Most often the mu rhythm is enhanced on the side of the lesion compared with the non-ischaemic side (Pfurtscheller *et al.* 1981). This may be explained by blocking of the afferents from the basal ganglia to the ventro-lateral part of the thalamus. Less frequently, small, deep infarcts cause attenuation of the mu rhythm on the side of the lesion. The so-called 'event-related desynchronization' (ERD), which includes attenuation or blocking of the mu rhythm during somatosensory stimuli (e.g. stroking of the skin or fist clenching), is a characteristic feature of the mu rhythm. An asymmetric loss of ERD can often be found in patients with small deep lesions (Pfurtscheller and Aranibar 1977, Pfurtscheller *et al.* 1981). A problem in the interpretation of the mu rhythm may be that this activity usually is not present in people in the fifth to the seventh decade. One might even wonder if the presence of such a rhythm in that age category should not be considered abnormal in itself.

A completely different approach of the application of qEEG concerns the peak frequencies of the alpha and mu rhythm. With small, deep infarcts, only minor frequency differences between these activities in the hemisphere with the lesion and the contralateral side may be important. Therefore, frequency resolution of the qEEG should be about 0.1 Hz, corresponding to an epoch of 10 s. An average of at least 10 of these epochs should be analysed, demanding a recording time of 100 s (Jonkman *et al.* 1986). Frequency asymmetries of both the alpha and mu rhythm have a constant character; the side with the slowest rhythm always indicates the ischaemic side (see Fig. 12.2) (van Huffelen *et al.* 1984, Jonkman *et al.* 1986). Such asymmetries were the major indication of lacunar infarctions in the study of Kappelle *et al.* (1990).

Changes in the beta activity are not very specific for the diagnosis of small, deep lesions. Also reactions to photic stimulation and to hyperventilation do not give much additional information. The use of medication, the quality of the EEG recording, and the experience of the electroencephalographer are all important in determining whether EEG abnormalities can be identified correctly (Jonkman *et al.* 1986). The age of the patient has to be taken into account, because old patients tend to have less specific EEG changes (Jonkman *et al.* 1986). Another important factor is the interval between onset of clinical features and investigation, because most abnormalities on the EEG are found more easily immediately after onset of the neurological deficits. The longer the patient has the neurological deficits, the less often EEG abnormalities can be found.

To summarize, absence of abnormal slow activity together with (minor) changes in the alpha and in the mu rhythms are very characteristic for small, deep ischaemic lesions. In only a few of the patients with these lesions is the EEG normal.

The EEG and the diagnosis of small, deep infarcts

The diagnosis of a small, deep infarct is based primarily on the history and neurological findings rather than on the results of any test. Nevertheless 'lacunar syndromes' may occasionally be caused by lesions other than these small, deep infarcts (Bamford *et al.* 1987, Kappelle *et al.* 1989, Sacco *et al.* 1991) and confirmation by ancillary studies is often important.

EEG findings in patients with small, deep infarcts have been reported in several series (Fisher and Curry 1965, Caplan and Young 1972, Caplan 1976, Haferkamp 1977, Mohr *et al.* 1978, Weisberg 1979, Otonello *et al.* 1980, Van der Drift *et al.* 1980, Pfurtscheller *et al.* 1981, Yanagihara *et al.* 1981, Donnan *et al.* 1982, Rascol *et al.* 1982, Soisson *et al.* 1982, Weisberg 1982, Dobkin 1983, Primavera *et al.* 1984, Dickmann and Müller 1985, Falcone *et al.* 1986, Loeb *et al.* 1986, Schaul *et al.* 1986, Zorzon *et al.* 1986, Janati *et al.* 1987, Ahmed 1988, Knibestöl *et al.* 1988, Macdonell *et al.* 1988, Abbruzzese *et al.* 1989, Kappelle *et al.* 1990). However, details about the alpha and mu rhythm are not mentioned in most of these studies. In addition, information about the clinical features and the CT or MRI scan in connection with relevant parameters of the EEG have been described rarely. In most studies, the EEG was found to be normal or non-specifically abnormal, probably because the presence of (focal) slow wave activity was considered the most characteristic abnormality.

One of the first studies about EEG and CT scan findings in patients with small, deep infarcts was reported by Otonello *et al.* (1980). They looked only for delta rhythm in patients with CT-proven infarcts and found this activity to be present in 55 per cent of their patients with small, deep infarcts and in 90 per cent of their patients with larger infarcts. Pfurtscheller *et al.* (1981) described the qEEG in 12 patients with

CT-verified subcortical infarcts, but did not mention the clinical features. All patients had some abnormalities of the mu rhythm; three had attenuation and seven enhancement, whereas in the other two patients reactivity to sensorimotor stimulation was abnormal. Furthermore, they found that an ipsilateral-enhanced mu rhythm in connection with symmetrical mu reactivity indicated a deep lesion with a 95 per cent probability versus a superficial lesion with only 5 per cent probability (Pfurtscheller *et al.* 1981).

In 1987, Janati *et al.* studied prospectively 50 patients with cerebral infarcts who all had both EEG and CT within the first 2 weeks after the onset of stroke. No information was given about the clinical features. Five patients had lacunar infarcts (<155 mm in diameter) in the basal ganglia, thalamus, or internal capsule; depression of the alpha rhythm was found in two, whereas some kind of 'focal slowing' was found in all of these patients. In two patients with lacunar infarcts, the EEG was assessed as normal. Seventeen patients had larger subcortical infarcts; an abnormal alpha rhythm was present in all, and 'focal slowing' was present in 14 patients. These authors did not describe the mu rhythm (Janati *et al.* 1987).

Ahmed (1988) described the EEGs of four patients with minimal weakness, no impairment of consciousness, and a relevant lacunar infarct on CT. He found lateralized slowing with persisting alpha rhythm, but no further details were given.

An important study dealing with the sensitivity and specificity of the EEG with regard to the distinction between cortical and subcortical infarcts in the acute phase was described by Macdonell *et al.* (1988). A late CT was used as the reference examination. They focused on the presence of theta or delta rhythms and on changes in the background rhythms, although details about the alpha and the mu rhythms were not mentioned. Lateralized slow wave activity had a sensitivity of 76 per cent and a specificity of 82 per cent when used as a marker of cortical infarcts. Its positive predictive value in diagnosing cortical infarcts was 0.62 and its negative predictive value in excluding subcortical infarcts was 0.9 (Macdonell *et at.* 1988).

In another series of 45 clinically well-defined patients with lacunar syndromes and a relevant lacunar infarct on CT, the EEG was abnormal in only 12 (Abbruzzese *et al.* 1989). EEG changes included lateral slow wave pattern in eight and discrete diffuse slowing in four patients. Details about the alpha and mu rhythms were not mentioned (Abbruzzese *et at.* 1989).

Kappelle *et al.* (1990) studied the EEGs and qEEGs of 12 patients with lacunar syndromes and relevant small, deep infarcts on CT and compared these with 12 patients with a recent cortical infarct and with 12 age-matched controls. The results of CT were not known during the interpretation of the EEGs. Abnormal delta and theta activities were not detected in any of the patients with small, deep infarcts, but were present in 10 patients with a cortical infarct. Asymmetric alpha rhythm was present in seven and asymmetric mu rhythm in 10 of the patients with small, deep infarcts. Absence of abnormal slow wave activity together with asymmetry of alpha or mu rhythms or both had both a specificity and a sensitivity of 0.8 in the diagnosis of small, deep infarcts. The positive predictive value of diagnosing a small, deep infarct by means of the EEG was 0.7 and chance-corrected agreement factor with CT was 0.75 (Kappelle *et al.* 1990).

EEG and prognosis of small, deep infarcts

Patients with small, deep infarcts usually improve rapidly and have a better functional outcome than patients with large vessel strokes (Bamford *et al.* 1991, Landi *et al.* 1991, Sacco *et al.* 1991). Survival after 1 year is better in patients with small, deep infarcts than in patients with large vessel strokes (Bamford *et al.* 1991, Sacco *et al.* 1991).

The literature about serial EEG recordings in stroke is limited. In general, EEG findings correlate well with the clinical course of patients with cerebral ischaemia (Kayser-Gatchalian and Neundorfer 1980, van Huffelen *et al.* 1980, Tolonen *et al.* 1980, Sainio *et al.* 1983). However, early prediction of the prognosis of patients with 'not further defined' ischaemia in the area of the middle cerebral artery by means of qEEG was of little value, if compared with clinical data in the study of De Weerd *et al.* (1988). Clinically well-documented studies in which the EEG was used to predict the functional outcome of patients with small, deep infarcts are lacking. Probably the same parameters that have been proven to be useful for diagnostic purposes are also useful for follow-up studies.

Conclusions

Refined qEEG analysis of mu and alpha rhythm in patients with recent small, deep infarcts usually shows rather characteristic abnormalities, although they are less specific than the clinical features. In clinical practice, CT and MRI are the preferred methods if the diagnosis has to be confirmed by ancillary studies. The diagnostic value of the qEEG in patients with clinical features of ischaemia in the area of small, deep perforating arteries, who have normal or non-specific findings on CT or MRI, is as yet unclear. Whether the qEEG can predict the long-term prognosis of these patients is also unknown. In order to make future studies of the qEEG applicable to clinical practice, additional information about how it can supplement both the clinical features and neuroradiological studies is needed.

Part V

Controversies and clinical syndromes

Chapter 13

About lacunes

C.H. Millikan

Introduction

'When I use a word,' Humpty Dumpty said in rather a scornful tone, 'it means just what I choose it to mean—neither more or less.' 'The question is,' said Alice, 'whether you can make words mean so many different things.' The word 'lacune' (dictionary definition—cavity, pit, hole, lake) exemplifies the inaccuracy presumed in Alice's comment! Bogousslavsky (1991a) wrote that the term 'lacunar infarct' is used for a least six different things. Phrases such as 'lacunar syndrome', 'lacunar stroke', 'lacunar dementia', or 'lacunar infarction' have become meaningless. The only common denominator found in the literature for the definition of lacune, whether used by a pathologist, clinician, or radiologist, is that it is small (Millikan and Futrell 1990). Faulty understanding of the fact that the size of the lesion is small has led C.M. Fisher (1991) to completely ignore the writings of Walter C. Alvarez about 'little strokes' (Alvarez 1946, 1948, 1955a,b). Beginning in 1946, Alvarez wrote extensively concerning what he referred to as 'little strokes, brief strokes, silent strokes, transient ischaemic attacks, and so on'. From that time on one can find any number of highly germane quotations from Alvarez's work. For instance, 'The first job for the gerontologist to tackle is that of identifying and learning to recognize quickly the symptoms that commonly go with a small infarct to the brain, especially when it comes in a comparatively "silent" area'. 'Often the pathognomonic point of a small stroke is that the illness dates from a peculiar attack, which came on at a certain minute of a certain day'. Illustrated in this article (Alvarez 1966) is a classic picture of coronal section of a brain showing small holes (lacunes). By 1966, Alvarez had found over 600 references in the literature to little strokes—references that have been essentially ignored! It is assumed that the modern literature about these little strokes contains no reference to Alvarez because none of his articles had the word 'lacune' in the title. He wrote such titles as *'Cerebral Atherosclerosis with Small Commonly Unrecognized Apoplexies'*, *'Small, Commonly Unrecognized Strokes'*, *'More About Little Strokes'*, and *'The Little Strokes'*. The title of his book (Alvarez 1966) was *'Little Strokes'*.

Fisher (1965a,b) originated the incorrect notion that small strokes are caused by a combination of hypertension and small vessel disease. Recently, Fisher has continued to write that 'the term lacune identifies a whole class of deep-lying infarcts that are the result of penetrating artery disease', and that 'unnecessary tests such as angiography may be avoided', also that 'the prognosis in lacunar infarction is often quite good, justifying optimism on the part of both physician and patient' (Fisher 1991). This incorrect notion about the cause of small strokes continues to be promulgated by a leading authority on stroke. Indeed, Caplan (1991) has stated: 'lacunes are caused by lipohyalinosis of the small penetrating arteries caused by high blood pressure or by microatheroma at the orifice of penetrating arteries', and that 'this condition is not likely to respond to either platelet-modifying agents or anticoagulants, and is far beyond the reach of the surgeon. If lacunar infarction is diagnosed the treatment is risk factor modification, that is, an attempt to optimize control of blood pressure and diabetes'.

The important facts about small strokes

These are as follows:

1. It is now established that small strokes are not caused by hypertension any more than any other type of cerebral infarct (Millikan and Futrell 1990). In general, approximately 60 per cent of patients with cerebral infarcts have hypertension, and the percentage of patients with hypertension is approximately the same regardless of the size of the infarct.

2. Atherosclerosis and lipohyalinosis are not necessarily the cause of, or even present in the small vessels supplying, small infarcts. The mortality rate for these lesion is so low that the nature of the arterial occlusion has not been studied within hours or a few days after the clinical event. Fisher (1979) reported his study of the appropriate artery leading into 10 small capsular infarcts. In two arteries there was an atheromatous plaque with a superimposed thrombus, in four there was severe stenosis from atherosclerosis, and in one instance the penetrating arteries were obstructed at their openings by an atheroma in the superior division of the middle cerebral artery. In only one was there lipohyalinosis. In another, the nature of the obstruction remained 'uncertain' and 'in two cases the vessels were patent, suggesting embolism'. The penetrating branches of the middle cerebral arteries of 14 brains from persons aged 31–65 years were examined, and the authors concluded that the size of the small infarcts depended upon the size and zone of supply of the occluded penetrating arteries (Marinkovic et al. 1985). It is apparent that the phrase 'small vessel occlusive disease' has been used without proof. The term should be 'small vessel occlusion', the occlusion caused by an embolus, a thrombus, or disease of the wall of the vessels.

3. These small infarcts are almost always caused by occlusion of a small primary artery (internal diameter generally <500 mm) or an occlusion in the collateral supply. Six basic causes have been identified previously for these small strokes (Millikan and Futrell 1990). These are the same causes as for any kind of ischaemic

stroke. Evidence is now accumulating that small emboli of various types are the most common of these causes. A few workers in the neurovascular area continue to be reluctant to accept the idea that tiny emboli can travel to the brain from the heart, arch of the aorta, or intra-arterial lesions (Mohr 1982, Bamford *et al.* 1987, Lodder *et al.* 1990, Boiten and Lodder 1991*a,b*, Caplan 1991, Fisher 1991) This reluctance has been generated by at least five phenomena.

(a) Little attention is directed to the history of onset of these little strokes. Most patients describe the onset as very sudden, which suggests that the small vessel has been occluded swiftly, as by an embolus.

(b) Some investigators do not understand that small, deep infarcts can cause dozens of clinical syndromes. They assume that small, deep strokes cause only four clinical syndromes—Fisher (1991) recently identified 62 syndromes— and have misclassified many small strokes as 'cortical' events because the patient has 'cortical dysfunction' such as aphasia, apraxia, neglect, visual field defect, or a sudden change in behaviour, and automatically placed such patients in a 'non-lacune' category. Since the invention of CT scanning, the literature has contained many reports that so-called 'cortical signs' are often caused by small deep infarcts. Impairment of memory, aphasia, anosognosia, neglect, amnesia, homonymous hemianopia, and many types of changes in behaviour have been caused by small, deep infarcts detected by CT or MRI scanning (Bogousslavsky *et al.* 1991*a*, Laloux and Brucher 1991, Cole *et al.* 1992, Malamut *et al.* 1992). This has been confirmed by an autopsy study (Tuszynski *et al.* 1989) (2859 autopsies) which disclosed that 6 per cent of the patients had small strokes (lacunes). In 33 out of 169 (20 per cent), aphasia plus right hemiparesis was the presenting neurological abnormality. The significance of faulty classification is exemplified in the reports about the Oxfordshire Community Stroke Project (Bamford *et al.* 1987) where four syndromes are labelled as 'lacunar infarction' in contrast to infarction involving the cortex (non-lacunar infarction). Infarction involving the cortex was defined as any unilateral motor and/or sensory disturbance if accompanied by ipsilateral higher cortical dysfunction (dysphasia, visual field defects, etc.). This faulty separation of patients into lacune and non-lacune categories without reporting CT or MRI scans, laboratory studies of the heart, aorta, cervico-cerebral arteries, or autopsies prevents drawing any valid conclusions about the pathogenesis of small strokes from these studies.

(c) Failure to examine the heart, aorta and cervico-cerebral arteries carefully is another cause of non-acceptance of the embolus hypothesis. Use of trans-thoracic echocardiography, trans-oesophageal echocardiography, and autopsy correlations has revealed many previously undetected cardiac and aortic sources of emboli (Robbins *et al.* 1983, Come *et al.* 1983, Tobler and Edwards 1988, Ono *et al.* 1989, Karalis *et al.* 1991). In the living patient, the nature of the material occluding the intracranial cerebral vessel cannot be proven (e.g. local thrombosis, embolus, etc.); instead, it must be inferred from the evidence provided in the clinical history, physical examination and by the laboratory. The frequency of strokes in patients with artificial heart valves (Kloster 1975) or atrial fibrillation (Cabin *et al.* 1990, Moulton *et al.* 1991) is generally accepted as evidence that embolization is the cause of the strokes.

Since CT scanning of the brain began in 1973, there has been much experience with CT detection of small strokes. Many of these CT lesions are associated with an 'appropriately' abnormal neurological examination. In addition to the 'appropriate' lesion, there are often one or more additional 'silent' lesions. There have been reports concerning CT scans on 'asymptomatic' patients with non-valvular atrial fibrillation. In one study (Feinberg *et al.* 1990), 36 out of 141 patients (25.5 per cent) had hypodense areas consistent with a diagnosis of cerebral infarction. Twenty-nine of these (29 out of 141, 20 per cent) were small (<1.0 cm) deep infarcts (lacunes). The mechanism was certainly embolic in most instances. Other investigators (Peterson *et al.* 1987) found 39 lesions in 14 out of 29 (48 per cent) patients with atrial fibrillation. The abnormal areas were thought to be small, clinically silent strokes. This is strong evidence that small emboli from a cardiac source can cause small strokes.

(d) That intra-arterial lesions are a source of emboli causing small brain infarcts is rejected by some neurovascular clinicians. In the Oxfordshire Community Stroke Project publication concerning the cause of 'lacunar infarction' (Bamford *et al.* 1987), the authors 'did not assess disease at the carotid bifurcation . . .' and 'excluded patients with symptoms and signs of brainstem or occipital disturbance'. These omissions are surprising as the evidence of an intra-carotid source of retinal cholesterol emboli was presented more than 30 years ago (Hollenhorst 1958). Occasionally at autopsy (Laloux and Brucher 1991) the material blocking a cerebral vessel contains cholesterol, which is convincing evidence that an ulcerated atheromatous arterial lesion was the source of the embolus. In another study (Soloway and Aronson 1964), atheromatous intra-cranial emboli were found in all of the 16 patients examined at autopsy. The size of the affected vessels was 17–585 mm. Recently there was the report of an autopsy that showed 'multiple cholesterol emboli occluding small arteries around lacunar infarcts and leptomeningeal arteries near cortical infarcts' (Laloux and Brucher 1991).

Another important investigation compared CT scans and carotid Doppler investigations in 115 patients with asymptomatic carotid stenosis (studied because of neck bruits), 203 with carotid transient ischaemic attacks (TIAs) and carotid stenosis, and 63 with TIAs but without carotid stenosis (Norris and Zhu 1992). The CT scans showed evidence of cerebral infarction in 137 out of 381 (36 per cent) patients. All the infarcts were small, less than 15 mm. Fifty-four (39 per cent) of the lesions were deep and 83 (61 per cent) were peripheral, located in the cortex or immediate subcortical areas. Patients with TIAs and carotid stenosis had significantly more infarcts than the other groups. The obvious inferred mechanism was embolic. In one large autopsy series of lacunes (Tuszynski *et al.* 1989), co-existent but non-contiguous cortical infarctions were present in 49 per cent of the patients with lacunes. The authors wrote, 'The high concurrence rate for cortical and subcortical infarction suggests shared risk factors and possibly shared pathogenesis'.

Data have been released from the North American Symptomatic Carotid Endarterectomy Study (Streifler *et al.* 1992) to document, with the aid of CT scans, the presence of many small silent infarcts distal to high-grade (70–90 per cent) stenosing carotid lesions. This is more objective evidence that emboli are causing small strokes (lacunes).

It should be obvious that if there is no search for cardiac, aortic or cervicocerebral arterial lesions, the lesions will not be found. Some (Fisher 1976, 1991) fail to understand that an embolus can be carried any place the blood goes and that an embolus may block a vessel and then fragment, lyse, or recanalize, ultimately leaving the vessel open. There are many kinds of small emboli including those made of platelets, atheromatous material, erythrocytes and fibrin, cholesterol, calcium, or their combinations. The size of each embolus determines where it stops and blocks the circulation, and the constituents of an embolus may determine whether each embolus is stable or relatively friable. The course of small emboli from a given source may be variable (as from the arch of the aorta) or may be remarkably consistent. The latter phenomenon occurs because of 'streamlined flow' which causes particles successively entering the same lamina of flow to take the same or a similar course through several branchings of the streamlined flow system.

(e) Many authors emphasize that small strokes are benign and that recovery from them is excellent. This myth has influenced some to write that 'unnecessary tests such as angiography may be avoided' or 'it is doubtful whether these patients should undergo extensive cardiac investigations or should be anti-coagulated in the presence of a cardioembolic source' and 'if lacunar infarction is diagnosed the treatment is risk factor modification, that is, an attempt to optimize control of blood pressure and diabetes' (Caplan 1991, Fisher 1991). As the maximum size of a small stroke is arbitrarily defined as 1.5 cm in diameter, the case fatality is close to zero. Follow-up of patients after the first small stroke reveals that one-third of the patients were not capable of independent living 1 month or 1 year after the stroke, and that the recurrent stroke rate in 1 year was 10–11 per cent (Bamford *et al.* 1987). In another study (Weisberg 1988), 16 patients with CT evidence of one small stroke were followed for 36 months. Seven patients had another small stroke, three developed a 'cerebral hemispheric stroke', two had myocardial infarction, and one died suddenly of an unknown cause. In a report from the Mayo Clinic (Sacco *et al.* 1991), 'the stroke recurrence rate of 4 per cent at 1 month, 11 per cent at 1 year and 27 per cent at 5 years in patients with lacunar infarcts in this study was not significantly different from the recurrence rate for those with non-lacunar infarcts'. The co-existence of large cerebral infarcts and cerebral haemorrhages with lacunes (Fisher 1965, Tuszynski *et al.* 1989, Adair and Millikan 1991) is evidence that small strokes often do not occur in isolation and that a small stroke is not a benign process. All of these studies coincide with my experience; a small stroke is a highly significant risk factor for subsequent stroke; with a greater than 10 per cent recurrence rate during the first year.

Summary

The word 'lacune' has been so distorted in the last 25 years that it has become meaningless and is often associated with incorrect assumptions about the pathogenesis of small cerebral infarcts. The number of patients not getting protective or preventive treatment after the first small stroke cannot be estimated but probably is several hundred thousand persons in the last two decades.

In 1955, the author generated the concept of pathogenesis of TIAs and small strokes as follows (Millikan *et al.* 1955):

> A thrombus begins to form in an area of diseased endothelium. This soft material may reach a size sufficient to produce enough alteration in blood flow to cause symptoms, break from its source, fragment and be carried away. More likely, however, appears the possibility that the newly formed clot becomes dislodged before symptoms occur, travels to a place where the vessels branch, lodges for minutes (symptoms produced) and then fragments and is carried away.
>
> *Millikan et al. 1955*

If the embolus continues to occlude the vessel, and collateral flow is not immediately established, infarction will result. The basic idea concerning pathogenesis of small strokes is built on several facts: the clinical manifestations depend on the site and size of the focal ischaemia; small or large cerebral infarcts are caused by failure of the primary and/or collateral blood supply to a local area of brain, an embolus can be carried any place the blood goes; and studies have identified many sites for the formation of emboli of variable size in the heart, aorta, cervical–cerebral arteries, and intracranial arteries. In animal stroke models, small strokes (lacunes) have been produced by embolic arterial occlusion in normotensive rats (Futrell *et al.* 1989). The use of the word lacune as an adjective (e.g. in lacunar syndrome, lacunar disease, etc.)

has caused 'only misleading confusion and should be abandoned' (Landau 1989). These lesions should be called small strokes. There are a variety of causes and the diagnostic evaluation of a person with a small stroke should be as thorough as for any patient with a recent TIA, a progressing stroke, or a recent stable stroke, in order to construct an appropriate plan for immediate and preventive treatment.

Chapter 14

Lacunar syndromes—are they still worth diagnosing?

J. Bamford

Introduction

In the past, the clinically defined lacunar syndromes (LACS) have been central to the debate about the importance of lacunar stroke. Nevertheless, the concept that a significant subgroup of strokes may be distinguished primarily by clinical means has always seemed to rest uncomfortably in the minds of many physicians, perhaps reflecting the increasing tendency in most branches of medicine to highlight the fallibility of clinical assessments, while being less critically accepting of the results of investigative techniques. Indeed, C.M. Fisher who, through his seminal clinico-pathological papers in the 1960s brought the issue of lacunar stroke into mainstream clinical practice, wrote that '... MRI has made dependence on clinical detail more or less obsolete' (Fisher 1991).

However, not everyone would agree with this view, and such clinical groupings should not be discarded lightly given their flexibility, economy, and ease of application to virtually all patients in all clinical environments. Clearly one needs to assess if these clinical patterns remain of any practical value both to cerebrovascular specialists and, perhaps more importantly, to the much larger number of non-specialists who care for the majority of patients with stroke worldwide, or are they simply the outdated product of clinical anecdote. This chapter seeks primarily to explore the issue of the clinical utility of LACS and does not attempt to be an exhaustive review of all cases reported under such a banner. Furthermore, the discussion is based on the premise that, in everyday clinical practice, the results of the clinical examination and subsequent investigations are used in a complementary fashion rather than in isolation from each other. Since the previous edition of this book, the utility of LACS in the hyperacute setting has become particularly important and therefore it will be discussed in a separate chapter.

General comments on definitions and methodology

Recognized limitations of LACS

Before embarking on a detailed consideration of individual LACS, it is worth addressing certain misconceptions that frequently are recycled in the lacunar debate.

First, it is important to remember that several pathological and radiological studies have shown that up to 80 per cent of lacunes (or radiological small, deep infarcts) are clinically 'silent' and therefore clinical syndromes are an insensitive way of detecting the pathological entity of the lacune (Tuszynski *et al.* 1989). Consequently, studies that select their cases on the basis of an imaged abnormality on computed tomography (CT) or conventional magnetic resonance imaging (MRI) that is thought to equate to a lacune, and then consider the presenting clinical features (often by retrospective case-note review) are likely to include a significant number of asymptomatic lesions. For most clinicians dealing with patients presenting with focal neurological deficits, the lacunar debate is mostly about the specificity of the correlation between clinically defined LACS and small, deep infarcts. Most of the studies that will be reviewed in this chapter have used the clinical features as the primary method of case selection and some have then refined their groups using the results of various imaging modalities, in much the same way that would occur in clinical practice (Mead *et al.* 1999).

The second misconception concerns the underlying pathological process. Most proponents of the value of LACS in current practice do not suggest that any of the clinical patterns by themselves help in the distinction of stroke from non-stroke pathologies. In general neurological practice, one frequently sees patients with, for example, pure motor deficits. Occasionally, such focal deficits will be of sudden onset, but the majority are not. In an Italian study in which 97 consecutive patients with LACS were identified in the emergency room, 5 per cent were the result of non-stroke pathologies (Anzalone and Landi 1989), while a Spanish study of 286 consecutive patients with LACS reported a non-stroke pathology rate of 1 per cent (Arboix and Marti-Vilalta 1992). Noorving and Staaf (1991) did not find any non-vascular pathologies among 180 consecutive patients with pure motor hemiplegia. Thus, the rates of 'false positive' diagnosis are very similar to those quoted for stroke in general (Sandercock *et al.* 1985) although whether such accuracy can be replicated with patients presenting in the hyperacute phase remains to be seen. Nevertheless, isolated case reports of non-stroke pathologies presenting with restricted clinical deficits should not divert the discussion of the clinical utility of LACS in patients with ischaemic stroke.

In similar vein, it has been shown repeatedly that any of the 'classical' LACS (see below) may be caused by a small haemorrhage. Large community-based series have reported that the proportion caused by haemorrhage is less than 5 per cent (Bamford *et al.* 1987, Bamford and Warlow 1988). In the pre-CT era, this fact may have been of some clinical utility, and it may still be the case in countries with limited access to CT where therapeutic decisions have to be made on the basis of probability rather than absolute evidence. However, the remaining part of this chapter will assume that cerebral haemorrhage and non-stroke pathologies have been excluded.

Care must be taken in interpreting the results of studies (often from very detailed hospital-based data banks) where the patients are grouped according to the putative mechanism of infarction. In such classifications, there is often a group identified as 'penetrating artery disease' (e.g. Chimowitz *et al.* 1991) or 'hypertensive arteriolo-pathy' (e.g. Bogousslavsky *et al.* 1988*b*). Although a presentation with a LACS may be part of the definition, the likely pathological mechanism is allocated after a series of investigations. Thus, patients in these series do not exactly equate with those seen with LACS in the emergency room or in large community-based studies. Some concern has also been expressed about the hierarchical nature of some of these pathologically based classifications, which tend not to acknowledge the possibility that small, deep infarcts due to penetrating artery disease may co-exist with, rather than be caused by, either a potential cardiac source of embolism or disease of the internal carotid artery (ICA).

Radiological investigations

The ability to image brain parenchymal abnormalities in life with CT and, latterly, MRI scanning added a new dimension to the original clinico-pathological debate. Unfortunately, at the same time, there was a precipitous decline in pathological reports of the underlying vascular pathology. The overall effect has been that radiological investigations have been used, at times uncritically, as a surrogate for the autopsy. The rash of reports purporting to describe clinico-anatomical relationships in this manner has been one of the major factors that has fuelled the debate about the clinical utility of LACS. Indeed, it has been pointed out that with the newer imaging modalities one is able to correlate the existence of lacunes (or at least small, deep infarcts) 'with a host of clinical syndromes previously obscured by their very rarity' (Orgogozo and Bogousslavsky 1989); however, this practice requires some comment. First, since most clinicians dealing with stroke still rely on CT, up to 50 per cent of symptomatic small, deep infarcts will not be visible without using special techniques or repeated scanning, neither of which is very practical in everyday practice. In the context of hyperacute stroke, this figure will be even lower. Even with MRI, cases are being described where infarcts seen at post-mortem have not been imaged. In addition, one must remember that even in experienced centres, there is some interobserver variability in the reporting of small, deep infarcts. Another potential problem that is common to both radiographic and autopsy studies arises when there are multiple abnormalities and it is difficult to decide which (if any) is the symptomatic lesion, and even if the imaged abnormality is truly ischaemic, for example Virchow–Robin spaces. The more sensitive imaging modalities become the more this dilemma is likely to arise, although newer MRI techniques such as diffusion-weighted imaging (DWI) may be of value in this situation.

Having accepted the presence of a lesion and the fact that it is 'symptomatic', one then has to consider whether it is confined to the territory of a single perforating artery. Measuring the size of an infarct, particularly acutely, can be very difficult, and there is evidence that the size of an infarct on a scan does not equate exactly with the dimensions at autopsy. There is also considerable variation in the area of supply of individual penetrating arteries (Kappelle and Van Gijn 1986, van der Zwan *et al.* 1992) and the number of cases where the detailed vascular supply of a lacune has been determined pathologically remains pitifully small. Hence, using the size (either diameter or volume) of a small, deep infarct on a scan is a questionable method of distinguishing lacunar from non-lacunar strokes. For the present, one may have to accept rather vague terms such as infarcts 'compatible with the occlusion of a single perforating artery'.

Which clinical syndromes should be called lacunar?

It might be argued that this is one of the key issues of the lacunar debate and, undoubtedly, the lack of any agreed definition of a LACS has been a major hindrance to constructive discussion of the subject. However, it is easy to see how this state of affairs has occurred because an individual physician or scientist's view as to what might be called a LACS will vary according to their potential use of the category. For example, if one starts with the pathological lesion of infarcts caused by occlusion of a single penetrating artery (or its convincing radiological equivalent) and documents the clinical features associated with them, the number of LACS is both daunting and of questionable value, particularly to the non-specialist clinician. Conversely, to the neuro-anatomist, isolated reports of very restricted clinical deficits that are convincingly associated with a lacune can be of the utmost interest in helping to trace neural pathways, even if most other patients with this syndrome have 'non-lacunar' pathology. Researchers in the field often strive to produce criteria that will 'guarantee' an exact clinico-anatomical correlation and may be tempted to reject less perfect associations. However, clinicians are used to coping with a lack of absolute certainty in all aspects of clinical medicine. To them, a classification that identifies subgroups of stroke that usually have a distinctive pathogenesis and prognosis can still be of clinical utility even though the specificity of the clinico-pathological correlation may be less than 100 per cent. In this context, the number of clinical syndromes that are usually caused by a lacune is much smaller and they are potentially of much more use in everyday clinical practice. These differing uses of LACS are rarely articulated in the lacunar debate.

One feature that should not vary between studies, however, is the rule that the clinical syndrome described should be the maximum deficit from a single vascular event. It is surprising how infrequently this is mentioned in the methodology of studies that purport to describe either a new LACS or equally those that cast doubt on the utility of the hypothesis. It is a particular problem with studies based on retrospective case-note reviews, and one has to accept that the accuracy of clinico-pathological or clinico-radiological correlations based on cases of first-ever stroke might not be so good when applied to cases of recurrent stroke. Furthermore, we know that of patients who are first seen within 12 h of the onset of symptoms and

Table 14.1 Types of lacunar syndromes

Classical LACS	Syndromes described in the original clinico-pathological studies	Pure motor stroke, pure sensory stroke, ataxic heiparesis[a], sensorimotor stroke
Partial LACS	Similar to classical but slightly less extensive deficits and less pathology	Brachio-crural and facio-brachial deficits
Extended LACS	Similar to classical LACS but with additional brainstem signs	e.g. Pure motor stroke + IV palsy
Occasional LACS	Infrequent syndromes or more often due to cortical ischaemia	e.g. Hemiballism e.g. monoparesis
Multiple LACS	Consequences of multiple lacunar infarcts	e.g. Pseudobulbar palsy

[a]Includes homolateral ataxia and crural paresis, and dysarthria–clumsy hand syndrome.

then re-assessed, 21 per cent will develop cortical symptoms or signs over the next few days, whilst in other cases cortical symptoms and signs will disappear (Toni *et al.* 1994). The latter problem can be overcome to some extent by taking a detailed history of the symptoms up to the time of assessment if that is outside the hyperacute phase, as was the case in the OCSP (Bamford *et al.* 1987), but the former may only be overcome by repeated assessment.

For practical purposes, one can identify five broad groups of syndromes that have been labelled as LACS (Table 14.1). First, there is the group that might best be described as the 'classical LACS'. They are those that were described originally in clinico-pathological studies and, if one accepts ataxic hemiparesis as a composite group, have all been demonstrated to occur (at least once) from occlusion of a single perforating artery. Secondly, there is a group of 'partial LACS' where the clinical deficits are similar to, but slightly less extensive than, the classical syndromes. Thirdly, there is the 'extended LACS' group with deficits that are similar to classical LACS but with some additional features (particularly brainstem signs). Fourthly, there is the group that might be described as 'occasional LACS'. Here associations have been reported between small, deep infarcts and certain clinical syndromes, which, in most cases, are either relatively uncommon in clinical practice (e.g. hemiballismus) or almost certainly occur more frequently as a result of cortical ischaemia (e.g pure motor monoparesis; Boiten and Lodder, 1991*b*). Finally, although the original definition of LACS was that they represented the maximal clinical deficit from a single 'stroke', for completeness, a final category of 'multiple lacunar states' should be included to account for presentations such as pseudobulbar palsy (which are beyond the scope of this chapter).

Classical LACS

Although reports linking specific clinical patterns with lacunes appeared in the late 19th and early 20th century literature, the clinico-pathological relationships were crystallized in the seminal papers of C.M. Fisher and colleagues in the 1960s. They described pure motor hemiplegia (PMH) (Fisher and Curry 1965), pure sensory stroke (PSS) (Fisher 1965*b*), dysarthria–clumsy hand syndrome (DCHS) (Fisher 1967), and homolateral ataxia and crural paresis (HACP) (Fisher and Cole 1965). Naturally, at this point, all clinico-anatomical correlations were based on autopsy examinations, albeit of relatively few patients. The fact that a lacune causing each syndrome (with the exception of HACP) had, on at least one occasion, been correlated with occlusion of a single perforating artery lent credence to the view that one was dealing with a distinct subtype of cerebral infarction. However, it is important to stress that these papers were essentially hypothesis generating and no prospective studies had been performed to examine the sensitivity and specificity of the clinico-pathological correlations.

Pure motor hemiplegia

In many respects PMH is the archetypal LACS. Fisher and Curry's original definition of PMH was 'a paralysis complete or incomplete of the face, arm and leg on one side unaccompanied by sensory signs, visual field defect, dysphasia, or apractagnosia. In the case of brainstem lesions, the hemiplegia will be free of vertigo, deafness, tinnitus, diplopia, cerebellar ataxia, and gross nystagmus'. The definition allowed sensory symptoms but not signs to be present, and in the Stroke Data Bank study (Chamorro *et al.* 1991) such symptoms were present in 9 per cent of cases of PMH. It was stressed that 'this definition applies to the acute phase of the vascular insult and does not include less recent strokes in which other signs were present to begin with, but faded with the passage of time' (Fisher and Curry 1965). In these cases, two-thirds of the lacunes were in the internal capsule and the remainder were in the basis pontis. Since then, cases have been reported with lacunes in other sites, including the corona radiata, the cerebral peduncle, and the medullary pyramid (Bamford and Warlow 1988). In virtually all large series, PMH is the most frequently encountered LACS (Orgogozo and Bogousslavsky 1989), although the actual proportion varies quite considerably because of different inclusion criteria. Furthermore, accepting the limitations of CT imaging, particularly in the posterior fossa, the distribution of the site of the lesions seems to be broadly in keeping with Fisher's original observations. The clinical presentation of capsular and pontine PMH may be identical. The clinico-radiological correlations of PMH in a number of large series are shown in Table 14.2, although it must be appreciated that most studies combined classical PMH with partial PMH syndromes (see below).

Pure sensory stroke

In essence, this is the sensory equivalent of PMH, but most studies suggest that it is much less frequent, for example 6 per cent of all LACS in the OCSP (Bamford *et al.* 1987) and 7 per cent in the Stroke Data Bank (Chamorro *et al.* 1991). Although the

Table 14.2 Clinico-radiological correlation in patients with pure motor hemiplegia

Study	Setting	Imaging	n	Non-lacunar lesion (%)
Bamford *et al.* (1987)	Community	CT	49	1 (2)
Hommel *et al.* (1990*a*)	Hospital	MR	35	0 (0)
Arboix and Marti-Vilalta (1992)	Hospital	CT/MRI	137	12 (9)
Melo *et al.* (1992*a*)	Hospital	CT	121	6 (5)
Norrving and Staaf (1991)	Hospital	CT	123	0 (0)
Gan *et al.* (1997)	Hospital	CT/MRI	101	7 (7)

Table 14.3 Clinico-radiological correlation in patients with pure sensory stroke

Study	Setting	Imaging	n	Non-lacunar lesion (%)
Bamford *et al.* (1987)	Community	CT	7	0 (0)
Hommel *et al.* (1990*a*)	Hospital	MRI	12	1 (8)
Arboix and Marti-Vilalta (1992)	Hospital	CT/MRI	45	3 (7)
Gan *et al.* (1997)	Hospital	CT/MRI	15	0 (0)

definition in the original paper (Fisher 1965*b*) suggested that there should be objective sensory loss, in a later paper (Fisher 1982*a*) Fisher recognized that there would be cases with persistent sensory symptoms in the absence of objective signs. Of course, it is well recognized that the sensory examination is probably the least reliable part of the neurological examination. Most studies have reported lesions in the thalamus in keeping with the original pathological studies, but the Stroke Data Bank also reported a lesion in the anterior limb of the internal capsule. Although there may have been another unimaged infarct in the thalamus, one notes the occurrence of sensorimotor deficits from lesions in this area and it was argued that this could arise by disruption of the anterior thalamic radiation (Chamorro *et al.* 1991). Most authors agree that infarcts causing PSS are the smallest of the symptomatic small, deep infarcts (Hommel *et al.* 1990*a*, Chamorro *et al.* 1991). The clinico-radiological correlations of PSS in a number large studies are shown in Table 14.3.

Sensorimotor stroke

At this point, it seems appropriate to discuss SMS even though it was not one of the original LACS described by Fisher and colleagues. For many years, it was considered that this syndrome could not occur from occlusion of a single perforating artery because of the different vascular supply of the internal capsule and the thalamus. Given the increasing evidence of considerable variability in the vascular supply to this area (van der Zwan *et al.* 1992), one might question why this combination should be any less acceptable than cases of PMH that have sensory symptoms. The inclusion of SMS as a classical LACS is based on a single case with autopsy (Mohr *et al.* 1977). This case was the result of a lacune in the ventro-posterior nucleus of the thalamus but there was also pallor of the adjacent capsule. Although there were marked sensory and motor signs that both persisted, the sensory symptoms preceded the motor symptoms. There is also autopsy support for an infarct primarily within the internal capsule being able to cause SMS (Tuszynski *et al.* 1989). This supports a previous report (Groothuis *et al.* 1977) although this SMS was caused by a small haemorrhage. The authors made the point that a sensory deficit can occur from lesions of the posterior limb of the internal capsule presumably by interruption of the thalamo-cortical pathways. Allen *et al.* (1984) reported 12 cases of SMS examined soon after onset, 11 of whom had low attenuation areas on CT. When superimposed, they were slightly larger and extended more medially than cases with PMH, abutting the postero-lateral aspect of the thalamus, but were still considered to be within the usual territory of a single perforating artery. In an MRI study (Hommel *et al.* 1990*a*), the infarcts in cases of SMS were larger than for other lacunar syndromes although still thought to equate with lacunes. In the Stroke Data Bank (Chamorro *et al.* 1991) where SMS was the most frequent LACS after PMH, 31 per cent had a lesion in the posterior limb of the internal capsule, 22 per cent had a lesion in the corona radiata, 7 per cent in the genu of the capsule, 6 per cent in the anterior limb of the capsule, and only 9 per cent in the thalamus. An interesting point was that the lesions in the corona radiata were on average almost twice as large as those in the capsule, but both were larger than the corresponding values for the PMH group.

There are three anatomical arguments running here. The first is that the motor and sensory disturbance occurs from a lacune that is primarily in the thalamus but extends into the posterior limb of the internal capsule, the second is that a lacune that is primarily in the capsule may interrupt thalamo-cortical sensory fibres, and the third is that it has been pointed out that the close anatomical and vascular relationship between the motor and sensory rolandic cortices may actually make the possibility of a pure SMS from cortical infarction more likely than a cortical PMH (Orgogozo and Bogousslavsky 1989).

In a prospective study of consecutive first-ever ischaemic strokes presenting to an emergency room (Landi *et al.* 1991), 34 out of 225 (15%) had a sensorimotor deficit without visual field, brainstem, or higher cortical dysfunction and involving at least two areas of face, arm, and leg. Of the 19 (56%) who had infarcts visible on CT in the appropriate hemisphere, 16 (84%) had lesions compatible with the occlusion of a single perforating artery, while the other three had large cortical or subcortical infarcts. Additionally, the risk factor profile and natural history of the SMS group were compared with a group of 'non-lacunar' infarcts and a group comprising the other classical LACS. The SMS group was found to be very similar to the classical LACS group. Lodder *et al.* (1991) reported very similar results from a

Table 14.4 Clinico-radiological correlation in patients with sensorimotor stroke

Study	Setting	Imaging	n	Non-lacunar lesions (%)
Bamford *et al.* (1987)	Community	CT	43	2 (5)
Hommel *et al.* (1990*a*)	Hospital	MRI	8	1 (12)
Landi *et al.* (1991)	Hospital	CT	34	3 (11)
Lodder *et al.* (1991)	Hospital	CT	47	5 (11)
Huang *et al.* (1987)	Hospital	CT	37	8 (21)
Arboix and Marti-Vilalta (1992)	Hospital	CT/MRI	42	8 (19)
Gan *et al.* (1997)	Hospital	CT/MRI	46	1 (2)

hospital-based series [47 patients with SMS of whom five (11%) had a 'non-lacunar' infarct on CT].

The clinico-radiological correlations of SMS in some large studies are shown in Table 14.4. If one calculates the number of 'non-lacunar' lesions among the non-haemorrhagic cases of SMS in a large study dedicated to the subject (Huang *et al.* 1987), the proportion was eight out of 37 (21%). However, one should note that in this study a 'lacune' could not be diagnosed if the volume of the lesion on CT was over 4 ml. Contrast this with the Stroke Data Bank study (Chamorro *et al.* 1991) where the average infarct volume for cases of lacunar SMS was 4.3 ml. However, further information about sensitivity and specificity is not available from the Stroke Data Bank publication since cases were excluded if imaging showed relevant non-lacunar lesions. Nevertheless, the result of the Hong Kong study is similar to one from Spain (Arboix and Marti-Vilalta 1992) where eight out of 42 (19%) ischaemic strokes presenting with SMS had 'non-lacunar' lesions.

The relative frequency of SMS and PMH in large series varies quite considerably. This is not surprising and, to an extent, will be related to the time after the onset at which patients are seen. Patients with a motor deficit at the time of examination and only a history of sensory symptoms will be called PMH, while patients with sensory signs and a history of a motor deficit will be called SMS rather than PSS.

Homolateral ataxia and crural paresis, dysarthria–clumsy hand syndrome, and ataxic hemiparesis

There has probably been most debate about this group of syndromes. One suspects this is mainly because of the difficulty of interpreting some physical signs. The original cases of homolateral ataxia and crural paresis (HACP) were described as having weakness of the lower limb, especially the ankle and toes, a Babinski sign, and 'striking dysmetria of the arm and leg on the same side' (Fisher and Cole 1965). In DCHS, although the deficit was described as being 'chiefly of dysarthria and clumsiness of one hand', closer examination of two of the three original cases shows that they had signs suggestive of pyramidal dysfunction in the ipsilateral leg and that both had an ataxic gait (Fisher 1967). Indeed, in his later paper in which he reported three further patients who had prominent vertical nystagmus as well as pyramidal weakness and cerebellar signs, Fisher drew the cases together under the new term 'ataxic hemiparesis' (AH) (Fisher 1978b). The lesions were all in the basis pontis and he attributed the variable distribution of the weakness in different cases to the involvement of motor fibres where they are relatively dispersed by the pontine nuclei.

It has been reported that if 'rigid' clinical criteria for DCHS are used, the syndrome predicts a lesion in the contralateral basis pontis (Glass et al. 1990). Conversely, Bogousslavsky et al. (1992) suggest that true HACP may be seen most frequently from partial anterior cerebral artery infarcts. They make the point that many other cases reported with CT evidence of corona radiata lacunes of similar size have had much more extensive deficits.

Fisher (1978b) discussed the question of whether weakness by itself could account for the incoordination. He stressed that there is a difference between the 'wavering' that is seen in slightly weak limbs and true dysmetria on finger–nose testing, which is not seen 'at least not of the severity in the present cases'. It is my opinion that this is the area that causes most confusion. In clinical practice, one encounters very striking cases that clearly fit the classical descriptions, although they seem to be relatively uncommon. However, there are also a significant number of other patients who have clinical syndromes that could be considered loosely under these groups. Some seem to be in the recovery phase from what otherwise would be considered PMH (perhaps they are seen later). This problem has been recognized by others (Hommel et al. 1990a). In their study, they classified many more patients as AH rather than PMH but stated that they were considered as AH even if the 'ataxia' appeared during the recovery phase of an otherwise typical PMH.

Additionally, it is noteworthy that sensory variants of AH have been reported but there is no evidence that the anatomical and clinical issues raised are significantly different from those concerning PMH and SMS (for a detailed discussion of these cases, see Orgogozo and Bogousslavsky 1989).

The alternative explanations for the syndrome that are proposed include cases of anterior cerebral artery infarction as already discussed, and, particularly when a supratentorial small, deep infarct is imaged, the possibility that there was a tandem, non-imaged lesion in the pons. The most detailed MRI study to date (Hommel et al. 1990a) argues against these causes being common. In their study, two out of 28 cases (7%) had 'non-lacunar' infarcts (Table 14.5). There were no such cases in the CT-based OCSP (Bamford et al. 1987). In the Grenoble MRI series, 19 per cent of cases of AH due to small, deep infarcts had more than one such lesion, but for cases with PMH the figure was 18 per cent. Additionally, in the Stroke Data Bank (Chamorro et al. 1991), a history of previous clinically apparent stroke was no more common in the AH/DCHS group than in those with other LACS.

Table 14.5 The clinico-radiological correlation in patients with ataxic hemiparesis

Study	Setting	Imaging	n	Non-lacunar lesions (%)
Bamford *et al.* (1987)	Community	CT	9	0 (0)
Hommel *et al.* (1990a)	Hospital	MRI	28	2 (7)
Gan *et al.* (1997)	Hospital	CT/MRI	41	1 (1)

Partial lacunar syndromes

This term usually refers to clinical deficits that are less extensive anatomically than in the classical syndromes. Although one might take this to its logical conclusion and include any pure motor (or sensory) deficit no matter how restricted in anatomical terms, by common usage it is usually understood to mean only facio-brachial and brachio-crural deficits. The term 'partial' should not be confused with the statement in the original definition of PMH, where the deficit was described as 'complete or incomplete'—this was referring to the severity of the motor deficit not its extent (Fisher and Curry 1965). It was the paper by Rascol *et al.* (1982) that brought the issue of partial LACS to the fore. Among 29 cases of pure motor stroke, 27 of whom had a small, deep infarct within the territory of a single perforating artery, 16 had the classical PMH while 13 had only facio-brachial weakness. Donnan *et al.* (1982) reported a series of 69 CT-positive cases of whom 32 per cent had incomplete syndromes, most frequently brachio-crural. Such lesions tended to occur in the corona radiata or junctional zone between it and the capsule, and were on average smaller than the infarcts with the classical PMH. A rather opposite pattern was reported from the Stroke Data Bank (Chamorro *et al.* 1991) where of pure motor syndromes with lesions in the corona radiata, nine out of 16 had involvement of the face, arm, and leg, four out of 16 had facio-brachial involvement, and one each had brachio-crural, pure face, and pure arm weakness.

Norrving and Staaf (1991) reported in detail their findings for patients with pure motor deficits. During a 4-year period, they saw 196 patients with pure motor stroke. Among patients with small, deep infarcts or no relevant lesion on CT, the face, arm, and leg were affected in 120, the arm and leg in 37, and the face and arm in 15, while eight had only one part affected. During the same period, 11 other patients with a monoparesis were seen who had cortical infarcts (i.e. the proportion of cases with a monoparesis and a cortical lesion was 58%) while only five cases with more extensive motor deficits had cortical infarcts (3%). In another study (Boiten and Lodder 1991*b*), out of 252 consecutive stroke patients with supratentorial infarcts, seven (3%) had isolated monoparesis of whom six had CT evidence of cortical infarction, and in the other case no lesion was visible on CT.

It is noteworthy that Fisher considered that partial syndromes of PSS were possible (Fisher 1965*b*) and such a case subsequently was verified pathologically (Fisher 1978*a*).

Many studies include these partial syndromes, although their validity as LACS is based on radiological rather than pathological data. Even then there is still room for confusion because few studies have stipulated what extent of involvement of the affected parts is required to call it a partial LACS. The large cortical representation of the hand was one of the reasons why in the OCSP it was stated explicitly that, in the case of the limbs, there should be evidence that the whole of the limb is affected and not, for example in the upper limb, just the hand (Bamford *et al.* 1987). In the end, it is a question of going back to first principles since it would be expected that the more restricted the clinical deficit becomes, the greater is the chance that it could arise from a cortical lesion that was small enough not to interfere with either visual or higher cortical functions. This is not to say that these more restricted deficits cannot ever be caused by lacunar infarction, just that it is an infrequent occurrence and they would be classed more appropriately under 'occasional LACS'. There may be specific exceptions to this. For example, there is still debate about the somatotopic organization within the internal capsule, but some reports suggest an antero-posterior face–arm–leg pattern. Restricted syndromes around the face may be due to selective involvement of corticobulbar fibres in the genu, but there is no study comparing the frequency of capsular and cortical infarcts with such a presentation.

Extended LACS

Much of the confusion surrounding the clinical utility of LACS stems from the review paper published by Fisher (1982*a*). In it he listed 23 clinical syndromes that might be caused by lacunar infarcts. As mentioned above, by the time of his more recent review (Fisher 1991), this figure had increased substantially. What is often overlooked is that he was neither suggesting that all these syndromes were usually caused by a lacune nor, for that matter, that an intrinsic small vessel vasculopathy was the cause of those that were. Indeed, much evidence has been presented about basilar branch occlusion from atheroma in the parent artery (Caplan 1996). Whether clinical syndromes that are essentially one of the 'classical LACS', most commonly PMH with the addition of an upper cranial nerve palsy or disorder of conjugate gaze, should be considered separately is a matter of debate (Orgogozo and Bougousslavsky 1989). Such cases usually have not been included in the major studies which have reported the sensitivity and specificity of clinico-radiological correlations and, therefore, at the present time, they are probably best considered as a group separate from the classical and partial LACS. However, in the major MRI study of this group (Hommel *et al.* 1990*a*), all 21 cases of such syndromes had infarcts compatible with the occlusion of a single perforating artery, although it is worth stressing again that this does not say anything about the pathological cause or, for that matter, site of the occlusion. The ratio of classical (plus partial) LACS to extended LACS in this study was about 4:1 although in the larger Stroke Data Bank study (Chamorro *et al.* 1991) the ratio was 15:1.

Occasional LACS

A vast constellation of clinical 'syndromes' have been reported in association with small, deep infarcts. Readers are referred to other texts for detailed references (e.g. Orgogozo and Bogousslavsky 1989). One gets the impression, however, that certain of these syndromes may, in the course of time, come to be regarded as much more valid LACS than others. Mention has already been made of isolated facial paresis, and Orgogozo and Bogousslavsky (1989) highlighted cases with isolated central disorders of eye movement control. The other group of syndromes are the lateralized movement disorders such as hemiballism/hemichorea. Nevertheless, in clinical practice, these syndromes seem to be relatively uncommon and certainly rarely are included in the larger studies of LACS.

Clinical utility of LACS—personal views and potential pitfalls

It is the author's view that the diagnosing of LACS remains a useful clinical skill. From the data presented, it is obvious that, although the correlation between LACS and small, deep infarcts is usually very good, errors do arise. This should not be a signal to discard the whole concept but rather it should prompt examination of the reasons for these errors. The relationship between LACS and vascular pathology is a separate and tremendously underinvestigated issue, although my prejudice is that, particularly in the carotid territory, such infarcts are not usually caused by large vessel atheroma or cardiogenic embolism. In everyday clinical practice, I encourage the use of a simple, clinically based classification of stroke, which includes LACS. This can be used by even the most junior doctor seeing patients acutely (Bamford et al. 1991). In the International Stroke Trial, clinical data were collected acutely by junior doctors and given over the telephone at the time of randomization. From these data, cases were identified who would fulfil the criteria for classical or partial LACS. A preliminary analysis has shown that this group have a distinctive natural history which is very similar to that of the patients with LACS in the OCSP (R. Lindley, personal communication). However, it is vital that, as a method of personal education, one reviews all clinical diagnoses systematically both before and after the results of investigations are known, since it has been shown that the specificity of the clinical diagnosis of LACS improves quite significantly when applied by clinicians with an interest in cerebrovascular disease (Lodder et al. 1994).

As mentioned earlier, in everyday clinical practice, a degree of uncertainty represents the norm and the clinician needs to be alert to situations where errors in the purely clinical diagnosis are most likely to occur. From the data presented above, one can see that of the classical LACS, most care should be taken with the AH group and, in particular, cases of HACP and also with SMS. On balance, it seems reasonable to consider that partial LACS are most likely to be caused by small, deep infarcts but, as the anatomical extent of the deficit decreases, so does the strength of this correlation.

There are certain clinical symptoms that may be difficult to assess, particularly in the acute phase. The well-known limitations of the sensory examination have been mentioned. The two other areas that have been shown to cause difficulty are the assessment of whether a patient is dysphasic or severely dysarthric and whether they have signs of non-dominant hemisphere higher cortical dysfunction (Lodder *et al.* 1994). In the end, this will come down to a question of individual clinical acumen and it is by no means clear that the involvement of either speech and language therapists or neuropsychologists actually helps this process.

Finally, one should always be cautious when there are features on clinical examination which occur less frequently in patients with small vessel disease (e.g. atrial fibrillation) or when there appears to be a discrepancy between the clinical and radiological findings (Mead *et al.* 1999).

Conclusions

The ability to recognize LACS remains a valuable clinical skill. For reasons set out in the following chapters, certain inferences may be made about the mechanism and prognosis that may influence clinical management. However, it cannot and should not stand in isolation from the others pieces of information that will become available in the hours, days, or weeks after a patient has had a stroke.

> Schemes of classification in biology are no more than mnemonics, mere skeletons upon which to hang information

Singer 1959

Chapter 15

The capsular warning syndrome and lacunar TIAs

G.A. Donnan, H.M. O'Malley, L. Quang,
S. Hurley, and P.F. Bladin

Should transient ischaemic attacks be subcategorized?

Transient ischaemic attacks (TIAs) were recognized quite early as a distinct clinical entity but, since then, in historical terms, there has been only modest development in their classification. They have been categorized broadly into either carotid or vertebrobasilar territory groups by earlier workers, but little further characterization has been attempted apart from the classification of carotid territory symptoms into retinal and hemispheric subsets. It was well known that TIAs as a group may herald subsequent stroke in the same vascular territory, hence the clinical recognition of these events assumed considerable importance. Because of various methodological difficulties with many earlier studies, the true annual stroke risk associated with TIAs was difficult to determine, the main problems being with TIA definition and end point definition (Brust 1977). For example, Acheson and Hutchinson used 1 h as the duration criterion for TIA and the events had to be repetitive for study entry; any event longer than 1 h was used as a stroke end point in the analysis (Acheson and Hutchinson 1964). So varied and methodologically unacceptable have studies of prognosis among TIA patients been that an appraisal of 60 studies performed after 1950 failed to identify any studies that adhered to six general research principles, although several did adhere to the three most important ones (Kernan *et al.* 1991). In spite of this, an average of around 5–7 per cent stroke risk per year became generally accepted by the mid to late 1970s (Toole *et al.* 1975) and this figure was used to calculate sample sizes for a series of studies of stroke prevention in patients with TIA using antiplatelet agents (Antiplatelet Trialists' Collaboration 1988).

It has been generally assumed that the stroke risk was fairly uniform for most presentations of TIA, and this was supported by the observation that there were similar stroke rates among hemispheric and vertebrobasilar ischaemic attacks in the majority of studies (Brust 1977). However, the results from recent trials of prophylactic carotid endarterectomy in patients with TIA suggest that subsets of TIA with higher and lower stroke risk exist, in these cases related to the degree of carotid artery stenosis ipsilaterally [European Carotid Surgery Trialists' Collaborative

Group 1991, North American Symptomatic Carotid Endarterectomy Trial (NASCET) Investigators 1991]. For example, in the NASCET trial, control patients with an ipsilateral carotid stenosis of 70 per cent or greater had a subsequent stroke rate of approximately 16 per cent annually on best medical treatment [North American Symptomatic Carotid Endarterectomy Trial (NASCET) Investigators 1991]. While control patients in the MRC European Carotid Endarectomy Trial with a similar ipsilateral degree of stenosis did not have such a high stroke risk (~6% annually), the subset of patients with carotid stenosis of less than 30 per cent had a negligible subsequent stroke risk (<1% annually) (European Carotid Surgery Trialists' Collaborative Group 1991). Based on this information, a useful classification of patients with TIA may be one related to the degree of ipsilateral carotid artery stenosis. However, this does not integrate adequately the clinical features of TIAs, which may make this classification even more relevant.

In view of the fact that TIAs and minor stroke have a similar risk profile for the development of subsequent stroke (Wiebers et al. 1982) and that if a subsequent infarct develops it is usually within the same territory of the preceding TIA, it seems reasonable to assume that similar pathophysiological mechanisms are operative for both transient ischaemia and infarction in the same patient. The multitude of different cerebral infarct patterns that are now recognized in cortex, subcortex, and brainstem are, therefore, most likely to be represented by TIAs of similar pathophysiological type. The challenge before clinicians is to subcategorize TIAs clinically, as has been done for ischaemic stroke syndromes. Such subcategorization is more difficult for TIAs as often only historical evidence is available. In some fortunate circumstances, patients may be examined during the course of a TIA and the precision of clinical categorization of the TIA is therefore improved. If the mechanisms and natural history of TIA subgroups were better understood, research into the development of more specific secondary prevention strategies might be possible.

The problems associated with a non-specific unimodal therapeutic approach for all TIAs is well illustrated by the meta-analysis of all trials of patients with TIA where antiplatelet agents were used to reduce the subsequent likelihood of stroke (Antiplatelet Trialists' Collaboration 1988). While an overall 22 per cent reduction in stroke rate was shown and this does suggest that platelet mechanisms are involved in a large proportion of cases of TIA and stroke, it also suggests that other mechanisms may be operative which are resistant to antiplatelet agents.

With these points in mind, the recognition of subcortical and/or lacunar transient ischaemic attacks may be a reasonable refinement of clinical TIA subclassification, particularly since lacunar syndromes may form up to 23 per cent of all cerebral infarcts (Mohr et al. 1978, Chambers et al. 1983) and are pathophysiologically distinct. Lacunar infarcts are usually due to in situ single penetrator atheromatous or lipohyalinotic disease, rather than large vessel disease; brief expressions of lacunar syndromes (lacunar TIAs) are therefore likely to differ pathophysiologically from other forms of TIA.

Lacunar transient ischaemic attacks: is the concept clinically useful?

Given that lacunar TIAs may be a pathophysiologically distinct group, can they be identified in a clinically useful way? For this to occur, an acceptable predictive value of this group for its clinical template would need to be demonstrated. This has been done by Hankey and Warlow who studied 130 patients with TIAs, 71 of whom underwent carotid angiography (Hankey and Warlow 1991). Lacunar TIA syndromes were defined as transient unilateral motor and/or sensory symptoms that involved at least two of three body parts (right face, arm, leg) in fully conscious right-handed patients who attempted to speak during the episode and who reported no disturbance of language, cognitive, or visual function. Symptoms were associated with a 50 per cent or greater stenosis in only one of 17 patients with presumed lacunar TIAs, but 36 (67%) of 54 patients with presumed cortical TIAs ($P <0.0001$). Using these clinical criteria, therefore, they have described a reasonably accurate predictive mechanism of identifying patients in whom the transient ischaemic attack was less likely to be related to large extracranial occlusive vascular disease.

Kapelle *et al.* (1991) studied 79 patients who had a clinically relevant lacunar infarct documented on CT who were a subset of 3050 patients with TIA or minor ischaemic stroke who had been randomized in a Dutch TIA trial. Lacunar symptoms were defined as unilateral dysfunction of face, arm, or leg, singularly or in combination in the absence of symptoms suggestive of cortical dysfunction (any of: visual field defects, spacial neglect, and disorder of language, writing, reading, memory, or orientation). Using these criteria, among 46 patients who were found to have a relevant recent lacunar infarct, 32 had a history of a unilateral neurological deficit without cortical symptoms consistent with a lacunar TIA. This gave a positive predictive value of these lacunar symptoms of 0.74 (95% confidence interval 0.59–0.87) and a negative predictive value of 0.61 (95% confidence interval 0.44–0.77). Using a different approach, therefore, this study also demonstrates that use of a set of parameters to identify the subcortex as the region of the ischaemia has a reasonable predictive value in detecting patients who are likely to have lacunar infarcts and, hence, by inference, ischaemic mechanisms restricted to small single penetrating vessels.

The criteria for subcategorization of transient ischaemic attack

Practical criteria need to be laid down for categorization of TIAs generally and subcortical TIAs specifically. As mentioned earlier, the precision of localization of the site of ischaemia is likely to increase significantly if the patient happens to be examined during the attack. However, this is unlikely to occur often. In developing these criteria, therefore, consideration needs to be given to the most likely site of ischaemia under a certain set of conditions. In the case of patients with subcortical ischaemia, this would include transient representations of the classical lacunar syndromes, particularly pure motor hemiparesis, pure sensory stroke, and sensorimotor stroke if these patients could be shown not to have cortical symptoms. This point was emphasized by Hankey and Warlow (1991) who, for this reason, restricted their subject group to right-handed individuals in whom left cerebral ischaemia occurred so that speech could be used as an index of cortical or subcortical involvement. To do this, the patient would need to have spoken during the event and clearly not have demonstrated any dysphasia. Other principles involving the prediction of the site of ischaemia based on clinical grounds include that of arm monoparesis which has been shown to be most probably of cortical origin, although this may not be absolute (Boiten and Lodder 1992). Based on these considerations, we have developed the following criteria to subcategorize all TIAs:

(1) Probably subcortical: involvement of the face, arm, and leg simultaneously with no cortical signs such as neglect, dyspraxia, or dysphasia, or involvement of any two of these if also: (a) the patient was examined during the event, and/or (b) a fresh infarct was seen in the subcortex appropriate to the clinical findings, and/or (c) ischaemia was in the left hemisphere in a right-handed person who spoke with no evidence of dysphasia.

(2) Probably cortical: typically, the presence of cortical symptoms such as dysphasia, neglect, or dyspraxia with or without hemiparesis involving the face, arm, and leg, or: (a) brachiofacial weakness with or without sensory involvement, (b) monoparesis with or without cortical signs, (c) the patient was examined during the event and cortical signs documented, (d) amaurosis fugax occurred within the study period in the same vascular territory.

(3) Probably vertebrobasilar: evidence of brainstem involvement by documentation of more than one of the symptoms of diplopia, visual blurring bilaterally, dysarthria, alternating hemiparesis, crossed hemisensory loss, vertigo, nausea, vomiting, or examination during the event confirming these findings.

(4) Retinal: an episode of sudden onset of total blindness in one eye or a shading effect moving vertically as a 'blind' or partial obscuration. Preferably the patient will have closed or covered one eye to avoid confusion with homonymous defects, although this is not essential.

(5) Uncertain: acute onset of focal neurological events which fall outside the above guidelines. Common situations may include hemiparesis involving the arm and leg during which no cortical symptoms were documented. Also lower limb monoparesis, isolated facial paresis with or without dysarthria.

The 'uncertain' group deserves special comment. Because the criteria are reasonably stringent, this group should be relatively large and investigators should avoid placing all patients in 'best guess' categories. By using this approach, the number of false positives in each group is likely to be minimized.

We have categorized all TIA patients in our own Stroke Unit population from 1977 to 1992 using the above criteria. Of a total number of 1093 patients who presented with a TIA, we found that 429 (39%) were probably cortical, 153 (14%) probably subcortical, 114 (10%) probably vertebrobasilar, 124 (11%) retinal, and 273 (25%) were in the unknown category. The majority of patients with subcortical ischaemia were categorized prospectively because of our interest in this group, but the remainder were categorized retrospectively. Although the majority of subcortical TIAs may be due to involvement of single penetrators, it must be realized that other subcortical ischaemic syndromes may also be represented. This includes restricted forms of striatocapsular ischaemia where sometimes few or no cortical signs are present (Bladin and Berkovic 1984, Donnan *et al.* 1991), anterior choroidal artery territory ischaemia where the clinical expression may be sometimes pure motor hemiparesis only (Helgason *et al.* 1988), and some forms of restricted internal watershed infarction which occasionally may have few, if any, cortical manifestations (Bladin and Chambers 1993). Since these other subcortical transient ischaemic syndromes may be due to large vessel involvement, this may reduce the predictive value of a lacunar TIA in identifying a pathophysiological subgroup where *in situ* small vessel disease is the only ischaemic mechanism. However, based on the work of Kapelle *et al.* (1991) and Hankey and Warlow (1991), the predictive power of the classification described above and interobserver reliability of the diagnosis of lacunar TIAs (Landi *et al.* 1992) is great enough for it to be clinically useful.

The capsular warning syndrome: crescendo subcortical transient ischaemic attacks

When TIAs are subclassified as described above and the subcortical group is considered separately, a proportion of these have multiple stereotypic events which often occur in brief clusters. The total duration of the episodes is usually quite brief, for example 72 h. These patients also appear to have a high risk of early stroke, although whether this is quantitatively different from other forms of TIA remains to be established. Because of its dramatic presentation and its early risk of capsular infarction, we have termed this the 'capsular warning syndrome' (Donnan 1980, Donnan *et al.* 1982, Donnan and Bladin 1987, 1988). Arboix and Marti-Vilalta (1991) also noted the stereotypic nature of the TIAs preceding lacunar infarction. When we considered 41 cases in which three or more events had occurred within 48 h, 16 of these (40%) had developed cerebral infarction and stroke during their in-patient stay (Donnan and Bladin 1987). The presentation occasionally may be so dramatic, with brief 10 min bursts of hemiplegia, hemisensory loss, or other transient expressions of the five classical lacunar syndromes and with complete resolution between events, that physicians may doubt the veracity of the patient's story. Indeed, one of our cases had been referred to a psychiatrist because of this concern. When the patient was examined later during an attack and the pure left hemimotor hemiparesis without cortical signs and an extensor left plantar was documented, there was little doubt of the genuine nature of his condition. Two typical cases are well represented by the following examples.

Case 1

A 74-year-old woman who had had a previous episode of left arm and leg weakness 2 years before, which left her with minimal weakness in her left hand, stepped out of the shower after washing her hair at 9.00 a.m., felt light headed and lost her balance. She noted her speech was slurred, following which she developed right arm and leg weakness without sensory symptoms. She was able to sit down and the symptoms passed in about an hour. At about 10.15 a.m. she was taken by ambulance to hospital and, while lying, noticed speech slurring again for a few minutes. At 10.40 a.m. in the emergency room, she had a further episode while being examined. She suddenly developed right face, arm, and leg weakness with profound dysarthria. During this period, there were no cortical signs present and a profound face, arm, and leg loss of power was documented without any sensory change. Blood pressure was 160/90 mmHg, pulse 76 beats/min and regular. She had bilateral cervical bruits. A CT scan was performed, which showed an old right posterior limb of internal capsule infarct (Fig. 15.1). Streptokinase $(1.5 \times 10^6 \, \text{U})$ was given intravenously, which was commenced at 1.40 p.m. Complete resolution of symptoms occurred over the next hour, but then at 5.30 p.m. she again developed a dense right hemiplegia affecting face, arm, and leg equally without cortical signs but again with profound dysarthria. This persisted with minimal recovery over subsequent weeks. A repeat CT scan 9 days later showed the presence of a small new left internal capsule infarct (Fig. 15.2). Routine examinations including chest X-ray, ECG, and full blood examination were

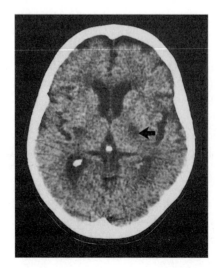

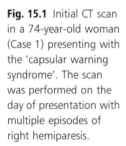

Fig. 15.1 Initial CT scan in a 74-year-old woman (Case 1) presenting with the 'capsular warning syndrome'. The scan was performed on the day of presentation with multiple episodes of right hemiparesis.

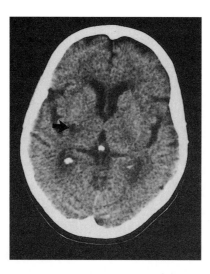

Fig. 15.2 Late CT scan after one episode of hemiparesis persisted and a dense right hemiplagia developed in the same woman (Case 1). The scan was performed 9 days after presentation. The left internal capsule is now visible.

within normal limits, although creatinine was slightly elevated at 0.17 mmol/l. Duplex scan of internal carotids revealed minimal change bilaterally.

Case 2

A 49-year-old business executive with a past history of hypercholesterolaemia (7–8 mmol/l) and common migraine was seated at a meeting at around 12 noon when his left face, arm, and leg felt numb and weak such that he was unable to get out of the chair. When he tried to speak, his speech was slurred and his tongue felt large and immobile. However, there were no visual symptoms and he had no headache. The episode resolved in about 5 min but over the next 2 h he had four or five identical episodes each lasting for 5 or 10 min. He described the onset of symptoms as sudden 'like a bang'. He was taken to the local community hospital where at around 4.00 p.m., while being examined by a physician, power in his left face, arm, and leg was reduced to approximately 3/5 and no cortical signs were recorded. A dull headache developed later in the day. He was transferred to our hospital where neurological examination was normal and blood pressure was 150/100 mmHg. Intravenous dextran and plasma expander was commenced and, on the next day, he had a further event during which he was examined and no cortical signs were found. Two days later, he had a further in-patient event involving the face, arm, and leg, with arm weakness predominating (0/5). No cortical signs were demonstrated. Bilateral carotid angiography was performed which revealed no abnormalities, and gradual recovery of function occurred over the next month. There was no history of hypertension, and subsequent readings were in the order of 140/80 mmHg without treatment. A CT scan showed the presence of a small right striatocapsular infarct (films since destroyed).

In keeping with the hypothesis that these events relate to small vessel disease, angiography was normal in 15 of the 17 cases we studied (Donnan and Bladin 1987) and only two showed moderate internal carotid stenosis. When carotid endarterectomy was performed on these, no active lesions with ulceration or clot formation were found. In the majority of instances, the stroke syndromes which developed were lacunar in type, although two were striatocapsular and one was in the territory of the anterior choroidal artery (Helgason *et al.* 1988). Interestingly, pontine infarction has been reported in cases of capsular warning syndrome, thus emphasizing that the precise subcortical location of cerebral ischaemia is difficult to predict clinically (Farrar and Donnan 1993, Benito-Leon *et al.* 2000).

Mechanism of subcortical transient ischaemic attack and the capsular warning syndrome

From the above discussion, it seems likely that the majority of subcortical TIAs relate to single penetrator vessel disease without evidence of large vessel arterial involvement. This assumes that the majority of subcortical TIAs are 'lacunar' in nature, while those with restricted presentations of striatocapsular, anterior choroidal artery territory, and internal watershed ischaemia, which may mimic the lacunar syndromes, are relatively uncommon. This is also supported by the two studies of lacunar TIAs: when angiography was performed in 17 lacunar TIAs in Hankey and Warlow's study, more than 50 per cent stenosis was found in only one case and the median level of stenosis was 15 per cent (Hankey and Warlow 1991). When this was compared with 54 cortical TIA patients, the median degrees of stenosis was found to be 50 per cent. These figures are similar to our own earlier study of the capsular warning syndrome (Donnan and Bladin 1987) where angiography revealed significant carotid artery disease in only two cases and no active atheromatous lesions were found at endarterectomy. Rothrock *et al.* (1988), in a study of crescendo TIAs, described nine patients who would fit the description of the capsular warning syndrome and in none of these were angiographic abnormalities detected.

If the infarct is restricted to small penetrating arteries, what is the mechanism in this region? The careful pathological studies of Fisher would suggest that either *in situ* atheromatous or lipohyalinotic change is responsible in the majority of cases (Fisher 1969, 1979) although, in his latter study, two lacunar infarcts were found with normal vessels, from which it was inferred that embolism may be responsible (Fisher 1979). However, Waterston *et al.* (1990) pointed out the infarcts were in the borderzones between the deep-perforating arteries and the internal branches of the middle cerebral artery, and haemodynamic ischaemic mechanisms should also be considered. They presented two cases of lacunar infarction of their own associated with ipsilateral high grade extracranial carotid occlusive disease and hypothesized that in these cases cerebral infarction may have a haemodynamic basis. The possibility that haemodynamic phenomena are responsible for the repetitive nature of clinical presentation of patients with capsular warning syndrome seems to be quite likely, perhaps due to high grade *in situ* small penetrator vessel stenosis or large vessel atheroma lipping over the penetrator origins (Waterston *et al.* 1990). This clinical pattern of the capsular warning syndrome is similar to incipient large vessel occlusion, as is seen with internal carotid thrombosis, but without the cortical symptoms or signs usually seen in the latter (Fisher 1951, Fisher and Caplan 1971). It was of interest that Terai *et al.* (2000) found a two-layered ischaemic lesion on MRI in a case of progressing lacunar infarction. They interpreted this as suggesting a haemodynamic mechanism, but involving sequential levels of a large perforating vessel and its ramifying branches (Marinkovic *et al.* 1985). The mechanism of artery-to-artery microembolism within the small penetrating vessels seems less likely because of the more widely separated clinical events usually seen in large vessel artery-to-artery embolism.

Vasospasm has been postulated as a mechanism of cerebral ischaemia by some workers (Bornstein and Norris 1989, Friberg and Olsen 1991). The recent description of retinal artery spasm seen during attacks of classical amaurosis fugax (Burger *et al.* 1991) would certainly support this contention, as would the repetitive nature of migrainous hemiplegic events on some occasions. In spite of the absence of migranous stigmata in our case 2, the possibility that vasospam was responsible remains a distinct possibility. However, *in situ* lipohyalinotic or atheromatous disease, or even atheroma in the middle cerebral artery causing a high grade obstruction at the origin of a local penetrating vessel (Waterston *et al.* 1990), appears to be the most likely mechanism in the majority of cases of capsular warning syndrome and many lacunar TIAs.

A further mechanism has been postulated recently by Norrving *et al.* (2000). They discussed five patients who presented with the capsular warning syndrome involving sensorimotor symptoms. In spite of the motor context of the symptoms in three and no permanent fixed deficit, diffusion-weighted MRI (DWI) abnormalities on MRI were seen adjacent to but not involving motor tracts (external thalamus in two and medial globus pallidus in one). They postulated that the transient symptoms may be due to an intermittent metabolic dysfunction affecting long tracts in deep white matter adjacent to the lesion.

Concluding remarks

Progress in prophylaxis against subsequent stroke after TIA over the last few decades has been immense. Carotid endarterectomy is now of proven benefit [European Carotid Surgery Trialists' Collaborative Group 1991, North American Symptomatic Carotid Endarterectomy Trial (NASCET) Investigators 1991] and antiplatelet agents reduce the risk of subsequent stroke by an overall value of around 20 per cent (Antiplatelet Trialists' Collaboration 1988). However, these studies have shown, first, that a single medical therapy is inadequate to cope with the multitudinous mechanisms whereby cerebral ischaemia and infarction may develop and, secondly, that high and low risk subgroups of TIAs may exist. The challenge before physicians, therefore, is to identify clinical patterns which may be associated with specific mechanisms in patients with TIAs so that a more appropriate therapeutic modality may be developed for each group. The identification of subcortical TIAs and the capsular warning syndrome makes modest progress in this area, but a further classification of TIA subtypes undoubtedly is possible. Close attention to clinical patterns coupled with the introduction of better non-invasive means of investigating the cerebrovascular system, such as magnetic resonance angiography, is likely to result in the recognition of a series of useful clinico-radiological TIA syndromes.

Chapter 16

Hyperacute diagnosis of subcortical infarction

D. Toni

Introduction

The differential diagnosis between stroke subtypes has many implications in terms of prognostic estimates, therapeutic approaches aimed at preventing stroke recurrence (Toni and Falcou 1999), and emergent treatment aimed at saving brain tissue. This last point, in particular, becomes of utmost importance following the demonstration of the efficacy of thrombolytic revascularization (Hacke *et al.* 1995, 1998, NINDS 1995) and its introduction into clinical practice (Grond *et al.* 1998, Trouillas *et al.* 1998, Hamilton *et al.* 1999). In fact, the effectiveness of thrombolytic agents is flawed by a relatively low therapeutic index since they are responsible for symptomatic haemorrhagic transformation in 3–9 per cent of patients even in the series with the best results (NINDS 1995, Grond *et al.* 1998, Hacke *et al.* l998, Trouillas *et al.* 1998, Hamilton *et al.* 1999). Hence, neurologists treating acute stroke patients need to bear in mind that their therapeutic choices may have different risk–benefit ratios in different stroke subtypes. In particular, given the reported spontaneous better outcome in patients with lacunar infarcts (Mohr and Martì-Vilalta 1998, Adams *et al.* 1999), it would be illogical to expose these patients to the risks of potentially harmful drugs such as thrombolytics. Moreover, even from the point of view of the pathophysiological mechanisms involved, lacunar infarcts might not represent the most appropriate target for thrombolysis. In fact, pharmacological revascularization may not be effective regardless of whether the vascular pathology underlying lacunes is 'segmental arterial disorganization' consequent to hypertension, also known as lipohyalinosis or fibrinoid degeneration, first described by Fisher (1969) or, as more recently suggested by Fisher himself (1991), lipohyalinosis is the pathological process underlying smaller asymptomatic lacunes with a diameter of 2–5 mm, and microatheroma and only rarely embolism are the causes of symptomatic lacunes over 5 mm.

In contrast to this general belief, the results of the National Institute for Neurological Disorders and Stroke trial with recombinant tissue plasminogen activator (rt-PA) have suggested that thrombolysis may also be effective in patients with small artery disease (NINDS 1995). However, both points of view (i.e. the one requiring

Table 16.1

Author(s)	N° of pts.	Type of syndrome	ΔT O/E	Gold standard	Definition of lacune	PPV
Bamford (1987)	93*	PMS, SMS, PSS, AH	4 days	CT	descriptive[†]	80.5%
Norrving (1989)	77[‡]	PMS, SMS	1 week	CT	descriptive[†]	79%
Ghika (1989)	62[§]	PMH, SMS, PSS, AH	N.R.	CT	$\varnothing < 1.5$ cm	53%
Boiten (1991)	109[¶]	PMH, SMS, PSS, AH/DCH	> 24 h	CT	$\varnothing < 2$ cm or no lesion	90%
Chimowitz (1991)	81	PMH, SMS, PSS	N.R.	CT (85%) MR (15%)	$\varnothing < 2$ cm or no lesion	54%
Arboix (1992)	286	PMH, PSS, SMS, AH, DCH Other	48 h	CT (80%) MR (20%)	$\varnothing < 3.2$ cm[#] or no lesion	80%
Landi (1992)	88**	PMH, PSS, AH, DCH, other (hemicorea/hemiballism)	72 h	CT	$\varnothing \leq 1.5$ cm or no lesion	100%
Melo (1992)	224[††]	PMH	N.R.	CT/MR ("selected patients")	$\varnothing < 1.5$ cm or no lesion	70%
Blecic (1993)	167	SMS	N.R.	CT/MR ("selected patients")	$\varnothing < 1.5$ cm or no lesion	57%
Lodder (1994)	147[‡‡]	PMH, PSS, SMS, AH, DCH	> 24 h	CT	$\varnothing < 2$ cm or no lesion	85%
Toni (1994)	219[§§]	PMH, SMS	≤ 12 h	CT (90%) autopsy (10%)	$\varnothing \leq 1.5$ cm or no lesion	56%
Madden (1994)	184[¶¶]	N.S.	< 24 h	CT (70%) MR (30%)	$\varnothing < 1.5$ cm or no lesion	66%
Gan (1997)	225[##]	PMH, PSS, SMS, AH	1 week	CT	≤ 1 cm or no lesion	87%
Staaf (1998)	32***	SMS	> 24 h ?	CT and MR	$\varnothing < 1.5$ cm or no lesion	53%
Mead (1999)	173[†††]	LACS	4 days	CT	$\varnothing < 1.5$ cm	80%
Tei (1999)	103[‡‡‡]	LACS	< 24 h	CT/MR	$\varnothing < 2$ cm or no lesion	73%
Toni (2000)	88[§§§]	PMH, SMS	< 6 h	CT	$\varnothing \leq 1.5$ cm or no lesion	29%

PMH = pure motor hemiparesis; SMS = sensorimotor stroke; PSS = pure sensory stroke; AH = ataxic hemiparesis; DCH = dysarthria-clumsy hand; N.S. = not specified; LACS = lacunar syndrome (not further specified).
ΔT O/E = interval time between stroke onset and first evaluation.
$\varnothing$ = diameter.
*out of 108 patients (15 patients without CT are not included).
[†]see text.
[‡]out of a total of 122 patients (with negative predictive value (NPV) 100%, sensitivity 100%, specificity 85%).
[§]out of 100 patients with subcortical infarction.
[¶]out of a total of 245 patients (7 patients without CT are not included) (with NPV 97%, sensitivity 95%, specificity 93%).
[#]see text.
**out of 191 patients (NPV 62%, sensitivity 69%, specificity 100%).

exclusion of lacunar infarcts from thrombolysis and the other indicating that this exclusion is not justified) imply that emergent diagnosis of lacunar infarcts is feasible and reliable.

The seminal works by Fisher and colleagues had suggested that lacunes were a nosological entity, characterized not only by the aforementioned specific vascular pathology, but also by stereotyped clinical presentations which consequently were called lacunar syndromes: pure motor hemiplegia (PMH) (Fisher 1965*d*), pure sensory stroke (PSS) (Fisher 1965*b*), ataxic hemiparesis (AH) (Fisher 1965*c*), dysarthria–clumsy hand (DCH) (Fisher 1967), and sensorimotor stroke (SMS) (Mohr *et al.* 1977). It is of interest that owing to the benign course of most cases, fewer than 20 per cent of the patients in Fisher's clinical series underwent an autopsy, and conclusions were inferred thanks to a unique capability of clinical observation. Subsequently, by inverting the perspective, Tuszynski and colleagues (1989) studied a large series of autopsy reports and found 169 patients with lacunar infarctions. By retrospectively reviewing patients' charts, they found that in 20 per cent of cases the clinical picture had been right hemiparesis plus aphasia, i.e. a non-lacunar syndrome. However, the relatively low reliability of retrospective data collection, in particular with regard to the clinical picture, is well known.

In this chapter, I will review the studies in which an attempt was made to test the accuracy of the clinical diagnosis of lacunar infarcts '*in vivo*', using cerebral computed tomography (CT) and/or magnetic resonance (MR) as the 'gold standard'. This entails calculating the positive predictive value (PPV) of the clinical presentation, which represents the percentage of all the patient with lacunar syndrome who actually have an index lacunar infarct at brain imaging. With regard to the studies in which data on both lacunar and non-lacunar syndromes are reported, I will also specify: (i) the negative predictive value (NPV), i.e. the percentage of patients with a non-lacunar syndrome who have a non-lacunar infarct; (ii) the sensitivity, i.e. the percentage of patients with lacunar infarct who appear to have a lacunar syndrome at admission; and (iii) the specificity, i.e. the percentage of patients with a non-lacunar infarct who at hospital admission have a non-lacunar syndrome (Table 16.1).

Table 16.1 (continued)

[††]out of 255 patients (31 patients with monoparesis are not included); data refer to the whole group; PPV in patients with 3 areas involved and hypertension (HT) was 87%, in patients with 2 areas and HT was 71%, in patients with 3 areas and no-HT was 71% and in patients with 2 areas and no-HT was 47%.

[‡‡]out of 350 patients (NPV 91%, sensitivity 87%, specificity 89%).

[§§]out of 517 patients (NPV 84%, sensitivity 72%, specificity 72%).

[¶¶]out of 479 patients (NPV 91%, sensitivity 81%, specificity 81%).

[##]out of 591 patients (NPV 78%, sensitivity 71%, specificity 90%).

[***]including 6 patients with normal findings/non relevant infarction at MR.

[†††]out of 536 patients (NPV 83%, sensitivity 69%, specificity 89%).

[‡‡‡]out of 250 patients (NPV 94%, sensitivity 89%, specificity 83%).

[§§§]out of 514 patients (NPV 88%, sensitivity 34%, specificity 86%).

From the (sub)acute to the emergent clinical diagnosis of lacunar infarcts

The first papers on '*in vivo*' studies of lacunes with CT were published between the late 1970s and the early 1980s (Nelson *et al.* 1980, Pullicino *et al.* 1980, Donnan *et al.* 1982, Weisberg 1982), but we are particularly indebted to Bamford and colleagues for their worthy effort to revive this field of research in the CT era. In their report on the natural history of lacunar infarction in the Oxfordshire Community Stroke Project published in 1987 (Bamford *et al.* 1987), they proposed the use of the terms PMH, SMS, and PSS syndromes when the deficit involves at least two of three areas (face, arm, and leg), and added that in cases of faciobrachial or brachiocrural symptoms the deficit should involve the whole limb. In PSS, the sensory deficit may include all modalities or may spare proprioception. AH is defined by the presence of a corticospinal and cerebellar-like dysfunction without other features clearly localizing to the posterior circulation; cases with predominantly dysarthria and clumsiness of the hand (DCH) are included in this subgroup. According to their definition, the presence of signs and symptoms such as dysphasia, visual field defect, visuospatial disturbance, and predominantly proprioceptive sensory loss suggest a cortical involvement, while gaze palsies or crossed deficits localize the lesion in the verte-brobasilar distribution, both thereby excluding a diagnosis of lacunar syndrome.

By applying this definition to a series of 93 patients presenting a lacunar syndrome at neurological examination performed within 4 days of stroke onset, Bamford and colleagues observed a PPV of 80.5 per cent. Although the original series was actually made up of 108 patients, in this calculation I have not included 15 patients not submitted to a control CT whose probable infarcts were defined according to the Allen score (Allen 1983). It is worth noting that the authors gave a descriptive definition of CT lacunes as 'CT compatible with cerebral infarction due to primary disease of a single perforating artery of the brain', including the negative CT scans (Bamford *et al.* 1987).

After this observation, other researchers confirmed the high PPV of lacunar syndromes, with figures ranging from 79 to 100 per cent (Norrving and Cronqvist 1989; Boiten and Lodder 1991*a*, Arboix and Martì-Vilalta 1992, Landi *et al.* l992, Lodder *et al.* 1994, Mead *et al.* 1999), despite some differences in the definition of lacunes at brain imaging. In fact, with the exception of Norrving and Cronqvist (1989), whose descriptive definition of lacunes was 'CT disclosing either an appropriate infarction within the territory of the lenticulostriate vessels or normal findings', all other authors provided a quantitative definition of lacunes based on their maximum diameter which, however, was set at < 1.5 cm (Mead *et al.* 1999), ≤1.5 cm (Landi *et al.* 1992), <2 cm (Boiten and Lodder 1991, Lodder *et al.* 1994), and <3.2 cm (Arboix and Martì-Vilalta 1992). The authors who chose this last limit, which doubles the maximum diameter of 1.5 cm suggested by Fisher's studies (Fisher 1965*a*), justified this choice by stating that 'CT scan in the acute phase of stroke may overestimate the diameter of a lacune by as much as 100 per cent

(Donnan *et al.* 1982). Unfortunately, the authors do not specify how many of their patients underwent CT within 72 h of stroke onset, and how many up to 3 weeks after, when caution might have been less warranted. 'Normal' or 'negative' brain imaging in patients with lacunar syndrome was considered compatible with a lacunar infarct in all the studies (Norrving and Cronqvist 1989, Boiten and Lodder 1991*a*, Arboix and Martì-Vilalta 1992, Landi *et al.* 1992, Lodder *et al.* 1994) except that by Mead and colleagues (1999) who decided to limit the analysis to patients with CT visible infarcts. In two studies (Boiten and Lodder 1991, Lodder *et al.* 1994), the Allen score (Allen 1983) was again adopted to classify stroke in patients not submitted to CT, though the number of these patients is not reported.

A common denominator of all these studies is that patients were first seen more than 24 h (Boiten and Lodder 1991*a*, Arboix and Marti-Vilalta 1992, Landi *et al.* 1992, Lodder *et al.* 1994) and up to 7 days (Bamford *et al.* 1987, Norrving and Cronqvist 1989, Mead *et al.* 1999) after stroke onset. This may be deduced from the definition that 'patients with a first brain infarct of >24 h' duration were entered' into the study (Boiten and Lodder 1991*a*, Lodder *et al.* 1994), inferred from previous (Bamford *et al.* 1987, Mead *et al.* 1999) or subsequent (Arboix and Martì-Vilalta 1992, Martì Vilalta and Arboix 1999) reports on the same populations, or is clearly stated (Norrving and Cronqvist 1989, Landi *et al.* 1992). This is not a negligible point, since the observations made in those studies led to the conclusion that 'lacunar syndromes are highly predictive of a small lacunar infarct' and since 'most lacunar infarcts are thought to be caused by a disease of a single basal perforating artery' (Bamford *et al.* 1991), a lacunar syndrome is almost synonymous with a lacunar infarct consequent to a small vessel disease. This is the 'lacunar hypothesis' according to which a simple bedside neurological examination is sufficient to identify accurately a lacunar stroke even in the emergency setting (Lodder *et al.* 1994). However, if this statement may apply to patients first seen many hours or days after stroke onset, its extension to the acute phase is an extrapolation.

On the other hand, a PPV of 80–85 per cent (Bamford *et al.* 1987, Norrving and Cronqvist 1989, Arboix and Martì-Vilalta 1992, Lodder *et al.* 1994, Mead *et al.* 1999) means that there is a non-negligible 15–20 per cent of patients presenting a lacunar syndrome who turn out to have a non-lacunar infarct or even a primary parenchymal haemorrhage (Bamford *et al.* 1987, Arboix and Martì-Vilalta 1992). This has been stressed recently in the paper by Mead and colleagues (1999) who compared 173 patients with lacunar syndrome with 363 patients with a clinical picture of partial involvement of the anterior circulation, and found that 20 per cent of the former had cortical infarcts and 17 per cent of the latter had lacunar infarcts. They also found that the misdiagnosis influenced the distribution of risk factors for stroke as well as the prognostic estimates, both of which were related more to the actual site and size of the infarct at CT than to the clinical presentation. Hence they concluded that 'brain imaging should modify the clinical classification and influence patient investigation' (Mead *et al.* 1999).

This is what our group had already pointed out in two papers on a series of 517 patients first seen within 12 h of stroke onset (Toni *et al.* 1994, 1995*a*). Previous observations on smaller samples of patients had reported a PPV of between 50 and 60 per cent for the various lacunar syndromes (Ghika *et al.* 1989, Chimowitz *et al.* 1991, Blecic *et al.* 1993). A PPV of 70 per cent for PMH as defined according to Bamford's criteria (i.e. involvement of at least two of three areas) had been observed by Melo *et al.* (1992*a*), though this was the mean of a PPV of 83 per cent in the case of simultaneous involvement of the face, upper and lower limb, and a PPV of 52 per cent in the case of involvement of only two areas. Hence, they proposed a reappraisal of the definition of PMH, suggesting that the term 'lacunar syndrome' should be applied only to cases presenting involvement of all three areas (Melo *et al.* 1992*a*). All the aforementioned studies provided a quantitative definition of lacunes by setting the maximum diameter either at < 2 cm (Chimowitz *et al.* 1991) or at <1.5 cm, (Ghika *et al.* 1989, Melo *et al.* 1992*a*, Blecic *et al.* 1993) and in no study was the interval time between stroke onset and the first neurological evaluation specified. The object of our studies (Toni *et al.* 1994, 1995*a*) were patients with PMH or SMS, since patients admitted to our Stroke Unit must have at least a moderate to severe motor deficit, which excludes not only patients with PSS, but also those with AH or DCH syndromes, owing to the very slight motor impairment. Moreover, PMH and SMS account for approximately 80 per cent of all classical lacunar syndromes (Bamford *et al.* 1987, Chamorro *et al.* 1991, Chimowitz *et al.* 1991, Arboix and Martì-Vilalta 1992, Landi *et al.* 1992). We found that PMH or SMS syndromes at entry corresponded in 56 per cent of cases to a lacunar infarct at CT or autopsy performed 15 ± 2 days after stroke onset. We did not find any differences in predictivity between PMH patients with two and those with three areas involved. However, as we were aware that the time frame we adopted prevented us from comparing our data with those of previous studies, and considering that changes in the clinical picture can occur over the first days after stroke, with the appearance or disappearance of 'cortical' signs and symptoms, we decided to test the predictivity of the clinical picture every day until the end of the first week of hospital stay. We observed a daily increase in the PPV up to a maximum of 66 per cent for PMH or SMS syndromes described 7 days after stroke onset (Toni *et al.* 1994). We also observed that both the distribution of risk factors for stroke and the 30 day outcome were related to the type of infarct and not to the clinical syndrome (Toni *et al.* 1995*a*).

More recently, we again tested the feasibility of the clinical diagnosis of lacunar infarct by exploiting the data gathered in the first European Cooperative Acute Stroke Study with t-PA (Toni *et al.* 2000). Complete data for this analysis were available for 514 of the 620 patients enrolled in that study. At the first neurological examination, performed on average within 4.2 ± 1 h of stroke onset, PMH or SMS with involvement of at least two areas were described in 17 per cent of the patients, and with involvement of all three areas in 13 per cent of patients. The 7-day CT was compatible with a lacunar infarct, which means that CT detected a lacune with a diameter

≤1.5 cm or was negative, in 15 per cent of patients. Hence, PMH/SMS involving at least two areas had a PPV of 29 per cent, while the involvement of three areas had a PPV of 27 per cent. After 24 h of stroke onset, PMH/SMS had a PPV of 44 per cent. Given this very low predictivity of the clinical diagnosis, we tried to look for surrogate instrumental predictors. In particular, considering that in patients with an index lacunar infarct leukoaraiosis, previous lacunes or both are reported more frequently (Hijdra *et al.* 1990, Hier *et al.* 1991, Miyao *et al.* 1992, Nadeau *et al.* 1993, Sacco *et al.* 1994, Salgado *et al.* 1996, Samuelsson *et al.* 1996*a*, van Zagten *et al.* 1996) and early CT signs of the infarct less frequently (Fiorelli *et al.* 2000) than in patients with non-lacunar infarcts, we tested the PPV of these CT variables. The PPV of the absence of early signs was 26 per cent and that of leukoaraiosis and/or previous lacunar infarcts was 22 per cent. Finally, the PPV of PMH/SMS involving at least two areas combined with the absence of early CT signs was 35 per cent, while that of PMH/SMS plus leukoaraiosis or previous lacunes was 19 per cent. Hence, we concluded that a lacunar infarct cannot be identified accurately on clinical grounds in the emergency setting and CT findings add little to the differential diagnosis (Toni *et al.* 2000).

A last example of these attempts of clinical diagnosis of lacunar infarct is the study by Staaf and colleagues who reported a PPV of 53 per cent for SMS syndrome described after 24 h of stroke onset (Staaf *et al.* 1998).

A clinical–pathogenetic diagnosis of lacunar infarcts

One attempt to improve the accuracy of the clinical diagnosis of lacunar infarcts has been made by also taking into account risk factors considered as specific for lacunar strokes. In the aforementioned paper on reappraisal of PMH, Melo and colleagues observed that by adding a history of hypertension to PMH involving three areas, the PPV rose to 87 per cent (Melo *et al.* 1992*a*).

This kind of clinical–pathogenetic classification has been developed particularly by the researchers of the Trial of Org 10172 in Acute Ischemic Stroke (TOAST). According to them (Adams *et al.* 1993*b*), a diagnosis of lacunar infarct is suggested by its clinical presentation as one of the classical lacunar syndromes combined with the presence of diabetes or hypertension in past medical history and with the absence of cardiac sources of emboli and of internal carotid stenosis higher than 50 per cent. On the contrary a clinical picture other than a lacunar syndrome combined with the presence of either cardiac sources of emboli or internal carotid stenosis higher than 50 per cent would suggest respectively a cardioembolic and a large artery atherosclerotic stroke. The detection of brainstem or subcortical hemispheric lesions with a diameter less than 1.5 cm or normal findings at CT or MRI would then confirm the diagnosis of lacunar stroke, while the finding of cortical or cerebellar lesions or of brainstem or subcortical hemispheric infarcts larger than 1.5 cm in diameter would confirm the diagnosis of cardioembolic or large artery atherosclerotic stroke

(Adams *et al.* 1993*b*). Unfortunately, when the TOAST researchers tested the accuracy of this clinical–pathogenetic subtype classification made within 24 h of stroke onset using CT or MRI as gold standards, they found that none of the three clinical subtypes corresponded to the final diagnosis in more than two-thirds of the cases and particularly the PPV of the initial diagnosis of lacunar strokes was 66 per cent (Madden *et al.* 1995). This might explain the apparent paradox of the NINDS trial, which reported an even higher benefit from thrombolysis in patients with small vessel occlusive stroke (i.e. a 23 per cent absolute increase in good outcome in treated versus placebo patients) as compared with patients with large vessel occlusive stroke (who had an 18 per cent increase in good outcome) and particularly to patients with cardioembolic strokes (who had a 10 per cent absolute increase in good outcome) (NINDS 1995). In that study, the diagnosis of stroke subtype before treatment, i.e. within 3 h of stroke onset, was based on the TOAST criteria, whose unreliability when applied to patients seen within 24 h has been clearly evidenced by the TOAST researchers themselves. In fact, in a recent paper on predictors of 7- and 90-day outcome, the TOAST researchers included in the multivariate analysis the stroke subtype diagnoses made after the acquisition of the results of ancillary tests, and not those made at baseline which they define as totally unreliable (Adams *et al.* 1999).

A similar approach was adopted by Gan and colleagues (Gan *et al.* 1997), the main differences from the TOAST group consisting of setting the maximum diameter of lacunes at ≤ 1 cm, the threshold of internal carotid artery stenosis which is still compatible with the diagnosis of lacunar stroke at 60 per cent, and above all in seeing patients within 1 week of stroke onset. The global PPV of the lacunar syndromes they described was 87 per cent, but ranged from 79 per cent for PMH to 100 per cent for PSS. When they considered as PMH only patients with all three areas involved, the PPV fell to 72 per cent. Moreover, a history of hypertension or diabetes did not increase the PPV of lacunar syndrome as a group. Interestingly, after completion of ancillary diagnostic tests and pathogenetic classification of the infarct, only 75 per cent of the cases with lacunar syndrome and brain imaging consistent with lacunes were ascribed to small vessel disease, again with a variation of between 69 per cent for PMH and 100 per cent for PSS.

More recently, following the same diagnostic steps in a series of 103 patients presenting with a lacunar syndrome within 24 h of stroke onset, Tei and colleagues (1999) found that the clinical picture predicted small subcortical infarctions with a maximum diameter less than 2 cm in the territory of deep perforators in 70 per cent of cases, whereas a small artery disease mechanism was confirmed in only 60 per cent of patients (Tei *et al.* 1999).

What are the possible causes of misdiagnosis?

From this review, it emerges that the clinical or clinical–pathogenetic diagnosis of lacunar infarcts is misleading in 20–60 per cent of cases (Bamford *et al.* 1987,

Norrving and Cronqvist 1989, Ghika *et al.* 1989, Chimowitz *et al.* 1991, Melo *et al.* 1992*a*, Blecic *et al.* 1993, Toni *et al.* 1994, Madden *et al.* 1995, Arboix and Martì-Vilalta 1996, Mead *et al.* 1999, Staaf *et al.* 1999, Tei *et al.* 1999, Toni *et al.* 2000).

There are a number of possible explanations for this misdiagnosis. First of all, it appears that the earlier patients are seen, the lower the PPV of the clinical picture. This may be attributed in part to reduced patient participation during the neurological evaluation in the emergency setting, consequent to fear, anxiety, and sometimes confusion, which makes the identification of 'cortical' signs and symptoms more difficult. Secondly, the dynamic course of the ischaemic damage may lead to spontaneous impairment or improvement over the initial 2–7 days (Toni *et al.* 1995*b*, 1997), and hence 'cortical' signs and symptoms may emerge or disappear. The disappearance of these signs and symptoms may be consequent to the recovery of the initially ischaemic tissue or to the reversal of an initial functional disconnection between subcortical infarcted areas and their cortical projections (Ferro and Kertesz 1984, Takano *et al.* 1985, Alexander *et al.* 1987, Basso *et al.* 1987, Perani *et al.* 1987, Bogousslavsky *et al.* 1988, Lazzarino *et al.* 1991). In contrast, the persistence of this disconnection might account for the lacunar infarcts underlying non-lacunar syndromes even days after stroke onset. In this regard, Fisher himself, in a review on lacunar infarcts published in 1991 (Fisher 1991), stated that 'the number of clinical patterns or syndromes linked to penetrator occlusion has grown to at least 70', thereby indicating that among the signs and symptoms may also be included Broca's aphasia, anosognosia, homonymous hemianopia, constructional apraxia, visual neglect, and gaze palsy, i.e. signs and symptoms which, according to the lacunar hypothesis, would exclude a diagnosis of lacunar infarct.

Another point of interest is the difficulty in adequately testing non-dominant higher functions, as clearly demonstrated by the fact that the PPV of lacunar syndromes related to right hemisphere lesions is lower than that related to left hemisphere lesions. (Lodder *et al.* 1994, Toni *et al.* 1994). This is particularly true for PMH which, in fact, is the syndrome with the lowest PPV in most of the studies we have reviewed.

Hence, the clinical differentiation of lacunar infarcts in the emergency setting is not reliable. This differential diagnosis requires additional data provided by CT or MRI, whereas extra- and intracranial ultrasound examinations, echocardiography, and sometimes angiography are also needed to attribute small subcortical infarcts to small vessel disease. However, since most of these techniques are not usually available in the emergency setting, the complete work-up necessary for subtype differentiation is at present not feasible.

Is there a future for emergent diagnosis of lacunar infarcts?

It could be argued that the correct question should be: is there a need for this diagnosis? This is the doubt expressed by Adams and colleagues (Adams *et al.* 1999), who stated that 'at present the usefulness of the emergent diagnosis of subtype of ischemic stroke in swaying decisions in early treatment is unknown', and since 'the trial of rt-PA' (that of the NINDS) 'did not demonstrate a difference in response to treatment between persons with different subtypes of stroke', they concluded that 'until definitive data show the usefulness of subtype diagnoses in emergent management, the rapid diagnosis of subtype should not be mandated'. However, the tautology in this statement is evident, since we have seen that stroke subtypes in the NINDS trial were diagnosed using unreliable criteria. I would like to add that if we are not able to differentiate lacunar infarcts before treatment, we will never be able to test a treatment hypothetically aimed at counteracting the underlying pathogenetic mechanisms.

One way out of this vicious circle might be provided by the latest imaging techniques. Diffusion-weighted imaging (DWI) and haemodynamically weighted imaging (HWI), with the calculation of relative cerebral blood volume, relative cerebral blood flow, and relative mean transit time, are likely to offer the most complete set of data on brain tissue viability and perfusion in the very first hours after stroke onset (Sorensen *et al.* 1996). It has been suggested recently that this also applies to subcortical lacunar and non-lacunar infarcts, (Noguchi *et al.* 1998, Singer *et al.* 1998, Ay *et al.* 1999*a,b*) though few of these patients have been studied so far in the hyperacute phase (Singer *et al.* 1998, Noguchi *et al.* 1998, Ay *et al.* 1999*b*). At present we know that the DWI of lacunar infarcts may be normal (Ay *et al.* 1999*a*) or may show a hyperintense signal of typical size and site (Singer *et al.* 1998). However, we also know that up to 17 per cent of cases with an initially normal DWI subsequently may show a cortical infarct (Ay *et al.* 1999*a*). Moreover, DWI reveals that up to 16 per cent of patients with lacunar syndrome and subcortical infarcts may have, in addition to the index lesion, subsidiary subcortical infarctions and harbour an underlying embolic source more frequently than patients with a single lesion (Ay *et al.* 1999*a*).

From the point of view of the emergent therapies, however, it could be argued that, irrespective of the clinical picture, it may be sufficient to detect ischaemic tissue at risk of infarction with the most sensitive imaging techniques available, with the corollary information on arterial patency provided by conventional or magnetic resonance angiography, or by ultrasound techniques.

Only prospective studies on large series of patients with subcortical infarcts, evaluated in the very first hours after stroke onset with the aforementioned techniques, will allow us to determine whether a lacunar infarct and its individual underlying pathogenetic mechanism may be diagnosed reliably in the emergency setting.

Acknowledgement

I gratefully acknowledge Professor Cesare Fieschi for his advice and criticism in reviewing the manuscript.

Chapter 17

Striatocapsular infarcts

C. Weiller

Introduction

Striatocapsular infarcts can be defined as large (>20 mm) subcortical infarcts in the territory of the lenticulostriate arteries, sometimes extending into the territory of the adjacent deep perforators, for example Heubner's recurring artery or the anterior choroidal artery. They do not usually present with a lacunar syndrome and are typically caused by a middle cerebral artery (MCA) mainstem lesion, and thus result from large vessel disease. Straitocapsular infarcts represent the prototype embolic brain infarction frequently are found in cases after successful thrombolysis. Collected evidence to support this hypothesis is reported in this chapter.

Pathogenesis

The lenticulostriate arteries (LSAs) (Salamon *et al.* 1966) are *functional* end arteries without collaterals with the other basal ganglia arteries, although small anatomical links do exist (Kaplan and Ford 1966, Salamon *et al.* 1966). They arise at an acute angle from the main trunk (Ml segment) of the MCA, its terminal or collateral branches (insular branches, M2 segment), form curves or real loops and end in certain parts of the basal ganglia and internal capsule (Marinkovic *et al.* 1985). Sometimes a medial and a lateral (larger) group has been differentiated (Takahashi *et al.* 1985, Ghika *et al.* 1990). The LSAs irrigate the putamen with some extension into the external capsule and the claustrum, the lateral part of the globus pallidus, and the head of the caudate nucleus, the anterior limb of the internal capsule, and the anterior part of the periventricular corona radiata (Roßerg *et al.* 1992) (Fig. 17.1). All structures from approximately 1 mm lateral to the putamen and the frontal deep white matter are supplied by the pial branches of the MCA. The fronto-caudal border of the LSA territory is irrigated by Heubner's recurrent artery and the medio-posterior border by the anterior and posterior choroidal arteries.

Lacunes also occur in the territory of the LSAs, but they are smaller (usually 0.5–1 cm diameter) than striatocapsular infarcts. According to the 'lacunar hypothesis', they are most often caused by a distinct vasculopathy of the small perforating arteries related to arterial hypertension, for example lipohyalinosis, fibrinoid necrosis, microatheroma formation, or local thrombosis (Fisher 1965*a*,

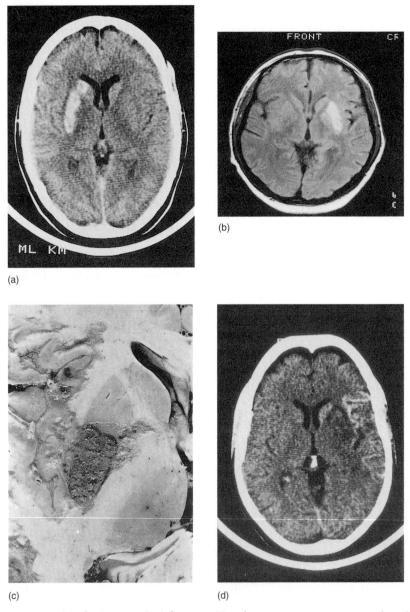

Fig. 17.1 Examples of striatocapsular infarcts on CT and post-mortem transverse sections. Note the typical comma-shaped form with sparing of the white substance in (a). The infarct strictly adheres to the lenticulostriate artery territory, not respecting the anatomical boundaries of the deep structures. Sparing of the head of the caudate is illustrated in (b), probably caused by an unaffected recurrent artery of Heubner. In (c), only the posterior part of the lenticulostriate artery territory was infarcted, while (d) (the patient presenting with aphasia) illustrates contrast enhancement of the insular cortex in a purely subcortical striatocapsular infarction on native scanning. Modified with permission from Weiller *et al.* (1992).

Miller 1983, Bamford and Warlow 1988), although there is increasing evidence that a lacune may occasionally be produced by embolic occlusion of a single perforator. In the basal ganglia, they are considered to result typically from blockage of a single, small, deep perforator of the MCA in its intracranial course, rather than from occlusion of the MCA itself or of the internal carotid artery (ICA) (Fisher 1969, 1979).

In his early papers on lacunar infarctions, Fisher designated large infarcts in the LSA territory ('putamino-capsulo-caudate infarcts') larger than 1 mm as 'giant' or 'super' lacunes. This term implicates a similar pathogenesis to common lacunes and large subcortical infarcts, i.e. small vessel disease. However, these large subcortical infarcts are too large to be caused by occlusion of a single deep perforator. Fisher himself realized that 'the deep territories may become infarcted because of the blockage of the mouth of the penetrating vessels and the absence of collateral channels by an embolus into the first bifurcation of the middle cerebral artery, where the largest lenticulostriate arteries arises' (Case 10 in Fisher and Curry 1965), thus they may be due to large vessel disease. Large subcortical infarcts in the territory of the LSA have long been recognized (Foix and Levy 1927, Schwartz 1930, Fisher 1965a). In several more recent studies, these large subcortical infarcts have been distinguished as an entity apart, different from lacunes regarding size, clinical presentation, prognosis, and pathogenesis. They have been described as 'putamino-capsulo-caudate' or 'capsulo-putamino-caudate infarcts' (Foix and Levy 1927, Fisher 1965a, Rascol et al. 1982), 'lateral striate artery infarcts' (Takahashi et al. 1985), 'extended lentiform nucleus infarcts' (Ringelstein et al. 1983), and 'striatocapsular infarctions' (Bladin and Berkovic 1984, Weiller et al. 1990, Donnan et al. 1991, Boiten and Lodder 1992) and correspond to type 1 of Rascol (Rascol et al. 1982), type 3 of Radue and Moseley (Radue and Moseley 1978) and the 'lateral type of capsular infarcts' of Kashihara and Matsumoto (Kashihara and Matsumoto 1985). They account for approximately 1 per cent of strokes and transient ischaemic attacks (TIAs) and for about 6 per cent of supratentorial brain infarcts in prospective stroke registries (Bladin and Berkovic 1984, Levine et al. 1988, Boiten and Lodder 1992). The incidence has increased considerably, coinciding with the more routine application of recombinant tissue plasminogen activata (rt-PA) in the treatment of stroke.

The author has studied 57 cases of such striatocapsular infarcts; these will be reported in this chapter (for demographic data see Table 17.1). When these infarcts were compared with the territory of the LSA derived from the post-mortem selective angiograms (Fig. 17.2) (Roßerg et al. 1992), they were found to cover the entire LSA territory, affecting all the structures that are supplied by the LSA as outlined already. Typically they had the comma-shaped appearance on transverse computed tomography (CT) sections as reported before (Ringelstein et al. 1983, Bladin and Berkovic 1984), with the rostral aspects in the lateral part of the head of caudate and the anterior limb of the internal capsule and the tail in the lateral and posterior part of the putamen (see Fig. 17.1). The size ranged from 2 cm to nearly 7 cm maximal diameter. The infarcts strictly adhered to the vascular territories and did not respect

Table 17.1 Meta-analysis of the most important findings in 10 studies on 177 cases of straitocapsular infarctions

	Rascol et al. (1982)	Ringelstein et al. (1983)	Adams et al. (1983)	Santamaria et al. (1983)	Bladin and Berkovic (1984)	Levine et al. (1988)	Weiller et al. (1990)	Donnan et al. (1991)	Boiten and Lodder (1992)	Weiller et al. (1993)	Total (%)[a]
Demographic data											
No. of patients	15	6	2	8	11	24	29	50	15	57	177 (100)
M/F ration			1/1	1/7	5/6	18/6	20/9	27/23	10/5	31/26	
Mean age (years)			33	48	63	59	55	63		53	
Age range (years)			24–42	34–65	50–84	26–88	22–86	24–88		16–89	
Clinical data											
Lacunar syndromes	15		1	1	2	5	6		3	19	46/132 (35)
Hemiparesis	15		2	8	11	24	29	49	14	57	169/17 (99)
Hemi-hypoaesthesia	0		1	6		15	23	30	10	40	102/171 (60)
Aphasia/neglect	0		1	4	8	17	8	35	11	26	93/156 (60)
Prognosis[b]											
No recovery	5/13			2	6	6	9	12		22	46/156 (29)
Moderate restitution			1	4	3	4	4	23		12	44/156 (28)
Complete restitution	8/13		1	2	2	14	11	15		19	60/156 (38)
Pathogenesis											
Cardiac source of embolism	2	4	0	8	5	5	14/24	7	7	25	58/177 (33)
ICA[c]	0/6		0		6/8	17	9	12/27	4	17	50/131 (38)
MCA[c]	2/6		2		2/8	5	15	3/27		25	37/116 (32)

[a] The cases of the study by Bladin and Berkovic (1984) are included in the study by Donnan et al. (1991) as are the cases of Weiller et al. (1990) in the study by Weiller et al. (1993). Empty cells indicate missing values.

[b] Prognosis of motor function only.

[c] Including high-degree stenoses, as well as complete obliteration.

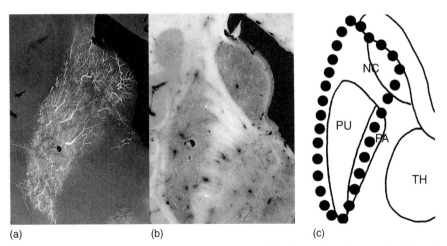

(a)   (b)   (c)

Fig. 17.2 Selective post-mortum angiographic picture of the lenticulostriate arteries (a) and macroscopic aspect of the corresponding brain slice of approximately 4 mm thickness (b), with a diagram of the same view (c); NC = caudate nucleus, PU = putamen, PA = pallidum, TH = thalamus. From Christine Roßerg, MD, Department of Neuropathology, University of Marburg, with kind permission).

the anatomical boundaries of the subcortical structures. On only six occasions was the grey matter within the LSA territory infarcted and the white substance spared, illustrating the comparatively low vulnerability to ischaemia of the white substance. In 12 per cent, the ventral portion of the head of the caudate nucleus was spared. This may be explained by Heubner's recurrent artery that, in these cases, may have supplied the ventral part of the head of caudate, reflecting the variability of vascularization of this area that phylogenetically is supplied by an anastomotic channel between the anterior cerebral artery (via Heubner's recurrent artery) and the MCA (via the LSA) (Abbie 1934). When the territory of the anterior choroidal artery was also involved, the infarctions extended into the medial pallidum, the genu or posterior limb of the internal capsule and sometimes affected the rim of the thalamus. In 60 per cent, the complete LSA territory was infarcted, in 12 per cent only the anterior part of the territory, and in 28 per cent only the posterior part was infarcted (see Fig. 17.1). No infarction was found that might have correlated with the presumed medial and lateral subdivision of the LSA (Kashihara and Matsumoto 1985). In summary, striatocapsular infarcts may be seen as infarcts of the territory of the LSA.

It seems unlikely that all the LSAs would occlude separately but simultaneously. It is more likely that a lesion of the M1 segment where most of the LSAs arise may cause an acute and simultaneous occlusion of the orifices of these arteries, whereas the superficial territory of the MCA may be largely spared because of the influx of blood from the anterior cerebral artery via the subarachnoid inter-arterial anastomoses. This would place striatocapsular infarcts, in contrast to lacunes, in the group of ischaemic cerebral infarcts from large vessel disease.

Angiographic demonstration of acute Ml occlusion and retrograde filling of the cortical branches of the MCA by leptomeningeal anastomoses has been reported repeatedly in association with striatocapsular infarcts and sparing of the superficial cortex (Fisher 1979, Okuno et al. 1980, Adams et al. 1983, Santamaria et al. 1983, Bladin and Berkovic 1984, Caplan et al. 1985, Ringelstein et al. 1985, Takahashi et al. 1985, Weiller et al. 1990, Bogousslavsky et al. 1991a). The author was able to demonstrate exactly this mechanism in 13 of the 57 patients in our recent series. The overall frequency of MCA pathology of the Ml segment was 44 per cent (25 out of 57). In seven cases, the ICA was occluded simultaneously leading to larger infarcts that often also involved the territory of the anterior choroidal artery. The duration of the MCA occlusion was monitored by repetitive angiography in cases with rt-PA treatment or by repetitive transcranial Doppler sonography examination at short intervals. Recanalization of the occluded MCA was observed in 13 cases within the first week and in 10 cases within 8 h after the stroke (Table 17.2). In patients without clinical cortical features, a rapid recanalization of the occluded MCA within hours was found (mean 5.9 h; median 4 h) along with excellent leptomeningeal anastomoses. One year after the even, all the MCAs were recanalized. In another series, the site and duration of the MCA occlusion were compared with the type of resulting infarction. Occlusion of the proximal MCA, thereby blocking the orifices of the LSAs, almost always lead to striatocapsular infarction (Ringelstein et al. 1992). This confirms that the LSAs are end arteries with no possibility of anastomotic collateral blood flow. However, the combination of early recanalization and good leptomeningeal collateral blood flow correlated with restriction of the infarction to the LSA territory; in others words, it prevented the superficial, cortical MCA territory from infarction in MCA occlusions. It was speculated that the leptomeningeal collateral flow may have maintained a certain degree of cortical perfusion, preventing the cortical neurons from irreversible cell death for the period until recanalization occurred (Ringelstein et al. 1992).

Several features suggest that MCA occlusion leading to striatocapsular infarction may be due to an embolus from the heart. Striatocapsular infarcts are a frequent cause of stroke in children and young adults (Okuno et al. 1980). Embolic occlusions tend to recanalize more frequently and within a shorter time than occlusions from local atherosclerosis and thrombosis. Haemorrhagic transformation occurs in 74 per cent of cardioembolic strokes (Lodder et al. 1990). Thus the frequent haemorrhagic transformation of striatocapsular infarcts (Bladin and Berkovic 1984, Ringelstein et al. 1985, Weiller et al. 1990) favours a cardioembolic genesis. Potential sources of cardiac embolism are often found in striatocapsular infarcts (13–100% of cases, mean: 33%, see Table 17.1). This is a much higher percentage than the 21–33 per cent seen in cortical territorial infarctions (Ringelstein et al. 1985, Boiten and Lodder 1992). Cardioembolic MCA occlusion was the most likely single mechanism in 10 of our cases. As early as 1930, Schwartz reported a series of striatocapsular infarcts, often haemorrhagic, in young individuals occurring as typical sequelae of rheumatic heart disease. Thus striatocapsular infarcts may be caused by a large embolus from the heart arresting in the trunk of the MCA thereby occluding the mouth of the LSA.

Approximately 38 per cent of striatocapsular infarcts in the pooled data of nine studies (see Table 17.1) were associated with tight ICA stenoses. This percentage is much higher than in a more recent series of lacunes (13%) (Boiten and Lodder 1992), and comparable with the incidence of ICA stenosis in cortical territorial infarcts (Ringelstein *et al.* 1985, Boiten and Lodder 1992). With the exception of the cases when ICA occlusion was found along with simultaneous cardioembolic MCA occlusion, 10 cases had tight ipsilateral ICA stenosis, two of them the result of arterial dissections, as the only evident pathogenetic factor. Secondary embolic MCA occlusion from tight ICA stenoses *(occlusio supra occlusionem)* has been suggested as a mechanism for the production of striatocapsular infarcts in these cases (Ring 1971, Ringelstein *et al.* 1983).

Local atherosclerosis of the Ml segment in the absence of cardiac or extracranial occlusive disease is a rare cause of striatocapsular infarcts (Ringelstein *et al.* 1985, Caplan *et al.* 1985, Weiller *et al.* 1990). Six cases with high-grade stenoses of the MCA at the Ml segment were found, and these did not change during follow-up; this may suggest that these were atherosclerotic in nature. All this makes striatocapsular infarcts the prototype embolic infarct; they are found frequent in child hood stroke, which is almost always due to cardiac embolism (Brückmann *et al.* 1989). A striato-capsular infarct is always suspicious for arterial or cardiac embolism. Striatocapsular infarcts have increased considerably in freqency with the advent of rt-PA and were often seen in the ECASS trials (von Kummer *et al.* 1995). Their pathogenesis of short-lasting M1 occlusion makes them a typical result of successful thrombolysis and are mirrored in sequential perfusion/diffusion MRI. Early ADC changes in diffusion-weighted, MRI often reveal an ischaemia in the form of striatocapsular infarcts during the first couple of hours after stroke onset, along with a large perfusion deficit in perfusion-weighted imaging, which covers large parts of the MCA territory (Röther *et al.* 2001). Depending on recanalization, this scenario may develop in complete MCA territory infarct in the worst case (no recanalization in time) or into a sole striatocapsular infarct in the case of more rapid recanalization. Striatocapsular infarcts often represent what we can gain when applying thrombolysis in M1 occlusion, thereby preventing complete MCA territory infarction.

Striatocapsular infarcts must be differentiated from haemodynamically produced subcortical low-flow infarcts due to extracranial ICA occlusion and insufficient intracranial collateral blood supply via the circle of Willis. While the former cover the entire ventral and rostral part of the LSA territory, the latter typically are located in the rostral terminal supply area of the LSA territory in the deep white matter (Ringelstein *et al.* 1985, Weiller *et al.* 1991*a*). Differentiation is possible by careful assessment of the infarcted area compared with the known distribution of the LSA territory (Kastrup *et al.* 1992). Differentiation may be helped by assessment of the cerebral perfusion reserve by estimating the ratio of the cerebral blood flow divided by cerebral blood volume with single photon emission computed tomography (SPECT) in the non-infarcted ipsilateral MCA territory (Weiller *et al.* 1991*a*). Another option is the measurement of the reactivity of the velocity of the blood in the MCA during hyper- and hypocapnia by transcranial Doppler sonography (Ringelstein *et al.* 1988). Both values are normal in striatocapsular infarcts and usually severly reduced in low-flow infarcts (Weiller *et al.* 1991*a*).

Clinical features

In nine clinical studies, 177 cases of striatocapsular infarcts have been reported including the 57 reported here. These studies are very inhomogeneous regarding selection criteria and methods. The pooled data are presented in Table 17.1. The onset was sudden in almost all cases. Preceding TIAs in the ipsilateral carotid artery territory are reported in 10–20 per cent of striatocapsular infarcts (Adams *et al.* 1983, Bladin and Berkovic 1984, Levine *et al.* 1988, Donnan *et al.* 1991). TIAs were noted in 10 of our 57 cases, often with identical symptomatology to the subsequent completed strokes. No amaurosis fugax was reported. Eleven of our patients presented with a progressive stroke, slightly more than in other series (Bladin and Berkovic 1984, Levine *et al.* 1988, Donnan *et al.* 1991) but consistent with stroke due to MCA occlusion (Caplan *et al.* 1985). In two out of the 11 patients with a progressive stroke, aphasia supervened an initial hemiparesis after some hours. Acute ipsilateral eye deviation and altered consciousness were present initially in three instances, as previously reported by Bladin and Berkovic (1984). The pooled data in Table 17.1 illustrate that striatocapsular infarcts do not present typically with lacunar syndromes (35% of cases) although the most common presenting symptom in striatocapsular infarcts is a motor hemiparesis.

In our own series, similarly to the report of Donnan *et al.* (1991), the pattern of weakness was mainly of the upper limb with facial weakness and only moderate leg weakness. In one case there, was only facial weakness. Hemi-hypoaesthesia and cortical symptoms are frequent (Adams *et al.* 1983, Bladin and Berkovic 1984, Weiller *et al.* 1990). Hemianopia was found in only one case. One patient had several generalized tonic clonic seizures. Although striatocapsular infarction affects several structures that are typically involved in movement disorders, dystonia is a rare finding in striatocapsular infarcts (Demierre and Rondot 1983). One patient had hemiballismus and one had dystonic posture of the paretic hand in our series. A possible explanation may be that the lesions are too large to allow specific neurotransmitter systems to be affected selectively.

Prognosis after striatocapsular infarcts has been placed somewhere between the excellent prognosis of lacunar infarcts (Bamford *et al.* 1987, Gandolfo *et al.* 1986) and the relatively poor prognosis of patients with large cortical MCA territory infarcts (Ringelstein *et al.* 1985). Two patients in our series died of coronary heart disease, another from a haemorrhagic brain infarct. Three developed a cortical MCA territory infarct within 1 year of the index stroke. The clinical course of the remaining 51 cases was followed up after 1 year. Hemi-hypoaesthesia had an excellent prognosis. Twenty-four patients had a complete restitution of motor function with return to work or to the same activity of daily living score (Barthel index) as before the stroke. In 12 patients, recovery was substantial and in 15 there was no or only marginal improvement, leaving the patient with a severe disability. These values are comparable with the data of the other two larger studies (Levine *et al.* 1988, Donnan *et al.* 1991).

Aphasia or neglect in striatocapsular infarcts

The most striking feature of these subcortical infarcts is the frequency of cortical symptoms such as aphasia or neglect (in 30–80% of cases, cf. Table 17.1). Four mechanisms have been put forward as explanations for aphasia or neglect after subcortical lesions, these are:

(1) participation of the dominant striatum or associated systems in language processing (Naeser *et al.* 1982, Damasio *et al.* 1982);

(2) disruption of connecting fibres between input/output or semantic and phonematic centres (A. Galaburda; see Damasio *et al.* 1982);

(3) functional de-activation of cortical language processing centres by the subcortical lesion (diaschisis) (Metter *et al.* 1983, Perani *et al.* 1987); and

(4) temporary ischaemic penumbra (Olsen *et al.* 1986) or selective neuronal loss of the cortex due to prolonged ischaemia (Weiller *et al.* 1990, 1991*b*).

In (1) and (2), the occurrence of aphasia or neglect was directly attributed to the subcortical lesion; (3) and (4) have been mentioned to explain the decreased cortical regional Cerebral blood flow (rCBF) reported in these cases. In our study of 57 patients with striatocapsular infarcts, 26 with aphasia or neglect and 31 without 'cortical' symptoms, the presence of aphasia or neglect was correlated with the anatomical distribution of the lesions, the duration of embolic MCA occlusion, cortical cerebral blood flow (estimated with ^{99m}Tc-HMPAO and SPECT), and the development of focal cortical atrophy. After subtraction of the lesioned grids of patients without neuropsychological deficits from those of patients with aphasia or neglect, no particular structure was predominantly infarcted in those with 'cortical' symptoms. Subtypes of aphasic syndromes were not related to the anatomical structures infarcted (Table 17.3). Thus it was not possible to identify a certain subcortical structure, for example the head of caudate, that might participate in language processing, nor any area possibly responsible for the occurence of diaschisis that may have induced aphasia or neglect in striatocapsular infarcts.

However, there was a strong correlation between the presence of cortical symptoms and the duration of MCA occlusion and collateral blood flow. In patients without aphasia or neglect, a rapid recanalization of the MCA or extensive and obviously sufficient cortical leptomeningeal anastomoses were found. Patients with cortical

Table 17.2 Duration of MCA occlusion and leptomeningeal cortical collaterals

Patients without aphasia or neglect			Patients with aphasia or neglect		
Patient no.	Duration of MCA occlusion[a]	Collaterals	Patient no.	Duration of MCA occlusion[a]	Collaterals[a,b]
24	1 h	Good	53	4.5 h (TIA)	(T)
12	1.5 h	Moderate	31	4.5 h (TIA)	(T)
13	4 h	Good	31	8 h (TIA)	Poor
52	4 h	Good	23	8 h (partial)	Poor
25	7 h	Good	8	18 h (partial)	Moderate
22	18 h	Gooid	34	37 h	(T)
			51	156 h	Poor
			5	> 10 days	Poor
			6	> 10 days	Moderate

[a] Occulsion of the MCA was monitored by repetitive transcranial Doppler sonography (for details also for judgement of collaterals, see Ringelstein *et al.* 1992) or by repetitive selective arterial angiography.
[b] In three Patients, no angiography was available. Transcranial Doppler sonography (T) did not allow assessment of cortical collaterals. (Modified, with permission from Weiller *et al.* 1993.)

Table 17.3 Lesion size as a percentage of model anatomical areas covered by the lesions for the patients with aphasia (method described in Willmes and Ratajczak 1987)

Aphasia subtype[b]	Aphasia syndrome points (ALLOC)[c]	Basal ganglia				White[a] matter	Total hemisphere
		Putamen	Pallidum	Head of caudate	Total		
Global	6	42	36	25	34	1	4
	44	38	30	11	53	1	4
	3	44	11	27	33	1	4
Wernicke	32	34	49	37	37	2	6
	39	8	9	1	5	0	1
	2	38	4	19	55	26	4
Broca	34	19	0	18	35	35	5
	42	35	17	33	28	31	5
	53	23	23	0	87	87	2
	8	42	17	33	35	1	5
Amnesic	48	16	0	10	12	1	2
	49	25	0	0	12	0	1
	54	32	23	0	35	0	2
Unclassifiable	36	16	4	4	9	1	2
Residual symptoms	50	46	28	25	35	2	5

[a] Only the deep periventricular white matter without the internal capsule is regarded.
[b] Differentiation of aphasia subtypes according to the Aachen Aphasia Test (AAT) (Huber *et al.* 1984).
[c] ALLOC (for allocation) is a non-parametric discriminant analysis procedure using Kernel density estimation [for reference, see Willmes and Ratajczak 1987).

symptoms showed only partial, late, or no recanalization within 10 days and mostly poor cortical collateral blood flow (see Table 17.2). In the two patients in whom recanalization of the MCA took place approximately 4 h after the event, cortical symptoms lasted for only a few hours. The rCBF in the cortical MCA territory, overlying the subcortical lesion was significantly lower in the patients with aphasia or neglect than in those without. The hypothesis was that decreased cortical rCBF may be the result of the prolonged MCA occlusion rather than functional deactivation (Weiller *et al.* 1990, 1993). Supporting evidence has come from a positron emission tomography study by Sgouropoulos *et al.* (1985) who have shown that a persistent MCA occlusion can indeed lead to a chronic decrease of rCBF and increase of oxygen extraction fraction in non-infarcted cortex.

A complete SPECT and MRI follow-up was made after 1 year in 19 patients of our group (14 with aphasia or neglect, five without). The MCA was now fully recanalized. In four patients of the aphasic group, a cortical infarction corresponding to an MCA branch occlusion was found after 1 year on MRI; these patients were excluded from further analysis. In nine of the remaining patients, who presented initially with aphasia or neglect, the cortical rCBF remained low and correlated with a marked focal cortical atrophy on MRI. In one patient, in whom the initial aphasia had lasted for only hours, the cortex was normal both on MRI and in terms of blood flow. No focal cortical atrophy or decreased cortical rCBF was found in any of the five patients who initially presented without cortical symptoms. These findings cannot easily be explained by pure functional deactivation. It is therefore suggested that, in striatocapsular infarcts, aphasia or neglect is due to selective neuronal loss (selective parenchymal necrosis) of the cerebral cortex from prolonged occlusion of the MCA along with, at least for the duration of the occlusion, insufficient leptomeningeal collateral blood supply. The reduced perfusion with decreased cortical blood flow is insufficient to keep the cortical neurons with a high metabolic demand alive, resulting in cortical symptoms. It is, however, sufficient to save the comparatively robust cortical glial cells, thus preserving the intact shape of the cortex seen in initial structural imaging. In the chronic state, the decreased cortical rCBF may represent an adaption to the decreased demand of the fewer number of cortical neurons, reflected by a focal atrophy on structural imaging. Post-mortem proof of this hypothesis has come from Lassen *et al.* (1983) who showed a loss of more than 50 per cent of the cortical neuron population in strictly subcortical striatocapsular infarcts on CT scanning from MCA occlusion and a critically low rCBF (20–25 ml/l00 g/min) in the superficial MCA territory.

None of our patients showed signs of neglect at 1 year post-stroke. Aphasia had improved considerably or recovered completely in 12 out of the 15 aphasics in our 57 cases. The usually good prognosis is in agreement with other studies (Adams *et al.* 1983, Olsen *et al.* 1986, Levine *et al.* 1988, Donnan *et al.* 1991), and is expected in 'subcortical' aphasia (Damasio *et al.* 1982). However, the presence of persisting disabling speech disturbances in 25 per cent of our cases and in some of Bladin and

Berkovic's (1984) and of Levine *et al.*'s patients (Levine *et al.* 1988) is remarkable. In terms of our hypothesis, the prognosis of aphasia in striatocapsular infarcts may be related to the degree of relative sparing of cortical neurons. There is further evidence for the involvement of the cortex in striatocapsular infarcts. Focal EEG abnormalities suggesting focal cortical dysfunction are common in striatocapsular infarcts (Santamaria *et al.* 1983, Bladin and Berkovic 1984, Donnan *et al.* 1991). In three out of our 57 cases with strictly subcortical striatocapsular infarcts on plain CT scanning, contrast enhancement was found in the insular cortex, indicating that the cerebral cortex is indeed not always completely spared in striatocapsular infarcts (see Fig. 17.1).

Remote effects

These findings in aphasic patients with striatocapsular infarcts do not exclude the possibility of functional deactivation. In a study (Weiller *et al.* 1992) of rCBF in 10 patients with striatocapsular infarcts without aphasia or neglect and 10 normal controls using positron emission tomography (PET), 3 months or longer after the stroke, a significantly decreased rCBF in the striatum and internal capsule corresponding to the site of the lesion was found (Fig. 17.3). In addition, there were significant decreases in rCBF in the insula, primary sensorimotor and dorsolateral cortices, thalamus, midbrain/cerebral peduncle, and contralateral cerebellum. A trend to decreased rCBF in the anterior cingulate cortex was not significant. None of these areas appeared infarcted on structural imaging. Hypoperfusion in the insula might be caused by partial neuronal attrition short of frank infarction, as mentioned already, but this cannot be true for the more distant areas (e.g. dorso-lateral prefrontal cortex) and those lying outside the territory of the feeding artery (e.g. thalamus). There are at least five parallel circuits involving the basal ganglia and the thalamus that have cortical projections to the primary motor, premotor, dorso-lateral prefrontal, and anterior cingulate cortices (Alexander and Crutcher 1990). It was suggested that disruption of these circuits at the level of the basal ganglia may result in deactivation of other parts of these circuits reflected by a decreased rCBF, although structural changes at a microscopic level from trans-synaptic or retrograde degeneration cannot be excluded. The hypoperfusion in the midbrain/peduncular region can be interpreted as the result of degeneration of the pyramidal tract. Some of these effects may be responsible for the subtle, persisting neuropsychological deficits found in striatocapsular infarcts (Donnan *et al.* 1991). They also may influence the potential for recovery of function.

Recovery of function

Further perspectives deal with the recovery of function after striatocapsular infarcts and its impact on the reorganizational changes of the cortex.

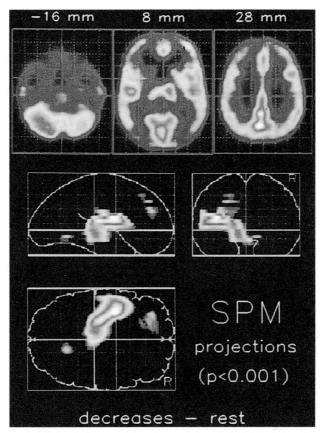

Fig. 17.3 Functional deactivation in striatocapsular infarcts. Regional cerebral blood flow (rCBFI was measured using an integral/dynamic $C^{15}O_2$ inhalation technique and PET (for details, see Weiller *et al.* 1992) at rest in 10 patients with striatocapsular infarcts (without aphasia or neglect) compared with 10 normal controls. The top row represents mean rCBF scans of the 10 patients averaged into the standard, proportional, stereotactic space of Tailarach and Tournoux (1988). The numbers refer to the distance of the plane from the intercommissural plane. The lower part of the figure shows sagittal, coronal, and transverse projections of the statistical parametric maps obtained from a group to group comparison of patients and normals in the grid of the standard stereotactic space. Only pixels with a significantly decreased rCBF in the patients at $p < 0.001$ (omnibus significance) are displayed on an arbitrary colour scale. In patients, there were significant decreases in rCBF in the left striatum and internal capsule, corresponding to the site of the lesion, and in the insula, lateral prefrontal and primary sensorimotor cortices, the thalamus, cerebral peduncle/midbrain, and right cerebellum (modified, with permission, from Weiller *et al.* 1992).

Our findings following striatocapsular infarcts and subsequent motor recovery with functional activation studies using rCBF changes detected by PET as an index of synaptic function are reported in Weiller *et al.* (1992). These observations compared the rCBF during sequential finger opposition in 10 patients with striatocapsular infarcts and 10 normal controls, and showed common patterns of reorganization that follow striatocapsular infarcts with motor recovery. During movement of the recovered hand, patients activated the appropriate contralateral cortical motor areas and ipsilateral cerebellum to the same extent as normal subjects. However, activation was greater than in normal subjects in both insulae; in the inferior parietal (area 40), prefrontal, and anterior cingulate cortices; in the ipsilateral premotor cortex and basal ganglia; and in the contralateral cerebellum. Some of these areas showed a decreased rCBF at rest in the patients, suggesting a chronic functional deactivation that is overcome during the task. It is suggested that bilateral activation of motor pathways and the recruitment of additional motor areas are systematic components of the pattern of cortical reorganization associated with motor recovery from stroke. Activation of anterior and posterior cingulate and prefrontal cortices may indicate that selective attentional and intentional mechanisms play a role in the recovery process. Almost identical patterns of reorganization have been reported in cases with acquired dystonia with subcortical lesions (Ceballos-Baumann *et al.* 1995).

Chapter 18

Caudate infarcts

L.R. Caplan

Historical background and perspective

Knowledge about the clinical consequences of infarction of the caudate nucleus and its incoming and outgoing fibre connections is still evolving. Most information about clinical signs and symptoms, physiology, and aetiology come from recent reports and case series.

Pierre Marie (1901*b*), at the beginning of the 20th century, recognized that small, deep infarcts often involved the head of the caudate nucleus. Foix and Hillemand (1925) and Foix and Levy (1927) described the blood supply of the caudate nucleus from both the anterior cerebral artery (ACA) and the lenticulostriate branches of the middle cerebral artery (MCA). In Fig. 18.1, taken from Foix and Levy (1927), the deep territory of the MCA, which includes supply of the caudate nucleus, internal capsule, and putamen, is illustrated. Neither of these two neurologists were able to correlate caudate infarcts found at post-mortem examination with clinical symptoms and signs because, at autopsy, infarcts were often multiple and involved more widespread ACA and MCA territory infarction. The author, during a year of neuropathology during the late 1960s, performed autopsies on several patients who had acute and old caudate infarcts but had no known recorded relevant symptoms during life. Figure 18.2 shows some examples of these infarcts.

The first major reports of clinical findings in patients with caudate vascular lesions followed the introduction and widespread dissemination of computed tomography (CT) scanning in the 1970s and early 1980s. Stein *et al.* (1984) and Weisberg (1984) reported series of patients with intracerebral haemorrhages that began in the caudate nucleus but often spread to the adjacent lateral ventricle and the white matter surrounding the caudate nucleus. Some of the haemorrhages spread into the hypothalamic region and some into the internal capsule. The high frequency of cognitive and behavioural abnormalities surprised the authors since prior concepts had always emphasized the motor functions of the striatum. CT also showed that caudate atrophy was an early finding in patients with Huntington's chorea, a disorder characterized by cognitive and behavioural abnormalities and abnormal movements.

A decade ago, Caplan *et al.* (1990) reported the clinical and CT findings in 18 patients with infarcts involving the caudate nucleus, the adjacent anterior limb of the internal capsule, and the anterior portion of the putamen. Only patients with single

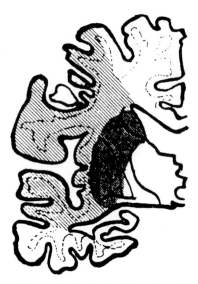

Fig. 18.1 Diagram showing middle cerebral artery territory. The dark shaded area, including the caudate nucleus, is supplied by lenticulostriate branches according to Foix and Levy (1927), used with permission.

infarcts were included. Behavioural abnormalities and dysarthria were common findings and motor weakness was often absent, minor, or transient. Some patients had non-pyramidal types of motor dysfunction resembling those found in Parkinsonism. Others have also reported prominent alterations in behaviour after unilateral (Caplan and Helgason 1995, Mendez *et al.* 1989, Markowitsch *et al.* 1990, Bokura and Robinson 1997), unilateral and bilateral (Kumral *et al.* 1999), and bilateral (Richfield *et al.* 1987, Trillet *et al.* 1990) caudate infarcts. In single case reports and small series, various movement disorders have been reported in patients with caudate infarcts (Schwarz and Barrows 1960, Goldblatt *et al.* 1974, Lodder and Baard 1981, Saris 1983, Tabaton *et al.* 1985, Kawamura *et al.* 1988, Midgard *et al.* 1989, Destee *et al.* 1990, Lownie and Gilbert 1990, Kim 1992, Broderick *et al.* 1995, Caplan and Helgason 1995). Other clinical signs and the causative stroke mechanisms have been less well analysed and discussed. Abnormalities in saccades are often present but seldom have been studied in detail (Vermersch *et al.* 1999). These past reports will be reviewed in this chapter.

Clinical findings

Cognitive and behavioural abnormalities

Mendez *et al.* (1989) reported 12 patients who came to their attention because of acute behavioural abnormalities who had caudate infarcts on CT. Lesions were confined to the caudate nucleus in six and the remainder had extension into the

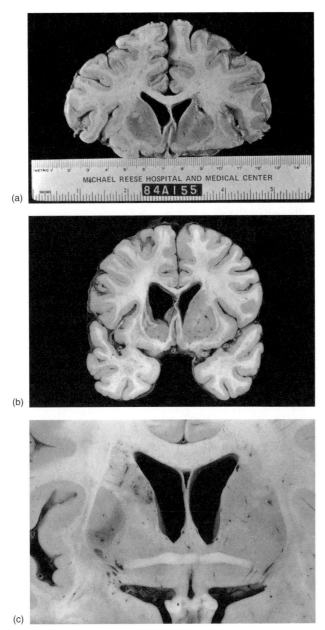

Fig. 18.2 Brains at autopsy. (a) Old infarct, cavitated on the right of the figure, involving the caudate nucleus and the anterior limb of the internal capsule (black arrow). (b) Very old infarct on the left of the figure. The caudate nucleus, anterior limb of the internal capsule, and the anterior putamen are shrunken compared with the same structures on the right of the figure. The lateral ventricle is grossly dilated on the side of the infarct. (c) A relatively acute infarct on the left of the figure (black arrows) showing some patechial haemorrhage and colour changes in the caudate nucleus, anterior limb of the internal capsule, and the putamen.

adjacent anterior limb of the internal capsule. Six lesions were right-sided, five left-sided, and one was bilateral. The authors divided the patients into three groups with different patterns of behavioural abnormalities. Group I patients were apathetic and had diminished verbal and motor activity. Group II patients were disinhibited, impulsive, and inappropriate, while Group III patients had affective changes such as anxiety and depression. All patients showed abnormalities on formal neuropsychological tests. They had difficulty especially with so-called executive functions such as analysing novel tasks, establishing and then following plans, organizing sequential activities, and starting and inhibiting various behaviours. These types of abnormalities have been described often in patients with frontal lobe lesions. Patients with caudate infarcts also had poor recall on immediate and delayed memory tests, and had decreased ability to sustain attention to tasks. The single patient with bilateral caudate nucleus infarcts had severe cognitive and behavioural abnormalities and was institutionalized. Two patients had minor left-sided weakness. Deficits did not correlate with the side of the lesion, but patients with affective abnormalities (Group III) tended to have the largest infarcts.

Caplan *et al.* (1990) found cognitive and behavioural abnormalities in 14 out of 18 (78%) unselected patients with unilateral caudate infarcts. Figure 18.3 shows cartoons of these lesions as found on CT scans. The infarcts often extended into the adjacent anterior limb of the internal capsule and anterior putamen. The commonest abnormality was abulia—an inactive, slow, apathetic state identical to the

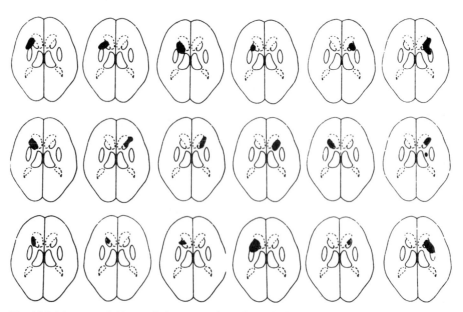

Fig. 18.3 Montage of CT scan lesions at a plane through the superior thalamus charted on Stroke Data Bank grids. The left hemisphere is on the left of the figure. From Caplan *et al.* (1990) with permission.

abnormality described in the patients in Group I of Mendez *et al.* (1989). These patients had decreased spontaneity, prolonged latencies in responding to queries and directions, and tended to respond verbally with short terse replies. They had difficulty persevering with tasks. The next most frequent abnormality was restlessness, hyperactivity, and agitation, with decreased ability to direct sustained attention to tasks. They were very easily distracted by visual and auditory stimuli. Two patients with left caudate infarcts had minor aphasic abnormalities, and three patients with right-sided infarcts showed left neglect. In this series, only four patients had lesions limited to the caudate nucleus; in the rest, the lesion extended to the anterior limb of the internal capsule (50%) or into the anterior limb and the putamen (28%).

Markowitsch *et al.* (1990) studied a 15-year-old adolescent boy with an infarct in the head of the left caudate nucleus, internal capsule, and putamen caused by occlusion of the internal carotid artery (ICA) intracranially. The major finding was poor recall of long-term verbal memory items. Defective recall had also been noted by Mendez *et al.* (1989).

Trillet *et al.* (1990) reported three patients with bilateral caudate infarcts who had severe abulia. They had apathy, disinterest, flattened affect, and lack of initiative for usual daily activities. One patient had prolonged akinetic attacks. Stereotyped behaviours were common. The single patient of Richfield *et al.* (1987) who had bilateral caudate nucleus lesions also showed inattention, disinterest, and lethargy. She also showed impulsivity, disinhibition, and violent attacks. The mix of apathy and inertia with hyperactivity and agitation had also been noted by Mendez *et al.* (1989) and Caplan *et al.* (1990). Patients with bilateral infarcts had more severe and more persistent behavioural abnormalities.

Among 21 patients with caudate infarcts reported by Caplan and Helgason (1995), 12 (57%) had some cognitive or behavioural abnormality. Figure 18.4 shows a cartoon of the CT scans in 34 patients in whom 21 had sufficient clinical data for correlation. Abulia was the most common abnormality, occurring in 10 patients— two with left-sided infarcts, seven with right caudate infarcts, and one with bilateral infarcts. Agitation was also common, occurring in three patients with left and three with right caudate infarcts. Apahasia was present in one patient with a left caudate infarct, and neglect was found in two patients with right-sided infarcts.

Kumral *et al.* (1999) analysed the clinical findings among 31 Turkish patients with acute caudate strokes, including 25 patients with caudate infarcts and six with haemorrhages originating in the caudate nucleus. As in other series, cognitive and behavioural abnormalities predominated. Among the patients with caudate infarcts, nine were abulic (five with right-sided infarcts, three with left, and one who had bilateral infarcts). Three patients had 'psychic akinesis'—one with right-sided infarction and two patients with bilateral infarcts. The authors characterized psychic akinesis as 'severe mental and affective stagnation and lack of initiative for action and speech' (Kumral *et al.* 1999). One of their patients had a flat affect

CAUDATE + INFARCTS

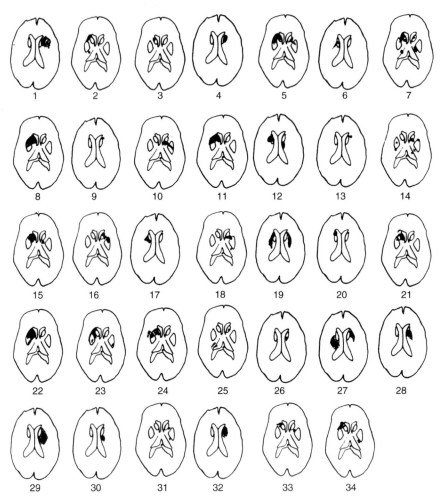

Fig. 18.4 Montage of caudate infarcts taken from the Illinois series and drawn from CT and MRI scans. From Caplan and Helgason (1995) with permission.

and had such severe impairment of mental activity and movement that they would not move unless asked to eat or stand up. The authors considered abulia, bradykinesia, psychic akinesia, and 'akinetic mutism' as terms that described a continuum from minor to major decreased observable behaviour. The four patients with caudate infarcts who were very restless during the acute phase had lesions confined to the caudate nucleus (three right, one left caudate). Patients who were abulic or had psychic akinesia tended to have larger lesions that extended outside the caudate nucleus. Eight of the patients had frontal lobe-type test impairment on formal neuropsychological test batteries. It is of interest that a quarter of the patients were considered depressed. Depression had also been mentioned by Caplan *et al.* (1990) as an occurrence in patients with caudate infarction. Some patients who are abulic are considered depressed because of their lack of activity; however, the patients with abulia most often do not mention or acknowledge sadness or feeling discouraged. Five patients with left caudate lesions were aphasic. One patient with a large lesion had a global aphasia, three had a non-fluent Broca-type aphasia with preserved comprehension, and one patient had minor word-finding difficulty and perseveration during writing. The patients with aphasia had lesions that extended outside the caudate nucleus. One patient with bilateral infarcts also had a non-fluent aphasia. Three patients with right caudate lesions had 'motor-exploratory neglect'.

In most of the reports cited, the authors studied acute behavioural and cognitive abnormalities but did not report long-term findings. Bokura and Robinson (1997), in contrast, studied long-term cognitive impairment among 21 patients with caudate infarcts (nine left and 12 right) and compared the findings with 70 other patients with subcortical lesions that did not involve the caudate nucleus (27 left and 43 right). Patients with caudate infarcts could have extension outside the caudate, but at least 50 per cent of the lesion had to be within the caudate. Patients were studied at 3, 6, 12, and 24 months after their strokes using formal neuropsychological test batteries. Patients with either left or right caudate lesions had lower scores on the Mini-mental State Examination than the patients with other subcortical lesions, and some patients with caudate infarcts had deterioration in their test scores (despite no new strokes) during the 1–2 year follow-up, in contrast to the subcortical group who improved. Depression was common in all groups acutely but had disappeared on follow-up in nearly all patients.

Table 18.1 summarizes the cognitive and behavioural changes found in the three largest series of patients with caudate infarcts (Caplan *et al.* 1990, Caplan and Helgason 1995, Kumral *et al.* 1999).

Cognitive and behavioural changes have been attributed to loss of function of cortical zones caused by loss of striatal efferent projections from the caudate nucleus.

Table 18.1 The most common cognitive and behavioural abnormalities among the 64 patients with caudate infarcts in three large series

Abnormality	Total	Left	Right	Bilateral
Abulia	33 (52%)	12	16	1
Restlessness/agitation	16 (25%)	7	9	3
Aphasia	9 (14%)	8		1
Neglect	9 (14%)		8	1

Extracted from the series of Caplan *et al.* (1990), Caplan and Helgason (1995), and Kumral *et al.* (1999).
Among 43 patients, there were 21 left, 19 right, and three bilateral infarcts (for 21 patients, the locations were not stated).

The caudate nucleus participates in a number of cortico–striato–pallido–nigral–thalamic–cortical circuits (Alexander and DeLong 1985, Alexander *et al.* 1986, Caplan *et al.* 1990). The prefrontal, orbitofrontal, anterior cingulum, and temporal lobe limbic cortex are all included in the circuitry.

Movement disorders

During the past four decades and in several case reports, patients with abnormalities of tone and movement after infarcts involving the caudate nuclei have been described. These various reports are listed in Table 18.2. In most patients, the lesions were unilateral and the contralateral arm and leg exhibited abnormal movements. Slight hemiparesis and dysarthria often accompanied the movement disorder, which usually occurred at the time of the stroke. In some patients, the disorder included proximal flinging movements that the authors called 'ballistic'. In others, the movements were more unpredictable and distal and were called 'choreic'. Some had a mixture of ballistic and choreic movements. Most reports contained little detailed description of the abnormal movements; however, Goldblatt *et al.* (1974) described their patient's

Table 18.2 Published cases of movement disorders among patients with caudate infarcts

Reference	Movements	Infarct site
Schwarz and Barrows (1960)	Right hemiballism	Left caudate, putamen, anterior limbic
Goldblatt *et al.* (1974)	Left hemichorea	Right caudate, putamen
Lodder and Baard (1981)	Bilateral ballism	Bilat caudate, putamen, anterior limbic
Kase *et al.* (1981)	Left hemichorea, hemiballism	Right caudate, putamen, anterior limbic
Saris (1983)	Left hemichorea	Right caudate, anterior limbic
Tabaton *et al.* (1985)	Bilateral chorea	Right putamen; left caudate, putamen, anterior limbic
Kawamura *et al.* (1988)	Right hemichorea	Left caudate
Midgard *et al.* (1989)	Left hemidystonia	Right caudate, putamen, anterior limbic
Destee *et al.* (1990)	Right hemiballism	Left caudate, putamen
Lownie and Gilbert (1990)	Left hemiballism	Right caudate, thalamus
Kim (1992)	Left arm tremor	Right caudate, putamen, anterior limbic
Kim (1992)	Left arm tremor	Right caudate, anterior limbic
Caplan and Helgason (1995)	Left arm ballism	Left caudate, anterior limbic
Caplan and Helgason (1995)	Right hemichorea	Right caudate, putamen, anterior limbic
Broderick *et al.* (1995)	Left hemichorea	Left caudate, putamen, anterior limbic
Broderick *et al.* (1995)	Bilateral hemichorea	Left caudate, putamen, anterior limbic; right putamen

limb abnormalities in detail:

> The upper limb moved chiefly at the shoulder (shrugging and rotation), at the proximal inter-phalangeal joints, and at the wrist (flexion, extension, rotation); flexion at the elbows was less frequent, but, on occasion, the arm would be flung across the chest. The lower limb showed hip rotation, occasional involuntary crossing of the legs, and undulating movements of the ankle and foot exaggerated at attempts at running the foot down the shin. Knee flexion was less frequent. The face was also active with pursing of the lips and protrusion of the tongue.

In this description, both ballistic flinging movements and distal choreic movements were observed.

The patient of Midgard *et al.* (1989) had an infantile stroke and had the delayed onset of abnormal movements and dystonia more than a decade later. 'Minor muscular effort would elicit alternating slow and involuntary movements of flexion and extension of the left shoulder girdle, arm, and fingers. Plantar flexion and inversion of the left foot became prominent on walking'. The two patients of Kim (1992) with caudate infarcts had delayed onset of a rest tremor of the left arm and hand months after recovery from a left hemiparesis caused by caudate infarction. In two reports (Lodder and Baard 1981, Tabaton *et al.* 1985), the infarcts and movement disorders were bilateral, beginning at once in all limbs. The two patients described by Broderick *et al.* (1995) were poorly controlled insulin-dependent diabetics who had choreic movements related to haemorrhagic infarcts involving the caudate nucleus that ocurred during severe hyperglycaemia. In one of the patients, the caudate infarcts and chorea were bilateral.

The report of Caplan and Helgason (1995) contains a description of two patients seen by Helgason who had movement disorders. A 62-year-old diabetic man with hyperlipidaemia and angina pectoris developed the acute onset of choreic movements of the left shoulder and arm and twisting movements of the mouth. Magnetic resonance imaging (MRI) showed multiple infarcts, the largest involving the right caudate, anterior limb of the capsule, and putamen. A 49-year-old hypertensive man with hyperlipidaemia and coronary artery disease had transient right facial weakness and dysarthria lasting 15 min. After recovery, he soon developed frequent uncontrollable flinging and twisting movements of the right arm and hand. MRI showed a large infarct in the left caudate nucleus and anterior limb of the capsule.

The striatum and subthalamic nucleus both project to the globus pallidus. The caudate nucleus has inhibitory projections to the lateral globus pallidus, which, in turn, projects to the subthalamic nucleus. Loss of inhibitory input to the subthalamic nucleus may allow release of abnormal movements. Abnormalities of movement and tone can follow acute lesions of either the striate nuclei or the subthalamic nucleus (Lownie and Gilbert 1990).

Dysarthria and motor dysphonia

Dysarthria and dysphonia were prominent findings in the series of Caplan *et al.* (1990). Eleven out of the 18 patients had an articulatory abnormality. In the series of

Caplan and Helgason (1995), 18/21 (86%) patients had dysarthria and/or dysphonia. In the series of Kumral *et al.* (1999), 12 caudate infarct patients had dysarthria, evenly divided between left and right caudate lesions. Most of the dysarthric patients in this series (80%) had lesions that extended into the anterior limb of the internal capsule and/or the anterior putamen. Patients reported by Kim (1992) and Saris (1983) also had dysarthric speech, but this abnormality was not mentioned in the other reports of patients with caudate infarcts and movement disorders. Dysarthria is probably explained by interruption of cortico–striato–cerebellar pathways, which influence the bulbar muscles involved with speaking. Dysarthria and dysphonia are prominent in all degenerative conditions affecting the basal ganglia (e.g. Wilsons disease, Parkinsonism, progressive supranuclear palsy, Huntington's disease, and so on).

Motor abnormalities of face and limbs

Motor weakness was present in 13 of the 18 (72%) patients in the series of Caplan *et al.* (1990) and was also noted in three out of 12 patients reported by Mendez *et al.* (1989), in 16/25 (64%) of the patients reported by Kumral *et al.* (1999), in two patients reported by Kim (1992), and the single patient described by Markowitsch *et al.* (1990). In the series of Caplan and Helgason (1995), all 21 patients had some motor weakness but the weakness was judged severe in only one patient. In this series, patients were identified mostly because of motor findings.

In some patients with dystonia and abnormal movements, weakness may have been overshadowed by involuntary movements and abnormal tone. Among 95 patients reported to date with caudate infarcts, 56 (59%) had motor weakness. This may not represent the frequency of motor involvement since, in some series, patients were selected because of specific abnormalities such as behavioural disorders or abnormal movements, and in other series, patients were selected mostly because they had motor weakness. Weakness, when present, was usually slight and relatively transient, rarely leaving any persistent motor handicap. The motor abnormality often was non-pyramidal and consisted of less use of the limbs, clumsiness, altered tone, etc. Weakness is explained by interruption of striato-pontine fibres projecting in the anterior limb of the internal capsule, and by involvement of the putamen. Patients with weakness invariably had lesions that extended into the anterior limb of the internal capsule and sometimes also into the putamen. Lesions confined to the caudate nucleus are not known to cause weakness.

Eye movement abnormalities

Although animal studies show convincing oculomotor effects of caudate nucleus lesions (Alexander *et al.* 1986), few clinical patients with caudate infarcts have had thorough testing of eye movements. Patients with diseases that affect the striatum (Parkinson's disease, Huntington's disease, Wilson's disease, progressive supranuclear palsy, and so forth) often have abnormalities of saccades or smooth pursuit when tested. The caudate nucleus has connections with the frontal eye fields and the posterior parietal cortex, regions known to be involved in generating conjugate eye movements (Alexander *et al.* 1986). The caudate nuclei and substantia nigra contain several neuronal populations that have saccade-related activity that is context dependent (Wurtz and Hikosaka 1986).

Vermersch *et al.* (1999) studied memory-guided saccades in a hypertensive patient with bilateral caudate nucleus infarcts. The left striatal infarct was acute and involved the body of the caudate nucleus and the putamen. An older infarct was also present in the right striatum involving the same structures. The mean latency and the gain of rightward memory guided saccades. The memory-guided leftward saccade gains were also abnormally low. At the same time, memory-guided pointing was normal and visually guided saccades were also within two standard deviations of normal.

In monkeys that had a unilateral infusion that depleted one caudate nucleus of dopamine, spontaneous saccades (Kato *et al.* 1995) and visual- and memory-guided saccades (Kori *et al.* 1995) were abnormal, especially toward the contralateral side. The deficits described in conjugate lateral gaze are relatively subtle and would not be mentioned by patients. They are probably detectable if carefully sought.

Vascular supply and location of infarcts

Accounts of the vascular supply of the caudate nucleus often vary (Kaplan 1965, Gillilan 1968, Dunker and Harris 1976, Gorczyca and Mohr 1987, Ghika *et al.* 1990). The main feeding arteries are branches of the ACA and MCA. The ACA gives rise to Heubner's arteries, a series of 2–4 vessels that usually arise from the A2 portion of the ACA near the anterior communicating–ACA junction (Gorczyka and Mohr 1987). These vessels supply the inferior part of the head of the caudate nucleus, the adjacent anterior limb of the internal capsule, and the subfrontal white matter. Direct penetrating arteries from the ACA (variously called 'medial striate' or 'anterior lenticulostriate' arteries by some authors) supply the anterior portion of the head of the caudate nucleus. The MCA gives rise to medial lenticulostriate arteries, which branch from the proximal M1 portion of that artery and supply a small portion of the lateral border of the caudate head and the adjacent internal capsule. The lateral lenticulostriate arteries branch from the mainstem MCA or its superior division branches to supply the major portion of the head of the caudate nucleus, as well as the adjacent internal capsule and the anterior half of the putamen. Figure 18.5, from Kumral *et al.* (1999), shows cartoons illustrating the location of Heubner, medial, and lateral lenticulostriate artery territory infarcts.

The reported series includes 108 patients with 119 caudate infarcts. Among these, 34 (29%) infarcts were confined on CT or MRI to the caudate nucleus. The lesion involved the caudate nucleus and the adjacent anterior limb of the internal capsule or corona radiata in 30 infarcts (25%). The remainder, 55 (46%) infarcts, involved the caudate nucleus, anterior limb of the capsule, the putamen, and sometimes the

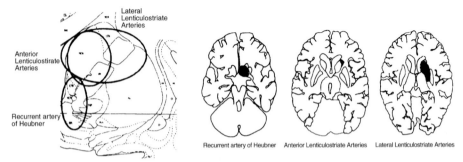

Fig. 18.5 Templates through the caudate nucleus depicting infarcts in three arterial territories. Shown are coronal views (left) and a horizontal view (right) of the caudate arterial territories. CG, cingulate gyrus; SCS, subcallosal striatum; bcc, body of corpus callosum; aic, anterior limb of the internal capsule; CFR, caudate fundus (body) region; EGP, external globus pallidus; Pu, putamen; IG, insular gyrus; ex, extreme capsule; ec, external capsule; Cl, claustrum; PuV, ventral putamen; NA, nucleus accumbens; pirT, piriform cortex, temporal area. From Kumral *et al.* (1999) with permission.

adjacent corona radiata. The most common pattern of infarction fits best the supply territory of the lateral lenticulostriate branches of the MCA, not with supply by Heubner's arteries. The only study that attempted to localize the infarcts to vascular territory was that of Kumral *et al.* (1999). In that series, which included 28 infarcts among 25 patients, 13 infarcts were considered to be in the territory of the lateral lenticulostriate arteries, 14 in the territory of medial lenticulostriate arteries, and only one in the supply of Heubner's artery. Infarcts in the portion of the caudate nucleus supplied by Heubner's arteries are described quite rarely.

Aetiology of infarcts

Unfortunately, in most instances, the data reported are insufficient to define the precise stroke mechanism. Most patients had risk factors for penetrating artery disease and intracranial branch atheromatous disease and no cardiac or large artery lesion or, alternatively, no satisfactory evaluation of the heart and large arteries. Risk factors for penetrating artery disease were very common. Hypertension was noted in 73/108 (68%) patients, and 33/108 (30%) were diabetic. Some patients had both hypertension and diabetes. However, some patients with caudate infarcts had potential cardiac and intra-arterial sources of emboli and some had occlusions of the ACA and MCA. Two patients seen in Boston are examples of patients with caudate nucleus and adjacent deep structure infarcts due to intracranial large artery occlusive disease. A 65-year-old black woman who had a history of hypertension developed an acute stroke. Her CT scan showed an infarct in the left caudate nucleus. She was noted to be abulic with reduced speech output and slight dysnomia after an automobile accident. After lowering of her blood pressure, she developed a right hemiparesis and became mute. The lesion responsible was a very tight stenosis of the ACA. A Chinese patient with a caudato-capsular-putaminal infarct had an occlusion of the MCA on angiography.

One report described a patient studied clinically and at autopsy (Nishida *et al.* 2000). This diabetic man developed aphasia and right hemiparesis 9 days after a myocardial infarct. At autopsy, he was found to have an acute thrombosis of the distal portion of the left MCA which decreased flow in six lateral lenticulostriate branches. The resultant infarct involved the head and anterior aspect of the body of the caudate nucleus, the adjacent anterior limb of the capsule, and the anterior portion of the putamen. Thrombus in the MCA was engrafted upon an atherosclerotic plaque.

MRI now shows the location and distribution of infarcts quite well. Figure 18.6 shows MRIs from two patients with caudate infarcts. Diffusion-weighted MRI (DWI) can show ischaemia soon after symptom onset and can differentiate acute from chronic infarcts. In some patients, perfusion-weighted MRI can show the extended region of hypoperfusion which may encompass more than the region of infarction shown by DWI. Since treatment should be determined by aetiology, if neuroimaging shows infarction of the caudate, with or without involvement of the adjacent anterior limb of the capsule and putamen, both cardiac and vascular non-invasive evaluations are indicated. Duplex scans of the ICA in the neck, and transcranial Doppler ultrasound of the intracranial ICA and its ACA and MCA branches, and/or magnetic resonance angiography (MRA), or CT angiography should be sufficient when screening for the presence of important occlusive vascular lesions.

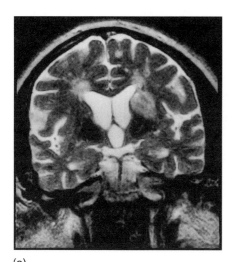
(a)

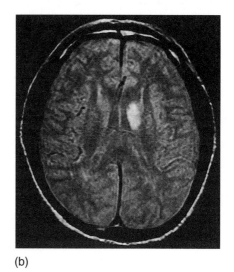
(b)

Fig. 18.6 Representative MRI scans from patients with caudate infarcts. (a) Large infarct on the right involving the caudate nucleus and the adjacent white matter. There are prominent caps surrounding the lateral ventricles. The lateral and third ventricles are dilated. (b) Acute infarct involving the caudate nucleus on the right of the figure.

Final comments and conclusions

Knowledge about the functions of the caudate nucleus and its connections is still evolving. Also, as yet, very little is known about the underlying stroke mechanisms and vascular aetiology. These points are well illustrated by a consultation by the author. A neurologist in his fifties presented with no known vascular risk factors but had been having frequent attacks during a period of over 20 years of a transient abnormality affecting the right side of his body. He would suddenly become aware that the right limbs were different from the left but could not characterize the difference as either sensory or motor. There were no paraesthesias and no numbness, and the limbs were neither weak, ataxic, nor stiff. Examinations by other neurologists during attacks were completely normal. More recently, this abnormal perception would persist for months at a time but yet would sometimes clear. While the author found no abnormalities on neurological examination, MRI defined two lesions involving the left caudate nucleus and the adjacent white matter Angiography was completely normal. The aetiology of these lesions, which look like cavitated old infarcts, is unknown. The nature of his perceived different right-sided feeling is obscure, and the presence of these large, subcortical, strategically placed cavities without clinical signs is daunting. Also obscure is why the symptoms continue to come and go despite the presence of fixed cavities. We still have much to learn.

The most recent clinical experience and review of published cases leads to the following conclusions:

(1) Most patients with caudate infarcts have multiple brain infarcts.

(2) Most often infarcts involve the caudate nucleus, anterior limb of the internal capsule, and the anterior part of the putamen. Pure caudate nucleus infarcts are recognized less often clinically.

(3) The caudate nucleus has multiple supplying arteries: Heubner's artery from the ACA (inferior caudate head), lateral lenticulostriate branches of the MCA (major part of the caudate head), and direct penetrating artery branches from the ACA and ICA (anterior caudate head).

(4) The most common pattern of infarction (caudate, anterior limb, putamen) suggests involvement of lateral lenticulostriate MCA branches.

(5) The most common cause of caudate infarcts is probably penetrating artery/ intracranial branch atheromatous disease. Large artery intracranial occlusive disease and cardiac and intra-arterial emboli also can cause caudate infarcts.

(6) The most common clinical signs are:

  (a) dysphonia;

  (b) slight contralateral hemiparesis;

  (c) behavioural abnormalities especially abulia, agitation, and loss of frontal lobe executive abilities. Neglect and aphasia occur less often;

    (d) movement disorders such as hemichorea, ballism, and tremor occur but less often than other clinical signs.

(7) Behavioural changes are more severe and more persistent after bilateral infarcts involving the caudate nucleus and its projections.

Chapter 19

Anterior choroidal artery territory infarcts

L.R. Caplan

Introduction and historical background

Charles Foix and his colleagues Chavany, Hillemand, and Schiff-Wertheimer (Foix *et al.* 1925) are usually given credit for describing the first case of anterior choroidal artery (AChA) territory infarction. The patient that they described developed the sudden onset of a severe right hemiplegia accompanied by severe sensory loss in the right limbs to all sensory modalities, and a right hemianopia. There was no decrease in alertness, no aphasia, and no cognitive or behavioural abnormality. At autopsy, the patient had an infarct in the teritory of the left AChA. Actually Kolisko (1891) had reported two patients with AChA territory infarction who had infarcts in the internal capsule before Foix and his colleagues, but his report has seldom been acknowledged. Long before computed tomography (CT) became available, a number of single case reports described patients with AChA territory infarcts shown at necropsy (Poppi 1928*a,b*, Abbie 1933). In these early reports, the patients' deficits generally conformed to the formula cited by Foix *et al.* (1925), i.e. a contralateral hemiplegia, hemisensory loss, and hemianopia without important cognitive or behavioural signs. All had infarcts at autopsy. These early authors defined the anatomical regions supplied by the AChA. After the report of these authors, clinicians considered the syndrome of hemiplegia, hemisensory loss, and hemianopia without cognitive abnormalities to be pathognomonic for AChA territory lesions. Steegmen and Roberts (1935) reported the case of a 17-year-old boy who had this syndrome associated with subarachnoid haemorrhage. These authors reported the case under the title 'the syndrome of the anterior choroidal artery' despite the lack of corroborative anatomical evidence.

During the middle years of the 20th century, experience concerning infarction in the territory of the AChA was gained mostly from purposeful ligation of the artery to treat Parkinsonism (Cooper 1955, Morillo and Cooper 1955, DuBois-Poulson *et al.* 1956, Rand *et al.* 1956). In the first patient, bleeding occurred during an attempt to make a brain lesion to treat Parkinsons disease, and Cooper had to tie the AChA to stop the bleeding. Cooper was surprised that, after surgery, the patient's tremor and Parkinsonism improved and he had no severe paralysis. Subsequently, the AChA was ligated intentionally by Cooper and his colleagues and also by French surgeons

(DuBois-Poulsen *et al.* 1956) as a treatment for Parkinson's disease. The neurological signs that resulted proved very variable. Some patients seemed to develop little or no deficits.

When CT became available and newer generation scanners were able to define regions of brain infarction accurately, reports began to appear about the usual CT locations of anterior choroidal territory infarcts (Sterbini *et al.* 1987). A plethora of case series of patients with AChA territory infarcts defined by brain neuroimaging scans appeared (Masson *et al.* 1983, Decroix *et al.* 1986, Helgason *et al.* 1986, 1988, Hupperts *et al.* 1994). In some of these reports, the infarcts were mostly limited to the deep capsular territory supplied by perforating artery branches of the AChA (Decroix *et al.* 1986, Helgason *et al.* 1988).

More recently, reports have emphasized specific features of AChA territory infarction, e.g. visual field abnormalities (Hoyt 1975, Frisen 1978), eye movement abnormalities (Viader *et al.* 1984), and cognitive and behavioural findings (Cambier *et al.* 1983, Hommel *et al.* 1985, Bogousslavsky *et al.* 1988c, Derex *et al.* 1997, Nagaratnam *et al.* 1998, Sarangi *et al.* 2000).

Anatomy of the AChA and its region of supply

Usual arterial anatomy and brain regions supplied

The AChA is a relatively small artery that originates from the internal carotid artery just after the origin of the posterior communicating artery. The size of the artery varies from 7 to 20 mm, with an average of 5 mm at its origin. (Gillilan 1968). Occasionally the AChA takes origin from the middle cerebral or posterior communicating artery. The AChA takes a posterolateral direction course. Figures 19.1–19.4 show the artery and its relationships: Fig. 19.1 is a drawing of a lateral view showing the course of the artery; Fig. 19.2 is a cartoon showing the AChA as it appears in antero-posterior and lateral angiographic views; Fig. 19.3 shows the relationships of the AChA as it courses posterolaterally; and Fig. 19.4 shows potential anastamoses with other adjacent arteries. At first the artery lies inferior and lateral to the optic tract. It then courses to the medial side of the optic tract, at which time the cerebral peduncle and the thalamus lie medial to the AChA and the medial temporal lobe lies on the lateral side of the artery. As the AChA courses caudally, it lies dorsal to the optic tract and gives off two branches; the smaller anterior branch supplies the medial temporal lobe uncus region and the amygdaloid nucleus and the larger posterior branch goes through the choroid fissure to supply the choroid plexus of the lateral ventricle entering it at the temporal horn (Gillilan 1968, Stephens and Stilwell 1969, Rhoton *et al.* 1979, Graff-Radford *et al.* 1985, Marinkovic *et al.* 1999).

In its proximal portion, the AChA gives off penetrating branches to the optic tract and to the medial portion of the globus pallidus. The anterior branch gives supply branches to the uncus, pyriform cortex, amygdaloid nucleus, and the anterior portion of the hippocampus and its dentate gyrus. Medial branches of the AChA penetrate the

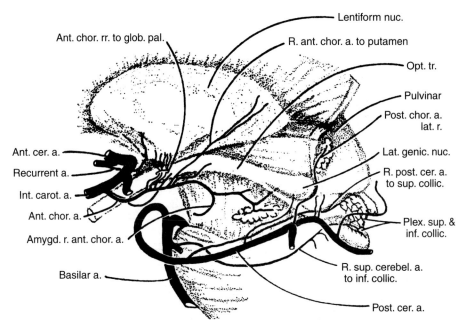

Fig. 19.1 Diagram showing the origin, course, and distribution of the anterior choroidal artery to various forebrain sites. ant.chor.a-anterior choroidal artery; Ant. cer. a-anterior cerebral artery; Int. carot. a-internal carotid artery; Recurrent a-recurrent artery of Heubner; Post. cer. a-posterior cerebral artery; Ant. chor.rr to glob pal-anterior choroidal artery rami to the globus pallidus; R. ant. chor. a to putamen-anterior choroidal artery rami to the putamen; Post. chor. a. lat. R-posterior choroidal artery lateral rami; Opt. tr-optic tract; Lat. genic. Nuc-lateral geniculate nucleus; Plex. sup and inf. collic-plexus of the superior and inferior colliculi; R. sup. cerebel. a. to inf. collic.-ramus of the superior cerebellar artery to the inferior colliculus; R. post. cer. a to sup collic-ramus of the posterior cerebral artery to the superior colliculus; Amygd.r.ant.chor.a-amygdaloid ramus of the anterior choroidal artery Reprinted from Gillilan (1968) with permission.

cerebral peduncle supplying its medial third, and branches extend quite variably to supply the substantia nigra and red nucleus within the midbrain, regions of the subthalamus, and portions of the ventral anterior, ventral lateral, pulvinar, and reticular nuclei within the thalamus. In the most posterior segment of the artery, penetrating artery branches supply the posterior limb of the internal capsule, the tail of the caudate nucleus, and portions of the retrolenticular portion of the internal capsule including a part of the geniculo-calcarine visual radiations and auditory radiations emanating from the medial geniculate body (Gillilan 1968, Helgason *et al.* 1986, Marinkovic *et al.* 1999). The terminal portion of the AChA can be traced by dissection to the anterolateral aspect of the lateral geniculate body. In this region, the lateral choroidal artery branch of the posterior cerebral artery interdigitates with branches of the AChA (Gillilan 1968, Frisen *et al.* 1978, Frisen 1979). The two arteries form a plexus oriented along the long axis of the lateral geniculate body. From this

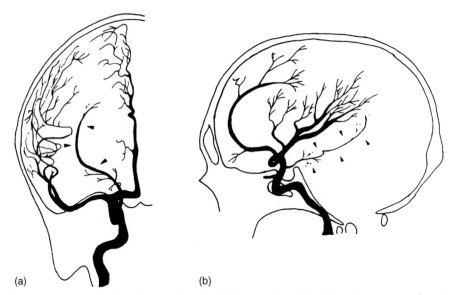

(a)   (b)

Fig. 19.2 Cartoon showing the anterior choroidal artery (arrowheads) as it appears on frontal anterior–posterior (a) and lateral (b) angiographic views. From Sterbini *et al.* (1987) with permission.

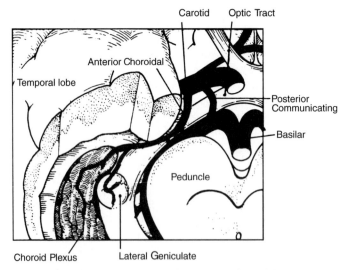

Fig. 19.3 Artist's drawing of the relationships of the anterior choroidal artery. From Helgason *et al.* (1986) with permission.

plexus, many fine straight arterial branches fan upward and supply the cellular layers of the nucleus. The lateral choroidal branch of the posterior cerebral artery supplies mostly the medial and posterior segments of the nucleus, while branches from the AChA supply mostly the hilum and anterolateral portions of the lateral geniculate

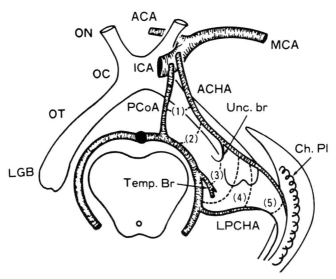

Fig. 19.4 Anastamoses of anterior choroidal artery (AChA) with posterior communicating artery (PCoA)–posterior cerebral artery (PCA) system. AChA has anastamotic channels (1) over the optic tract with branches from the PCoA; (2) over the cerebral peduncle with the proximal PCA; (3) over the pyriform cortex (uncal branches) with temporal (Temp. Br) and hippocampal branches of the PCA; (4) over and around the lateral geniculate body (LGB) with PCA branches including the lateral posterior choroidal artery (LPCHA); and (5) in the choroid plexus (Ch. Pl) with posterior choroidal artery branches. ON-optic nerve; OC-optic chiasm; OT-optic tract; ICA-internal carotid artery. From Takahashi *et al.* (1990) with permission.

body. The blood supply to the lateral geniculate body has been used to explain the patterns of visual field defect that occur in patients with AChA and posterior cerebral artery occlusions that result in infarction within the lateral geniculate body (Frisen *et al.* 1978, Frisen 1979).

There is much overlap of supply arteries to the temporal lobe and to the rostral brainstem. The supply of the AChA to these areas is very variable. Probably the most consistent supply of the AChA is the penetrating arteries to the optic tract, medial globus pallidus, posterior limb of the internal capsule, and to the choroid plexus and the lateral geniculate bodies.

Controversy over the supply of periventricular regions of the corona radiata

Considerable debate still surrounds the issue of the contribution of the AChA to the supply of the superior posterior periventricular region of the white matter of the corona radiata. Figure 19.5 shows diagrammatically the regions generally accepted as supplied by the penetrating branches of the AChAs and those that are controversial. Some authors (Van den Bergh and Van der Eecken 1968, Van den Bergh 1969, Van der Eecken 1969) have taken the view that the periventricular white matter is supplied

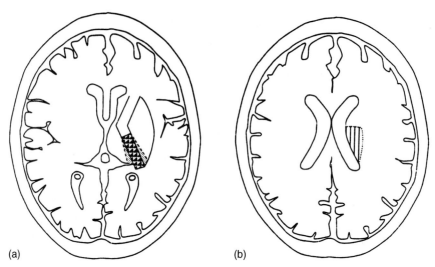

(a) (b)

Fig. 19.5 Schematic CT templates of presumed AChA territories. In (a), triangles show the area generally agreed upon; dots are located in areas in which there is some disagreement, and in (b) vertical lines outline contentious areas. From Hupperts *et al.* (1994) with permission.

by subependymal ventriculofugal branches arising from the choroidal arteries. After the AChA supplies the choroid plexus within the temporal horn of the lateral ventricle, it then continues within the ventricle to curve dorsally and forward above the thalamus to supply the choroid plexus of the lateral ventricle sometimes as far forward as the foramen of Monroe (Theron and Newton 1976, Rhoton *et al.* 1979, Helgason 1995). The intraventricular portion of the AChA is thus in a position where ventriculofugal branches could penetrate into the more superior periventricular region. The opposing view is that this region of the periventricular corona radiata is supplied by ventriculopetal branches of the deep penetrating medullary arterial branches of the middle cerebral artery (Mohr *et al.* 1991). Although this issue remains controversial, there are some reported patients with otherwise typical AChA territory infarcts in whom the infarct seems to extend from inferiorly into this superior periventricular region.

Anatomical vascular variations

On occasion, a well-developed artery other than the posterior communicating artery and the AChA originates from the internal carotid artery and supplies the medial temporal lobe and other structures usually supplied by the AChA and the posterior cerebral artery (Takahashi *et al.* 1990). There are four regularly recognized hyperplastic anomalies of the AChA: (1) a hypertrophic uncal branch that supplies tissue ordinarily supplied by the anterior temporal branch of the posterior cerebral artery; (2) a hypertrophic AChA branch that supplies most of the territory ordinarily supplied by the anterior and posterior branches of the posterior cerebral artery; (3) an

AChA branch that supplies an occipitoparietal artery which supplies the calcarine region and adjacent occipital cortex usually supplied by the occipitoparietal branch of the posterior cerebral artery; and (4) the entire posterior cerebral artery territory is supplied by branches of the AChA (Takahashi *et al.* 1990, Chen and Barkovich 1998, Abrahams *et al.* 1999).

Unilateral AChA territory infarcts

Clinical findings

The clinical signs related to AChA territory infarcts are variable mostly because the area of infarction is quite variable. The region most often infarcted is the posterior limb of the internal capsule (Poppi 1928*a,b*, Abbie 1933, Buge *et al.* 1979, Decroix *et al.* 1986, Helgason *et al.* 1986, 1988, Hupperts *et al.* 1994). The medial globus pallidus, the lateral geniculate body, and the proximal portion of the geniculo-calcarine tract are also involved relatively commonly. Infarction of the optic tract and the midbrain and thalamus are quite rare. Only occasional patients with AChA territory infarcts have important involvement of the medial temporal lobe.

The onset of symptoms is most often abrupt, but some patients have had the gradual development of neurological signs. Some patients have had headache before onset of neurological symptoms and others have had headache at onset.

Motor abnormalities

In the two largest series of patients with AChA territory infarcts studied clinically and with CT, motor symptoms were common and prominent (Decroix *et al.* 1986, Hupperts *et al.* 1994).

In the series of Decroix *et al.* (1986), 14/16 patients (87.5%) had prominent motor signs. Severe and moderate hemiplegia was present in six patients each (37.5%) and in two patients there was facio-brachial weakness. All of the patients with motor weakness had hemisensory abnormalities except three (two with severe hemiplegia and one with brachiofacial weakness) in whom the deficit was 'pure motor' (Decroix *et al.* 1986). Six of the 14 patients (37.5%) were considered dysarthric. In the series of Huppert *et al.* (1994), 35/77 (45%) of patients with AChA territory infarcts had 'pure motor' deficits, while an additional 21 (27%) had sensorimotor abnormalities. Dysarthria was also a common symptom in this series of patients.

The motor weakness is usually accompanied by hyperreflexia and a Babinski sign. Occasional patients are described as clumsy or ataxic but not paralysed.

Sensory abnormalities

Sensory symptoms and signs are quite variable. Sensory loss can be isolated (Derouesne *et al.* 1985, Decroix *et al.* 1986). The sensory loss is often incomplete and can be temporary. The AChA supplies the sensory radiations within the posterior limb of the internal capsule and at the level of the sensory nuclei within the ventrolateral thalamus. All sensory modalities are usually involved, but proprioception can be spared (Pertuiset *et al.* 1962, Graff-Radford *et al.* 1985, Helgason *et al.* 1986). Formications, a feeling of swelling of the involved limbs, and painful paresthesias are sometimes noted. Some patients later develop a thalamic pain syndrome after AChA territory infarcts (Abbie 1933). Most often the sensory abnormalities improve rapidly and seldom leave a residual sensory loss.

Among the 16 patients with AChA territory infarcts studied by Decroix *et al.* (1986), only three had no sensory deficit; five (31%) had severe sensory loss and eight (50%) were judged to have a moderately severe sensory loss. Two patients had a pure sensory syndrome (Decroix *et al.* 1986). Among 77 patients with AChA territory infarcts studied by Hupperts *et al.* (1994), 21 (27%) had sensory and motor deficits and none had a pure sensory syndrome.

Visual field loss and oculomotor signs

Visual symptoms and signs are probably the most variable feature of AChA territory infarction. The AChA supplies visual fibres at three separate locations: the optic tract, the lateral geniculate body, and the proximal portion of the geniculo-calcarine tract. In patients with hyperplastic AChAs, this artery can be the supply of the calcarine cortex. Foix and Schiff-Wertheimer (1926) reviewed the blood supply of the optic tract, the lateral geniculate body, the geniculo-calcarine tract, and the occipital visual cortex. A diagram from their review is reprinted as Fig. 19.6. However all of these visual perceptual regions are often spared in patients with AChA territory infarcts.

Among 12 patients in one series in whom the AChA was ligated, one had a transient homonymous hemianopia but only one patient developed a visual field defect that persisted—an upper quadrantanopia (Morillo and Cooper 1955). Among the 16 patients studied by Decroix *et al.* (1986), three (19%) had a homonymous hemianopia and one had visual extinction only; 12 had no visual abnormalities.

Although, in theory, infarction of the optic tract related to AChA occlusion could cause an incongruent hemianopia accompanied by a failure of the pupil to react when light is shown from the hemianopic side (a Wernicke's hemianopic pupil), such a patient has not been reported. The most common visual field defect in patients with AChA territory infarction is a congruous hemianopia. This visual defect can be transient. Upper quadrantanopia sometimes with sparing of the macula has also been reported (Abbie 1933, Pertuiset *et al.* 1962, Helgason *et al.* 1986).

Lars Frisen, a Swedish ophthalmologist, and his colleagues in two articles clarified the nature of visual field deficits found in patients with infarction of the lateral geniculate body (Frisen *et al.* 1978, Frisen 1979). The lateral choroidal artery, a branch of the posterior cerebral artery, supplies the medial and posterior portions of the lateral geniculate body. The AChA branches to the lateral geniculate enter inferiorly and laterally and supply the hilum and anterolateral portions of the nucleus.

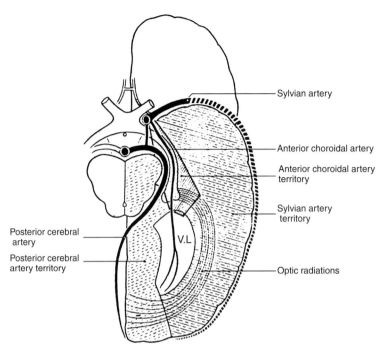

Sylvian artery

Anterior choroidal artery

Anterior choroidal artery territory

Sylvian artery territory

Posterior cerebral artery

Posterior cerebral artery territory

V.L

Optic radiations

Fig. 19.6 Diagrammatic representation of visual perceptual areas and their blood supply. From Foix and Schiff-Wertheimer (1926) with permission.

The upper quadrant of the visual field is located anterolaterally in the lateral geniculate body. Frisen and colleagues (1978) reported two patients with isolated horizontal sector visual field deficits probably attributable to occlusion of branches of the lateral choroidal artery branch of the posterior cerebral artery. In 1979, Frisen reported a patient who had the converse visual field defect, i.e. a defect in the upper and lower visual field that spared a horizontal sector along the meridian. He called this defect a quadruple sectoranopia because it was characterized by congruous defects in both the upper and lower quadrants of each eye. Others have described patients with AChA territory infarcts with identical field defects. This quadruple sector defect, illustrated in Fig. 19.6, is probably specific for AChA territory infarction.

Hoyt (1975) emphasized that visual field defects related to lesions of the lateral geniculate body are often incongruous, but Luco *et al.* (1992) disagreed and emphasized their usual congruity. Luco *et al.* reported five patients with strokes that involved the lateral geniculate body and confirmed the patterns emphasized by Frisen, i.e. horizontal sectoranopia, quadruple sectoranopia, and an upper quadrantanopia. All of their described lesions were congruent. Only one patient had an infarct in the territory of an AChA and that patient had a quadruple sectoranopia. The visual field from this patient is shown in Fig. 19.7.

The three most common visual field defects in patients with AChA territory infarction are: a homonymous hemianopia sometimes with macular sparing; an

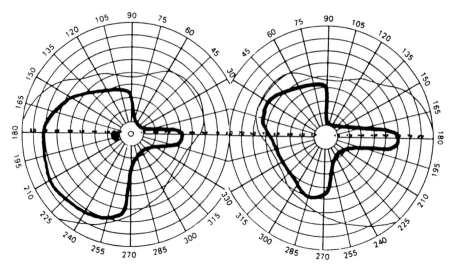

Fig. 19.7 Quadruple sector anopia due to presumed AChA territory infarction of the lateral geniculate body. From Luco *et al.* (1992) with permission.

upper quadrantanopia, again often with macular sparing; and a quadruple sectoranopia

Occasionally patients with an AChA territory infarct that involves the midbrain may have an oculomotor abnormality. Viader *et al.* (1984) reported a patient who presented with a right hemiplegia and hemisensory loss without a hemianopia who also had vertical diplopia. He had a defect in looking upward with the left eye. A patient reported by Buge *et al.* (1979) with bilateral AChA territory infarcts had defective upward gaze.

Cognitive and behavioural abnormalities

Although Foix and colleagues and subsequent authors felt that a key feature of AChA territory infarction was the absence of cognitive or behavioural abnormalities, many patients with AChA territory infarcts have been reported who have had abnormalities of higher cortical function.

Two of three patients reported by Helgason, myself, and our colleagues had left visual neglect and one patient also had difficulty drawing and copying (Helgason *et al.* 1986). Cambier *et al.* (1983) reported four patients with AChA territory infarcts who had cognitive abnormalities. Three patients with right AChA territory infarcts had visual neglect, constructional apraxia, anosognosia, and motor impersistence. The fourth patient had a left AChA territory infarct and had diminished speech fluency, made semantic paraphasic errors and perseverated in speech (Cambier *et al.* 1983). Graff-Radford *et al.* (1985) reported eight patients with AChA territory infarcts involving the posterior limb of the internal capsule and the lateral thalamus on CT scans. Two of these patients had angiographically documented AChA occlusions.

The patients with left thalamic infarcts had dysarthria and minor language abnormalities detected mostly by difficulty making word associations and in comprehending a written paragraph. They also had defective verbal memory. The patients with right thalamic infarction had defective visual memory (Graff-Radford *et al.* 1985). Hommel *et al.* reported a patient with a left AChA territory infarct involving the posterior limb of the internal capsule who had decreased speech fluency and abnormal drawing abilities. The lesion spared the thalamus on CT scan, but cerebral blood flow as measured by xenon inhalation showed diminished cerebral cortical blood flow especially in the left frontoparietal region (Hommel *et al.* 1985).

Bogousslavsky *et al.* (1988c) reported two patients with right AChA territory infarcts who had severe multimodal left neglect. One of the patients who had a severe left hemiparesis, left hemisensory loss, and a left hemianopia died, and, at autopsy, the infarct destroyed the lateral half of the retrolenticular portion of the internal capsule and also extended into the globus pallidus, putamen, the body of the caudate nucleus, and into the area surrounding the inferior horn of the lateral ventricle next to the choroidal fissure (Fig. 19.8). A single photon emission computed tomography (SPECT) scan in this patient showed marked right parietal lobe hypoperfusion. A second patient with an infarct of the right posterior limb of the internal capsule had spatial hemineglect, and abnormal drawing and copying and abnormal visual–spatial

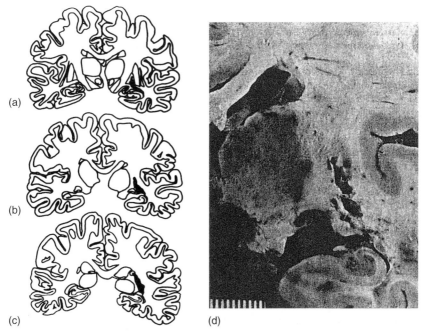

Fig. 19.8 Schematic drawing of the autopsy findings in a patient with an AChA territory infarct (a–c). (b) The infarct at the level marked in (b). From Bogousslavsky *et al.* (1988) with permission.

abilities. A SPECT scan showed decreased right parietal and right frontal lobe blood flow (Bogousslavsky *et al.* 1988*c*).

A patient with poor memory and a reportedly progressive mental decline had an AChA territory infarct that involved the parahippocampal cortex on magnetic resonance imaging (MRI). SPECT scanning in this patient showed a medial temporal decrease in metabolism and blood flow (Sarangi *et al.* 2000). Two reports concern individual patients with pathological crying after infarction of the AChA territory posterior limb of the internal capsule (Derex *et al.* 1997, Nagaratnam *et al.* 1998). A 55-year-old man had an infarct in the left posterior capsular limb that extended upward into the posterior periventricular corona radiata region. He had frequent fits of crying—up to eight times a day—during which there was no affective feeling of sadness, and he was not depressed (Derex *et al.* 1997). Naratnam *et al.* (1998) reported a 79-year-old man, with an infarct shown on MRI to involve the posterior limb of the internal capsule and the posterior paraventricular corona radiata, who had emotional lability and frequent bursts of crying; he would also at times become aggressive and hostile without apparent provocation.

Bilateral AChA territory infarcts

Buge *et al.* (1979) described a patient who developed the sudden onset of lingual, pharyngeal, and laryngeal functions accompanied by dysarthria, facial diplegia more severe on the right, limited vertical eye movement, and bilaterally brisk deep tendon reflexes. At autopsy, there was a fresh infarct that involved the posterior limb of the internal capsule and the medial portion of the globus pallidus. An old, presumably silent, infarct involved the same structures on the right side (Buge *et al.* 1979).

Helgason *et al.* (1988) reported eight patients with bilateral deep AChA territory infarcts. All had the sudden onset of inability to speak or swallow. Facial diplegia and hemiplegia with hemisensory loss were often found. The bilateral infarcts involved the posterior limb of the internal capsule and the medial portion of the globus pallidus. Pseudobulbar mutism has also been described in patients with unilateral AChA territory infarcts involving the posterior limb of the capsule on one side and infarction involving the internal capsule on the contralateral side, but not in the territory of the AChA (Helgason *et al.* 1988).

Imaging and angiography

CT and MRI most often show infarcts in the territory of penetrating artery branches of the AChA. The lesions are usually in the posterior limb of the internal capsule and may extend into the medial globus pallidus. Figure 19.9 from Decroix *et al.* (1986) is a schematic representation of these deep infarcts. The lesions are usually near the lateral geniculate body just above and medial to the temporal horn of the lateral ventricle. Figure 19.10 shows CT scans of typical AChA territory deep infarcts. The medial

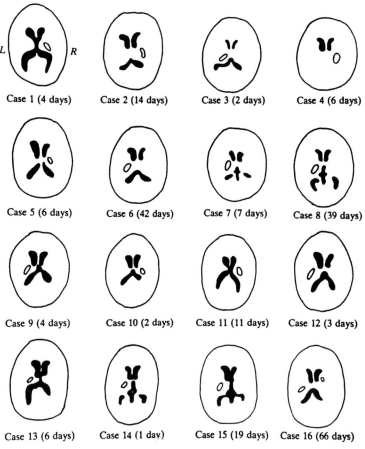

Fig. 19.9 Diagrams showing the lesions on CT scans among 16 patients with AChA territory infarcts. The interval between the onset of neurological symptoms and the CT scans are noted in parentheses. From Decroix *et al.* (1986) with permission.

temporal lobe and the lateral thalamus occasionally are involved. At times the infarcts extend to the periventricular region of the corona radiata.

In many patients, AChA territory infarction is accompanied by other infarcts in the distribution of carotid artery branches. Levy *et al.* (1995) performed a clinico-pathological study of 35 patients who were found at autopsy to have AChA territory infarcts. Most patients had CT scans that showed deep middle cerebral artery territory striatocapsular infarcts. Large hemispheral middle cerebral artery territory infarcts were common, and sometimes infarction extended into anterior cerebral artery territory. At autopsy, only two patients had infarcts limited to AChA territory, one bilateral; the remainder (94%) had AChA territory infarcts accompanied by middle cerebral and sometimes anterior cerebral artery territory infarcts. The commonest arterial finding was occlusion of the internal carotid artery (74%). The occlusion

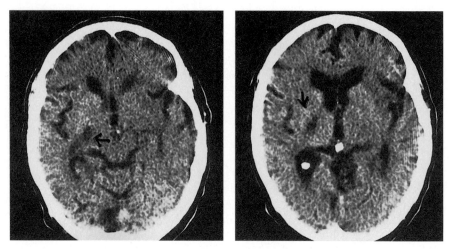

Fig. 19.10 CT scans show typical AChA territory deep infarcts (black arrows).

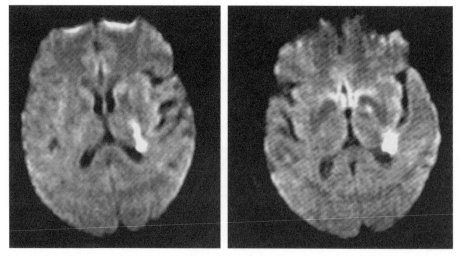

Fig. 19.11 Diffusion-weighted MRI scans from a patient with an AChA territory infarct caused by an occlusion of the internal carotid artery in the carotid siphon.

often involved the entire internal carotid artery or the intracranial portion, and often extended into the middle cerebral artery. Embolism (77%) was the most common mechanism of the carotid artery occlusions (Levy *et al.* 1995). AChA infarcts on neuroimaging always suggest the likelihood of internal carotid artery occlusion involving the intracranial portion of the artery. Figure 19.11 is an MRI of an AChA territory infarct in a patient with an internal carotid artery occlusion at the level of the carotid siphon.

In the angiographic study of Takahashi *et al.* (1990), the origin of the AChA was identified in all 216 patients studied. The origin was always just proximal to the intracranial termination of the internal carotid artery and distal to the origin of the posterior communicating artery. In some patients the internal carotid artery is occluded or stenosed intracranially. In others, the AChA is missing and presumably occluded. Sometimes an aneurysm of the internal carotid artery–AChA junction is accompanied by AChA territory infarction. In many cases of infarction limited to the penetrating artery branch territories of the AChA, the artery is patent on angiography.

Stroke mechanisms and treatment

The causes of AChA territory infarcts vary. The most common posited mechanism of infarction, especially when the infarcts are limited to the posterior limb of the internal capsule and the medial globus pallidus, is intrinsic disease of small penetrating artery branches of the AChA (Helgason *et al.* 1986, Bruno *et al.* 1989). Most patients have had hypertension and/or diabetes. Smoking has also been a common risk factor. Among 31 cases studied by Bruno *et al.* (1989), 28 (90%) infarcts were attributed to penetrating artery disease while one patient had intracranial carotid artery stenosis and two patients probably had cardiac origin embolism. Among 12 cases reviewed by Helgason *et al.* (1986) culled from the literature, seven were attributable to penetrating artery disease, four to cardiogenic embolism, and one to an aneurysm of the supraclinoid internal carotid artery. Helgason *et al.* (1986) also described two patients in whom the AChA had been injured during temporal lobectomy surgery for epilepsy, resulting in a post-operative hemiplegia.

Others have emphasized the frequency of embolism and internal carotid artery disease in the aetiology of AChA territory infarcts (Fisher *et al.* 1989, Mayer *et al.* 1992, Leys *et al.* 1994*a*, Levy *et al.* 1995). Carotid artery disease and brain embolism are especially likely when neuroimaging shows AChA + infarcts in one cerebral hemisphere (Levy *et al.* 1995). Leys *et al.* (1994*a*) studied stroke mechanisms among 16 patients with AChA territory infarcts, eight of which were limited to the deep territory of the AChA and eight which extended into the medial temporal lobe. Among the eight patients with medial temporal lobe infarction, seven had a deter-mined cause of stroke—cardioembolism in three, large artery atherosclerosis in two, and carotid artery dissection in two. Only two of the patients with deep infarction had stroke mechanisms defined by the evaluation. Among the eight with infarction limited to the deep territory, six were hypertensive. Hypertension was also present in four of the six patients whose stroke was attributed by the authors to cardiac origin embolism or large artery atherosclerosis (Leys *et al.* 1994*a*). Mayer *et al.* (1992) reported two patients with AChA territory infarcts who had an ipsilateral carotid artery occlusion. In one of these patients, the infarct was limited to the posterior limb of the internal capsule, while the other patient had a posterior limb capsular infarct as well as involvement of the medial temporal lobe. Fisher *et al.* (1989) reported two patients with AChA territory infarction who had carotid artery disease. One patient had a large ulcerated plaque located at the origin of the internal carotid artery and the AChA was occluded on angiography. The second patient had an internal carotid artery occlusion.

When infarction is limited to the posterior limb of the internal capsule and adjacent medial globus pallidus, the likelihood is high that the cause is small artery disease, especially if the patient is or has been hypertensive. When the infarct extends to the medial temporal lobe, and especially if there are co-existent infarcts in the territory of other carotid artery branches in the same hemisphere, then the likelihood of embolism or carotid artery disease is high. Some diabetics and those with hyperlipidaemia may have atheromatous branch infarcts (Caplan 1989).

Treatment should depend on the stroke mechanism found. Trouillas *et al.* (2000) studied the effectiveness of intravenous recombinant tissue plasminogen activator (rt-PA) thrombolysis among nine patients with AChA territory infarcts who were treated within 7 h of the onset of neurological symptoms. Seven of the nine had early recoveries within 6 h of the rt-PA infusion; recovery was complete in five and partial in two patients. Three patients developed recurrent symptoms and infarction 12, 25, and 48 h after treatment. Four of the patients reported by Trouillas *et al.* (2000) had potential cardiac sources of embolism, one had bilateral internal carotid artery stenosis in the neck, and one patient had an intracranial internal carotid artery stenosis within the siphon.

Heparin, coumarin, and antiplatelet aggregants have all been used, but the effectiveness of these drugs has not been formally studied.

Chapter 20

Internal watershed infarction

B.R. Chambers and C.F. Bladin

Introduction

Watershed infarction occurs in the borderzone between adjacent arterial perfusion beds and generally results from a critical reduction in perfusion pressure (Zülch 1961a, Romanul and Abramowicz 1964, Adams et al. 1966, Torvik and Jørgensen 1966, Torvik 1984). Other terms include 'borderzone', 'borderline', 'subcortical junctional', 'extraterritorial', 'distal field', 'terminal zone', and 'low-flow' infarction. Bilateral watershed infarction may occur following prolonged severe hypotension after cardiac arrest, but more commonly one sees unilateral infarction in association with carotid occlusive disease. In such patients, regional perfusion failure may result from myocardial infarction, cardiac arrhythmia, cardiac failure, orthostatic hypotension, blood loss, or other disorders producing systemic hypotension. Watershed infarction has also been associated with microemboli arising from carotid occlusion (Jørgensen and Torvik 1969, Torvik and Skullerud 1982), and there is experimental evidence that emboli of a certain size will find their way preferentially to arterial borderzones (Pollanen and Deck 1990).

Whilst most clinicians are familiar with the cortical borderzone regions of the cerebral and cerebellar hemispheres, some may not be aware that there are also internal borderzone regions. Although internal watershed infarction was described in the German literature decades ago (Zülch 1961b), it is only in recent years that attention has been drawn to this relatively common stroke syndrome (Ringelstein et al. 1983, Bogousslavsky and Regli 1986a,b, Bozzao et al. 1989, Angeloni et al. 1990, Waterston et al. 1990, Weiller et al. 1991, Bladin and Chambers 1993b, 1994), due largely to the advent of modern imaging techniques.

Vascular anatomy

Blood flow to each cerebral hemisphere derives mainly from three vessels, the anterior (ACA), middle (MCA), and posterior (PCA) cerebral arteries, and there are several excellent atlases illustrating their territories of supply (Salamon 1973, Matsui and Hirano 1978, Damasio 1983). The proximal segment of each vessel gives off a number of small-calibre, perforating arteries which supply the internal capsule and basal ganglia regions. The MCA trunk, with average length 16 mm (range 3–50 mm) and diameter 3–5 mm, has 6–20 small perforators of diameter less than 1 mm

(Herman *et al.* 1963, Jain 1964). Lateral lenticulostriate arteries supply the globus pallidus externa, body of caudate nucleus, putamen, and superolateral two-thirds of the anterior and posterior limbs of the internal capsule. Medial lenticulostriate arteries supply the globus pallidus interna. These vessels are end arteries, having no anastomotic connections.

The ACA, MCA, and PCA each course to the external surfaces of the cerebral hemisphere, to supply a branching network that constitutes the pial–arachnoidal circulation. The territories of supply of each of the major cerebral arteries are connected by anastomoses between arteries and arterioles (Van der Eecken and Adams 1953). From pial arteries, another system of penetrating vessels arises, plunging into the parenchyma of the cerebral hemisphere to supply subcortical white matter. Like the deep perforators arising from the proximal segments of the basal cerebral arteries, these medullary arteries and arterioles are long (20–50 mm), and have no anastomotic connections (Moody *et al.* 1990). The longest converge centripetally toward the angles of the lateral ventricles. The lower portion of the centrum semiovale therefore represents a borderzone between medullary vessels penetrating inward from the pial–arachnoidal circulation and deep penetrating arteries arising from the basal cerebral arteries. A reduction in perfusion pressure will compromise blood flow not only in cerebral cortex lying between the territories of supply of adjacent cerebral arteries, but also in this internal borderzone (Moody *et al.* 1990).

Classification of watershed infarcts

The most familiar watershed regions are the strips of cerebral cortex lying between the territories of supply of the major cerebral arteries. These are best referred to as external watersheds, and infarction that affects this territory as external watershed infarction (Table 20.1). Infarction in the watershed between the ACA and MCA produces a thin fronto-parasagittal wedge of infarction extending from the anterior horn of the lateral ventricle to the cortex (Romanul and Abramowicz 1964), so-called anterior watershed infarction (Fig. 20.1a), or a linear strip of infarction on the superior convexity of the cerebral hemisphere close to the sagittal sulcus, superior watershed infarction (Fig. 20.1b). Posteriorly, infarction in the watershed between the ACA, MCA, and PCA produces a temporo-parieto-occipital wedge of infarction extending from the occipital horn of the lateral ventricle to the cortex (Gastaut *et al.* 1971), posterior watershed infarction (Fig. 20.1a). The classical total watershed infarct involves a continuous strip of cerebral cortex, and underlying white matter, extending from the frontal pole and back along the convexity of the cerebral hemisphere in a parasagittal line to the occipital pole and then forward again along the inferior surface of the temporal lobe.

More commonly, watershed infarction involves the internal watershed region, lying in the centrum semiovale between the territories of supply of the medullary branches

Table 20.1 Classification of watershed infarcts

Type	Vessels involved
Hemisphere	
External	
Anterior	ACA, MCA
Superior	ACA, MCA
Posterior	MCA, PCA
Extensive	ACA, MCA, PCA
Internal	Medullary, deep
Confluent	
Partial	
Cerebellar	SCA, AICA, PICA

ACA = anterior cerebral artery; MCA = middle cerebral artery; PCA = posterior cerebral artery; medullary = penetrating branches of thr pial–arachnoidal plexus; deep = penetrating branches of basal cerebral arteries; SCA = superior cerebellar artery; AICA= anterior inferior cerebellar artery; PICA = posterior inferior cerebellar artery.

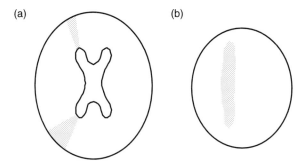

Fig. 20.1 Diagram of axial brain slices showing typical locations of (a) anterior and posterior watershed infarction and (b) superior watershed infarction.

of the superficial pial–arachnoidal plexus and the deep penetrating (or perforating) branches of the basal cerebral arteries. This zone includes the white matter lying alongside and slightly above the body of the lateral ventricles. Deep grey matter is spared. Some authors refer to these as terminal supply-area, low-flow, subcortical junctional, or subcortical watershed infarcts (Ringelstein *et al.* 1983, Weiller *et al.* 1991). Two patterns of infarction are recognized; confluent internal watershed infarction (CIWI) where there is an extensive area of involvement, and partial internal watershed infarction (PIWI) where there is a small discrete area of involvement (Fig. 20.2).

Watershed zones are also recognized between the territories of supply of the superior cerebellar artery (SCA), and the anterior (AICA) and posterior (PICA) inferior cerebellar arteries.

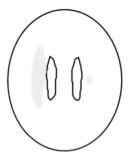

Fig. 20.2 Diagram of an axial brain slice at the level of the superior portions of the lateral ventricles showing typical locations of confluent and partial internal watershed infarction.

Frequency of occurrence

In autopsy series, watershed infarcts account for about 10 per cent of all brain infarctions (Jørgensen and Torvik 1969), but this is likely to underestimate the true incidence given that unilateral watershed infarction is seldom fatal.

In patients with stroke associated with carotid occlusion, computed tomography (CT) of the brain demonstrates a comparatively high proportion of cases with watershed infarction. Ringelstein *et al.* (1983) studied 107 patients with 111 carotid occlusions and 87 relevant infarcts on CT. There were eight (9%) with external watershed infarcts, and 36 (41%) with internal watershed infarcts. On the other hand, Bogousslavsky and Regli (1986*b*) found only eight cases of watershed infarction including two (1.3%) with internal watershed infarction in their series of 154 patients with symptomatic internal carotid artery (ICA) occlusion. However, during follow-up, 25 patients had a further CT-confirmed stroke, of whom 18 had watershed infarcts including four with internal watershed infarction (16%).

In our own study (Bladin and Chambers, 1993*b*, 1994), 18 (6%) of 300 consecutive stroke admissions had internal watershed infarction, including six with CIWI and 12 with PIWI. However, our stroke population was comprised mainly of war veterans and widows, and was therefore an older group compared with patients treated at most general hospitals.

Gandolfo *et al.* (1998) studied 383 consecutive patients with acute stroke and found a total of 725 infarcts of which 90 (12%) were in the internal borderzone. However, many of these infarcts were clinically silent and internal borderzone infarction as an isolated finding was only found in 13 (3.4%) patients. It is probable, however, that internal borderzone infarction was the incident event in at least some of those with multiple lesions.

Shuaib and Hachinski (1991) reviewed 116 published articles on stroke and found that watershed infarction was more common in the elderly, attributing this to increased postural hypotension, cardiac arrhythmias, and over-medication.

Imaging characteristics

Cranial CT shows internal watershed infarcts as paraventricular or supraventricular low density lesions in the white matter of the centrum semiovale (Wodarz 1980,

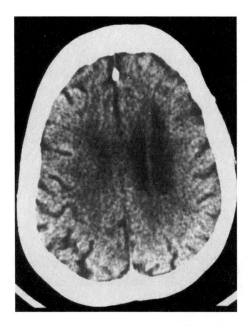

Fig. 20.3 Axial CT scan showing a confluent internal watershed infarction in the left coronal radiata.

Zülch 1985). Two main types are distinguished. Confluent internal watershed infarction (CIWI) represents a large cigar-shaped infarct extending the length of the lateral ventricle (Fig. 20.3). Partial internal watershed infarction (PIWI) produces smaller, single or multiple, discrete infarcts in the same zone (Fig. 20.4a). Multiple PIWIs form a linear chain of lesions in the internal watershed zone (Fig. 20.4b). Magnetic resonance imaging (MRI) scans (Fig. 20.5) show similar changes (Weiller *et al.* 1991, Yamauchi *et al.* 1991), and Krapf *et al.* (1998) emphasized the significance of multiple small rosary-like infarctions in the centrum semiovale, as a sign of haemodynamic failure due to severe carotid disease. However, MRI often shows discrete high intensity abnormalities in subcortical white matter on T_2-weighted images not corresponding with CT abnormalities (Yamauchi *et al.* 1991). In the acute setting, diffusion-weighted imaging is helpful in differentiating acute infarcts from ischaemic white matter hyperintensities.

PIWI is sometimes lumped together with other types of small centrum ovale infarction (Bogousslavsky and Regli 1992, Lammie and Wardlaw 1999) and is commonly mistaken for corona radiata lacunar infarction. Lacunar infarction, resulting from occlusion of a single perforating artery, generally occurs in the basal ganglia and internal capsule but may also occur in the corona radiata (Donnan *et al.* 1982). PIWI generally occurs at a slightly higher plane (Fig. 20.6) and the lesions are usually larger with indistinct margins (Read *et al.* 1998*a*).

White matter medullary infarcts are small immediately subcortical infarcts due to occlusion of medullary penetrators arising from the pial–arachnoid plexus

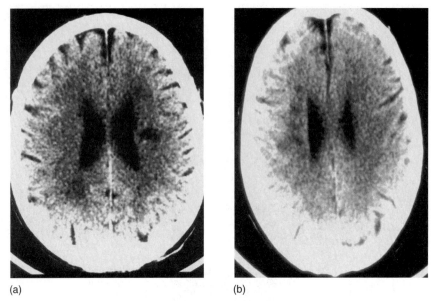

(a)   (b)

Fig. 20.4 Axial CT scans showing partial internal watershed infarction: (a) a single PIWI in the left coronal radiata; (b) multiple PIWIs lying in a chain in the right corona radiata.

(Bogousslavsky and Regli 1992). These can be difficult to distinguish from PIWI but are generally more superficial (Fig. 20.6) and smaller (Read *et al.* 1998*a*).

Striatocapsular infarction also occurs at a deeper plane to PIWI, involving both the internal capsule and deep grey matter in the distribution of multiple deep perforating arteries, in both proximal and distal parts of their territory. On CT, the lesion frequently is comma shaped. These infarcts are caused by embolic occlusion of the MCA trunk (Bladin and Berkovic 1984, Weiller *et al.* 1990, Donnan *et al.* 1991), but overlying cortex remains viable because of effective pial collateral. On CT and MRI, the margins are usually well defined.

PIWI must also be distinguished from periventricular lucency (PVL), or leukoaraiosis (Hachinski *et al.* 1987), representing chronic, diffuse white matter ischaemia, which produces a more diffuse white matter change. PIWI and PVL may co-exist, however, particularly in the elderly.

Clinical features

Most patients with CIWI present with a fluctuating but progressive neurological deficit (Bladin and Chambers 1993*b*). Dizziness and collapse are prominent prodromal symptoms. The clinical deficit consists of either hemiparesis, hemisensory loss, or both, and focal cortical signs. Focal limb shaking may occur (Baquis *et al.* 1985, Yanagihara *et al.* 1985).

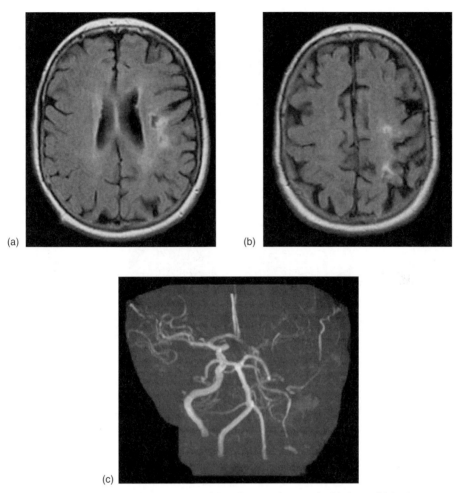

Fig. 20.5 MRI flare images showing PIWIs (a) and external watershed infarcts (b) in the same patient in association with MRA showing trickle flow in the left ICA (c).

In contrast, only two-thirds of patients with PIWI describe dizziness or give a history of collapse (Bladin and Chambers 1993*b*). The clinical features are more diverse. The predominant picture is a facio-brachial motor and sensory deficit with focal cortical signs on either clinical examination or neuropsychological assessment (Bogousslavsky and Regli 1986*a,b*, Waterston *et al.* 1990, Bladin and Chambers 1993*b*, Staaf *et al.* 1998). The motor deficit can vary from mild clumsiness to overt paresis. Dominant hemisphere lesions produce language disorders, and non-dominant lesions produce hemineglect. Transcortical aphasia is an interesting association (Bogousslavsky *et al.* 1988*d*).

Many patients with PIWI present with features similar to the 'dysarthria–clumsy hand' lacunar syndrome (Fisher 1967). However, dysarthria and hand incoordination

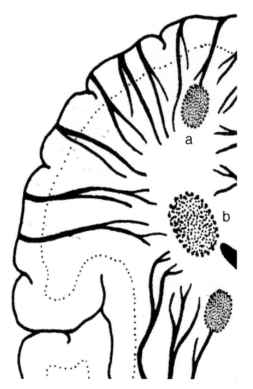

Fig. 20.6 Diagram illustrating the distinction between white matter medullary infarction (a), partial internal watershed infarction (b), and lacunar infarction (c). From Read *et al.* (1998*a*) with permission.

are accompanied by sensory symptoms and signs of focal cortical dysfunction (Bladin and Chambers 1993*b*). If such a clinical deficit is encountered in a patient who also describes syncopal symptoms at the time of stroke, then PIWI should be strongly considered and the patient investigated for carotid pathology or haemodynamic problems.

Internal watershed infarction may be clinically silent. Ringelstein *et al.* (1983) noted that of 36 cases of CT-diagnosed internal watershed ('terminal supply area') infarcts, two had no deficit, 18 had one or more transient ischaemic attacks (TIAs) or minor strokes, four had progressive stroke, five had completed stroke with premonitory attacks, and seven had completed stroke without premonitory attacks. Motor deficit was absent in two, slight in 24, and major in 10.

Pathogenesis

Internal watershed infarction usually results from haemodynamic insufficiency due to vascular obstruction and superimposed systemic hypotension (Bladin and Chambers

1993*b*, 1994). The reduction in perfusion pressure can be transient and seemingly benign, for example orthostatic hypotension. Prolific vomiting accounts for some cases. Valsalva during vomiting produces a temporary fall in venous return to the heart with a fall in cardiac output. Vomiting may also cause vagal atrio-ventricular blockade, as with cough and micturition syncope. More common are cardiac arrhythmias, often paroxysmal, and cardiomyopathies that prevent a rise in cardiac output during exertion. Internal watershed infarction also occurs in association with operative hypotension and may complicate carotid endarterectomy (CEA). There were two cases of internal watershed infarction among the 34 cases of CT-confirmed post-CEA cerebral infarction in the series of Krul *et al.* (1989), assumed to be haemodynamic in origin on the basis of EEG changes during carotid clamping.

In our series (Bladin and Chambers 1993*b*, 1994), we demonstrated vascular obstruction (occlusion or severe stenosis) and factors causing systemic hypotension in 33 per cent of patients. Another 28 per cent had vascular obstruction without a demonstrable haemodynamic insult, and 39 per cent had a haemodynamic insult but no significant vascular pathology. Subsequent experience suggests that up to 25 per cent have neither vascular obstruction nor demonstrable systemic hypotension. In the study by Gandolfo *et al.* (1998), 62 per cent of patients with internal borderzone infarction had carotid strenosis or occlusion compared with 31 per cent for other stroke subtypes.

Watershed infarction has been studied in the two large symptomatic carotid endarterectomy trials, ECST (Hupperts *et al.* 1997*a*) and NASCET (Del Sette *et al.* 2000). Pre-randomization CT scans were examined for watershed infarcts which were correlated with ipsilateral carotid stenosis. In ECST, all categories of watershed infarcts were included and the trend for watershed infarction to occur more often distal to severe carotid disease was not significant. In NASCET, 413 patients had visible ischaemic lesions ipsilateral to their symptomatic carotid stenosis. Of these, 138 had perforator infarcts, 108 had internal borderzone infarcts, 122 had cortical infarcts, and 45 had a combination. Sixty-three per cent of patients with internal borderzone infarcts had 70–99 per cent carotid stenosis, compared with 42 per cent of patients with perforator infarcts. Patients with carotid occlusion were not included in either study. Hennerici *et al.* (1998) also found a relationship between subcortical borderzone infarction and carotid stenosis in their retrospective review of cases selected from the Nimodipine European Stroke Trial; however, they questioned the concept that stroke mechanisms can be inferred from infarct patterns. Internal watershed infarction has also been associated with carotid artery dissection (Steinke *et al.* 1996).

What is the pathogenesis in patients without carotid obstruction or systemic hypotension? Embolic occlusion of the MCA beyond the origin of the lenticulostriate arteries accounts for some cases (Bozzao *et al.* 1989, Angeloni *et al.* 1990, Baird *et al.* 1991). This is uncommon in our experience, and Ringelstein *et al.* (1989) had no cases of internal watershed infarction among their 60 cases of cardioembolic stroke.

Patency of the lenticulostriate arteries ensures the viability of the internal capsule and basal ganglia. ACA- and PCA-derived pial collateral preserves overlying cortex and a variable part of the subcortical white matter. In the Italian study (Bozzao *et al.* 1989, Angeloni *et al.* 1990), seven of 36 patients with MCA occlusion demonstrated by angiography within 6 h of ictus had internal watershed infarction. One had occlusion of the MCA just distal to the lenticulostriate origins, three distal to the temporal pial branch origin, and three affecting peripheral pial branches. All had good pial collateral. None had more proximal stenoses. Increasing application of transoesophageal echocardiography to detect cardiac embolic sources (Pop *et al.* 1990) may increase the number of cases of internal watershed infarction attributed to emboli. Caplan *et al.* (1985) illustrated that PIWI can occur with proximal MCA stenosis, and Horowitz *et al.* (1991) showed that it can occur with proximal MCA occlusion.

Small vessel disease caused by hypertension, diabetes, or amyloid accumulation, and involving both deep penetrating arteries and pial-derived medullary arteries, is possibly the most frequent cause of internal watershed infarction not associated with carotid obstruction and systemic hypotension. CT and MRI may reveal associated findings of PVL (leukoaraiosis) or lacunar infarction in some patients. Diffuse small vessel disease is the postulated mechanism for leukoaraiosis (Hachinski *et al.* 1987) and PVL embraces the internal watershed zones. Patchy involvement of small vessels could give rise to internal watershed infarction without CT appearances of diffuse ischaemia.

Regionally impaired autoregulation probably plays an integral role in pathogenesis of all cases of internal watershed infarction. In normals, autoregulation maintains reasonably constant cerebral blood flow (CBF) despite changes in perfusion pressure, within mean arterial blood pressure (MABP) limits of 60–150 mmHg (Strandgaard and Paulson 1984). In chronic hypertension, the autoregulation curve is right-shifted. Whereas normals tolerate a drop in MABP from 100 to 60 mmHg, chronic hypertensives may suffer a fall in CBF. In the presence of small vessel disease secondary to hypertension, diabetes, or amyloid angiopathy, the limits of autoregulation are likely to be narrower, and, in the worst cases, autoregulatory responsiveness may be abolished. Minor falls in MABP, easily tolerated by healthy individuals, can produce symptomatic cerebral ischaemia in elderly patients with impaired autoregulation (Wollner *et al.* 1979).

Bogousslavsky and Regli (1986*a,b*) examined risk factors in patients with unilateral watershed infarcts and emphasized the importance of vascular obstruction, highlighting a high prevalence of contralateral carotid stenosis, and heart disease. Forty-two per cent had syncope at the time of stroke. They also cited elevated haematocrit and smoking as other important factors. Smoking, in addition to accelerating atherogenesis, causes nicotine-mediated vasoconstriction, increased viscosity through elevation of haematocrit, and a reduction in the oxygen-carrying capacity of the blood, all of which may be factors contributing to subcortical ischaemia (Donnan *et al.* 1989).

Diabetes was also prevalent in our series (Bladin and Chambers 1993*b*). Diabetic autonomic neuropathy produces orthostatic hypotension, and diabetic small vessel disease involving both deep and superficial perforating arteries causes chronic ischaemia and autoregulation failure, as discussed above.

In another series of 493 consecutive stroke or TIA cases (Mounier-Vehier *et al.* 1994), 26 had external and 18 had internal watershed infarcts. Patients with external watershed infarcts were more likely to have severe carotid stenosis and hypertension than those without watershed infarcts, whilst those with internal watershed infarcts were more likely to have heart disease. However, these findings are not supported by other studies.

Blood flow studies

Investigation of intracranial haemodynamics with inhaled 133Xe, positron emission tomography (PET), single photon emission computed tomography (SPECT), transcranial Doppler (TCD), and, more recently, MRI, distinguishes internal watershed infarction associated with carotid occlusion from other forms of ischaemic stroke including cerebral embolism and lacunar infarction. Several studies (Skyhoj Olsen *et al.* 1986, Perani *et al.* 1987, Hojer-Pedersen and Petersen 1989, Baird *et al.* 1991, Weiller *et al.* 1991) have shown reduced regional cerebral blood flow (rCBF) and cerebral perfusion reserve (Gibbs *et al.* 1984), involving an area far greater than the area of CT abnormality, consistent with the clinical presentation of combined motor, sensory, and focal cortical involvement.

Weiller *et al.* (1991) studied 17 patients with internal watershed infarction ('low-flow infarcts'), selected on the basis of CT patterns, and severe stenosis or occlusion of the ICA (or MCA in one patient) using SPECT and TCD. They compared the results with 20 patients with territorial infarcts (12 with occluded ipsilateral carotid artery, eight with cardiogenic embolism), and controls. Blood flow, measured 3–4 weeks after onset of symptoms, was reduced in patients with territorial and internal watershed infarcts, to the greatest degree in territorial infarcts with carotid occlusion. Perfusion reserve was normal in territorial infarcts due to cardiac embolism, reduced 14 per cent in territorial infarcts with vascular occlusion, and reduced 30 per cent in patients with internal watershed infarcts, again in an area far greater than the area of CT abnormality. Carbon dioxide (CO_2) reactivity, measured 5–6 weeks after onset of symptoms by TCD, revealed almost a 60 per cent reduction in reactivity in patients with internal watershed infarcts.

Yamauchi *et al.* (1991) used MRI and SPECT to study 16 patients with TIA or stroke and carotid stenosis or occlusion. All patients had abnormalities on T_2-weighted MRI but only five had a confluent high-intensity area in the middle centrum semiovale consistent with discrete ischaemic damage. PET studies revealed significantly decreased rCBF, oxygen metabolism ($CMRO_2$), and CBF/CBV ratio, and increased oxygen extraction (OEF) in this subgroup. Increased OEF is regarded as a sign of misery perfusion. Earlier, they had shown that nine patients with minor strokes and carotid occlusion had decreased rCBF and CBF/CBV ratio and increased OEF in the distribution of the MCA and surrounding watershed areas compared with eight control subjects (Yamauchi *et al.* 1990*b*). The same group showed that the confluent high-intensity area on T_2-weighted MRI images contained increased CBV consistent with compensatory vasodilatation (Yamauchi *et al.* 1990*a*). More recently (Yamauchi *et al.* 1996), this group has studied 40 patients with symptomatic ICA or MCA occlusive disease with PET, and shown that those patients with an ipsilateral increase in OEF had a higher incidence of recurrent stroke, mostly watershed infarction, within the next 12 months.

Weiller *et al.* (1991) claim that internal watershed infarcts do not occur in a haemodynamically intact hemisphere, but they selected cases with carotid or MCA occlusion. In our experience, there is a subset without significant compromise of flow in major supply arteries. This subset has not been formally evaluated with PET or SPECT. Our own experience with TCD reveals normal MCA velocity, pulsatility index, and CO_2 responsiveness (unpublished data).

Sorteberg *et al.* (1996) used TCD to assess 63 patients with symptomatic carotid obstructive disease, dividing them into watershed and other infarct groups. The watershed infarct group showed lower MCA velocity and pulsatility index (compared with the PCA), U_{hem} index ($U_{hem} = V_{MCA} \times PI_{MCA}/V_{PCA} \times PI_{PCA}$), and CO_2 vasomotor reactivity than the other infarct group. In individual patients, a reduced U_{hem} index was the only differentiating factor.

Moriwaki *et al.* (1997) assessed rCBF and perfusion reserve with SPECT coupled with acetazolamide in 29 patients with supratentorial watershed infarcts among 96 patients with severe carotid stenosis occlusion. The 22 patients with internal watershed infarcts had significantly lower perfusion reserve compared with the seven patients with external watershed infarcts. Furthermore, perfusion reserve was lower in those patients with deeper infarcts.

Van der Grond *et al.* (1999) used MRI, magnetic resonance angiography (MRA), and magnetic resonance spectroscopy (MRS) to study 34 patients with borderzone infarcts, 16 patients with territory infarcts, and 16 patients with no infarcts. Patients with borderzone infarcts had reduced flow in the ICA and MCA and decreased *N*-acetyl-L-aspartate (NAA)/choline in non-infarcted regions, consistent with chronic hypoperfusion, compared with controls and patients with territorial infarcts. There was no comparison made between external and internal borderzone infarcts.

Chaves *et al.* (2000), in their MRI diffusion-weighted (DWI) and perfusion-weighted (PWI) study of 17 patients with borderzone infarction, were able to divide them into three groups based on PWI patterns. Seven patients had extensive perfusion deficits and all had severe stenosis or occlusion of a large feeding vessel. Five had normal perfusion and most of these had transient systemic hypotension at the time of stroke. Five had PWI deficits corresponding to localized DWI deficits and, in this group, there were two patients with a proximal embolic source, and none with carotid obstruction. Although this study included patients with external and internal watershed infarcts, the proportions of patients in each pathogenic category were similar to our study (Bladin and Chambers 1993*b*).

Prognosis

The neurological deficit in CIWI is usually severe, and many patients are left with major motor disability. Only three of six patients in our series (Bladin and Chambers 1993*b*) achieved independence in self-care. In contrast, the majority of patients with PIWI make an excellent recovery with minor or no residual incapacity. Ten of 12 patients in our series recovered to full independence.

Long-term prognosis depends upon the underlying pathological mechanisms, and whether or not these can be corrected. Without interventions, these patients are prone to repeated events, and in some of our patients with repeated events, sequential CT showed progression from single to multiple PIWI, and from PIWI to CIWI.

Bogousslavsky and Regli (1986*b*) found that their group of patients with carotid occlusion and unilateral watershed infarcts had a similar rate of recurrent stroke but higher mortality compared with patients with carotid occlusion and other types of stroke. All deaths were cardiac.

Prophylaxis

As with all forms of stroke, successful prophylaxis depends upon identification and treatment of the underlying pathological mechanisms. Carotid duplex scanning should be performed routinely and, where severe carotid stenosis is identified, CEA merits consideration. However, in many cases, the ICA is occluded or the stenosis is surgically inaccessible, as in carotid siphon or MCA stenosis. One should assume that there is also intermittent systemic perfusion failure, for example caused by orthostatic hypotension, or other problems such as paroxysmal arrhythmias. For most of the time, these patients have adequately compensated cerebrovascular disease. They become symptomatic when transient systemic hypotension drops the CBF below threshold.

Twenty-four hour Holter monitoring identifies clinically occult cardiac arrhythmias, preventable by anti-arrhythmic drugs or electrical pacing. Sick sinus syndrome is of particular importance, giving rise to tacchyarrhythmias and bradyarrhythmias. A 2 or 3 day chart of lying and standing blood pressure identifies patients with orthostatic hypotension. In addition, 24 h blood pressure monitoring may prove enlightening. Orthostatic hypotension without a change in pulse rate should prompt further investigation for autonomic failure. Salt loading, fludrocortisone, indomethacin, caffeine, elasticized stockings, and sleeping in the head-up position are among a number of symptomatic treatments. In most patients, however, orthostatic hypotension is iatrogenic. Drugs most commonly implicated are diuretics, calcium antagonists, methyl dopa, vasodilators especially prazosin, tricyclic antidepressants, and prochlorperazine. Prochlorperazine ironically exacerbates the dizziness for which it is erroneously prescribed.

Angiotensin-converting enzyme inhibitors are the antihypertensive drugs of choice for patients with chronic cerebral ischaemia and hypertension, having the least propensity to orthostatic hypotension. Particularly in the elderly, a compromise between optimal blood pressure control and adequate cerebral perfusion is often necessary in the acute phase.

Tilt-table testing with isoprenaline challenge (Almquist *et al.* 1989) is often diagnostic in patients with a typical history of syncope or near syncope, without obvious explanation. This detects hyperactive myocardial mechanoreceptor reflex activity, treated effectively by vagolytic or β-blocker drugs (Abboud 1989).

Advice to quit smoking is especially important in this group. Cessation of smoking improves oxygenation of the blood, lowers haematocrit, reduces blood viscosity, reduces fibrinogen levels, increases CBF, and may allow repair of vessel damage. Binge drinkers should moderate their alcohol consumption, as a contracted blood volume predisposes to cerebral ischaemia. All our patients are prescribed antiplatelet therapy unless there is some contraindication.

Patients with demonstrated potential sources of embolism also require specific therapy. CEA should be considered for significant carotid arterial lesions, particularly those with radiological evidence of ulceration or thrombus. Anticoagulation is recommended for chronic atrial fibrillation and suspected left atrial clot, rheumatic valvular disease, mural thrombus post-myocardial infarction, and other cardiac pathology that may give rise to emboli.

Chapter 21

Thalamic infarcts

G.R. de Freitas and J. Bogousslavsky

Introduction

Infarcts restricted to the thalamus account for 11 per cent of vertebrobasilar infarcts, and the thalamus is involved in 27 per cent of vertebrobasilar infarcts (Bogousslavsky *et al.* 1988*b*). While the thalamus is involved in about one-third of patients with basilar artery occlusion (Labauge *et al.* 1981), 10–20 per cent of patients with embolism distal to the middle third of the basilar artery may have isolated thalamic infarcts (Goto *et al.* 1979, Fisher 1986). In 1958, Façon *et al.* reported the 'syndrome of the basilar artery bifurcation' or 'top of the basilar syndrome' resulting from distal basilar artery occlusion, and emphasized that it was always associated with thalamic involvement, a finding that has since been confirmed (Caplan 1980, Sato *et al.* 1987, Barkhof and Valk 1988, Mehler 1989). In addition, about one-third of patients with occipital infarction show associated thalamic infarction (Bogousslavsky *et al.* 1981, Georgiadis *et al.* 1999), which can be in any of the arterial territories of the thalamus (Henderson *et al.* 1982, Louarn *et al.* 1986, Hommel *et al.* 1990*b*, Chambers *et al.* 1991).

In contrast to most other deep infarcts, thalamic infarcts can result in a multitude of diverse neurological disturbances, with the result that they are commonly misdiagnosed or overlooked before imaging. The first cases with appropriate clinical diagnoses verified by autopsy were probably reported by Jules Dejérine (Fig. 21.1) at the Société de Neurologie in Paris, 2 April 1903. This was before the publication in 1906 of the pioneering paper by Dejérine and Gustave Roussy and its discussion by Pierre Marie (Dejérine and Roussy 1906, Marie 1906), in which the term 'thalamic syndrome' replaced that of 'syndrome of the capsular sensory crossing of Charcot' (De Smet 1986). Although earlier reports had already addressed this issue (Dejérine and Long 1898, Dejérine and Egger 1903, Chinny 1904, Dide and Durocher 1904, Thomas and Chiray 1904), Dejérine and Roussy provided such a good description of the characteristics of the 'thalamic syndrome' that, since this time, the association of (i) slight and regressive hemiparesis; (ii) hemianaesthesia as the most common deep sensory change; (iii) hemiataxia and astereognosia; (iv) often persisting or paroxysmal pain and occasional hyperaesthesia; and (v) choreoathetotic movements has been referred to as Dejérine–Roussy syndrome. It is important to emphasize that, in the three clinico-anatomical cases reported by Dejérine and Roussy, the infarct was not

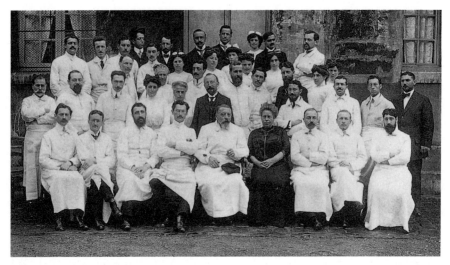

Fig. 21.1 Jules Dejérine (first row, fifth from the left) and his wife among his staff at La Salpêtrière in 1911. The author's great uncle Henri Laugier, fourth successor to Claude Bernard at the chair of General Physiology at La Sorbonne, is second left in the last row.

limited to the thalamus, but extended through the adjacent internal capsule toward the medial aspect of the putamen. Since the early descriptions, several other syndromes have been reported to result from thalamic infarction; these have been reviewed by Foix and Hillemand (1925), Martin (1970), Lapresle and Haguenau (1973), Cambier *et al.* (1982), Verret and Lapresle (1986), Graff-Radford *et al.* (1985*a*) and Bogousslavsky *et al.* (1988*a*).

Arterial supply to the thalamus

The arterial supply to the thalamus (Figs 21.2 and 21.4) can be divided into four main arterial territories, which are supplied mainly by the vertebrobasilar system (Duret 1874, Foix and Hillemand 1925, Gillilan 1968, Percheron 1973, Schlesinger 1976, Castaigne *et al.* 1981, Bogousslavsky *et al.* 1988*a*, Caruso *et al.* 1990):

(1) the polar (or tuberothalamic, anterior paramedian thalamo-subthalamic, premamillary or anterior internal optic) territory;

(2) the paramedian (or posterior paramedian thalamo-subthalamic, thalamo-perforate, or posterior internal optic) territory;

(3) the inferolateral (or thalamogeniculate or infero-external optic) territory; and

(4) the posterior choroidal territory.

Within the thalamus, there are rectangular ramifications of the larger branches, which run in parallel, mainly in the white matter, so that tracts in the white matter are likely to be affected by ischaemia (Büttner 1960, Plets *et al.* 1970).

(a)   (b)

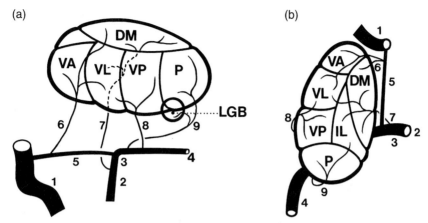

Fig. 21.2 Arterial supply to the thalamus: (a) lateral view; (b) view from above.
DM = dorsomedial nucleus; VA = ventral arterial nucleus; VL = ventral lateral nucleus;
VP = ventra posterior nucleus; P = pulvinar; IL = intralaminar nuclei; LGB = lateral geniculate
body; 1 = carotid syphon; 2 = basilar artery; 3 = P1 segment of the posterior cerebral artery; 4
= P2 segment of the posterior cerebral artery; 5 = posterior communicating artery; 6 = polar
artery; 7 = paramedian arteries; 8 = inferolateral arteries; 9 = posterior choroidal arteries.

Polar territory

There is usually one polar artery per hemisphere which originates from the middle
third of the posterior communicating artery or, more rarely (4%), from the P1
segment of the posterior cerebral artery (Percheron 1976, Pedroza *et al.* 1987*a,b*). A
hypothalamic–fornical branch and the peduncle-subthalamic artery originate from
the posterior communicating artery at the same level as the polar artery. However, in
approximately one-third of hemispheres, there is no polar artery, and the
corresponding territory is supplied by the paramedian arteries (Percheron 1976,
Castaigne *et al.* 1981).

Paramedian territory

There are mesencephalic branches, which supply the rostral midbrain at the level of
the posterior commissure, and thalamic branches, which originate from the P1
segment of the posterior cerebral artery. Usually, the paramedian branches originate
symmetrically (type I), but, in up to one-third of brains, there is a common unilateral
pedicle, which supplies both paramedian territories (type II) (Percheron 1976,
Castaigne *et al.* 1981).

Inferolateral territory

There are usually 5–6 small branches, which originate from the P2 segment of the
posterior cerebral artery, together with smaller thalamic branches (lateral geniculate
artery, medial geniculate artery, and inferior pulvinar artery). In fewer than

one-quarter of cases, their origin may be more distal along the posterior cerebral artery (Milisavljevic *et al.* 1991).

Posterior choroidal territory

The posteromedial and posterolateral choroidal arteries also originate from the P2 segment of the posterior cerebral artery. The posteromedial choroidal system can be divided into dorsal (medial pulvinar artery and superomedial artery) and ventral (lateral mesencephalo-thalamic artery, inferocentral artery, medial geniculate artery, posterocentral artery, and brachiopulvinar artery) portions, while the posterolateral choroidal system is less well characterized (lateral geniculate artery, inferolateral pulvinar artery, and superolateral artery) (Percheron 1977).

Nuclear supply

The respective distribution of the four main thalamic arterial groups to the thalamic nuclei and tracts is summarized in Figs 21.3 and 21.4.

Contribution of other arterial groups

The anterior choroidal artery provides very little supply, if any, to the thalamus (the most posterolateral region) (Percheron 1973, Castaigne *et al.* 1981). Since this artery

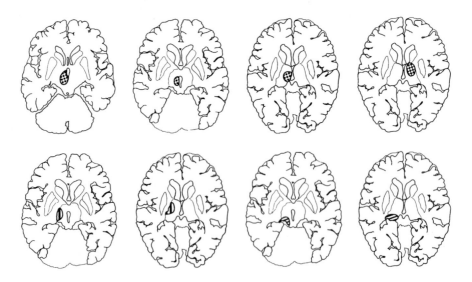

▦	Posterior thalamo-subthalamic paramedian arteries *thalamo-perforate*
▦	Anterior thalamo-subthalamic paramedian arteries *tuberothalamic or polar*
▥	Infero-lateral arteries *thalamo-geniculate*
▨	Posterior choroidal arteries

Fig. 21.3 Schematic transverse slices with arterial territories of the thalamus.

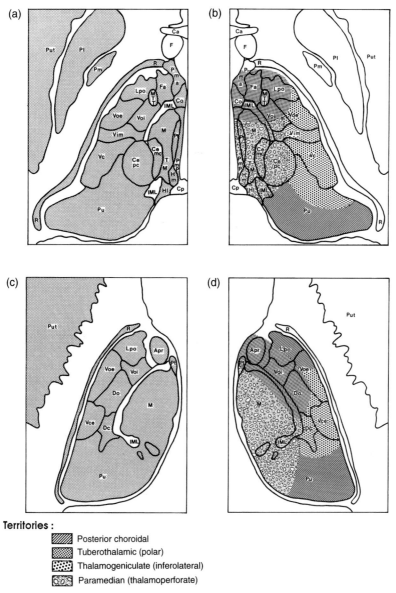

Territories :

▨ Posterior choroidal
▦ Tuberothalamic (polar)
▨ Thalamogeniculate (inferolateral)
▨ Paramedian (thalamoperforate)

Fig. 21.4 Detailed relationship between arterial territories and nuclear subgroups within the thalamus (after Von Cramon *et al.* 1985). R = reticular nuclei; Co = commissural nuclei; Lpo = N. lateropolaris; Vim = N. ventro-oralis intermedius; Voi = N. ventro-oralis internus; M = N. dorsomedialis; Pmp = N. paramedianus posterior; Cepc = N. centralis parvocellularis; MTM = tract of Meynert; Hl = N. habenularis lateralis; Pu = pulvinar; Pma = N. paramedianus anterior; Fa = N. fascicularis; Voe = N. ventro-oralis externus; Vc = N. ventrocaudalis; MTT = mamillo-thalamic tract; Pt = N. parataenialis; Cemc = N. centralis magnocellularis; IML = internal medullary lamina; Hm = N. habenularis medialis; Dc = N. dorsocaudalis; Apr = N. anterior principalis; Put = putamen; Pl = pallidum (lateral); Pm = pallidum (medial).

sometimes originates from the posterior communicating artery (instead of the carotid siphon), infarcts involving both the polar thalamic territory and anterior choroidal artery occasionally can occur (Bogousslavsky *et al.* 1988*a*). The middle cerebral artery gives off a few capsular branches, which irrigate the reticular nucleus of the thalamus and the external medullary lamina.

Collateral system

The thalamic arteries classically have been considered perforating end arteries without mutual anastomoses of functional importance (Plets *et al.* 1970). However, recent microsurgical work has suggested that up to two-thirds of cases may demonstrate well-formed anastomoses, especially between the inferolateral and posterior choroidal networks and between the inferolateral and paramedian networks (Marinkovic *et al.* 1986, Milisavljevic *et al.* 1991). These findings may be important in discussing the embolic versus microangiopathic aetiologies of thalamic infarction.

Aetiology of thalamic infarcts

The sex ratio, mean age, and age range do not differ from those seen in stroke in general (Bogousslavsky *et al.* 1988*a,b*). The prevalence of the main risk factors (hypertension, diabetes, cigarette smoking, and hypercholesterolaemia) is also similar.

Reported causes of thalamic infarcts are listed in Table 21.1. The relative proportion of the main causes in consecutive cases has been studied in only one report (Bogousslavsky *et al.* 1988*a*), in which the main cause was found to be small artery disease (14/40), followed by large artery atheroma (7/40), cardioembolism (5/40), and migraine stroke (4/40). This study confirmed that thalamic infarcts may often be 'lacunar' (i.e. due to *in situ* occlusion of a perforator), but it also showed that the proportion of lacunar strokes may have been overestimated in previous studies of thalamic infarct. Except in the case of bilateral paramedian infarcts, which were highly suggestive of cardioembolism, involvement of one of the main arterial territories of the thalamus was not associated with a particular cause of stroke. The higher frequency of cardioembolism and lower frequency of small artery disease seen compared with other topographical forms of subcortical infarct (deep middle cerebral artery territory) may result from the presence of reciprocal collaterals in the thalamic territory, but not in the other subcortical territories: several embolic occlusions often may be necessary to produce thalamic infarction, which might be less likely to develop when a single penetrator is occluded as a result of *in situ* disease. Thus, the rule that occlusion of a single penetrator will produce a small infarct corresponding to its specific territory may not apply to many thalamic infarcts, as a high proportion of thalamic arterioles are not end arteries. Transient ischaemic attack (TIA) prior to infarction is not very common (15%) and does not suggest a particular potential cause of stroke (Bogousslavsky *et al.* 1988*a*).

Table 21.1 Causes of thalamic infarction

Small artery disease	
associated with diabetes	Elghozi *et al.* (1979), Cohen *et al.* (1980), Jankovic and Patel (1983), Bogousslavsky *et al.* (1988a), Gorelick *et al.* (1988), Reilly *et al.* (1992)
or with hypertension with/without diabetes	Fisher (1969, 1978a), Mohr *et al.* (1977), Büttner-Ennever *et al.* (1982), Pierrot-Deseilligny *et al.* (1982), Guberman and Stuss (1983), Landi *et al.* (1984), Gorsselink and Lodder (1985), Gerber and Gudesblatt (1986), Roßberg and Mennel (1986), Meissner *et al.* (1987), Bogousslavsky *et al.* (1988a), Gutrecht *et al.* (1992), Baumgartner and Regard (1993), Kulisevsky *et al.* (1993b), Milandre *et al.* (1993), Ott and Saver (1993), Pepin and Auray-Pepin (1993), Sharp *et al.* (1994), Solomon *et al.* (1994), Ghika *et al.* (1995), Hashimoto *et al.* (1995), Sodeyama *et al.* (1995), del Mar Sáez de Ocariz *et al.* (1996), Kim (1996), Anastosopoulos and Bronstein (1999), Kim *et al.* (1999), Soler *et al.* (1999), Versino *et al.* (1999)
Cardioembolism	Halmagyi *et al.* (1978), Trojanowski and Wray (1980), Castaigne *et al.* (1981), Smith and Laguna (1981), Trojanowski and Lafontaine (1981), Kessler *et al.* (1982), Speedie and Heilman (1982), Bewermeyer *et al.* (1985), Biller *et al.* (1985), Gorelick *et al.* (1985), Powers (1985), Swanson and Schmidley (1985), Rondot *et al.* (1986), Bogousslavsky *et al.* (1988a, 1991), Graff-Radford *et al.* (1990), Levasseur *et al.* (1992), Reilly *et al.* (1992), Baumgartner and Regard (1993), Ceccaldi and Milandre (1994), Shuren *et al.* (1994), Clark and Alberts (1995), Bassetti *et al.* (1996), del Mar Sáez de Ocariz *et al.* (1996), Müller *et al.* (1999).
Large artery (BA or PCA) atherosclerosis	Castaigne *et al.* (1962, 1991), Sieben *et al.* (1977), Goto *et al.* (1979), Gorelick *et al.* (1985), Bogousslavsky *et al.* (1988a), Baumgartner *et al.* (1994), Nadeau *et al.* (1994), Clark and Alberts (1995), del Mar Sáez de Ocariz *et al.* (1996), Lee *et al.* (1998).
Toxic angiopathy (metamphetamine, ethyl -phenyl-isopropyl- amphetamine, cocaine)	Bogousslavsky *et al.* (1988a), Rowley *et al.* (1989), Sachdeva and Woodward (1989)
Radiation theraphy	Reilly *et al.* (1992)
Segmental necrotizing angiitis	Poirier *et al.* (1983)
Infectious angiitis	
acute meningitis	Bewermeyer *et al.* (1985)
syphilis angiitis	Bogousslavsky *et al.* (1988a)
Borrelia burgdorferi angiitis	Uldry et al. (1988)
Zoster angiitis	Geny *et al.* (1991)
Postpartum angiopathy	Barbizet *et al.* (1981)
Chronic meningitis	Angelergues *et al.* (1957)
Coronary angiography	Levasseur *et al.* (1992), Abe *et al.* (1993)

(continued)

Table 21.1 (continued) Causes of thalamic infarction

Cerebral angiography	Fung *et al.* (1997), del Mar Sáez de Ocariz *et al.* (1996)
Aortography	Kömpf *et al.* (1984)
Aneurysm surgery	Meissner *et al.* (1987), Fung *et al.* (1997)
Subarachnoid haemorrhage	Kulisevsky *et al.* (1993a), Kotila *et al.* (1994)
Oral contraceptives	Mills and Swanson (1978), Petit *et al.* (1981)
Lupus anticoagulants	Biller *et al.* (1984)
Hypo-plastic vertebro-basilar arteries	Szirmai *et al.* (1977)
Cogan syndrome	Karni *et al.* (1991)
Migraine stroke	Bogousslavsky *et al.* (1988a)
Marfan syndrome	Bogousslavsky *et al.* (1988a)
Arterial dissection	Bogousslavsky *et al.* (1988a), Metz *et al.* (1993), del Mar Sáez de Ocariz *et al.* (1997), Fukatsu *et al.* (1997)
Congenital factor V deficiency	Petiot *et al.* (1991)
Protein S deficiency	Baumgartner and Regard (1993), Masson *et al.* (1994)
Fibromuscular dysplasia	Levasseur *et al.* (1992)
Cerebral vein thrombosis	Rousseaux *et al.* (1998)
Vasculitis	del Mar Sáez de Ocariz *et al.* (1996)

Topographical forms of thalamic infarct

Clinico-radiological–anatomical studies suggest that it is appropriate to divide thalamic infarcts into four groups, based on the four main arterial territories. Inferolateral infarcts are the most common (45%), followed by paramedian (35%), polar (12.5%), and posterior choroidal (7.5%) infarcts (Bogousslavsky *et al.* 1988a).

Inferolateral infarcts (Fig. 21.5)

Cases with pathological studies are listed in Table 21.2. Several cases have been documented by computed tomography (CT) or magnetic resonance imaging (MRI) (Beasley *et al.* 1980, McFarling *et al.* 1982, Landi *et al.* 1984, Gorsselink and Lodder 1985, Bogousslavsky *et al.* 1984, 1988a, Graff-Radford *et al.* 1985a, Sacco *et al.* 1987, Caplan *et al.* 1988, Combarros *et al.* 1991, Gutrecht *et al.* 1992, Solomon *et al.* 1994, Kim 1996, 1997, Vuilleumier *et al.* 1998, Kim *et al.* 1999, Soler *et al.* 1999). Clinical syndromes may develop with involvement of the inferolateral nuclear groups, mainly the ventral posterior nucleus and the posterior part of the ventral lateral nucleus.

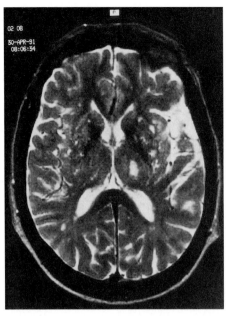

Fig. 21.5 Right inferolateral (thalamogeniculate) infarct (MRI transverse slice).

Pure sensory stroke

Fisher (1965*b*) reported this syndrome in a 75-year-old man, who had a 7 mm lacune in the ventral posterior nucleus on the opposite side. Paraesthesias, sometimes painful, on one side of the body are usually the first, and sometimes only, symptom. However, in most cases, these are followed by the development of a hemisensory deficit, which may involve the entire hemibody, but may also be partial, with cheiro-oral, cheiro-podo-oral or pseudo-radicular patterns (Sittig 1914, Garcin and Lapresle 1954, 1960, Fisher 1965*b*, 1978*a*, 1982, 1991, Haguenau 1965, Lapresle and Haguenau 1973, Ten Holter and Tijssen 1988, Lee *et al.* 1989, Kawakami *et al.* 1989, Kim 1994). Exceptionally, restricted non-acral sensory syndrome (Kim 1996) and inverse cheiro-oral syndrome (Kosner and Sparr 1992), i.e. a sensory deficit that spares the hand and the perioral regions, may be seen. All modalities of sensation can be affected, but dissociated loss with sparing of temperature and pain is rather common (Lapresle and Haguenau 1973, Graff-Radford *et al.* 1985*a*, Sacco *et al.* 1987, Caplan *et al.* 1988, Bogousslavsky et *al.* 1988*a*). In their initial report, Dejérine and Roussy (1906) mentioned that delayed (weeks to months) pain may develop ('anesthésie douloureuse'). This painful syndrome, which can occur in 15–20 per cent of infero-lateral infarcts (Bogousslavsky *et al.* 1988*a*), is not specific to thalamic stroke, although clinical and somatosensory evoked potential dysfunction is most severe with thalamic involvement (Schott *et al.* 1986, Mauguière *et al.* 1987, Mauguière and Desmedt 1988, Holmgreen *et al.* 1990). It seems that pain is produced preferentially by right thalamic lesions (Nasreddine and Saver 1997). In rare instances, the sensory

Table 21.2 Infarcts in the territories of the thalamogeniculate, tuberothalamic, and posterior choroidal arteries: pathological cases

Thalamogeniculate arterial territory		
Left	Fisher (1965)	M 72 years
	Fisher (1978a)	F 85 years
	Masdeu and Gorelick (1988)	F 72 years
Right	Bonhoeffer (1928)	F 61 years
	Kleist and Gonzalo (1938)	M 56 years
	Garcin and Lapresle (1954)	M 56 years
	Garcin and Lapresle (1960)	M 65 years
	Mohr et al. (1977)	M 61 years
	Fisher (1978a)	M 54 years
	Sunohara et al. (1984)	M 61 years
Other cases associated with more extensive infarction		
	Dejérine and Roussy (1906)	
	Schuster (1936)	
	Nadeau et al. (1994)	
Posterior choroidal artery territory		
	Walther (1945–1946)	M 52 years (left-sided infarct)
	Devic et al. (1964)	F 67 years (right-sided infarct)
Tuberothalamic artery territories		
Partial infarct sparing the polar region		
	Laplane et al. (1982)	F 64 years (right-sided infarct)
Infarcts combined with paramedian territory involvement		
See Table 21.3		

loss may show complete clinical recovery, while pain remains prominent (pure algetic syndrome) (Mauguière and Desmedt 1988). We have seen some patients in whom pain transiently recurred in the acute phase of certain diseases, such as viral infections and post-vaccine reactions.

Sensorimotor stroke

In a few instances, the infarct can involve the adjacent portion of the internal capsule, with corresponding hemiparesis associated with the sensory loss (Dejérine and Roussy 1906, Mohr et al. 1977, Caplan et al. 1988).

Ataxic syndromes

Hemiataxia is not uncommon in inferolateral infarcts. Even when impairment of position sense is present, the ataxia shows characteristics that also suggest a cerebellar type of dysfunction (oscillations, hypermetria, and dysdiadochokinesia) (Dejérine and Roussy 1906, Caplan et al. 1988, Masdeu and Gorelick 1988, Maraist et al. 1991, Gutrecht et al. 1992, Melo et al. 1992). Hemiataxia correlates well with involvement of the ventral lateral nucleus on the opposite side (Melo and Bogousslavsky 1992, Melo *et al.* 1992). It does not occur in isolation, and three main syndromes can be delineated:

(1) hemiataxia–hypoaesthesia: this association seems quasi-specific for inferolateral thalamic infarct (Melo and Bogousslavsky 1992) or haemorrhage (Heo and Choi 1996, Tatu *et al.* 1996*b*);

(2) hypoaesthesic ataxic hemiparesis;

(3) ataxic hemiparesis: in thalamic infarcts, ataxia is more common than hemiparesis (Bogousslavsky *et al.* 1984, Hommel *et al.* 1987, Masdeu and Gorelick 1988, Lee *et al.* 1989, Melo *et al.* 1992). Although ataxic hemiparesis is usually caused by a small infarct in the contralateral upper pons or internal capsule, when the syndrome is accompanied by pain, even without altered sensation ('painful ataxic hemiparesis'), it suggests a thalamic infarct (Bogousslavsky *et al.* 1984).

In thalamic astasia, the patients are unable to stand, they may not be able to sit unassisted and may fall, usually backwards or towards the side opposite to the infarct (Masdeu and Gorelick 1988). Rarely, a cerebellar syndrome may appear weeks to years after the stroke ('delayed onset cerebellar syndrome') (Louis *et al.* 1996).

Involvement of the dentatorubrothalamic tract is probably responsible for the cerebellar findings (Solomon *et al.* 1994), and this is supported by a positron emission tomography (PET) study (Tanaka *et al.* 1992). However, lesions of the ventrolateral thalamus cause different movement deficits from those caused by lateral cerebellar lesions involving the dentate nucleus, which suggests that the dentate nucleus may also influence movement by pathways other than the thalamic pathway (Bastian and Thach 1995).

Abnormal movements

Delayed (weeks) dystonia and jerks may develop in the hand contralateral to the infarct, usually in patients with marked sensory loss and ataxia (thalamic hand and unstable ataxic hand) (Lapresle and Haguenau 1973). These involuntary movements may take the form of action-induced dystonia and myoclonus (Sunohara *et al.* 1984), marked unilateral tremor (Mano *et al.* 1993, Mossuto-Agatiello *et al.* 1993, Soler *et al.* 1999), unilateral asterixis (Stell *et al.* 1994), or acute onset choreoathethosis or choreoballism (Milandre *et al.* 1993, Lee *et al.* 1998, Kim *et al.* 1999), probably when the infarct extends caudally toward the posterior choroidal territory.

Dystonia may be due to involvement of the ventrooralis intermedius and ventrocaudal nuclei, which, respectively, receive cerebellar and ascending lemniscal fibres (Lehéricy *et al.* 1996). Another mechanism that has been proposed is dysfunction of the cortico-striato-pallido-thalamo-cortical loop leading to overactivity in primary and accessory motor areas (Krystkowiak *et al.* 1998).

Acute onset and delayed involuntary movements probably have different mechanisms. In the former, movements may be secondary to loss of proprioception, hence the term 'pseudochoreoathethosis' (Sharp *et al.* 1994). This is supported by the observations that the onset of the movements temporally correlates with the onset of the sensory loss, i.e. acute stroke, and the movements disappear when the sensory loss resolves. Pseudochoreoathethosis may be aggravated by closing the eyes. Delayed involuntary movements may be due to late effects of the reorganizing process in the brain following deafferentation (Ghika *et al.* 1994).

Neuro-psychological dysfunction

This is characteristically absent (Bogousslavsky *et al.* 1988*a*), although dysphasia has been reported occasionally (McFarling *et al.* 1982).

Vestibular dysfunction

Although 11 out of 16 patients presented a tilt of internal representation of gravity, in only two was this associated with postural instability (Dieterich and Brandt 1993). The ventrooralis intermedius, ventrocaudal, and dorsocaudal nuclei have been proposed to have a 'vestibular function' (Dieterich and Brandt 1993). Others have argued that the tilt of gravity representation may be due to somatosensory dysfunction (Anastosopoulos and Bronstein 1999).

Paramedian infarcts (Figs 21.6 and 21.7)

These are the best autopsy-documented type of thalamic infarcts (Table 21.3). Several unilateral (Elghozi *et al.* 1978, Demeurisse *et al.* 1979, Massey *et al.* 1979, Smith and Laguna 1981, Bogousslavsky and Regli 1984, Feldmeyer *et al.* 1984, Friedman 1985, Graff-Radford 1985*a*, Powers 1985, Bogousslavsky *et al.* 1986*a*,

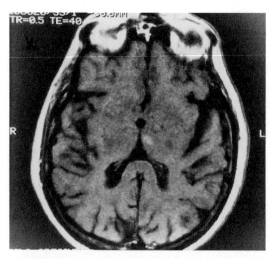

Fig. 21.6 Paramedian (thalamoperfurate) infarct (MRI transverse slice, gadolinium enhanced).

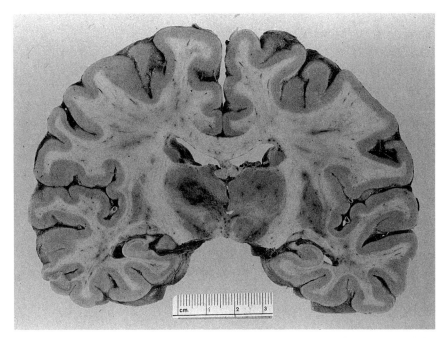

Fig. 21.7 Left paramedian infarct at autopsy (coronal slice at the level of the dorsomedial nucleus).

1988*a*,*e*, Franck *et al.* 1986, Mori *et al.* 1986, Fensore *et al.* 1988, Gorelick *et al.* 1988, Ghidoni *et al.* 1989, Mennemeier *et al.* 1992, Baumgartner and Regard 1993, Metz *et al.* 1993, Noda *et al* 1993, Clark and Albers 1995, Tatu *et al.* 1996*a*, Fung *et al.* 1997, Shuren *et al.* 1997, Van Der Werf *et al.* 1999) and bilateral cases with good clinico-topographical studies (Mills and Swanson 1978, Von Cramon and Zihl 1979, Petit *et al.* 1981, Dehaene 1982, Kessler *et al.* 1982, Graff-Radford *et al.* 1984, 1985*a*,*b*, 1990, Winocur *et al.* 1984, Bewermeyer *et al.* 1985, Biller *et al.* 1985, Karabelas *et al.* 1985, Swanson and Schmidley 1985, Gerber and Gudesblatt 1986, Vighetto *et al.* 1986, Wall *et al.* 1986, Gentilini *et al.* 1987, Kobari *et al.* 1987, Meissner *et al.* 1987, Bogousslavsky *et al.* 1988*b*, 1991, Ghidoni *et al.* 1989, Rowley *et al.* 1989, Eslinger *et al.* 1991, Kölmel 1991, Levasseur *et al.* 1992, Reilly *et al.* 1992, Abe *et al.* 1993, Ackermann *et al.* 1993, McGilchrist *et al.* 1993, Clark and Albers 1995, Otto *et al.* 1995, Rousseaux *et al.* 1996, van Domburg *et al.* 1996, Awada 1997, Fukatsu *et al.* 1997, Fung *et al.* 1997, Müller *et al.* 1999, Muroi *et al.* 1999, Versino *et al.* 1999) have also been reported. Neurological and neuro-psychological dysfunction is due mainly to involvement of the intralaminar formation, dorsomedial nucleus, and associated lesion of the uppermost midbrain at the level of the posterior commissure and rostral interstitial nucleus of the medial longitudinal fasciculus (Table 21.4). The classical syndrome of unilateral infarction associates acute loss or decrease of consciousness (usually transient), followed frequently by neuro-psychological

Table 21.3 Infarcts in the territories of the paramedian arteries: pathological cases

Left	Chiray *et al.* (1923)	F 43 years
	Balthasar and Hopf (1966)	F 84 years
	Sieben *et al.* (1977)	F 75 years (case 1)
	Castaigne *et al.* (1981)	M 64 years (case ?)
		M 61 years (case 26)
	Bogousslavsky *et al.* (1986e)	F 72 years
	Tuszynski and Petito (1988)	M 77 years
Right	Schuster (1936)	F 69 years (case 9)
		M 74 years (case 10)
	Sigwald and Monnier (1936)	M 67 years
	Garcin and Lapresle (1969)	M 78 years
	Castaigne *et al.* (1981)	F 75 years (case 1)
		M 72 years (case 21)
	Ranalli *et al.* (1988)	M 64 years
	Noda *et al.* (1993)	M 72 years
Other unilateral infarcts, but with extensive vertebrobasilar infarcts		
	Schuster (1936), Kleist and Gonzalo (1938), Gruner and Feuerstein (1966), Jakimowicz *et al.* (1968), Sieben *et al.* (1977)	
Bilateral	Schuster (1936)	F 49 years (case 11)
	Grünthal (1942)	F 61 years
	Brage *et al.* (1961)	F 44 years
	Segarra *et al.* (1970)	M 51 years (case 1)
	Jacobs (1973)	M 42 years
	Lechi and Macchi (1974)	F 72 years
	Csornai (1974)	M 57 years
	Halmagyi *et al.* (1976)	F 65 years (case 2)
	Szirmai *et al.* (1977)	F 48 years
	Trojanowski and Wray (1980)	M 58 years
	Trojanowski and Lafontaine (1981)	F 56 years
	Castaigne *et al.* (1981)	M 66 years (case 27, previously reported by Castaigne *et al.* 1962)
	Graff-Radford *et al.* (1985)	F 43 years (case 28, previously reported by Lhermitte *et al.* 1963)
		F 67 years (case 2, previously reported by Castaigne *et al.* 1966, case 2).
		M 70 years

disturbances, with upward gaze limitation, but very few motor or sensory abnormalities.

Impaired consciousness may erroneously suggest hypoxic or metabolic coma, especially in the absence of conspicuous findings, other than eye movement disorders, on neurological examination. It correlates with acute involvement of the intralaminar nuclei and rostral midbrain reticular formation. Lack of disturbed consciousness is exceptional at onset in this type of infarct (Karabelas *et al.* 1985).

Vertical gaze dysfunction

Conjugate disturbances arise from rostral midbrain involvement and include upgaze palsy or combined (up- plus downgaze) vertical gaze palsy, while pure downgaze palsy apparently requires a bilateral lesion (Bogousslavsky 1989, Hommel and Bogousslavsky 1991). A skew deviation may be present. Although vertical gaze palsy has been reported in patients with MRI-documented medial thalamic infarctions without midbrain involvement (Clark and Albers 1995), concomitant mesencephalic lesions, too small to be detected, could not be excluded.

Horizontal gaze dysfunction

This is much less common and less prominent, with hypometric contralateral saccades and low-gain ipsilateral pursuit with interposed saccades (Brigell *et al.* 1984, Rousseaux *et al.* 1985, Masdeu and Rosenberg 1987). It probably corresponds to involvement of transthalamic frontal and parietal brainstem horizontal gaze pathways. Occasionally, dysconjugate abnormalities, such as acute aesotropia (Gomez *et al.* 1988), may develop (Tatemichi *et al.* 1992). Lateral gaze sinkinesis on downward saccade attempts has been reported after bilateral lesions (Versino *et al.* 1999).

Vestibular dysfunction

Formal testing of vestibular function revealed an ocular tilt reaction, i.e. the triad of head tilt, skew deviation, and ocular torsion, in eight out of 14 patients (Dieterich and Brandt 1993). However, in all of these, the infarcted area extended to the brainstem, including the rostral interstitial nucleus of the medial longitudinal fascicle and the interstitial nucleus of Cajal. Patients may exhibit a lateral head tilt opposite to the side of the lesion, skew deviation with ipsilateral over contralateral eye, and binocular ocular torsion.

Sleep disturbances

Hypersomnia, defined as excessive daytime sleepiness and/or prolonged sleep, may be a chronic consequence of paramedian stroke. It has been attributed to disruption of activating impulses ascending from the brainstem reticular formation to the thalamus. However, sleep–wake studies suggested that it may be caused by disruption of both arousal and non-rapid eye movement sleep (Bassetti *et al.* 1996). Lesions of the dorsomedial nucleus may lead to sleep–wake disturbances, even without involvement of the ascending reticular activating system.

Neuropsychological dysfunction

This is summarized in Tables 21.4 and 21.5. It is usually discovered at the time when the consciousness disturbances resolve and may be difficult to differentiate from cortical neuropsychological dysfunction, although it is usually less severe and more rapidly resolved.

Table 21.4 Reported cases with unilateral infarct of the right paramedian thalamus

Reference	Patient	Thalamic lesion	Associated lesion	Initial state of consciousness	Neurological dysfunction	Neuropsychological disturbances[a]
Sigwald and Monnier (1936)	F 76 years	Central nuclei (+ pulvinar and lateral nuclei) (autopsy)	Lacunes	N	Transient hemiparesis, hemitremor, and ataxia with increased tone	NR
Schuster (1936)	F 39 years[b] (case 9)	Inferior part of medial nuclei and middle part of lateral nuclei (autopsy)	Cerebral and cerebellar hemispheres, right hypothalamus, and upper midbrain	Transient coma	Nearly complete ophtalmoplegia, hemiataxia, and hypoaesthesia, facial paresis	NR
Kleist and Gonzalo (1938)	M 69 years (case 1)	Intralaminar nucleus, ventral nuclei (autopsy)	Bilateral midbrain	N	Complex ophtalmoplegia, hemiparesis, hemiataxia, hemihypoaesthesia, dystonia	NR
Gruner and Feuerstein (1966)	M 65 years (case F)	Dorsomedian nucleus, centromedian nucleus (autopsy)	Right upper midbrain, lacunes	N	Hemiparesis, bilateral ataxia, dysphagia	NR
Jakimowickz et al. (1968)	F 72 years (case 3)	Dorsomedian nucleus, intralaminar nuclei, ventral posterolateral nucleus (autopsy)	Left upper midbrain, cerebellum, occipital lobe, hypothalamus	Somnolence	Faciolingual paraesthesias, vertical ophtalmoplegia, and partial third nerve palsy	Apathy, disorientation
Garcin and Lapresle (1969)	M 78 years	Dorsomedian nucleus, intralaminar nuclei (autopsy)	Right occipital lobe	N	Ataxic paresis in left lower limb	NR
Sieben et al. (1977)	M 67 years (case 1)	Posterior and lateral parts (autopsy)	Right temporal and occipital lobes, hypothalamus, and upper midbrain	N	Hemiparesis, opposite third nerve palsy (Weber's syndrome), dysarthria	NR
Cambier et al. (1980)	M 79 years[c] (case 1)	Dorsomedian and ventral posterolateral nuclei, pulvinar (autopsy)	Right fornix, occipital lobes, and temporal lobes	N	Hemiparesis and anaesthesia, syncinesia	Motor neglect and impersistence, anosognosia, hemi asomatognosia

Reference		Nuclei (method)	Lesion site	Consciousness	Neurological signs	Cognitive/behavioural
Castaigne et al. (1981)	M 75 years[c] (case 1)	Dorsomedian nucleus, intralaminar nuclei, ventrolateral nucleus (autopsy)	Right upper midbrain, lacunes	Obtundation	Hemiparesis with hypoaesthesia and hemianopia	NR
Castaigne et al. (1981)	F 73 years (case 18)	Dorsomedian nucleus, intralaminar nuclei, ventrolateral nucleus, polar nuclei (autopsy)	Right upper midbrain, cerebral hemispheres	Somnolence	Hemiparesis with hypoaesthesia and hemianopia, left VII palsy	Disorientation, impaired short-term memory
Castaigne et al. (1981)	M 72 years (case 21)	Dorsomedian nucleus, intralaminar nuclei, pulvinar, ventral posterior nucleus (autopsy)	Cerebral hemispheres, lacunes	N	Hemiparesis, incontinence	Apathy, disinterest, 'psychomotor retardation'
Watson et al. (1981)	M 62 years	Intralaminar nuclei, ventral posterior nucleus, pulvinar (CT)	—	N	Hemiparesis	Hemineglect
Pierrot-Deseilligny et al. (1982)	F 78 years (case 3)	Dorsomedian nucleus, intralaminar nuclei, ventrolateral formation (autopsy)	Right upper midbrain, cerebral hemisphere	Somnolence	Upgaze palsy	Impaired anterograde memory
Speedie and Heilman (1983)	M 64 years	Dorsomedian nucleus, pulvinar, anterior and posterior lateral formations (CT)	—	N	Hemiparesis, ataxia, dysarthria	Anterograde memory impairment for visuospatial material
Bogousslavsky and Regli (1984b)	M 68 years	Dorsomedian nucleus, intralaminar nuclei (CT)	Right upper midbrain and occipital white matter	Somnolence	Hemiataxia and asterixis, vertical one-and-a-half	Apathy, lack of motor spontaneity, impaired memory
Friedman (1985)	M 68 years	Paramedian part (CT)	—	Coma	Transient dysarthria	Confusional state

(continued)

Table 21.4 (continued) Reported cases with unilateral infarct of the right paramedian thalamus

Reference	Patient	Thalamic lesion	Associated lesion	Initial state of consciousness	Neurological dysfunction	Neuropsychological disturbances[a]
Franck et al. (1986)	M 55 years	Anterior paramedian part (CT)	–	N	Hemiparesis and hypoaesthesia	Dysmnesia, slight hemineglect, impaired visuospatial processing, apathy, loss of initiative, irritability
Bogousslavsky et al. (1988e)	F 72 years	Dorsomedian nucleus, intralaminar nuclei, internal part of ventral lateral nucleus (CT)	Lacune in the head of left caudate	Somnolence	Slight upgaze paresis (?)	Logorrhoea with inadequate comments, jokes and laughing, prefrontal-like disturbances during conflictual tasks, impaired non-verbal memory, mild impairment of visuospatial processing and hemineglect
Baumgartner and Regard (1993)	W 47 years (case 1)	Paramedian part (MRI)	–	Somnolence	Upgaze palsy, hemiparesis	Impaired verbal and non-verbal memory, reduced verbal and non-verbal fluency, dysfunction of conceptual thinking
Baumgartner and Regard (1993)	W 46 years (case 2)	Paramedian part (MRI)	–	–	–	Right hemispatial neglect, impaired verbal and non-verbal memory, reduced non-verbal fluency

Reference	Patient	Lesion location	Associated lesion	Consciousness	Oculomotor/neurological signs	Neuropsychological findings
Baumgartner and Regard (1993)	W 34 year (case 3)	Paramedian part (MRI)	–	Somnolence	Upgaze palsy, anisocoria	Dysfunction of conceptual thinking impaired non-verbal memory, reduced non-verbal fluency
Noda et al. (1993) (case 1)	M 72 years	Dorsomedian nucleus, intralaminar nuclei (autopsy)	–	Somnolence	Normal	Auditory and visual experimental hallucination
Clark and Albers (1995) (case 2)	M 47 years	Paramedian part (MRI)	–	Somnolence	Upgaze palsy, dysarthria.	NR
Clark and Albers (1995) case 3	M 72 years	Paramedian part (MRI)	Right medula (pontomedullary junction). Old cerebellar infarction (PICA)	–	Upgaze and downgaze palsy, dysarthria, VII palsy, ataxic gait	NR
Tatu et al. (1996a)	M 30 years	Paramedian part (MRI)	–	Somnolence	Upgaze palsy	Hallucinosis
Fung et al. (1997) (case 1)	M 62 years	Dorsomedian nucleus, ventral posterolateral (CT)	Right occipital lobe	Somnolence	Hemianopia, complete ophthalmoplegia except for abduction of left eye, hemiataxia and hemiparesis,	Right clonic perseveration, palilalia
Shuren et al. (1997)	M 25 years	Dorsomedian nucleus, internal medullary lamina (MRI)	–	Somnolence	–	Disorientation, impaired non-verbal memory and temporal order judgement
Van Der Werf et al. (1999)	M 44 years lamina (MRI)	Dorsal caudal medullary	–	–	NR	Apathia, lethargia, verbal and non-verbal memory impairment, slowness, lack of concentration.

[a]NR = not reported.

[b]Case 10 (74-year-old man) is not listed because of extensive associated cerebral atrophy.

[c]Also involving the posterior choroidal artery territory.

Table 21.5 Paramedian infarcts: neuropsychological disturbances

---

Left-side infarct

dysphasia, aphonia
decreased verbal memory
amnesia (Korsakoff-like)

. . . .

Right-side infarct

hemineglect and impaired visuospatial processing
decrease non-verbal memory
apathy, aspontaneity
acute confusional state
pseudo-maniac state

. . . .

Bilateral infarcts

amnesia and other disturbances listed above
thalamic dementia
akinetic mutism
loss of psychic self-activation
other: palilalia, hallucinosis, utilization behaviour, bulimia

---

Abnormal movements

Asterixis (Massey *et al.* 1979, Feldmeyer *et al.* 1984), hemiataxia with or without marked hemitremor contralateral to the infarct (Chiray *et al.* 1923, Sigwald and Monnier 1936, Garcin and Lapresle 1969, Speedie and Heilman 1983), blepharospasm (Powers 1985, Leenders *et al.* 1986, Kulisevsky *et al.* 1993*a*, Awada 1997), and head tremor (Otto *et al.* 1995) have been reported. Clonic perseveration, i.e. inappropriate repetition of an action, was present in two patients with bilateral paramedian infarctions and was ipsilateral to the lesion in one patient with a right paramedian infarction (Fung *et al.* 1997). Delayed (usually after 1–3 months) dystonia/chorea may also develop in a previously paretic limb contralateral to the infarct (Powers 1985, Bogousslavsky *et al.* 1988*a*, Reilly *et al.* 1992) and may correspond to posterior extension of the infarct toward the pulvinar region (posterior choroidal territory).

Motor weakness

Mild hemiparesis has been reported (Sigwald and Monnier 1936, Garcin and Lapresle 1969, Demeurisse *et al.* 1979, Smith and Laguna 1981, Speedie and Heilman 1983, Bogousslavsky *et al.* 1988*a*). The mechanism involved is not clear.

Sensory loss

This is uncommon, but can occur, as the ventral posteromedial nucleus and inner part of the ventral posterolateral nucleus may be supplied by the paramedian pedicle. In a detailed clinico-pathological study in a 72-year-old woman with a left paramedian infarct, there was hemihypoaesthaesia involving the right side of the face down to a sensory level at D10, which correlated well with involvement of these nuclei (Bogousslavsky *et al.* 1986*e*).

Bilateral paramedian infarcts are not uncommon and represent at least one-third of paramedian thalamic infarcts (Bogousslavsky *et al.* 1988*a*). The explanation is the common finding of a unilateral paramedian pedicle supplying the paramedian region on both sides.

Neurological and neuropsychological disturbances are usually more severe and long-lasting than in the case of unilateral involvement. Peculiar behavioural/neuropsychological disturbances include:

(1) akinetic mutism (Lhermitte *et al.* 1963, Segarra 1970, Szirmai *et al.* 1977, van Domburg *et al.* 1996);

(2) 'thalamic dementia' (Castaigne *et al.* 1966, De Boucaud *et al.* 1968, Chassagnon *et al.* 1969, Poirier *et al.* 1983, Kömpf *et al.* 1984, Gentilini *et al.* 1987, Katz *et al.* 1987, Muller *et al.* 1989);

(3) loss of psychic self-activation or robot syndrome (Bogousslavsky *et al.* 1991);

(4) other disturbances, such as palilalia (Yasuda *et al.* 1990), stuttering-like repetitive speech (Abe *et al.* 1993), hallucinosis (Feinberg and Rapcsak 1989, Kölmel 1991), a compulsive tendency to assume a sleeping position (Castman-Berrevoets and Van Harskamp 1988), Klüver–Bucy syndrome (Müller *et al.* 1999), utilization behaviour (Eslinger *et al.* 1991), or childish behaviour (Fukatsu *et al.* 1996, Muroi *et al.* 1999).

Polar infarcts (Fig. 21.8)

There is only one autopsy-documented case of an infarct limited to the polar territory (Table 21.2) and four with associated involvement of the paramedian territory

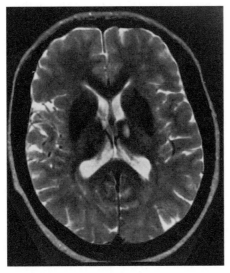

Fig. 21.8 Left polar (tuberothalamic) infarct (MRI transverse slice).

(Table 21.3). These infarcts, either unilateral (Goto *et al.* 1979, Archer *et al.* 1981, Speedie and Heilman 1982, Goldenberg *et al.* 1983, Biller *et al.* 1984, Gorelick *et al.* 1984, Graff-Radford *et al.* 1984, 1985*a*, Bogousslavsky *et al.* 1986*b*, 1988*a*, Franck *et al.* 1986, Laplane *et al.* 1986, Mori *et al.* 1986, Von Cramon *et al.* 1985, Geny *et al.* 1991, Rousseaux *et al.* 1991, Desmond *et al.* 1992, Lisovoski *et al.* 1993, Ott and Saver 1993, Pepin and Auray-Pepin 1993, Cohen *et al.* 1994, Kotila *et al.* 1994, Hashimoto *et al.* 1995, Sodeyama *et al.* 1995, Kim *et al.* 1998) or bilateral (Barbizet *et al.* 1981, Von Cramon *et al.* 1985, Muller *et al.* 1989, Bogousslavsky 1991, Kaplan *et al.* 1991), have therefore mainly been studied by CT or MRI. The occurrence of bilateral infarction without concomitant involvement of the paramedian territory suggests that, in a few instances, a single artery may supply both polar regions of the thalamus. In other instances, the polar territory may be supplied, together with the paramedian territory, through the paramedian branches, and infarcts then result in the involvement of both territories (autopsy results in Table 21.3; CT/MRI results: Schott *et al.* 1980, Michel *et al.* 1982, Dubois *et al.* 1986, Rondot *et al.* 1986, Gorelick *et al.* 1988, Graff-Radford *et al.* 1990, Malamut *et al.* 1992). Clinical dysfunction is mainly neuropsychological and seems to be related to involvement of the region of the mamillo-thalamic tract and ventral lateral nucleus, while most of the dorsomedial nucleus is usually spared. Left-sided infarcts are associated with the same dysphasic disturbances seen in 'subcortical' dysphasia in general, while right-sided infarcts are associated with hemineglect and impaired visuospatial processing (Bogousslavsky *et al.* 1986*b*, 1988*a*). In a few instances, unilateral left (Michel *et al.* 1982, Speedie and Heilman 1982, Goldenberg *et al.* 1983, Ott and Saver 1993, Clarke *et al.* 1994, Kotila *et al.* 1994) or right (Rousseaux *et al.* 1991), or, more often, bilateral (Schott *et al.* 1980, Barbizet *et al.* 1981, Von Cramon *et al.* 1985, Muller *et al.* 1989, Graff-Radford *et al.* 1990) infarcts can result in acute amnesia as the main dysfunction. Mild transient hemiparesis or hemisensory disturbances, when present, are usually the only neurological findings (Bogousslavsky *et al.* 1986*b*, 1988*a*). Facial paresis for emotional movements (Speedie and Heilman 1982, Bogousslavsky *et al.* 1986*b*), hemiataxia (Goto *et al.* 1979, Laplane *et al.* 1982, 1986, Melo *et al.* 1992), and the disappearance of hemi-Parkinsonian dysfunction (Dubois *et al.* 1986) have been reported. Micrographia has been reported after a thalamo-mesencephalic infarction, but was probably due to involvement of the substantia nigra (Kim *et al.* 1998).

Posterior choroidal infarcts (Fig. 21.9)

These were previously the least well characterized type of thalamic infarct, but, recently, several papers on this topic have been published (Bogousslavsky *et al.* 1988*a*, Besson *et al.* 1991, Luco *et al.* 1992, Serra Catafan *et al.* 1992, Baumgartner *et al.* 1994, Ghika *et al.* 1994, 1995, Shuren *et al.* 1994, Borruat and Maeder 1995, Gérald *et al.* 1998) and one detailed study of 10 cases (Neau and Bogousslavsky 1996). To our knowledge, only two autopsy cases compatible with this type of infarct have

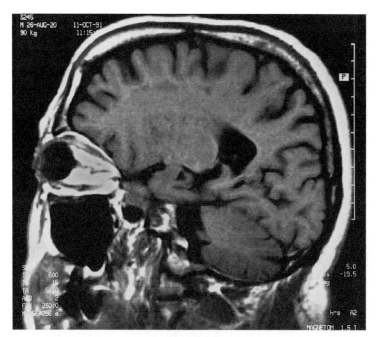

Fig. 21.9 Right posterior choroidal infarct involving the lateral geniculate body and responsible for horizontal sectoranopia (MRI, longitudinal slice).

been reported (Table 21.2); the first, a 52-year-old man, developed a confusional state with dysphasic disturbances (Walther 1945–1946), while the second, a 67-year-old woman, showed vertical eye movement dysfunction with nystagmus retractorius, an abolished photomotor response, and, later, hemiparesis (Devic *et al.* 1964). The three following neurological features are the most important symptoms of these infarcts.

(1) Visual dysfunction: CT- or MRI-documented cases have shown that visual field cuts resulting from involvement of the lateral geniculate body may be the most suggestive neurological symptom (Frisén *et al.* 1978, Shacklett *et al.* 1984, Rousseaux *et al.* 1985. Bogousslavsky *et al.* 1988*a*, Besson *et al.* 1991, Luco *et al.* 1992, Serra Catafan *et al.* 1992, Baumgartner *et al.* 1994, Borruat and Maeder 1995, Neau and Bogousslavsky 1996), and include upper or lower quadrantanopia or, more typically, horizontal sectoranopia. Pure stereoacuity has been reported as the manifestation of a small pulvinar haemorrhage (Takayama *et al.* 1994).

(2) Sensorimotor hemisyndrome (Bogousslavsky *et al.* 1988*a*, Besson *et al.* 1991): hemihypoaesthesia and slight hemiparesis were present respectively in five and six out of 10 patients (Neau and Bogousslavsky 1996). As with inferolateral infarcts, in rare cases, pain can develop a few months after the stroke (Neau and

Bogousslavsky 1996). Sensory loss may be due to involvement of the thalamic sensory radiations in the internal capsule (Ghika *et al.* 1994), but is probably often due to direct damage to the ventral posterior nucleus, which may often be supplied by the lateral posterior choroidal artery. The origin of weakness remains unclear, although it may be explained by damage to corticobulbar and corticospinal fibres in the adjacent posterior limb of the internal capsule.

(3) Neuropsychological disturbances can include amnesia (Rousseaux *et al.* 1986), hallucinosis in a visual hemifield (Serra Catafan *et al.* 1992), and transcortical aphasia (Neau and Bogousslavsky 1996). Since the most rostral part of the thalamus, including the anterior nucleus, can be supplied by the most distal branches of the posterior choroidal arteries after they loop around the superior part of the thalamus, it is conceivable that some of the neuropsychological disturbances seen in posterior choroidal infarcts are not caused by posterior thalamic lesions, but are due to anterior thalamic involvement.

Involuntary movements, such as acute onset choreoathethosis (Milandre *et al.* 1993, Neau and Bogousslavsky 1996), delayed choreathethosis associated with dystonia, myoclonus and action tremor ('jerky dystonic unsteady hand') (Ghika *et al.* 1994), focal myoclonus (Gatto *et al.* 1998), tremor (Miwa *et al.* 1996), and unilateral akathisia (Ghika *et al.* 1995), may develop.

Eye movement disorders, such as impaired ipsilateral pursuit and contralateral saccadic impairment, upgaze and horizontal gaze paresis, myosis, Horner's syndrome, rectratory nystagmus, and skew deviation, are uncommon (Oglen *et al.* 1984, Rousseaux *et al.* 1985, Neau and Bogousslavsky 1996, Gérald *et al.* 1998).

Neuro-psychological dysfunction

This is present mainly in paramedian or polar infarcts and can be classified into five main groups, dysphasia, hemineglect, mood dysfunction and delirium, amnesia, and dementia and related syndromes.

As with thalamic infarctions, disruption of thalamocortical pathways due to lower capsular genu (Moreaud *et al.* 1996, Schnider *et al.* 1996) or subthalamic infarctions (Trillet *et al.* 1995) may lead to neuropsychological dysfunction.

Dysphasia

This has been described (Elghozi *et al.* 1978, Demeurisse *et al.* 1979, Mazaux *et al.* 1979, Cohen *et al.* 1980, Cambier *et al.* 1982, McFarling *et al.* 1982, Michel *et al.* 1982, Wallesch *et al.* 1983, Gorelick *et al.* 1984, Mori *et al.* 1986, Puel *et al.* 1986, Fensore *et al.* 1988, Bruyn 1989, Nadeau *et al.* 1994). Speech is more often non-fluent rather than fluent, with decreased output in voice volume, sometimes as in parkisonian dysarthria (Ackermann *et al.* 1993), with more verbal than phonemic paraphasias, perseverations (only slight, if present), comprehension impairment, and spared repetition. Palilalia (Yasuda *et al.* 1990), stuttering-like repetitive speech (Abe *et al.* 1993), cessation of stuttering (Muroi *et al.* 1999), or isolated aphonia (Lazzarino and Nicolai 1988) can occur. Although the first reported autopsied case was in the left posterior choroidal territory with pulvinar involvement (Walther 1945–1946), all four subsequent pathological cases were in the left paramedian territory (Molnár 1958–1959, Davous *et al.* 1984, Bogousslavsky *et al.* 1986*a*, Tuszynski and Petito 1988). Involvement of the dorsomedial nucleus or the inner part of the ventral lateral nucleus has been proposed, and it is interesting that, in circumscribed infarction not extending into the most rostral region of the polar or paramedian territory, amnesia is not seen. Conversely, in an autopsy case of primary haemorrhage of the thalamus, the same region was involved as in Walther's (1945–1946) case (Crosson *et al.* 1986). This relative lack of unequivocal topographical correlates may result from the fact that more than one area in the thalamus may be involved in language processing, and that thalamo-frontal connections are not arranged topographically, but, instead, show a frontal rostrocaudal/thalamic mediolateral interrelationship that is not restricted to specific nuclei (Bruyn 1989). Dynamic involvement of reciprocal thalamo-cortical loops has been demonstrated both by cerebral blood flow studies (Rousseaux *et al.* 1990) and by the degenerate fibres technique at autopsy (Miklossy *et al.* 1987, Bogousslavsky *et al.* 1988*e*).

Other disturbances of language, namely mirror writing, may be linked to the thalamus (Tashiro *et al.* 1987).

Hemi-neglect

This has been described in several papers (Cambier *et al.* 1980, 1982, Watson *et al.* 1981, Henderson *et al.* 1982, Laplane *et al.* 1982, 1986, Louarn *et al.* 1986, Graveleau *et al.* 1986, Bogousslavsky *et al.* 1986*b*). It usually occurs on the left in patients with a right-sided infarct involving the ventral lateral and intralaminar nuclei, but the reverse may also occur (Bogousslavsky *et al.* 1986*b*, Baumgartner and Regard 1993). Hemineglect may take the form of:

(1) motor neglect or under-utilization behaviour, whichever space is involved;

(2) sensory extinction; or

(3) spatial neglect, either attentional or intentional (Graveleau *et al.* 1986).

In right-sided lesions, associated visuospatial disturbances, motor impersistence, asomatognosia, and anosognosia may also be present (Cambier *et al.* 1980, Henderson *et al.* 1982, Louarn *et al.* 1986, Hashimoto *et al.* 1995, Liebson 2000). Difficulty in judging emotional expressions, a disorder termed prosopoaffective agnosia, has also been reported in right-sided lesions (Vuilleumier *et al.* 1998). Ideomotor apraxia is seen occasionally after left thalamic infarcts (Nadeau *et al.* 1994, Shuren *et al.* 1994).

Mood dysfunction and delirium

Mood changes are more common in paramedian infarcts, usually with apathy/abulia (Gentilini *et al.* 1987, Katz et al. 1987, Bogousslavsky *et al.* 1988*e*, Starkstein *et al.* 1988). Less commonly, a disinhibition syndrome, with 'frontal-like' disturbances, utilization behaviour, childish behaviour, Vorboireden (i.e. approximate answers), bulimia, an acute confusional state, or manic-like delirium, may develop (Speedie and Heilman 1982, Friedman 1985, Gentilini *et al.* 1987, Bogousslavsky *et al.* 1988*e*, Eslinger *et al.* 1991, Kulisevsky *et al.* 1993*b*, McGilchrist *et al.* 1993, Hashimoto *et al.* 1995, Fukatsu *et al.* 1997, Vuilleumier *et al.* 1998, Muroi *et al.* 1999, Liebson 2000). Hallucinosis may be present after paramedian infarcts (Feinberg and Rapcsak 1989, Kölmel 1991, Noda *et al.* 1993, Tatu *et al.* 1996*a*) or, more rarely, after lesions in other thalamic territories (Danziger *et al.* 1997, Kim 1997). A transient fit of laugher has been described as the inaugural symptom ('le fou rire prodomique') of an infarct involving the left posterolateral thalamus and the adjacent part of the internal capsule (Ceccaldi and Milandre 1994). Disappearance of the hedonic character of olfactory and gustatory perceptions has also been reported (Rousseaux *et al.* 1996).

Amnesia

The thalamus may show hypoperfusion during episodes of transient amnesia (Goldenberg *et al.* 1981). In fact, thalamic strokes/tumours may well be the smallest lesions that can lead to amnesia in man. Amnesia may develop in isolation (Ziegler *et al.* 1977, Barbizet *et al.* 1981, Choi *et al.* 1983, Winocur *et al.* 1984, Brown *et al.* 1987, Gorelick *et al.* 1988, Moonis *et al.* 1988, Ott and Saver 1993, Clarke *et al.* 1994), although associated neurological/neuropsychological disturbances usually co-exist (Swanson and Schmidley 1985, Von Cramon *et al.* 1985, Rondot *et al.* 1986, Vighetto *et al.* 1986, Gentilini *et al.* 1987, Ghidoni *et al.* 1989, Graff-Radford *et al.* 1990, Kotila *et al.* 1994).

There are three major types of clinical onset of thalamic amnesia:

(1) mimicking transient global amnesia (Gorelick *et al.* 1988);

(2) after an episode of decreased consciousness; or

(3) simultaneously with other disturbances (Signoret and Goldenberg 1986).

The amnesia initially consists of total forgetfulness of actual events, as well as of immediately preceding (hours to weeks) events, associated with anxious perplexity and loss of temporal co-ordinates, leading to a confused chronology of events. There is severe impairment in explicit recall of new facts (Malamut *et al.* 1992), but several memory abilities may be preserved (Nichelli *et al.* 1988). Although not always the case (Rondot *et al.* 1986, Vighetto *et al.* 1986, Stuss *et al.* 1988, Desmond *et al.* 1992, Kotila *et al.* 1994, Müller *et al.* 1999), recovery is usually very good and occurs within a few months, and only moderate selective verbal or non-verbal memory disturbances, depending on the lesion side, may persist in isolation (Speedie and Heilman 1982, 1983, Akiguchi *et al.* 1983, 1987, Mori *et al.* 1986, Rousseaux *et al.* 1986, 1998, Fensore *et al.* 1988, Sodeyama *et al.* 1995). Selective amnesia for proper names has been reported (Cohen *et al.* 1994, Moreaud *et al.* 1995). Attentional deficit and executive disturbance have been proposed as the mechanism in some cases of thalamic amnesia (Mennemeier *et al.* 1992, Van Der Werf *et al.* 1999).

The role of the dorsomedial nucleus (its medial third or magnocellular part) has been both emphasized and questioned (Spiegel *et al.* 1956, Victor *et al.* 1971, Markowitsch 1982, 1986, Speedie and Heilman 1982, Von Cramon *et al.* 1985, Kritschevsky *et al.* 1987, Cole *et al.* 1992, Lisovoski *et al.* 1993). In the alcoholic Korsakoff syndrome, it is not always involved (Mayes *et al.* 1988). Similarly, a study of six infarct cases (Von Cramon *et al.* 1985), pooled with a review of five reported cases (Schott *et al.* 1980, Barbizet *et al.* 1981, Michel *et al.* 1982, Speedie and Heilman 1982, Goldenberg *et al.* 1983), failed to demonstrate involvement of this nucleus, except in its outermost ventrobasal portion, whereas there was constant involvement of the internal medullary lamina (which consists mainly of cortical afferents to the dorsomedial nucleus), the mamillo-thalamic tract, or part of the ventral lateral nucleus (internal ventro-oral nucleus). The authors also presented two cases with severe damage to the dorsomedial nucleus, but no amnesia. On the basis of animal experimental studies, damage involving both the dorsomedial nucleus and anterior thalamic nucleus has been proposed (Aggleton 1986). Selective involvement of the ventro-amygdalo-fugal pathway (immediately lateral to the mamillo-thalamic tract) has also been emphasized (Graff-Radford *et al.* 1990). Thus, thalamic amnesia might be considered a disconnection syndrome, corresponding to interruption of the Papez loop (with a mamillo-thalamic tract lesion) and amygdalo-fugo-thalamic tract fibres (with an internal medullary lamina lesion). Mamillo-thalamic tract involvement has been emphasized in another study of amnesia as a result of thalamic infarction (Gentilini *et al.* 1987), and other cases support this finding (Delay and Brion 1962, Castaigne *et al.* 1981, Mori *et al.* 1986, Stuss *et al.* 1988, Graff-Radford *et al.* 1990, Rousseaux *et al.* 1991, Malamut *et al.* 1992, Lisovoski *et al.* 1993, Ott and Saver 1993, Pepin and Auray-Pepin 1993, Clarke *et al.* 1994, Sodeyama *et al.* 1995). In contrast, there are well-documented cases of thalamic amnesia, sometimes very long-lasting, with infarction of the dorsomedial nucleus, but sparing of the mamillo-thalamic tract (Bogousslavsky *et al.* 1986a, Vighetto *et al.* 1986, Graff-Radford *et al.* 1990, Shuren *et al.* 1997). Moreover, monkeys with bilateral restricted lesions of the posterior portion of the mediodorsal nucleus exhibit marked memory deficit (Zola-Morgan and Squirre 1985). In addition, the internal medullary lamina may well be spared (Gentilini *et al.* 1987). Other thalamic nuclei that may play a role in memory include the medial nuclei of the mamillary bodies, the paratenial nucleus, the laterodorsal nucleus, and the anterior nucleus, but clear evidence of their involvement is lacking in thalamic amnesia (Markowitsch 1986).

These findings suggest that there are at least two main topographical correlates of amnesia from thalamic infarct:

(1) infarction with major involvement of the dorsomedial nucleus; and

(2) infarction with involvement of the mamillo-thalamic tract and internal medullary lamina, largely sparing the dorsomedial nucleus.

The first type corresponds to paramedian infarction (Bogousslavsky *et al.* 1986*a*, 1988*e*, Roßberg and Mennel 1986, Vighetto *et al.* 1986, Graff-Radford *et al.* 1990, Shuren *et al.* 1997), while the second corresponds to polar infarction (Barbizet *et al.* 1981, Michel *et al.* 1982, Speedie and Heilman 1982, Goldenberg *et al.* 1983, Von Cramon *et al.* 1985, Muller *et al.* 1989, Rousseaux *et al.* 1991, Lisovoski *et al.* 1993, Ott and Saver 1993, Pepin and Auray-Pepin 1993, Clarke *et al.* 1994, Kotila *et al.* 1994, Sodeyama *et al.* 1995). In the smallest autopsy-confirmed haemorrhagic stroke case, the haemorrhage selectively destroyed the region of the mamillo-thalamic tract/ anterior nucleus (Hankey and Stewart-Wynne 1988). There are also infarcts with concomitant paramedian and polar territory involvement (Schott *et al.* 1980, Michel *et al.* 1982, Pierrot-Deseilligny *et al.* 1982, Rondot *et al.* 1986, Gorelick *et al.* 1988, Graff-Radford *et al.* 1990, Malamut *et al.* 1992), but, in this case, the amnesia does not seem to be more severe than in the former case. In addition, the uni/bilaterality of infarction may not play a major role in the development of the acute amnestic syndrome, but it is likely that long-lasting amnesia resulting from thalamic infarction isassociated with bilateral lesions (Rondot *et al.* 1986, Vighetto *et al.* 1986). Amnesia resulting from posterior choroidal infarction may exist (Rousseaux *et al.* 1986), but the relative role of thalamic versus medial temporal involvement has not been decided in such instances. One of the unexplained issues is the occurrence of bilateral paramedian or bilateral polar infarction without the development of amnesia (Von Cramon *et al.* 1985, Bogousslavsky *et al.* 1991), suggesting that further studies are needed to refine our present concepts of the topographical correlates of amnesia in thalamic infarcts.

Dementia and related syndromes

Dementia is a feature of large bilateral paramedian or polar infarcts (Castaigne *et al.* 1962, De Boucaud *et al.* 1968, Chassagnon *et al.* 1969, Poirier *et al.* 1983, Kömpf *et al.* 1984, Katz *et al.* 1987, Bogousslavsky *et al.* 1988*e*, Muller *et al.* 1989), although the concept of thalamic dementia was emphasized initially in non-vascular cases (Stern 1939, Grünthal 1942). It is associated with impaired attention, slowed verbal–motor responses, apathy, poor motivation, and amnesia as its main features. A related syndrome, athymhormia (also called loss of psychic self-activation, robot syndrome, or psychic akinesia), is characterized by severe apathy, aspontaneity, and emotional indifference with loss of motor and affective drive, but without memory or other neuropsychological dysfunction; typically, this mental and motor inertia is readily reversible when the patient is stimulated by another person. This syndrome was first reported in basal ganglia or frontal lesions, but it may also be due to thalamic infarction with bilateral dorsomedial nucleus (non-magnocellular portion) and midline nuclei involvement (Bogousslavsky *et al.* 1991). It has also been reported after a left polar infarct, but, in this case, it was transient in comparison with the cases of bilateral thalamic infarcts (Lisovoski *et al.* 1993). Sparing of the magnocellular portion of the dorsomedial nucleus might explain the absence of amnesia in this syndrome, which may be related to dysfunction of the striatal–ventral–pallidal–thalamo-fronto-mesial–limbic loop (Haber *et al.* 1985) with corresponding hypoperfusion of the frontal cortex (Bogousslavsky *et al.* 1991). Athymhormia must be differentiated from akinetic mutism, which can also be a consequence of bilateral paramedian thalamic infarction (Lhermitte *et al.* 1963, Segarra 1970, Szirmai *et al.* 1977, van Domburg *et al.* 1996). The Klüver–Bucy syndrome, the main components of which are overattention to external stimuli or distractibility (hypermetamorphosis), hyperorality with oral exploration of objects and uncontrolled food intake, affective dyscontrol, and severe amnesia, has been reported after bilateral paramedian infarcts (Müller *et al.* 1999).

Hypoxic–ischaemic encephalopathy may lead to thalamic and basal ganglia involvement with relative preservation of the cortex and subcortical white matter (Kinney *et al.* 1994, Roland *et al.* 1998). Persistent vegetative state may be seen after extensive bilateral thalamic damage, with little, or only focal, damage to the cerebral cortex (Kinney *et al.* 1994). Similarly, extensive bilateral thalamic injury may be one pattern of perinatal hypoxic–ischaemic cerebral injury and is associated with a poor outcome (Roland *et al.* 1998).

Cerebral blood flow (CBF) and metabolic correlates of neuropsychological dysfunction have been evaluated by PET, single photon emission computed tomography (SPECT), and other CBF studies in patients with thalamic stroke (Bewermeyer *et al.* 1985, Baron *et al.* 1986, Franck *et al.* 1986, Viader *et al.* 1987, Rousseaux *et al.* 1989, 1990, 1998, Pappata *et al.* 1990, Bogousslavsky *et al.* 1991, Goldenberg *et al.* 1991, Kuwert *et al.* 1991, Szelies *et al.* 1991, Baron *et al.* 1992, Levasseur *et al.* 1992, Tanaka *et al.* 1992, 1996, McGilchrist *et al.* 1993, Pepin and Auray-Pepin 1993, Cohen *et al.* 1994, Hashimoto *et al.* 1995, Fukatsu *et al.* 1997, Müller *et al.* 1999, Van Der Werf *et al.* 1999). Although cortical diaschisis as a dynamic correlate to neuropsychological dysfunction, associated with infarcts limited to the thalamus, has been emphasized, these CBF or metabolic findings may represent the consequences of the interruption of cortical–subcortical loops, without implying that cortical deactivation is the cause of neuropsychological dysfunction *per se.*

Recovery and prognosis

Little is known about the long-term prognosis of patients with thalamic infarcts, because the literature is mainly anecdotal (Rondot *et al.* 1986, Vighetto *et al.* 1986). In a study of 40 patients with thalamic infarcts (Bogousslavsky *et al.* 1988*a*), one patient died in the acute phase from pulmonary embolism and myocardial infarct. During a mean follow-up of 45.6 months in the 39 survivors, the annual risk was 4.0 per cent for death and 3.8 per cent for recurrent stroke. Delayed symptoms from the initial infarct developed in six patients, with a delayed painful syndrome in three of the 27 patients with initial sensory dysfunction, and delayed abnormal movements of the dystonic–chorea type in three patients with paramedian infarction (always involving a previously paretic limb). Overall, two-thirds of the survivors could return to most, or all, of their previous occupations, while one-third remained disabled, mainly because of persisting neuropsychological dysfunction.

In two other studies, none of the 18 or 22 patients with thalamic infarcts died (Steinke *et al.* 1992, del Mar Sáez de Ocariz *et al.* 1996). However, most had persistent motor and sensory deficits (del Mar Sáez de Ocariz *et al.* 1996).

Treatment

General therapy for subcortical stroke is discussed in Chapter 24. Thalamic pain may persist as the most important stroke sequela. In our experience, tricyclic antidepressants, especially amitriptyline, relieve the pain in some patients. We often begin with a small dose (10–25 mg) and increase it up to 100 mg in patients who tolerate the side effects; in other patients, carbamazepine or serotonin re-uptake inhibitors may be of some value. Serotoninergic neurons are though to play a role in pain modulation, and development of pain 5 years after a thalamic infarct, following abrupt discontinuation of a serotonin re-uptake inhibitor antidepressant, has been reported (Lauterbach 1994). If the above medications fail to control the pain, the use of opioids or local application of lidocaine gel becomes necessary. If this is ineffective, the patient must be referred to a specialized pain clinic. Interestingly, relief of thalamic pain by a further thalamic infarct has been observed (Cordery and Rossor 1999), the mechanism probably being similar to that in stereotactic thalamic surgery for chronic pain treatment.

Haloperidol, in daily doses ranging from 2 to 10 mg, may be the most effective agent in suppressing choreoathetosis and other involuntary movements. Valproic acid may be effective in some patients. Treatment of thalamic tremor may be difficult, and experience comes mainly from anecdotal reports. The combination of propanolol and primidone (Soler *et al.* 1999), ceruletide (Mano *et al.* 1993), and levodopa (Lee *et al.* 1993) have given satisfactory results.

Thalamic infarctions versus haemorrhages

In two series of thalamic stroke, patients with either thalamic infarcts or restricted haematomas could not be distinguished by their neurological presentation (Steinke *et al.* 1992, del Mar Sáez de Ocariz *et al.* 1996). Indeed, small-size haemorrhages restricted to a limited portion of the thalamus have been classified into four groups, posterolateral, posteromedial, anterior, and dorsal, on the basis of the arterial blood supply, in the same way as thalamic infarcts (Chung *et al.* 1996). However, patients with ventricular bleeding or haemorrhages not restricted to the thalamus had a more severe motor deficit and a higher frequency of stupor or coma and death (Steinke *et al.* 1992, Chung *et al.* 1996, del Mar Sáez de Ocariz *et al.* 1996). A More detailed discussion of thalamic haemorrhages is provided in Chapter 26.

Thalamic infarctions in children

Thalamic infarcts were seen in eight of 36 children with deep subcortical infarction (Brower *et al.* 1996). The cause was unknown in three patients and was meningitis in three, trauma in one, and cardiac heart disease in one. The most common presenting symptoms were hemiplegia (5/8 patients), followed by seizures (3/8). Altered mental status and hemisensory syndrome were each present in one patient. All patients survived; no residual impairment was seen in four patients, while mild hemiparesis and severe residual impairment were each seen in two patients.

Conclusions

Thalamic infarcts lead to diverse neurological manifestations that can mimic superficial infarcts, other deep infarcts, and even other neurological and psychiatric diseases. In addition, thalamic infarcts can rarely be distinguished from thalamic haemorrhages on clinical grounds. The use of neuroimaging, especially MRI, is therefore essential for the diagnosis of the infarct and identification of the territory involved. Identification of the arterial territory is important for the prognosis and may also provide meaningful clues about stroke aetiology.

Further studies are required to delineate the clinical presentation and aetiology of combined thalamic infarcts. Moreover, the study of thalamic lesions and functional studies of the thalamus may shed some light on the physiology of important brain processes, such as memory, language, and consciousness.

Chapter 22

Acute infarcts in the white matter medullary artery territory of the centrum ovale

A. Tsiskaridze, G.R. de Freitas, P.-A. Uldry, and J. Bogousslavsky

Introduction

Patchy or diffuse abnormalities of the white matter (the core of which is formed by the centrum ovale), seen as areas of decreased attenuation on computed tomographic (CT) scans and signal hyperintensity on magnetic resonance imaging (MRI), are common findings in the elderly. To avoid pathological and aetiological confusion, the term 'leukoaraiosis' has been proposed (from leuko = white, and araiosis = rarefied) for this radiological phenomenon (Hachinski *et al.* 1987), which can easily be distinguished from infarction on the basis of the CT criteria proposed by Steingart *et al.* (1987) (Table 22.1). Although leukoaraiosis is sometimes associated with a decline in memory and intellectual function, its clinical significance remains largely undefined. These white matter changes are usually associated with an age of more than 60 years and a history of cardiac disorders and stroke (Pantoni and Garcia 1995). Repeated episodes of restricted perfusion in the centrum ovale may cause chronic injury resulting in 'partial or incomplete infarction' with oedema and demyelination, loss of oligodendrocytes, astrocyte gliosis, and dilatation of the perivascular spaces (Brun and Englund 1986), which may be clinically inconspicuous, but can be identified by MRI (Ransom *et al.* 1990). Conversely, most cases of leukoaraiosis are not associated with acute stroke syndromes, and acute infarcts selectively involving the centrum ovale are rarely reported, perhaps because they are often not recognized. The first case of centrum ovale infarct, a 74-year-old man presenting with left ataxic hemiparesis and hemihypoaesthesia and showing a large lesion in the right centrum ovale on autopsy, was reported by Souques in the Proceedings of the 'Société Francaise de Neurologie' (Roussy and Foix 1910).

Anatomy and blood supply

The common central mass of the supraventricular white matter containing commissural, association, and projection fibres has an oval appearance in horizontal

Table 22.1 Computed tomography criteria used to distinguish infarction from leukoaraiosis

Parameter	Infarct	Leukoaraiosis
Site	White matter and/or cortex	White matter only, without extension to cortex
Extent	Internal capsule, basal ganglia, or thalamus may be involved	No involvement of internal capsule, basal ganglia, or thalamus
Margins	Well demarcated	Ill defined, patchy, diffuse
Shape	Wedge-shaped, can follow a vascular territory	Diffuse white matter involvement
Other effects	Enlargement of ipsilateral ventricle or sulcus	Ventricle and sulcus unchanged locally

sections of the brain and is termed the 'centrum ovale' (or 'centrum semiovale of Vieussens'). Radiologically, its outermost and innermost limits, respectively, are the cortical ribbon and the lower corona radiata at the level of the deep perforators (Damasio 1983, Ghika *et al.* 1989). The vascularization of the centrum ovale is still debated (De Reuck 1971, Moody *et al.* 1990) and there is a lack of specific anatomic studies on the origin of the blood supply to the centrum. In general, this includes transcortical arterioles that have an exclusive territory and some terminal ramifications of certain deep perforating branches. The deep perforating branches from the distal internal carotid artery (ICA) or the middle cerebral artery (MCA) trunk are terminal branches which perforate the basal part of the cerebral hemispheres (Bogousslavsky 1991). The MCA is the origin of two main groups of deep perforators, the lateral and medial lenticulostriate arteries. The anterior cerebral artery (ACA) also gives rise to two groups of perforators, the anterior lenticulostriate arteries and the recurrent artery of Heubner (Ghika *et al.* 1990). These branches do not contribute markedly to perfusion of the centrum ovale. The core of the centrum is supplied from the brain surface by single-source, long (20–50 mm) perforating arteries and arterioles originating from the superficial 'pial' arteries and having exclusive territories that border smoothly on one another, rather than interdigitate. These medullary arteries are close to one other (i.e. they originate from the same pial distribution artery) and penetrate to different depths, the longest converging centripetally toward the angles of the lateral ventricules (Moody *et al.* 1990). Many vessels supplying the centrum ovale arise from distributing pial arteries at the cortical borderzones, between the MCA and the ACA or the MCA and the posterior cerebral artery (PCA); these zones are known to be positioned precariously and are vulnerable to hypoperfusion. Thus, there are at least two vascular borderzones of the white matter medullary arteries in the core of the centrum ovale itself. There is also another part of the white matter in the upper corona radiata and the lower portion of the centrum ovale which lies between irrigation. At this level, the medullary

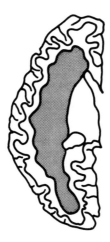

Fig. 22.1 Centrum ovale with the white matter medullary artery territory.

arteries form a junctional zone with the deep perforating branches of the MCA (lenticulostriate arteries) and anterior choroidal artery. This zone should be considered as 'junctional' rather than 'watershed' or 'borderzone', as all these networks are terminal, without collateralization or anastomoses (Bogousslavsky and Regli 1992). The centrum ovale and the white matter medullary arterial territory are shown in Fig. 22.1. In summary, the major part of the centrum ovale is supplied by superficial perforators (white matter long medullary branches), the territory of which is surrounded by two borderzones:

(1) a zone between the vascular territories of the long medullary arteries and short medullary branches ending in the arcuate fibres, which is present mainly at the level of the sulci and in which bending long medullary branches are absent;

(2) a junctional zone in the periventricular white matter of the corona radiata between the ventriculopetal long medullary branches and the ventriculofugal branches arising from the lateral striatal arteries in the anterior part of the brain and from the lateral posterior choroidal arteries in its posterior part (De Reuck 1971).

In this chapter, we only consider brain infarcts in the territory of the medullary arteries, so the terms 'centrum ovale infarcts' and 'white matter medullary infarcts of the centrum ovale' are considered synonymous.

Definition and frequency

There is no general agreement about the definition of centrum ovale infarcts. Some misunderstanding is caused by the fact that the small part of the centrum ovale in its lower portion represents the internal junctional zone between the medullary arteries and deep perforators of the MCA. This is the reason why some authors refer to internal junctional infarcts as centrum ovale infarcts, although, in fact, they are not 'pure' centrum ovale infarctions of the white matter medullary territory.

The criteria for a centrum ovale infarct are:

(1) acute stroke limited to the territory of the medullary branches, irrespective of its size;

(2) no involvement of the cerebral cortex or the territories of the deep perforators (lenticulostriate, anterior choroidal, and thalamic) or borderzone (junctional) territories adjacent to the territory of white matter medullary arteries; large infarcts in the core of the centrum ovale may extend to the border (junctional) zone between the superficial and deep perforators, but infarcts strictly limited to this zone should not be classified as centrum ovale infarcts, but as internal watershed (junctional) infarcts;

(3) the infarct seen on the CT scan or MRI must be consistent with the clinical picture and cannot be explained simply by leukoaraiosis or as the sequelae of haemorrhage.

It should be mentioned that it is sometimes difficult to classify the type of infarct accurately according to the vascular supply territories, as the cerebral vascular supply areas may vary and the use of rigid vascular templates may sometimes result in incorrect definition of the borderzones (Van der Zwan et al. 1992).

In the prospective Lausanne Stroke Registry (Bogousslavsky et al. 1988b), an infarct limited to the white matter territory of the centrum ovale was found in 36 (1.63%) of 2200 patients admitted for first-ever stroke (Bogousslavsky and Regli 1992). This percentage is lower than that for cerebral infarction in the watershed area, multiple territories, or the ACA territory (all 3%). The male:female ratio was 1.6:1, with a mean age of 65 ± 6 years. Some patients experienced previous transient ischaemic attacks, which were ipsilateral to the centrum ovale infarct. In another consecutive series of 225 first-ever stroke patients, 57 (22.4%) had small infarcts in the centrum ovale (Leys et al. 1994). However, in 34 of these 57 patients, the centrum ovale infarct were clinically silent, so only 23 (10%) patients actually showed a clinically manifested acute infarct in the centrum ovale. It is possible that there may have been overlapping of centrum ovale and internal junctional infarcts, which may explain the higher frequency of centrum ovale infarcts compared with the Lausanne series. The European Carotid Surgery Trialists' Collaborative Group (ECST) (Boiten et al. 1997) also reported a higher incidence of centrum ovale infarcts (7%) among first-ever stroke patients, which may be due to differences in patient selection and categorization of infarct type. In the most recent report on centrum ovale infarcts in which more strict definitions were used, 22 (1.2%) of 1800 consecutive acute stroke patients had a centrum ovale infarct (Read et al. 1998b).

Clinical features

Two types of centrum ovale infarct can be defined on the basis of infarct size and shape, clinical picture, risk factors, and associated vascular disease (Bogousslavsky and Regli 1992):

(1) small infarcts: round or ovoid infarct, maximal diameter less than 1.5 cm; and

(2) large infarcts: maximal diameter greater than 1.5 cm, with an irregular shape, the geographical margins following the inner border of the cortex.

Examples of small and large infarcts of the centrum ovale are shown in Figs 22.2 and 22.3.

Small infarcts

These represent the most common type of stroke limited to the centrum ovale (72.2%). They are small deep infarcts that may be considered as 'lacunes'. The relative frequency of lacunar stroke varies between 10.7 and 20 per cent of a stroke series (Orgogozo and Bogousslavsky 1989). The neurological deficit can develop over several hours (24–48 h) or within a few minutes, and is compatible with so-called 'lacunar syndrome' (Fisher 1965a, 1991), consisting of facio-bracio-crural or partial hemiparesis, sensorimotor stroke, and ataxic hemiparesis. In rare cases, the clinical syndrome includes speech disturbance (both dysarthria and dysphagia) (Lanoe et al. 1994, Read et al. 1998b). Small infarcts in the centrum ovale frequently are clinically silent and are detected accidentally (Leys et al. 1994).

The majority of patients with small infarcts (69.2%) have complete or partial motor dysfunction. Boiten and Lodder (1991b) reported seven patients with isolated

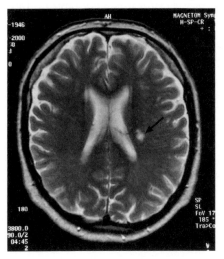

Fig. 22.2 Small infarct in the centrum ovale, close to the anterior choroidal artery territory.

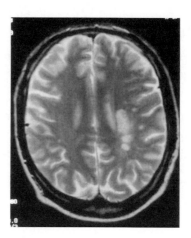

Fig. 22.3 Large infarct in the centrum ovale.

monoparesis (the arm in five cases and the leg in two). The CT scan showed a small infarct involving the subcortex in the superficial MCA territory. A small infarct involving the cortex can lead to monoparesis, but an infarction in the subcortex or centrum ovale may have the same effect, as the corticospinal tract converges from the rather extended sensorimotor cortex into a small tract running through the internal capsule to the medullary pyramid and spinal cord. The low frequency of sensorimotor strokes in cases of centrum ovale infarction can be explained in the same way. This syndrome may be present in the case of infarction in the white matter in the neighbourhood of the internal capsule where the motor and sensory fibres run close to each other. In a recent series of 32 patients with sensorimotor stroke, only one patient (3%) was shown by MRI to have a small (<1.5 cm) infarct in the centrum ovale (Staaf *et al.* 1998).

Ataxic hemiparesis is relatively uncommon in centrum ovale infarcts (Gutmann and Scherer 1989, Bogousslavsky and Regli 1992). This syndrome is characterized by weakness and ataxia (defective postural fixation and limb ataxia) on the same side of the body. The lesion usually lies in the pons, the posterior limb of the internal capsule, the corona radiata, or, occasionally, the centrum ovale (Fisher 1978*b*, Iragui and McCutchen 1982, Sage and Lepore 1983). However, CT may fail to identify a co-existing pontine lesion, and MRI should be performed to exclude this possibility (Helweg *et al.* 1988). To produce ataxic hemiparesis, the infarct must interrupt the fibres connecting the ventrolateral nucleus of the thalamus to the precentral cortex in the centrum ovale. Alternatively, a centrum ovale lesion may interrupt fibres arising from the prefrontal and precentral areas, subsequently forming the frontopontine tract or Arnold's bundle, or fibres from the temporal, occipital, and parietal areas, which subsequently unite to form the occipito-temporo-parietopontine tract or Türks bundle.

Hemichoreoathetosis is rare in centrum ovale infarcts, and only three cases have been reported (Barinagarrementeria *et al.* 1989, Bogousslavsky and Regli 1992,

Pelletier *et al.* 1997). The case reported by Barinagarrementeria *et al.* (1989) was a 66-year-old man who presented with acute onset of involuntary movements of the left arm and leg, without any motor or sensory deficit. CT and MRI showed an infarct in the right corona radiata without extension into the putamen or caudate nucleus. Pelletier *et al.* (1997) described a 17-year-old woman with subacute onset of slight hemiparesis and abnormal choreoid movements in the left extremities appearing 2 weeks after starting oral contraceptives. Cerebral angiography showed features resembling moya-moya disease, while MRI revealed a small (<1.5 cm) vascular lesion in the right centrum ovale. It is probable that an infarct in the centrum ovale would interrupt the excitatory corticostriate pathways, causing a decreased rate of firing in the striatum and liberating the pallidum from strial inhibition and resulting in the syndrome of chorea.

Large infarcts

This type of infarct involves the territory of more than one medullary branch. The maximal diameter is always greater than 1.5 cm and is usually greater than 2.5 cm. It accounts for a quarter of centrum ovale infarcts in the Lausanne Stroke Registry (Bogousslavsky and Regli 1992). In a consecutive series of 1800 admissions to a stroke unit, among the 22 patients with centrum ovale infarcts, there were only three (13%) with infarcts larger than 1.5 cm (Read *et al.* 1998*b*); this low frequency of large centrum ovale infarcts was explained by the authors as resulting from the use of stricter anatomo-topographical inclusion criteria by which large infarcts in the internal watershed (junctional) territory of the corona radiata were classified as internal watershed infarcts and therefore excluded, although it is noteworthy that the same approach was used in the Lausanne study (all study patients had large infarcts in the core of the centrum ovale itself and not at the junction of the deep and superficial territories of the MCA) (Bogousslavsky and Regli 1992). The reason for this discrepancy seems to be the lack of exact anatomo-topographical criteria for the zones supplied by the medullary arteries (Tatu *et al.* 1998) and the well-recognized interindividual variation in vascular territories (Van der Zwan *et al.* 1992), which may complicate classification of infarct type, with subsequent effects on the observed clinical and risk factor profiles. Nevertheless, Read *et al.* (1998*b*) provided rather simple and practical guidelines for distinguishing centrum ovale white matter medullary infarcts from internal watershed (junctional) infarcts (Table 22.2).

In terms of the clinical characteristics of large centrum ovale infarcts, stroke onset is usually sudden, and the neurological deficit stabilizes within a few minutes. The neurological signs are similar to those found in large superficial or extended MCA infarcts. The deficits are characterized by marked hemiparesis affecting the upper limb and face to a greater extent than the lower extremities, with an accompanying sensory deficit which follows a similar pattern of facio-brachial predominance. Additional elements include either aphasia (dominant hemisphere infarct) or visuospatial

Table 22.2 Features that distinguish white matter medullary infarcts of the centrum ovale from internal watershed (junctional) infarcts

Feature	Internal watershed (junctional) infarct	White matter medullary infarct
Location white	Deeper (more paraventricular; closer to deep perforator territory)	More superficial (immediate subcortical white matter)
Size	Typically larger (>1.5 cm)	Mostly smaller (<1.5 cm), occasionally larger (>1.5 cm)
Proposed pathological mechanism	Carotid occlusion, haemodynamic or embolic occlusion of the MCA	Usually *in situ* small vessel disease, occasionally embolic

MCA = middle cerebral artery.

disturbances (non-dominant hemisphere involvement). A visual field defect is encountered when the infarct affects the optic radiations which traverse the posterior part of the centrum ovale.

Pathogenesis

Based on analysis of the Lausanne Stroke Registry, chronic hypertension and diabetes are frequent in small infarcts, whereas carotid disease is rare (Bogousslavsky and Regli 1992). These findings suggest that small centrum ovale infarcts are related to small vessel disease involving the medullary branches in a way similar to lacunar infarction in the territory of the deep perforators of the MCA (Ghika *et al.* 1989). Leys *et al.* (1994) noted small artery disease in two-thirds of their patients with small centrum ovale infarcts and indicated that other mechanisms account for the other third. Classically, occlusion of a deep penetrating artery by a local primary process is included in the definition of a lacune. This *in situ* arteriopathy is considered to result from chronic hypertension or diabetes (Fisher 1965a). Later studies have disputed the role of small vessel disease as the sole contributor to small centrum ovale infarcts. Mull *et al.* (1997) have emphasized the importance of MCA occlusive disease in the development of small supraventricular white matter lesions. Krapf *et al.* (1998) found a strong association between multiple small rosary-like centrum ovale infarcts and both ipsilateral high-grade carotid disease (occlusion or stenosis) and diminished ipsilateral CO_2 reactivity, indicating haemodynamic failure. However, it is possible that these infarcts were referred improperly to the white matter medullary territory, as their extent, site, and multiplicity would seem to attribute them to the so-called partial internal watershed infarcts (Bladin and Chambers 1993a), which appear in the internal junctional zone and result from haemodynamic failure. Other studies, using stricter topographical inclusion criteria, also emphasized the role of ipsilateral large artery disease in the development of small centrum ovale infarcts. Thus, analysis of the ECST data has shown that classical lacunar infarcts and small centrum ovale infarcts have a similar vascular risk factor profile, but the latter is associated with a significantly higher degree of symptomatic carotid stenosis (or occlusion) of more than 50 per cent (Boiten *et al.* 1997). Actually, small infarcts in the centrum ovale and classical lacunes can be haemodynamic in origin, resulting from impaired blood flow in the long medullary and striatal branches due to several atherosclerotic stenoses throughout their long course. Moreover, studying small infarcts in the internal borderzones, Hupperts *et al.* (1997*b*) concluded that even borderzone small infarctions are compatible with occlusion of a single penetrator and that the stroke mechanism in the borderzones does not differ from that in small deep infarcts in general, i.e. small vessel disease. They supposed that reduced perfusion drop in distal supply areas is the most likely cause of such infarcts. Such perfusion drops may occur during periods of hypotension in the presence of a proximal (carotid) arterial obstruction in some or a more distal obstruction (small artery disease) in the majority of borderzone small deep infarcts. The same mechanism may be involved in small centrum ovale infarcts. However, the most recent large clinical series has shown the same incidence of ipsilateral carotid disease in cases of centrum ovale medullary infarcts as that seen in the Lausanne Stroke Registry (Read *et al.* 1998*b*).

The only systematic clinico-pathological study of small centrum ovale infarcts included 12 pathologically verified small centrum ovale infarcts, of which six were symptomatic (Lammie and Wardlaw 1999). Histologically, small centrum ovale infarcts were often mixtures of complete and incomplete infarcts. Incomplete infarction is now recognized to result from either global circulatory insufficiency, which may be due to atherosclerotic stenosis of small vessels (small vessel disease), sometimes co-existing with large artery disease, or from arterial occlusion of short duration and/or of moderate severity (Garcia *et al.* 1995). The majority of small centrum ovale infarcts have shown borderzone localization, i.e. they were found at the junction of the ACA and MCA territories (Lammie and Wardlaw 1999). According to the authors, such a distribution suggests haemodynamic mechanisms, ICA occlusive disease, or embolism. Indeed, 10 of the 12 patients had possible embolic sources. However, it must be emphasized that, in all 12 cases, there was evidence of co-existing small artery disease which was severe in five cases and moderate in seven. In two cases, the small vessel disease was considered as a definite or probable mechanism for infarction. The authors favoured a concept of pathogenetic heterogeneity or 'plurality' of small centrum ovale infarcts, in which embolic and/or haemodynamic mechanisms as well as small vessel disease are considered as being responsible for the development of this type of infarct. However, this observation was based on only a small series of cases and further pathological studies would be necessary to confirm the association of small vessel disease or other possible underlying causes with small deep infarcts in the centrum ovale.

The mechanisms of large infarcts are not clear. Ipsilateral carotid occlusion or greater than 50 per cent stenosis is common (80%), which may suggest distal haemodynamic failure (Bogousslavsky and Regli 1992). In a series of 38 patients with major arterial occlusive disease and newly developed large subcortical infarcts (Nakano *et al.* 1995), there were nine cases with infarcts greater than 2 cm in the centrum ovale, all of which showed evidence of occlusive disease in the ICA, which also points to distal haemodynamic insufficiency. This mechanism is supported by the facts that (i) borderzones between the ACA, MCA, and PCA also exist in the centrum ovale and are known to be vulnerable to hypoperfusion; (ii) deep medullary arteries, over their long course, may also undergo atherosclerotic obstruction and, in the case of the co-existence of ipsilateral high degree stenosis or occlusion of the ICA, show vulnerability to hypoperfusion, as indicated above (De Reuck 1971). However, artery-to-artery embolism or cardiac embolism cannot be formally excluded in many instances.

Evolution

Stroke patterns and evolution from acute infarction in the centrum ovale are still not well known. In general, these infarcts seem to have a good prognosis. Patients with small infarcts usually improve more quickly than those with large infarcts. Patients with isolated monoparesis recover within 2–4 weeks (Boiten and Lodder 1991*b*). In acute hemichorea, haloperidol (10 mg/day) can reduce the involuntary movements (Barinagarrementeria *et al.* 1989).

Chapter 23

Prognosis of patients with lacunar infarction syndromes

B. Norrving

Introduction

As more specific therapies are developed for the prevention and treatment of stroke, definition of the pathophysiological mechanism assumes greater importance in clinical practice. For different subgroups of patients, prognostic data are needed by clinicians for counselling and managing the individual patient. Also, for the planning of treatment trials, background data on prognosis from clinical series are essential. It should be recognized that almost no prognostic study on stroke patients reflects the true natural course, but rather the prognosis in patients given some form of treatment, such as active management of risk factors and antiplatelet therapy.

Basic data that need to be known include prognosis for survival, recurrence of stroke, residual disability, and quality of life, as well as predictive factors for the main outcome events. The long-term prognosis with regard to cognitive function also needs to be assessed, as well as the risk of asymptomatic progression of the underlying vascular process.

The present review analyses existing research on prognosis of patients with lacunar infarction syndromes. The main focus will be on studies with the primary purpose of providing long-term prognostic data in cases with first-ever lacunar stroke, describing the prognosis in this stroke subgroup either as a separate entity or together with other specific subtypes of stroke.

Baseline characteristics of available studies

Prognostic data are available from 18 studies, five of which are community-based (Bamford *et al.* 1987, Giroud *et al.* 1991, Sacco *et al.* 1991, Anderson *et al.* 1994a, Petty *et al.* 2000) whereas 13 studies are based on hospital series (Gandolfo *et al.* 1986, Hier *et al.* 1991, Brainin *et al.* 1992, Landi *et al.* 1992, Boiten and Lodder 1993, Nadeau *et al.* 1993, Clavier *et al.* 1994, Sacco *et al.* 1994, Salgado *et al.* 1996, Samuelsson *et al.* 1996a, Yamamoto *et al.* 1998, Staaf *et al.* 2000, Kazui *et al.* 2001). The principal features of these studies are summarized in Table 23.1. Of two reports from the Oxfordshire Community Stroke Project providing data on prognosis in lacunes (Bamford *et al.* 1987, 1991), data from the first report were used.

Table 23.1 Baseline characteristics of prognostic studies for lacunar infarction syndromes

Reference	No. of patients	Proportion with CT scan or MRI (%)	Mean age (years)	Male (%)	Hypertension (%)	Diabetes (%)	Proportion with carotid studies (%)	Proportion with major cardioembolic source (%)	Design
Hospital-based studies									
Gandolfo et al. (1986)	107	100	65.3	79.4	60.7	NR	NR	NR	Retrospective
Hier et al. (1991)[a]	337	98	65	50	75	26	18	NR	Prospective
Brainin et al. (1992)	107	100	67	NR	NR	NR	100	NR	Prospective
Landi et al. (1992)	88	100	63.5	62.5	64.8	19.3	100	12.5	Prospective
Boiten and Lodder (1993)[b]	103	93	67	55	50	27	83.5	14.6	Prospective
Nadeau et al. (1993)	59	100	NR	100	NR	NR	NR	NR	Prospective
Clavier et al. (1994)	172	100	NR	62.7	75.7	22.6	NR	NR	Retrospective
Sacco et al. (1994)	85	100	NR	NR	NR	NR	NR	NR	Prospective
Salgado et al. (1996)	145	100	64.8	64	72	25	100	10	Prospective
Samuelsson et al. (1996a)[c]	81	100	66	63.0	51.6	24.7	100	3.7	Prospective
Yamamoto et al. (1998)	105	100	68	68.6	66.7	23.8	NR	0	Prospective
Staaf et al. (2000)	180	57	72	58.5	52.2	15.6	42.2	2.8	Retrospective
Kazui et al. (2000)	60	100	64.6	35/60	43/60	9/60	80	3	Prospective
Community-based studies									
Bamford et al. (1987)[d]	102	96	71.8	41.2	44	13	NR	12	Prospective

Giroud et al. (1991)[e]	68	100	70.9	58.8	77	25	NR	NR	Prospective
Sacco et al. (1991)	78	76	70	48	81	14	NR	12	Retrospective
Anderson et al. (1994a)[f]	22	100	71	73	64	14	NR	0	Prospective
Petty et al. (2000)[g]	72	100	73	43	75	22	NR	6	Retrospective

NR = not reported.

[a] Also includes data from Chamorro et al. (1991).

[b] Also includes data from Boiten (1991).

[c] Also includes data from Samuelsson et al. (1994, 1996b).

[d] Also includes data from Lodder et al. (1990).

[e] Data on mean age, gender, hypertension, and diabetes refer to 165 cases with lacunes, 68 of whom was followed till 2 years.

[f] Includes data provided by C. Anderson (personal communication 2001).

[g] Also includes data from Petty et al. (1999).

Of the two reports from the Perth Community Stroke Study, one (Anderson *et al.* 1994*a*) used a strict definition of lacunar infarcts (lacunar syndrome and small or no visible ischaemic lesion on neuroimaging) whereas the other report (Anderson *et al.* 1994*b*) used the Oxfordshire classification system; data from the first report were used for this review. A study by Miyao *et al.* (1992) reported prognostic features for 215 patients with lacunar infarction, but data were subdivided into the subsets of patients who had presence or absence of leukoaraiosis on computed tomography (CT) scan, and not given in aggregate.

A prospective design was adopted in 12 of the studies. Inclusion criteria are, in general, patients with a first-ever stroke presenting with one of the five commonly recognized lacunar syndromes (pure motor hemiparesis, pure sensory stroke, sensorimotor stroke, ataxic hemiparesis, and dysarthria – clumsy hand syndrome). Exceptions are the study of Gandolfo *et al.* (1986) in which 25.2 per cent of the patients had 'pseudobulbar palsy' (a clinical presentation not generally accepted as a lacunar syndrome and uncertain if first-ever cases of stroke) and the study of Clavier *et al.* (1994) in which 26.6 per cent of the patients had a history of stroke or transient ischaemic attacks (TIAs). The study of Staaf *et al.* (2000) was limited to patients with pure motor stroke only, whereas in the study from the Mayo Clinic (Sacco *et al.* 1991) patients with a sensorimotor stroke were included only if there was CT evidence of an appropriate small, deep infarction. The proportions of patients examined with neuroimaging of the brain are variable; in several studies either CT or magnetic resonance imaging (MRI) was mandatory for inclusion into the study. MRI was performed in all patients in two of the studies (Clavier *et al.* 1994, Samuelsson *et al.* 1996*a*).

Data on the prevalence of risk factors (all items not available from all studies) differ markedly, from 50 to 81 per cent for hypertension, and 14 to 27 per cent for diabetes. The presence of a major cardioembolic source was an exclusion criterion in some studies, whereas others reported rates up to 14.6 per cent for this risk factor. The mean age of patients tends to be younger in hospital-based than in community-based studies.

Prognosis for survival

Data on prognosis for survival, available from 16 of the 18 studies, are summarized in Table 23.2.

A very low early case–fatality ratio (0–2% at 30 days) is a common finding in all reports which provide data on this issue (Bamford *et al.* 1987, Sacco *et al.* 1991, 1994, Landi *et al.* 1992, Boiten and Lodder 1993, Anderson *et al.* 1994*a*, Nadeau *et al.* 1993, Samuelsson *et al.* 1996*a*, Staaf *et al.* 2000, Petty *et al.* 2000, Kazui *et al.* 2001), the exception being the study by Giroud *et al.* (1991) which reported a rate of 10 per cent. Cases who died within 30 days after the onset were excluded from the study by Gandolfo *et al.* (1986). In total, only 21 out of 828 patients (2.5%) died within 30 days after onset, which illustrates that the possibility of obtaining timely pathological examinations in patients with lacunar syndromes is very limited.

The long-term risk of death varies markedly between the studies. At 1 year after stroke onset, between 2.4 (Sacco *et al.* 1994) and 15 per cent (Boiten and Lodder 1993) were dead. The annual death rate ranges from 3.1 (Sacco *et al.* 1991) to 15 per cent (Boiten and Lodder 1993), with an average of 2.8 per cent for these studies (Gandolfo *et al.* 1986, Giroud *et al.* 1991, Sacco *et al.* 1991, 1994, Landi *et al.* 1992, Nadeau *et al.* 1993, Clavier *et al.* 1994, Salgado *et al.* 1996, Samuelsson *et al.* 1996*a*, Staaf *et al.* 2000, Petty *et al.* 2000, Kazui *et al.* 2001). In the six studies reporting survival up to 4 years or more (Sacco *et al.* 1991, 1994, Clavier *et al.* 1994, Salgado *et al.* 1996, Petty *et al.* 2000, Staaf *et al.* 2000), the range is 2.8–7 per cent. No clear relationship between the survival rates and design or baseline characteristics of the studies is apparent.

The prognosis for survival generally has been found to be more favourable in patients with lacunar infarcts than in those with other stroke subtypes (Sacco *et al.* 1991, 1994, Brainin *et al.* 1992, Landi *et al.* 1992, Boiten and Lodder 1993, Nadeau *et al.* 1993, Anderson *et al.* 1994*a*, Petty *et al.* 2000). Sacco *et al.* (1991) even reported that survival in patients with lacunar infarcts was similar to an age- and sex-matched general population. However, the recent study by Staaf *et al.* (2000) showed that from age 4 years and onwards, patients with lacunar infarcts carried an excessive risk of death compared with the general population. In aggregate, about 60 per cent of deaths are due to cardiovascular disease.

Predictive factors for death determined by multivariate analysis have been reported in three of the studies (Clavier *et al.* 1994, Salgado *et al.* 1996, Staaf *et al.* 2000), and were found to be age, diabetes, and smoking (Clavier *et al.* 1994), age and disability score (Salgado *et al.* 1996), and age, sex, and non-use of aspirin (Staaf *et al.* 2000). Miyao *et al.* (1992) reported that leukoaraiosis was associated with an increased risk of death, but multivariate statistics were not adopted.

Prognosis for recurrence of stroke

The reported 1 year stroke recurrence rate, summarized in Table 23.2, ranges from 2.3 (Staaf *et al.* 2000) to about 10.7 per cent (Sacco *et al.* 1994) in hospital-based studies, whereas the rates are more uniform, ranging from 10 to 11.8 per cent, in the community-based studies. Twelve studies provide data for periods of follow-up longer than 1 year. When calculated as average risk per year, the range is from 2.4 to 7 per cent (mean value 4.8% per year). In most studies, the risk of recurrent stroke is approximately the same after the first year. However, in the study with the longest period of follow-up (Staaf *et al.* 2000), the annual rate decreased from about 5 per cent per during the first 5 years, to less than 1 per cent between 5 and 10 years after the index stroke.

There is considerable variation between studies on the subtype of recurrent strokes. Sacco *et al.* (1991) reported that only 17 per cent of recurrent strokes were lacunar

Table 23.2 Prognosis for survival and recurrent stroke: lacunar infarction syndromes

Reference	No. of patients	Time of follow-up	30-day case: fatality ratio (%)	Rate of death	Rate of recurrent stroke
Hospital-based studies					
Gandolfo et al. (1986)	107	47 months (mean)	NR	7.4% per year	4.7% per year
Hier et al. (1991)	337	2 years	NR	NR	12.3% at 2 years
Brainin et al. (1992)	107	1 year	0	11.3% at 1 year	NR
Landi et al. (1992)	88	31.1 months (mean)	0	9.1% at 2.6 years	7.9% at 1 year
					13.6% at 2.6 years
Boiten and Lodder (1993)	103	11 months (mean)	2	15% at 1 year	5.0% at 1 year
Nadeau et al. (1993)	53	36 months (mean)	2	25% at 3 years	21% at 3 years
Clavier et al. (1994)	172	35 months (mean)	NR	10% at 2 years	6% at 2 years
				20% at 4 years	15% at 4 years
Sacco et al. (1994)	85	3.3 years (mean)	0	2.4% at 1 year	10.7% at 1 year
				15.4% at 5 years	17.3% at 5 years
Salgado et al. (1996)	145	39 months (median)	NR	14% at 5 years	28% at 5 years
Samuelsson et al. (1996[a])	81	4 years (median)	0	6% at 4 years	21% at 4 years
Yamamoto et al. (1998)	105	3.2 years (mean)	NR	NR	14.3% at 3.2 years
Staaf et al. (2000)	180	77.9 months (mean)	NR	60% at 10 years	23.5% at 10 years
Kazui et al. (2001)	60	3.9 years (mean)	0	3.3% at 1 year	6.7% at 1 year
				Mean 2.8% per year	Mean 5.2% per year

Community-based studies

Bamford et al. (1987)	102	1 year	1	9.8% at 1 year	11.8% at 1 year
Giroud et al. (1991)	68	2 years	10	22% at 2 years	11% at 2 years
Sacco et al. (1991)	78	NR	0	3% at 1 year 25% at 5 years	4% at 1 month 10% at 1 year 26% at 5 years
Anderson et al. (1994a)	22	1 year	0	14% at 1 year	9% at 1 year
Petty et al. (2000)	72	3.2 years (mean)	1.4	6.9% at 1 year 12.5% at 2 years 35.1% at 5 years	7.1% at 1 year 11.6% at 2 years 24.8% at 5 years

infarcts, whereas other studies have reported proportions up to 84 per cent (Boiten and Lodder 1993). A recent study by Yamamoto and Bogousslavsky (1998) on pathophysiological mechanisms of second and further strokes in patients from the Lausanne Stroke Registry reported that about half of recurrent infarcts in patients with lacunes were of the same type as the index stroke. A substudy from the Dutch TIA Trial showed that patients with large vessel disease were more likely to have an ischaemic stroke of the same vessel type than patients with small vessel disease (Kappelle *et al.* 1995). In the detailed study on pathogenetic mechanisms of recurrent stroke after lacunar infarction by Samuelsson *et al.* (1996*a*), in which all patients with recurrent strokes were examined with MRI with gadolinium contrast, a heterogenous pattern was also found. In patients with recurrent lacunes, the clinical features were sometimes complex and included a parkinsonian type of gait disturbance, prominent pseudobulbar features, and somnolence, gaze disturbance, and progressive decline in cognitive functions. The proportion of intracerebral haemorrhage among recurrent strokes after lacunar infarction appears to be similar to that of stroke in general, i.e. about 10 per cent.

Predictive factors for recurrent stroke were analysed by multivariate statistics in five of the studies (Clavier *et al.* 1994, Salgado *et al.* 1996, Samuelsson *et al.* 1996*a*, Staaf *et al.* 2000, Kazui *et al.* 2001). Clavier *et al.* (1994) and Salgado *et al.* (1996) were unable to show any predictive variable, whereas Samuelsson *et al.* (1996*a*) found age, and Staaf *et al.* (2000) found hypertension and diabetes, to be independent factors. In the most recent study by Kazui *et al.* (2001), in which all patients were assessed by transoesophageal echocardiography, any source of embolism from the heart was the only factor which significantly enhanced the risk of recurrence. Miyao *et al.* (1992) reported that recurrent stroke was significantly associated with the presence of leukoaraiosis in a univariate analysis. Yamamoto *et al.* (1998), also adopting univariate comparisons, reported that a high average ambulatory blood pressure, especially during the night, increased the risk of new infarcts in patients with lacunar stroke.

Comparisons of the risk of recurrent stroke for lacunar infarcts versus other subtypes of stroke are available from several studies. In the Oxfordshire Community Stroke Project, patients with lacunar infarcts manifested a significantly lower risk of recurrence at 1 year (hazard ratio 0.5) than patients with partial and total anterior circulation infarcts or posterior circulation infarcts (Bamford *et al.* 1991). In contrast, the Mayo Clinic series reported that the actuarial risk of recurrence at 5 years among survivors was similar across stroke subtypes: 26 per cent for lacunar and 27 per cent for non-lacunar infarcts (Sacco *et al.* 1991). In the Stroke Data Bank, the 2-year stroke recurrence rates were similar for lacunar and embolic infarcts (12.3 and 12.4%, respectively), higher than in patients with infarcts of unknown cause (8.3%) and lower than in those with infarcts due to large vessel atherosclerosis (21.8%) (Hier *et al.* 1991). A lower rate of recurrence in lacunar infarcts was reported by Landi *et al.* (1992) and Nadeau *et al.* (1993), whereas Boiten and Lodder (1993) found no significant difference in the risk of recurrent stroke in patients with lacunar versus superficial infarcts. However, in the latter study, there were only a total of nine patients with recurrent stroke. Petty *et al.* (2000) found that ischaemic stroke subtype was not a significant predictor of long-term recurrence before or after adjusting for age, stroke severity, and diabetes mellitus.

Prognosis for disability, handicap, and quality of life

The long-term prognosis for functional outcome after lacunar infarction syndromes has received less attention than the prognosis for survival or recurrent stroke.

In the Oxfordshire Community Project (Bamford *et al.* 1987), functional outcome was assessed by the modified Rankin scale. Before the stroke, 11.8 per cent of the patients were dependent; at 1 year after the stroke, 10 patients (9.8%) were dead, 61 patients (59.8%) were independent, and 31 patients (30.4%) were dependent. Thus, of patients surviving at 1 year, fully one-third were dependent on other persons to some extent. A similar proportion (64%) was reported at 2 years by Giroud *et al.* (1991). A more favourable functional outcome, with 81.9 per cent of the patients being independent at 1 year according to the modified Rankin scale, was reported by Petty *et al.* (2000), and may be attributable to a higher proportion of patients (95.8%) being independent before the stroke in this study. Compared with the other stroke subtypes, patients with lacunar ischaemic stroke had milder maximal neurological deficits and better post-stroke Rankin scores. The proportions of independent patients in other studies varies from 58 per cent at 6 months (de Haan *et al.* 1995), 83 per cent at 3–6 months (Boiten and Lodder 1993), 74 per cent at 1 year (Clavier *et al.* 1994), to 71 per cent at 1 year and 58 per cent at 3 years (Samuelsson *et al.* 1996*b*). Yamamoto and Bogousslavsky (1998) reported that the excellent activities of daily living (ADL) score in the lacunar group after the first stroke decreased markedly in conjunction with recurrent strokes.

Using logistic regression analysis, the predictive factors of disability were age more than 70 years, diabetes, history of stroke or TIA, and type of lacunar syndrome (pure motor hemiparesis) in the study of Clavier *et al.* (1994). In the study of Samuelsson *et al.* (1996*b*), moderate to severe hemiparesis 1 month after stroke onset was the strongest predictor of dependence or death at 3 years, followed by white matter hyperintensities on MRI.

Samuelsson *et al.* (1996*b*) reported a high degree of consistency between disability and degree of handicap assessed by the Oxford Handicap Scale. However, about 10 per cent of the patients who were independent in ADL still had a handicap that restricted customary social relations, employment, or recreational activities.

Quality of life was determined by the Sickness Impact Profile in 82 patients with lacunar stroke in a study by de Haan *et al.* (1995). Compared with other types of supratentorial infarction and haemorrhage, patients with lacunar infarction reported significantly less dysfunction in all quality of life categories except for emotional discomfort, for which no difference was noted. However, 23 of the 82 patients with lacunar stroke had reported severely impaired quality of life overall or in the psychosocial life domains only. Life satisfaction after lacunar infarction was also assessed by Olsson *et al.* (1996), but the scales used were found to be too insensitive to allow reliable conclusions.

Prognosis for cognitive dysfunction

The association of cognitive impairments after stroke has been the subject of growing interest in the past decade. In lacunar infarction, it is a common view that cognitive functioning is spared in the acute phase, whereas the development of cognitive impairment and dementia is a matter of concern in the longer term. However, there are a number of case studies in the literature with remarkable focal neuropsychological impairments after single lacunar infarcts localized to the internal capsule or posterior putamen (Ferro and Kretesz 1984, Tanridag and Kirshner 1985, Kooistra and Heilman 1988, Tatemichi *et al.* 1992*b*, Pullicino *et al.* 1994, Schneider *et al.* 1996, Yamanaka *et al.* 1996). The neuropsychological deficits described in these cases include verbal fluency, verbal and visual memory, amnesia, word retrieval, and abulia. Some caution is needed in ascribing focal lesions identified by CT scan or MRI to cognitive impairments, because these techniques may fail to visualize acute co-existing cortical lesions, as recently demonstrated in a study based on diffusion-weighted MRI (DWI) (Ay *et al.* 1999*a*).

In clinical practice, patients with single lacunar infarcts often report non-specific symptoms on long-term follow-up. In the study by Samuelsson *et al.* (1996*b*), subtle subjective impairment of cognitive function, e.g. reduced speed of mental processing, was a frequent complaint even in patients with little or no disability. A detailed neuropsychological assessment was performed by Van Zandvoort *et al.* (1998) in 16 patients with single symptomatic supratentorial lacunar infarcts and in 16 healthy controls. Although lacunar infarct patients had a normal performance on most tasks, an impairment was found in tasks that were particularly strenuous and required the effective use of several capacities.

In the study by Samuelsson *et al.* (1996*b*), 5 per cent of surviving patients were considered demented at 1 year and 11 per cent at 3 years. Miyao *et al.* (1992) reported a similar poportion, about 11 per cent after a mean follow-up of 2.3 years. In both studies, the dementia often developed in conjunction with recurrent strokes. Miyao *et al.* (1992) found that the presence of leukoaraiosis implied an increased risk of dementia, a finding corroborated by van Swieten *et al.* (1996) who reported that diffuse lesions of the white matter were also related independently to intellectual dysfunction in patients with lacunar infarcts. A truly independent analysis was considered to be difficult because the most severe involvement of the white matter tended to be associated with the largest number of lacunar infarcts. There is growing evidence that progressive ischaemic white matter lesions affect mentation, with dementia corresponding to widespread demyelinitation and arteriolosclerosis

(Binswanger's disease) at the extreme end of the spectrum. Thus, the cognitive dysfunction and development of dementia after symptomatic lacunar infarcts may be due, at least in part, to co-existing leukoaraiosis and multiple clinically silent small, deep infarcts (Longstreth *et al.* 1998).

Asymptomatic progression of small vessel disease

Autopsy reports as well as neuroimaging studies indicate that a large proportion, possibly the majority, of lacunar infarctions are asymptomatic (Fisher 1991, Longstreth *et al.* 1998). Only few longitudinal studies on the evolution of silent small, deep infarcts and ischaemic white matter abnormalities/leukoaraiosis have been performed. Samuelsson *et al.* (1994) reproted a 10 per cent rate of new silent small, deep infarcts detected on MRI at 1 year after the index stroke, a proportion twice that of new symptomatic lacunar infarcts. A similar relationship between silent and symptomatic new lacunar infarcts was reported by Yamamoto *et al.* (1998): 25.7 per cent of the patients had developed new small, deep, silent infarcts and 14.3 per cent symptomatic infarcts after a mean follow-up of 3.2 years. An even higher rate of silent lesions was found in the study by Van Zagten *et al.* (1996): after 2.8 years, 51 per cent of patients with lacunar infarcts had developed new silent small, deep infarcts compared with an 8 per cent rate of symptomatic infarcts. Progression of leukoaraiosis was documented in 41.5 per cent of the patients.

Comments on methodological issues

Compared with several other subtypes of ischaemic stroke, there are fewer reports available on prognosis in patients with lacunar infarction syndromes. The prognosis reported in the various studies is relatively homogenous for some outcome variables, whereas vastly different results were obtained for other items. One obvious reason may be that several studies have limited precision because of the small number of patients and a limited number of outcome events. Only three of the studies were based on 150 or more patients (Hier *et al.* 1991, Clavier *et al.* 1994, Staaf *et al.* 2000). Another reason may be methodological differences between studies with respect to inclusion/exclusion criteria, referral patterns, conduct of follow-up, definitions and assessment of outcome events, use of life-table technique, and multivariate techniques to control for and evaluate prognostic factors. None of the available studies is methodologically complete in all aspects.

The pattern of patient referral is not clearly described in all hospital-based studies. Most, but not all (Gandolfo *et al.*1986, Clavier *et al.* 1994), of the studies included patients with first-ever strokes only. However, even in patients with a first-ever symptomatic lacunar infarct, there appears to be a large variation in the extent of ischaemic white matter lesions/leukoaraiosis and silent small, deep infarcts, indicating more or less advanced stages of cerebral small artery disease. Both factors have been found to influence the development of cognitive dysfunction (Miyao *et al.* 1992,

Samuelsson *et al.* 1996*b*, Van Swieten *et al.* 1996), and may also be of importance for other prognostic variables, although not yet well documented. There is also variation in the age composition and prevalence of vascular diseases and other risk factors which may contribute to differences in prognosis between studies.

The level of diagnostic work-up is also different between studies, and different definitions are used. Some studies use a clinical definition, based on recognized lacunar syndromes, whereas others use a combination of clinical and neuroimaging data, and only include patients in which a defined diagnostic work-up was performed. As discussed in previous chapters, the specificity of clinical features alone for single penetrating artery disease is probably only about two-thirds. If a CT scan is performed, as usually done routinely today, at least intracerebral haemorrhage is excluded as the underlying cause. However, in up to 50 per cent of cases, the CT scan is normal and no infarct is visualized. The sensitivity of MRI for identifying a small, deep infarct is higher than for CT (see Chapter 10), but for both methods the separation of recent symptomatic lesions from old infarcts is problematic and often not possible. Only DWI has the ability to identify small, deep infarcts with an accuracy approaching 100 per cent (Noguchi *et al.* 1998, Schonewille *et al.* 1999, Lee *et al.* 2000, Lindgren *et al.* 2000, Oliveira-Filho *et al.* 2000). However, a recent study showed that 16 per cent of patients presenting with a lacunar syndrome had a lesion both in a penetrator territory ('index lesion') and in leptomeningeal artery territories ('subsidiary lesions'), suggesting embolism as the underlying cause (Ay *et al.* 1999*a*). Although DWI is clearly superior to MRI and CT in the detection of small, deep infarcts in the acute phase, the technique is not available today on a routine basis for all stroke patients, and its use, for example, in a prospective population-based study covering all age groups would probably not be feasible.

Patients with potential cardioembolic sources or large artery stenotic disease are excluded in some studies, but accepted in others (provided clinical and radiological criteria are fulfilled) on the assumption that the cardiac disorder or large vessel disease is co-incidental (Lodder *et al.* 1990, Boiten *et al.* 1996). The distinction may, in the individual case, sometimes be clarified by DWI (if a lesion site incompatible with a single penetrating artery is demonstrated), but is more often a matter of speculation (e.g. if a single small, deep infarct is visualized). Small infarcts in the deep arterial borderzone area (subcortical low-flow, or internal borderzone infacts), generally associated with severe haemodynamically significant, extracranial carotid disease, may also be potentially difficult to separate from those related to *in situ* disease (Waterston *et al.* 1991). Such infarcts, which may present as a lacunar syndrome, presumably carry a different prognosis from that of lacunar infarcts. Few studies have consistently applied echocardiography or ultrasonography.

There is also considerable variation in presentation of prognostic data, hampering comparisons between studies. Actuarial methods were not always applied, and in some studies follow-up was incomplete. Multivariate statistics to identify prognostic variables were adopted in a few studies only.

Summary and directions for future research

From available reports, there is consensus that the prognosis for survival is excellent in the short term, with a minimal death rate at 1 month. This should not be unexpected: the risk of death from the primary brain lesion is likely to be minimal given the small infarct size, the rate of recovery is generally more rapid, decreasing the risk of death due to secondary complications, and the proportion of patients with cardiac co-morbidities is less than in most other stroke subtypes. The risk of death remains low for the first few years after stroke onset. However, from 5 years and onwards, the rate of death exceeds that of the general population—myocardial infarction is the most common cause of death.

Data on the risk of recurrent stroke within the first year after stroke onset are variable in hospital-based studies, with risks ranging from 2.3 to 11.8 per cent, whereas the rates reported in community-based studies are more uniform (10–12%). The risk of recurrent stroke during subsequent years averages 5 per cent per year. The pathophysiology of recurrent stroke is heterogenous, and in aggregate only about half of recurrent strokes are again lacunar, presumably because the major risk factors that predispose to vascular occlusions in small brain arteries also promote atherosclerosis in the coronary arteries, aorta, and cervico-cranial arteries.

Compared with other stroke subtypes, patients with lacunar infarcts tend to have a better functional outcome. There is also agreement that most patients do not have marked cognitive impairments or general cognitive deterioration, although impairments in particularly strenuous mental activities requiring the simultaneous use of several capacities may not be uncommon and correspond to frequent patient complaints of subjective impairment of cognitive function. Dementia sometimes develops in conjunction with recurrent stroke. Asymptomatic progression seems to outweigh new symptomatic ischaemic stroke several fold, although data on this issue are limited.

Although more favourable than other subtypes in the early phase and within the first few years, in the longer term there is an excess risk of death, continual occurrence of recurrent stroke, and development of cognitive dysfunction and new asymptomatic lesions. The commonly held view that lacunar infarcts are relatively benign is probably true only for the first few years; in the longer term, the prognosis appears to be worse than previously considered.

Aspects of prognosis that have not been investigated completely include prognosis over longer than a few years only, methods for estimating the outcome risk for individual patients, the risk of cognitive decline with time, and the rate of asymptomatic progression of the underlying vascular process. Future research is clearly needed and should target underinvestigated topics.

Part VI

Therapy

Chapter 24

Therapy for lacunar and subcortical stroke

P.M. Wright and G.A. Donnan

Introduction

Lacunar infarction, as discussed earlier, was first recognized by Fisher following his clinico-pathological observations. With sophisticated imaging techniques, there is now evidence that the classic lacunar syndromes are usually accompanied by a compatible acute small, deep white matter infarction, and each syndrome typically is associated with specific locations, most commonly the internal capsule or pons (Schonewille *et al.* 1999, Lindgren *et al.* 2000).

The pathology has been described elsewhere but, in summary, lacunar stroke probably results from occlusion of small single penetrator arteries that are affected by arteriolosclerotic lesions which include:

(1) Microatheroma: usually a small atheromatous plaque occluding the origin of the affected vessel, which tends to result in larger lesions (Fisher 1991).

(2) Lipohyalinosis: here, intrinsic vessel wall changes occur in even smaller vessels, with fibrinoid and collagen deposition replacing muscle fibres and hyaline connective tissue.

It has been shown earlier that the established lacunar stroke risk factors of age, hypertension, and diabetes are similar to those of atherothrombotic stroke. The exception is hyperlipidaemia which does not appear to be a risk factor for lacunar stroke (You *et al.* 1995). However, the broad commonality of risk factors allows speculation that secondary prevention strategies may be beneficial across these stroke subtypes, even though the exact mechanisms of their effect may differ between types. Most importantly, the final common pathway in both lacunar and atherothrombotic acute stroke is thought to involve platelet adhesion, aggregation, and recruitment, followed by thrombus formation. Therefore, it is reasonable to consider similar proven stroke therapies to prevent and reverse these mechanisms across the stroke subtypes if there is no specific evidence to show that lacunar stroke should be treated differently. This is the approach we have used in the current review of potential lacunar stroke therapies.

As discussed elsewhere in this volume, there is mounting evidence that the dominant mechanism for tissue responses to ischaemia may differ in subcortical white matter compared with cortical grey matter. Hence, it may be that more specific treatment options may become available specifically for white matter strokes. Within grey matter, ischaemic stress leads predominantly to excitotoxin release (Benveniste *et al.* 1984, Hansen 1985) and subsequent calcium flux (Siesjo and Bengston 1989), causing cellular damage. In white matter, the stress results predominantly in membrane depolarization through K^+ accumulation (Ransom *et al.* 1992) and reverse Na^+/Ca^{2+} ion exchange because of Na^+ pump dysfunction, and calcium influx through ischaemic voltage-gated Ca^{2+} channels. Fern *et al.* investigated therapies to interrupt these pathways, and have shown in addition that γ-aminobutyric acid (GABA) and the neuromodulaor adenosine can partially interrupt the anoxic cascade in white matter and are a means of autoprotection employed to minimize damage to white matter under tissue stress (Fern *et al.* 1996). Manipulation of these neurochemical processes holds some promise for the future treatment of acute white matter stroke.

First, we will examine those therapies which have been tested in the acute period following stroke, anticoagulants and intravenous thrombolysis. Then, the role of antiplatelet agents in acute therapy and in secondary prevention will be considered separately. Finally, the role of carotid endarterectomy after lacunar stroke will be examined.

It needs to be emphasized that there are much more data describing the treatment of lacunar stroke than the other subcortical stroke types. There is little information concerning treatment of anterior choroidal artery (AChA) territory, or striatocapsular strokes, to mention a few. While it is presumed that these non-lacunar stroke subtypes may be atherothrombotic in aetiology, this is far from certain. Hence, in this review, we have focused on the management of the lacunar aspects of subcortical strokes almost exclusively.

Acute stroke therapy for lacunar stroke

Anticoagulants and antiplatelet therapy in acute lacunar stroke

There are now two very large trials published whose authors have established the role of anticoagulant and antiplatelet therapy in acute stroke, and in each their effect on the lacunar stroke subtype has been reported. These two trials were designed prospectively for analysis both together and separately.

The International Stroke Trial (IST) investigators (IST 1997) showed that amongst almost 20 000 participants, defined by the Oxfordshire stroke clinical subtypes classification (Bamford *et al.* 1990), 24 per cent had lacunar cerebral infarction (LACI). For both aspirin and heparin, there was absolutely no direct evidence in this study to support any change in the likelihood of being dead or dependent at 6 months, when treatment was begun as soon as possible after lacunar stroke presentation. It should be noted that not all subjects had a computed tomography (CT) brain scan in this study, and that, during heparin therapy, the APTT was not monitored, even on the high dose regimen. For this reason, haemorrhagic complications of heparin therapy may have been more prevalent than could be expected when including these tests, and reduced the net potential benefit of this treatment.

In the Chinese Acute Stroke Trial of 21 000 participants (CAST 1997), 6102 (29.5%) were lacunar strokes. In these, the end points of death, dependency, or stroke were reached in 78 given aspirin and 88 on placebo, with an odds ratio similar to all the other stroke subtypes, perhaps suggesting a trend toward improvement on acute aspirin treatment, but confidence intervals were wide. Hence, despite very large patient numbers in these studies, no specific evidence to support the use of acute antiplatelet or anticoagulant therapy in lacunar stroke had been found.

In the prospectively planned meta-analysis of the two studies (Chen *et al.* 2000), early aspirin statistically significantly reduced, by seven per 1000, the risk of having a recurrent ischaemic stroke within 14–28 days. This occurred in 1.6 per cent of aspirin users versus 2.3 per cent on placebo. There was a trend towards an increase of two per 1000 in the risk of having a haemorrhagic stroke or haemorrhagic transformation. Aspirin reduced the rate of 'death without further stroke' by four per 1000. The combination of such outcomes putatively yields an overall risk reduction of nine per 1000 for the composite outcome of 'any further stroke or death', and of 12 per 1000 patients for the end point of 'death or dependency'.

For lacunar stroke, a similar outcome to those described above for all ischaemic strokes is found. The odds ratio is no different from that of the non-lacunar groups but the confidence intervals are wider due to the smaller sample size. Nevertheless, a statistically significant benefit is observed, with recurrent ischaemic stroke occurring in 1.1 per cent of the lacunar aspirin group and 1.7 per cent of the placebo group. The 95 per cent confidence interval for this difference of 0.6 per cent is 0.1–1 per cent (Fig. 24.1).

Results from other trials using heparinoids (TOAST 1998, FISS 1998) or low molecular weight heparin (FISS and BIS-FISS) have not been consistent with a benefit from either treatment type for the acute treatment of stroke in any stroke subtype.

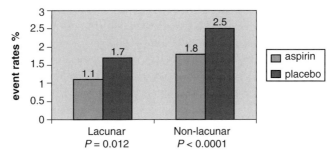

Fig. 24.1 Meta-analysis of the Chinese Acute Stroke Trial and the International Stroke Trial. Proportional effects of early aspirin on recurrent ischaemic stroke. Fatal and non-fatal events are included.

The TOAST study was a carefully conducted, double-blind, placebo-controlled study of an i.v. heparinoid, danaparoid sodium, in 1281 patients with acute ischaemic stroke. In this, 306 patients had lacunar strokes at presentation. The agent and dose adjustment were selected to maximize the chance of a favourable risk–benefit ratio, and compliance with the study protocol was excellent. Despite this, the trial did not provide evidence of a benefit. Irrespective of treatment, of all the subtypes, only lacunar stroke had a positive odds ratio for an excellent outcome at 3 months of 3.1 (95% CI, 1.5–6.4), which is consistent with previous reports that lacunar strokes tend to fare better than other subtypes. No analysis of the effect of heparinoid treatment on each of the various stroke subtypes has been reported from this study however (Adams *et al.* 1999). Considerable differences in the baseline National Institutes of Health Stroke Scale (NIHSS) scores among the various stroke subtypes were also seen. Here, large artery and cardioembolic strokes had an NIHSS score of at least 7 in about two-thirds of cases, contrasted with lacunar strokes where two-thirds had an NIHSS of less than 7. Predictably, the baseline NIHSS score strongly predicted subsequent outcomes.

Conclusion

There is evidence of a small but statistically significant benefit from the use of aspirin in all acute ischaemic stroke, and in the smaller lacunar stroke subgroup. Aspirin should therefore be used in acute lacunar stroke as soon as intracerebral haemorrhage can be excluded on CT brain scan. In contrast, there is strong evidence that acute anticoagulation is ineffective, and potentially harmful when given routinely in acute ischaemic stroke, although the lacunar subtype has not been analysed separately.

Thrombolysis

If lacunar infarcts can be diagnosed adequately before acute stroke thrombolysis, a decision about whether to include or exclude them from this potentially dangerous therapy could be made. An analysis of the accuracy of acute clinical presentation and early CT findings for identifying lacunar strokes in the ECASS trial has been performed recently (Toni *et al.* 2000). The repeat CT brain scan at 7 days was used as the gold standard by which the diagnosis of lacunar stroke was reached, and by this standard the positive predictive values of clinical and early CT findings (alone or in combination) were very poor. Unfortunately, the sensitivity of CT for detecting lacunar infarction is itself poor, in the order of 15–58 per cent documented in four studies comparing CT with magnetic resonance imaging (MRI). Within 5 days of lacunar stroke, the sensitivity of standard MRI sequences for detecting lacunar lesions is probably better than with later scans (92% versus 67%) (Rothrock *et al.* 1987). Without diffusion-weighted MRI, the sensitivity for detecting the lesion is 74–98 per cent in patients with symptoms and signs of ischaemic stroke syndromes (Salgado *et al.* 1986, Rothrock *et al.* 1987, Brown *et al.* 1988, Arboix *et al.* 1990*b*, Warach *et al.* 1995, 1996, Sorensen *et al.* 1996, Gonzalez *et al.* 1999). With the advent of diffusion-weighted imaging (DWI), the sensitivity has been improved and almost all lacunar syndrome strokes may be anticipated to be abnormal within 3 days of onset (Lindgren et al. 2000). DWI is a new technology, and no sensitivity nor specificity data are yet available in the setting of hyperacute lacunar stroke. The susceptibility artefact that is seen commonly in the brainstem and anterior temporal poles may be problematic, thereby making it less useful in lacunar than in atherothrombotic stroke. However, DWI lesions usually become visible in the hyperacute setting, making this a promising imaging tool to identify clinically relevant lacunar infarction.

Is there any evidence that lacunar or subcortical strokes are less likely to benefit from thrombolysis?

Barber et al. have shown that in 7/26 acute patients studied with DWI, white matter infarction was present. They found subcortical infarctions in six patients and the seventh had a lacunar infarct. The lacunar stroke had no perfusion deficit detected, although the resolution of perfusion techniques currently is too low to be able to see small deficits. Of the six patients with subcortical lesions on acute DWI, three had a patent proximal artery and normal perfusion imaging, one had a small perfusion lesion that corresponded to the DWI lesion, and two had cortical branch perfusion lesions distant to the subcortical DWI lesions. The proportion of subcortical strokes with mismatch between the diffusion and perfusion imaging lesions was much lower than that seen with cortical strokes, and the authors found that in those patients with no mismatch between perfusion and diffusion MRI lesion size, no significant increase in infarct size occurred, in direct contrast to the those with mismatch (Barber et al. 1999). Further studies are needed before real conclusions can be drawn on this issue.

The National Institute of Neurological Disorders and Stroke study investigators of acute thrombolysis for ischaemic stroke (NINDS 1995) established the efficacy of using recombinant tissue plasminogen activator (rt-PA) when given within 3 h of onset. A significant relative increase in the proportion of patients with minimal or no disability, of at least 30 per cent, with an absolute increase of 11–13 per cent was demonstrated, despite a 7 per cent absolute increase in symptomatic intracranial haemorrhage (3-fold relative increase), but no overall change in mortality.

The results of the ECASS I trial, however, were not conclusive (Hacke et al. 1995), suggesting a trend towards efficacy of thrombolysis in acute ischaemic stroke that was not statistically significant in the less than 6 h time window from stroke onset. In the ECASS II trial, a trend to improved outcome in patients treated within 6 h was also shown, but the primary end point (an increase in the proportion of patients with a modified Rankin score of 0–1, representing a favourable outcome) was not statistically significantly improved (Hacke et al. 1998). A post hoc analysis of the data dichotomizing the Rankin score differently from the pre-determined end point (to represent death or dependency) gave a statistically significant 8.3 per cent difference in favour of rt-PA. Obviously such analyses should be interpreted cautiously.

Table 24.1 Meta-analysis of death and disability at 3-month follow-up in patients given treatment less than 3 h from stroke onset in three rt-PA stroke studies

Comparison: tPA Vs Placebo

Outcome: Benefits: death/disability < 3 hours

Study	tPA n/N	Placebo n/N	OR (95% CI Fixed)	OR (95% CI Fixed)
ECASS I	28 / 47	28 / 37		0.49 (0.20–1.21)
ECASS II	47 / 81	48 / 77		0.84 (0.44–1.58)
NINDS	179 / 312	229 / 312		0.49 (0.35–0.69)
Subtotal (95% CI)	254 / 440	305 / 426		0.55 (0.41–0.72)
Chi-square 2.15 (df=2) Z=4.27				

0.1 0.2   1   5 10

A meta-analysis (Table 24.1) of the patients given rt-PA within 3 h in these three trials (Hacke *et al.* 1999) confirms the significant benefit from rt-PA for reducing death and disability by about one-third, despite increased symptomatic intracerebral haemorrhage.

Specifically focusing on the lacunar subgroups included in these three trials, only from the NINDS trial has data been analysed separately for each of the stroke subtypes to assess their impact on clinical outcome. The results are presented in the Table 2. Due to smaller sample sizes for the lacunar stroke subtype, separate statistical analyses were not performed by the investigators. However, we have tested each of the stroke subtypes listed for a difference in proportion with a favourable response as measured by the four clinical assessment tools at 3 months. It is evident that for lacunar stroke, on the Barthel Index, there are greater proportions who did well in the rt-PA treatment group than in the placebo group. No measure supported a trend to unfavourable outcome. This suggests that the risk of haemorrhage was no higher in this subtype, and that lacunar stroke also benefits from thrombolysis. Unfortunately, the risk of intracerebral haemorrhage was not given for each subtype either and, as a result, the relative benefits are difficult to assess. In spite of the small numbers within this 'small vessel' stroke subtype, it is also evident that overall they fared better than the other subtypes whether or not they were given rt-PA, perhaps leaving the most important inference: that they did not do worse, as originally feared (Table 24.2). This finding has been supported by a published 100 case r-tPA treatment series (Trouillas *et al.* 1998) wherein at 3-month follow-up it was found that stroke of small size vessels had a better outcome after thrombolysis in this series than those of large size vessels.

Other published reports of thrombolysis in subcortical ischaemic strokes are rare. The most significant is from a case series with thrombolysis for AChA territory ischaemia (Trouillas *et al.* 2000). AChA territory stroke is associated with hypodensity

Table 24.2 Outcome at 3 months after stroke for each stroke subtype in the NINDS stroke trial

Stroke subtype[a]	Stroke score[b]	OR	95% CI	P-value (raw)	P-value (corrected for the 12 inferences)
Small vessel occlusive (n = 51)	Barthel	2.92	1.01–8.44	**0.047**	0.470
	Mod. Rankin	2.53	0.91–7.09	0.079	0.632
	Glasgow	2.20	0.80–6.11	0.143	0.715
	NIHSS	1.78	0.64–5.12	0.330	0.672
Large vessel occlusive (n = 117)	Barthel	1.67	0.98–2.85	0.062	0.558
	Mod. Rankin	2.35	1.31–4.23	**0.003**	**0.036**
	Glasgow	0.89	0.51–1.54	0.751	0.751
	NIHSS	0.43	0.23–0.81	**0.007**	0.077
Cardioembolic (n = 136)	Barthel	1.46	0.87–2.43	0.161	0.715
	Mod. Rankin	1.61	0.94–2.78	0.086	0.632
	Glasgow	1.44	0.85–2.46	0.188	0.564
	NIHSS	1.64	0.90–3.00	0.112	0.672

[a] Eighteen patients (2.9%) with other stroke types were excluded from this analysis.
[b] Scores of 95 or 100 on the Barthel Index, ≤ 1 on the NIHSS and Modified Rankin scale, and 1 on the Glasgow outcome scale were considered to indicate a favourable outcome.
OR is the (odds for rt-PA favourable)/(odds for placebo favourable).
95% CI is the 95 per cent confidence interval of the odds ratio.
Bold type highlights results that are statistically significant.
Analysis used StatXact v3.1(Cytel Software Corporation, Cambridge, MA).
All estimations were done by the exact method (Agresti 1990).
P(corrected) values are determined using the Ryan–Holm stepdown Bonferroni procedure to control the family-wise type I error rate (Ludbrook 1998).

in the posterior two-thirds of the posterior limb of the internal capsule on CT brain imaging. The AChA is a relatively small vessel and the mechanisms of its occlusion are probably varied, but may include emboli of cardiac or carotid origin. Nine patients (7.9%) in a series of 114 consecutive hyperacute thrombolysed patients with ischaemic stroke in the internal carotid artery (ICA) territory had clinico-radiological evidence compatible with this subcortical stroke type. No patient had the complete classical presentation with hemiplegia, hemianaesthesia, and hemianopia, nor ataxia. Each had hemiplegia, with or without dysphasia or fluctuating course. The untreated prognosis of hyperacute AChA is not known, but in this series complete recovery in five patients and near complete recovery in two was observed during i.v. rt-PA thrombolysis. A re-infarct syndrome in three patients (33%) within 48 h was not seen in the large vessel strokes (Trouillas *et al.* 2000). The cause of the re-infarct syndrome remains speculative, and prevention is uncertain.

Conclusion

Hyperacute lacunar strokes can, in a high proportion of cases, be identified using DWI, and there are theoretical reasons why they might not benefit from thrombolysis.

However, thrombolysis with rt-PA is a proven therapy for ishaemic stroke overall, when presenting within 3 h of onset. The limited data available suggest a similar benefit for lacunar stroke. These patients should therefore routinely be considered for thrombolytic therapy if the NINDS trial criteria for entry are fulfilled (NINDS 1995).

Secondary prevention

Antiplatelet agents in secondary prevention after lacunar stroke

There are now a number of agents which can be given to prevent adhesion of platelets to the inner surface of injured arterial walls. This is the first step in intra-arterial thrombus formation and subsequent embolization which may be important in the formation and acute destabilization of hypertensive arteriopathy and microatheroma in the perforating arteries. However, such agents are known to carry modest but significant risk, not only from the systemic side effects, but also from an increased bleeding propensity. In a large case–control study, the investigators found an odds ratio of 3.05 ($P = 0.047$) for haemorrhagic stroke, with high dose aspirin usage in the preceding 2 weeks that was not seen with lower doses commonly used in stroke prophylaxis (Thrift 1999). The Physicians' Health Study investigators reported a 5-fold increased risk of brain haemorrhage on such treatment compared with placebo, although this trend did not reach statistical significance (Physician's Health Study 1988). It is important, in view of these potential risks, that antiplatelet clinical efficacy can be demonstrated prior to routine use for specific cerebrovascular disorders. There are several commonly used oral antiplatelet agents now available for stroke prevention therapy which should be considered in this context.

Aspirin, the first antiplatelet agent used in stroke prevention, acetylates the enzyme cyclooxygenase, and inhibits the formation of cyclic endoperoxidases and thromboxanes, hence inhibiting platelet aggregation irreversibly for the lifespan of the platelet. Ticlopidine, a thienopyridine, inhibits the platelet aggregation induced by collagen, platelet-activating factor, adrenaline, and adenosine diphosphate (ADP). The ADP-dependent effects include activation of the glycoprotein IIb–IIIa complex that is a major receptor for fibrinogen on the platelet membrane. Clopidigrel is a newer thienopyridine with fewer side effects. Dipyridamole inhibits platelet function through the cyclic AMP phosphodiesterase. Lotrifibran is an example of a specific oral inhibitor of platelet glycoprotein IIb–IIIa.

The nature of the evidence

While lacunar stroke represents about 25 per cent of all ischaemic strokes, there have been no specific studies where the subtype alone has been studied in the context of secondary stroke prevention. Hence, all data concerning the efficacy of antiplatelet agents in preventing further stroke after a lacunar event come from subgroup analyses of two larger trials. These two trials, together with other published trials relevant to the use of antiplatelet agents in stroke secondary prevention, will be described below.

Ticlopidine In a meta-analysis of 9840 patients with ischaemic stroke or transient ischaemic attack (TIA), secondary prevention with thienopyridine treatment (either ticlopidine or clopidigrel) resulted in an incidence of 'any vascular events' of 16.8 per cent for thienopyridine versus 18.3 per cent for aspirin (OR 0.90, 95% CI 0.81–1.00) and, in terms of 'any stroke', 10.4 per cent for thienopyridine versus 12.0 per cent for aspirin (OR 0.86, 95% CI 0.75–0.97) (Hankey *et al.* 2000).

Ticlopidine was assessed as an agent of secondary stroke prevention, and the stroke subtypes have been considered in the Canadian–American Ticlopidine Study (CATS) (Gent *et al.* 1989). Here, ticlopidine 250 mg twice daily was compared with placebo. Qualifying strokes were atherothrombotic in 74 per cent and lacunar in 26 per cent (275 lacunar strokes), with cardioembolic strokes being excluded. Of the lacunar group, approximately 80 per cent were within the carotid arterial territory and 20 per cent were in the vertebrobasilar territory. The reduction in relative risk of stroke, myocardial infarction, and cardiovascular death was 30.2 per cent (95% CI 7.5–48.3%) over all subgroups. The number of lacunar stroke patients enrolled was 275, and the benefits for atherothrombotic and lacunar subtypes of stroke were not significantly different for any of the defined end points. The odds ratio for the end point of 'stroke and stroke death' combined was 55 per cent from 11 per cent/year to 5 per cent/year in the lacunar group, and there was a 23 per cent reduction in the atherothrombotic stroke subtype, but the differences in this ($P=0.10$) and the other end points examined were not statistically significant (see Table 24.3 and Fig. 24.2) (M. Gent personal communication).

Table 24.3 Event rates in the lacunar stroke group per 1000 patient-years using efficacy data from the Canadian–American Ticlopidine Study (CATS)

CATS (n = 275)	Events/1000 patient-years		Odds ratio	95% CI	P (raw)	P (corrected for 5 inferences)
	Placebo	Ticlopidine				
Stroke MI VD	130.5	84.3	0.65	0.46–1.13	0.198	0.792
Stroke MI D	140.2	118.1	0.84	0.64–1.05	0.625	0.999
Stroke strD	111.1	50	0.45	0.23–0.94	**0.044**	0.220
VD	22.7	16	0.7	0.20–1.70	0.902	0.999
Death	31.8	48	1.51	0.93–2.00	0.563	0.999

From data in a personal communication from M. Gent to G. Donnan (1999).

MI = myocardial infarction; VD = vascular death; D = death any cause; StrD = stroke-related death; 95% CI = 95 per cent confidence intervals.

Odds ratio is the (odds for an event on treatment)/(odds for an event on placebo).

Bold numbers highlight statistically significant results. The same end point was, however, not significantly significant in the 'intention-to-treat' analysis.

Analysis used StatXact v3.P(Cytel Software Corporation, Cambridge, MA).

All estimations have been done by the exact method (Agresti 1990).

P (corrected) values are determined using the Ryan–Holm stepdown Bonferroni procedure to control the family-wise type I error rate (Ludbrook 1998).

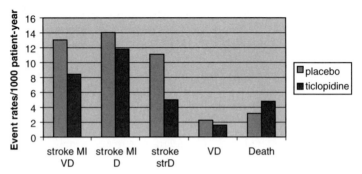

Fig. 24.2 Bar graph of efficacy data from the Canadian–American Ticlopidine Study (M. Gent personal communication).

Aspirin The other antiplatelet study in which an analysis of stroke subtypes was included is the French AICLA aspirin trial (Bousser *et al.* 1983). A total of 604 patients with atherothrombotic cerebral ischaemic events were included in this double-blind, well-randomized trial to determine whether high dose aspirin, or aspirin plus dipyridamole, would produce a significant reduction in the 3-year stroke recurrence rates compared with placebo. Adherence to protocol and follow-up rates were excellent. Ninety-eight participants had lacunar stroke as their presenting event, and aspirin or aspirin–dipyridamole reduced the relative risk of lacunar stroke recurrence by 70 per cent ($P<0.01$) from absolute rates of 26 per cent down to 7 per cent. This was a greater effect than the effect on non-lacunar stroke. The combination of aspirin and dipyridamole did not significantly improve outcomes in lacunar stroke compared with aspirin alone, but neither did it significantly improve outcomes for all strokes combined. With the benefit of hindsight, this was probably due to type II error.

Although not specifically exploring the role of aspirin in lacunar stroke, meta-analysis of aspirin trials confirms the role of this treatment in secondary prevention following recent ischaemic stroke of all subtypes combined. The authors of one such analysis assessed the 11 randomized, placebo-controlled trials with a total of 5228 patients on aspirin only and 4401 patients on placebo (Table 24.4). Aspirin at a wide range of doses decreased the risk of stroke by about 15 per cent (relative risk ratio, 0.85; 95% CI, 0.77–0.94) (Johnson *et al.* 1999).

The investigators from the Antiplatelet Trialists' Collaboration (APT 1994) found that among about 10 000 patients with a past history of stroke or TIA, 18 per cent taking antiplatelet therapy versus 22 per cent taking a placebo had a further vascular event, with an estimated 3-year benefit of about 40/1000 ($P<0.00001$). Taking all 'high risk' vascular patients (coronary, cerebro-, and peripheral vascular disease) together showed highly statistically significant reductions of one-third in non-fatal stroke and about one-sixth in vascular death by taking antiplatelet agents (each $P<0.00001$). There was no evidence that non-vascular deaths were increased. There was also a sigenificant ($P<0.00001$) benefit documented from taking this treatment for 3 years compared with just 1 year. No meta-analysis has been performed to

Table 24.4 Forrest plot of data from the meta-analysis of aspirin in the secondary prevention of stroke, compared with placebo control. (Johnson 1999)

Study	RR (95% CI Fixed)	OR (95% CI Fixed)
Diener 1996	0.82 (0.69,0.98)	
– SALT 1991	0.84 (0.65,1.08)	
– EAFT 1993	0.91 (0.71,1.18)	
– Farrell 1991	0.85 (0.66,1.09)	
Fields 1979; Lemak 1986	0.21 (0.05,0.91)	
Bousser 1983	0.59 (0.35,1.01)	
Sorensen 1983	1.77 (0.92,3.40)	
Farrell 1991	0.85 (0.66,1.08)	
Fields 1979; Lemak 1986	0.80 (0.39,1.67)	
Canadian Cooperative 1978; Gent 1980	1.06 (0.61,1.86)	
Reuther 1978	0.25 (0.03,2.10)	
– Britton 1987	1.00 (0.63,1.57)	
Total (95%CI)	0.85 (0.77,0.93)	

0.1 0.2   1   5   10

Aspirin better   Placebo better

RR = relative rise; OR = odds ratio.

investigate the role of aspirin in lacunar stroke alone, but the lacunar stroke group is assumed to have contributed greatly to the overall findings.

Dipyridmole The combination of dipyridamole and aspirin has been investigated on several occasions, but only in the AICLA study described above has the lacunar subtype been explored in its analysis for lacunar stroke alone. In that study, there was no evidence of a benefit from dipyridamole over and above that of aspirin. Considering the European Stroke Prevention Studies (ESPS I and ESPS II) (ESPS 1990, Diener *et al.* 1996), while the results of these studies have been somewhat contentious, there is a consistency revealed, which cannot be denied. In ESPS I, amongst patients with TIA or minor stroke, there was a 36 per cent relative risk reduction for those who received aspirin plus dipyridamole. Unfortunately, there was no aspirin-only treatment arm. This problem was corrected in ESPS II where for all stroke subtypes combined (there was no subgroup analysis of lacunar stroke), aspirin alone reduced the risk of stroke by 18 per cent over placebo, and the combination of dipyridamole plus aspirin versus placebo reduced the risk of stroke by 37 per cent. ESPS II is the only large study examining this treatment. The authors analysed 6602 participants, over 2 years follow-up, and the outcomes are shown in Table 24.5.

When the results of ESPS-II are added to earlier cerebrovascular trials of dipyridamole (Guiraud-Chaumeil *et al.* 1982, Bousser *et al.* 1983, ACCSG 1985), a statistically significant 25 per cent reduction in the odds of non-fatal stroke and a statistically significant 18 per cent reduction in the odds of all vascular events is seen (Wilterdink and Easton 1999).

The two greatest difficulties with accepting dipyridamole as being valuable in this setting are that, first, only ESPS II conclusively supports its efficacy out of 15 vascular

Table 24.5 Results from ESPS II

ESPS II trial Results	Stroke Events/1000 patients	OR	95% CI	Death Events/1000 patients	OR	95% CI	Stroke and/or death Events/1000 patients	OR	95% CI
Placebo	151			22			229		
DP + A versus placebo	95	0.59	0.48–0.73	112	0.9	0.73–1.12	173	0.71	0.59–0.84
DP versus placebo	128	0.81	0.67–0.99	113	0.92	0.74–1.13	194	0.81	0.68–0.96
A versus placebo	125	0.79	0.65–0.97	110	0.88	0.71–1.09	200	0.84	0.71–0.99
DP + A versus A		0.97	0.95–0.992		0.999	0.998–1.002		0.973	0.95–0.9998

From Diener et al. (1996).

Events are recorded as events per 1000 patients studied

Each arm had approximately 1650 patients.

DP = dipyridamole 200 mg sustained release formulation twice daily; A = aspirin 50 mg daily.

Bold type highlights results that are statistically significant.

trials including three cerebrovascular secondary prevention trials (PARIS 1980, Schoop and Levy 1983; Brown *et al.* 1985, Goldman *et al.* 1988, 1989). Secondly, its effect on stroke, and its surprising lack of effect on myocardial infarction and vascular death, is somewhat inconsistent.

Once again, however, without direct evidence for a role for dipyridamole in lacunar stroke, we can only extrapolate from these less specific studies that lacunar strokes are assumed to have contributed greatly to the total recruitment.

Clopidigrel The Clopidogrel versus Aspirin in Patients at Risk of Ischaemic Events (CAPRIE) investigators conducted a randomized, double-blinded trial of antiplatelet therapy comparing these two therapies (CAPRIE 1996). In this study, the combined vascular end point of ischaemic stroke, myocardial infarction, and death from vascular disease (vascular death) occurred with similar rates among the 2543 patients with lacunar stroke compared with those with atherothrombotic stroke. Comparing the efficacy of clopidigrel versus aspirin for lacunar stroke presentations shows no significant efficacy from the newer treatment, and a similarly non-significant effect in atherothrombotic stroke subtype on an intention-to-treat analysis. In addition, there was no statistical difference between these two stroke subtypes, although a modest trend to benefit was seen only in the atherothrombotic group. These were, however, *post hoc* analyses in a study not powered to analyse stroke as an isolated end point, let alone specific stroke subtypes at entry, or whether fatal or non-fatal strokes were seen at follow-up. Overall, patients actually treated with clopidigrel had a 8.7 per cent/ year reduction in combined vascular risk compared with aspirin therapy ($P=0.043$) (M. Gent personal communication).

Of interest is that Benavente *et al.* plan the Secondary Prevention in Small Subcortical Strokes pilot study (SPS3) wherein a comparison of the efficacy of aspirin plus clopidigrel and aspirin alone will be made. The investigators will also consider the issue of the effect of blood pressure lowering as a means of secondary stroke prevention in this group. The anticipated completion of the pilot study and analysis is 2003 (Benavente personal communication).

Conclusion

There is now compelling evidence that antiplatelet therapy is efficacious in the secondary prevention of ischaemic stroke. Within these trials, there is reasonable evidence that lacunar stroke is afforded a similar protection, although this would need to be tested by further randomized controlled trials in order to be established with greater certainty. A further need is to find more effective antiplatelet treatments or combinations of treatments through well-established large clinical trials.

Anticoagulants in secondary prevention

The investigators of the ongoing Warfarin–Aspirin Recurrent Stroke Study (WARSS) are comparing warfarin with aspirin in patients with recent ischaemic stroke.

The clacunar stroke subtype will be analysed separately for relative benefit, and the study is scheduled to be completed in 2000. No other evidence is available regarding the use of anticoagulants in lacunar strokes. Another trial that is designed to address the role of anticoagulants is the European/Australian Stroke Prevention in Reversible Ischaemia trial (ESPRIT). In this, the therapeutic International Normalised Ratio (INR) will be 2.0–3.0, and there will be an aspirin–dipyridamole and an aspirin-alone arm to the study. The planned 4500 subjects will have transient ischaemic attack, or non-disabling stroke at presentation, including lacunar stroke, and will be followed for approximately 3 years (ESPRIT 2000).

Carotid endarterectomy

It has been shown that with carotid Doppler, severe (70–99%) ipsilateral carotid stenosis was found in none of a series of 80 patients with clinically defined lacunar infarct (LACI). Severe carotid stenosis or occlusion in the ipsilateral carotid artery was not more frequent than contralateral disease in the LACI stroke patients, suggesting that ipsilateral carotid disease is not an important cause of stroke for those with LACI (Mead *et al.* 1998).

Hence, carotid artery stenosis in patients presenting with lacunar stroke may be coincidental or, on rare occasions, possibly causal. The role of carotid endarterectomy in cases of lacunar TIA or minor stroke as a form of secondary prevention is, therefore, problematic. Inzitari *et al.* reanalysed the North American Symptomatic Carotid Endarterectomy Trial (NASCET) data to determine the role of carotid endarterectomy in lacunar stroke presentations (Inzitari *et al.* 2000). Strokes were divided into three groups, non-lacunar, possible lacunar (clinical syndrome, but a negative CT brain scan), and probable lacunar (both clinical syndrome and a lacunar CT lesion appropriate to the symptoms). Thus, radiological evidence alone was considered insufficient to define the stroke as lacunar. Of 1158 patients with hemispheric stroke, 493 had features of lacunar stroke (283 possible and 210 probable). In the patients with stenosis of less than 50 per cent, none of the three groups showed benefit of surgery over medical therapy, as shown in Fig. 24.3.

In contrast, in the 50–99% stenosis group, the conclusive benefit from surgery seen in non-lacunar cases [24.9% versus 9.7% risk of ipsilateral stroke at 3 years (relative risk reduction = 61%, $P = 0.003$)] was not seen in the possible nor probable lacunar groups, as shown in Fig. 24.4.

For patients with 50–99 per cent ICA stenosis, the relative risk reductions in stroke from carotid endarterectomy were 35 per cent when the presenting stroke was probable lacunar, 53 per cent with possible lacunar, and 61 per cent when the stroke was non-lacunar. Although this trend is suggestive, the confidence intervals were wide for the possible and probable lacunar groups, leaving this as an unproven therapy. Unfortunately, although this way of interpreting the NASCET results is helpful, because of the small sample size, and the *post hoc* nature of the analysis, it does not

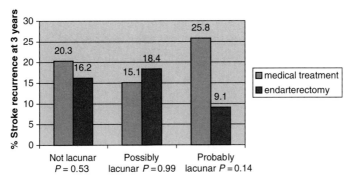

Fig. 24.3 Analysis of the NASCET stroke subtypes' outcome data in those with less than 50 per cent stenosis of the internal carotid artery (Inzitari *et al.* 2000). *P*-values are for the null hypothesis that there is no difference between the two treatments.

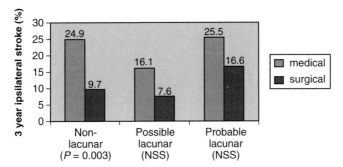

Fig. 24.4 NASCET analysis of the stroke subtypes outcome data in those with 50–99 per cent stenosis of the internal carotid artery (Inzitari *et al.* 2000). *P*-values are for the hypothesis that there is no difference between the two treatments. NSS, not statistically significant.

answer the question of whether the 70–99 per cent stenosis in the probable or possible lacunar subtypes would benefit from carotid endarterectomy.

Conclusion

There is no strong evidence at present to recommend carotid endarterectomy for lacunar stroke. However, recurrent stroke is more likely to be of atherothrombotic than lacunar type, and each stenotic artery ipsilateral to a lacunar stroke may be assessed for high risk features. This issue has not been resolved satisfactorily at this time.

Risk factor management

An essential component of stroke treatment is to identify and treat risk factors. For lacunar stroke, advancing age, hypertension, and diabetes are well-established risk factors (You *et al.* 1995). Analysis of data from the NASCET study reveals that a history of diabetes and hyperlipidaemia was associated independently with lacunar stroke more than with non-lacunar stroke, even after accounting for the degree of carotid stenosis, and arterial hypertension was a similarly important risk factor across stroke types (Inzitari et al. 2000). Petty et al., in contrast, found that there was no difference in diabetes frequency with lacunar than other subtypes of stroke (Petty et al. 1999). The untreated annual risk of stroke recurrence of any stroke type has been shown to be around 8–9 per cent following a lacunar stroke (Bousser et al. 1983, Gent et al. 1989), although a wide range has been reported, and the efficacy of management of these risk factors for secondary prevention needs to be determined.

Hypertension

Despite its great importance as a risk factor for stroke, there are many unanswered questions about the optimum treatment for blood pressure in stroke patients, and even less is known about the lacunar stroke subtype. It is reasonable to examine the literature on the treatment of hypertension in all stroke types as a starting point, particularly as about 70 per cent of patients with lacunar stroke in recent studies have a convincing history of hypertension, thus making this the most prevalent modifiable risk factor (You et al. 1995, Lammie et al. 1997, Petty et al. 1999, Lodder et al. 1990). In addition, from the NASCET study, it is shown that even in those lacunar stroke patients with less than 50 per cent carotid stenosis, the most frequent stroke subtype at recurrence was atherothrombotic rather than lacunar, thus making treatment of risk factors for both subtypes important. This may not, however, be true for those with no carotid atheroma.

The primary prevention of stroke by reducing blood pressure with medication is well documented by studies showing that, for example, a 5 mmHg reduction in diastolic blood pressure is associated with a reduction of almost 40 per cent in the incidence of stroke (Collins et al. 1990). A similar effect is seen with the treatment of isolated systolic hypertension.

The issue is not as simple when secondary prevention of stroke is considered. However, meta-analysis of the available studies reveals that antihypertensive treatment of stroke and TIA patients reduces the risk of recurrent stroke by about 28 per cent ($P<0.01$), although stroke mortality and total mortality showed a trend to reduction that was not statistically significant (Gueyffier et al. 1996, 1997). The blood pressure goals for systolic and diastolic pressures are also not well established. Whether to aim for as low as possible or to treat all stroke patients regardless of the presence or absence of hypertension is not proven. The latter has, however, been shown to be safe in a Dutch TIA trial (Dutch 1993), although more elderly patients with diseased cerebral arteries and poor vascular autoregulation may not receive the same benefits from antihypertensive treatment as younger patients. There is also evidence from subgroup analysis of stroke survivors that isolated systolic hypertension should be treated for secondary prevention of stroke with a relative risk reduction of about 30 per cent (O'Brien et al. 1999).

In addition, the investigators for the ongoing international Perindopril Protection Against Recurrent Stroke Study (PROGRESS) trial have already finished recruiting about 6000 participants with stroke during their prior 5 years (Chalmers *et al.* 2000). In this cohort, about one-third have lacunar infarcts which will be analysed independently. Angiotensin-converting enzyme inhibitor-based blood pressure lowering as secondary prevention of stroke or TIA will be assessed in this double-blind, placebo-controlled randomized trial of both hypertensive and non-hypertensive participants (PROGRESS 1996).

The effects of an angiotensin-converting enzyme inhibitor (ACEI), ramipril, on stroke incidence in patients with atherosclerotic diseases, prior stroke, or diabetes with another cardiovascular risk factor have been assessed in the Heart Outcomes Prevention Evaluation (HOPE) study (Yusuf *et al.* 2000). These patients were at least 55 years old, and did not have a specific indication for ACEI therapy, nor uncontrolled hypertension. There were over 9000 participants, after exclusion at the run-in phase of the 10 per cent intolerant or poorly compliant subjects, and there were about 30 per cent who later discontinued the study treatment in each arm. In this study, there was an impressive impact on all vascular end points. When the prevention of stroke was considered in these high vascular risk patients, 156 (3.4%) in the treatment arm suffered stroke, as compared with 226 (4.9%) on placebo, a relative risk reduction of 32 per cent ($P < 0.001$). These effects were seen in those with and without a prior history of stroke, and are in addition to the effects of antiplatelet and lipid treatments. The effect on blood pressure was a mean reduction of 3/2 mmHg, which is likely to effect no more than 40 per cent of this reduction in stroke incidence, although a recent review of large epidemiological studies suggests that the impact of hypertension may be higher than initial estimations (Hansson *et al.* 1998, Clarke *et al.* 1999). Most patients did not have conventionally defined hypertension at enrolment.

Of particular interest is the analysis of the stroke secondary prevention data from this study. The 1013 participants with a prior history of stroke ($\sim$11% of the total) had a significant reduction in the composite end point of myocardial infarction, stroke, and death from cardiovascular causes from the 25.9 per cent in the placebo group (OR <0.8, P<0.05). Stroke secondary prevention was not a pre-determined end point, and stroke subtypes were not reported separately, so lacunar stroke can only be considered as part of the total stroke pool.

Conclusion There is no evidence that specifically describes the efficacy of blood pressure management in the primary or secondary prevention of lacunar stroke. Lacunar stroke is included as a significant proportion of the subjects in most studies on hypertension management in stroke that indicate efficacy in both primary prevention, and by meta-analysis in secondary prevention. Therefore, it is likely that managing hypertension, a known risk factor for lacunar stroke, will be similarly effective, and hence it is likely to reduce the risk of stroke recurrence by about

28 per cent. Furthermore, there is now evidence from a single large trial that ramipril, an ACEI, can significantly prevent vascular events in stroke patients, irrespective of prior hypertension, despite very modest mean reductions in blood pressure. Specific information on lacunar stroke therapy is awaited from the ongoing PROGRESS trial.

Diabetes

Again, there are no studies in which a specific analysis of the effect of diabetes management on the secondary prevention of lacunar stroke has been undertaken. Hence, all stroke subtypes will be considered together. The roles of tight glycaemic and blood pressure control will both be considered in this section, as there is evidence for their efficacy specifically in the diabetic population.

Glycaemic control Cardiovascular disease including stroke is the most important cause of mortality and morbidity among patients with type 2 diabetes. Increasing glucose is associated with an increased risk for cardiovascular disease in non-diabetic subjects even below 6.1 mmol/l, and many prospective studies have shown that hyperglycaemia contributes to cardiovascular disease in type 2 diabetes. In the Diabetes Control and Complications Trial (DCCT 1993), intensive treatment of type 1 diabetes reduced the relative risk of all major macrovascular events combined from 0.8 to 0.5 events per 100 patient-years (relative risk reduction 41%, 95% CI 10–68%). No subgroup analysis of an effect on stroke was possible. In the Kumamoto study, the number of major cerebrovascular, cardiovascular, and peripheral vascular events in the intensive treatment group was half that of the conventional treatment group (0.6 versus 1.3 events per 100-patient years). Event rates in this small trial were low and the results were not statistically significant (Ohkubo *et al.* 1995). The UK Prospective Diabetes Study (UKPDS; Turner *et al.* 1998) of type 2 diabetic patients has shown a definite but limited effect of glycaemic control on the prevention of cardiovascular events, but treatments were not ideally effective in reducing glucose, thus weakening their potential influence on outcomes. Finally, the balance between benefits and harms of intensive treatment may be less favourable in children under 13 years or adults over 70 years and in people with repeated severe hypoglycaemia or unawareness of hypoglycaemia.

Blood pressure control Tight blood pressure control compared with 'less tight' control in diabetics has been associated with a reduction in risk of subsequent stroke of 44 per cent (11–65%; $P = 0.013$). Using captopril or atenolol as first-line agents, and aiming for both a systolic blood pressure of less than 150 mmHg and a diastolic pressure of less than 85 mmHg, the authors of the UKPDS achieved a mean 144/82 mm Hg compared with 154/87 mmHg in a control group of type 2 diabetic patients. Twenty-nine per cent of patients in the tight control group required three or more hypotensive treatments (Turner *et al.* 1998).

In the HOPE study, an analysis of the subgroup of 3577 subjects with diabetes plus one other vascular risk factor, but not macroscopic albuminuria, was also undertaken. The investigators found that stroke incidence was reduced from 6.1 to 4.2 per cent ($P = 0.0074$) with ramipril treatment. The initial blood pressures were lower and the mean reduction in blood pressure was less in this study compared with the UKPDS, and the authors postulated a separate vascular mechanism of effect for ramipril than simply its effect on blood pressure (HOPE 2000). No separate analysis of lacunar stroke patients at entry was undertaken.

Conclusion For the primary prevention of macrovascular complications including stroke in patients with type 1 and, to a lesser degree, type 2 diabetes tight glycaemic control is effective through intensive management. In addition, intensive hypotensive therapy is considerably more effective than less intensive therapy for the prevention of stroke, and no lower limit of treatment goal has been established. Ramipril may provide additional benefits over and above any hypotensive effects. No secondary prevention data are available for stroke in diabetes. No specific data for lacunar stroke are yet available, but since this subtype forms a part of most studies, it is reasonable to extrapolate until further data are presented.

Hyperlipidaemia

As mentioned elsewhere in this volume, hypercholesterolaemia has not been identified by investigators as a major risk factor for stroke, although in most studies no distinction is made between haemorrhagic and ischaemic stroke. The possibility that hyperlipidaemia is a risk factor for lacunar stroke is discussed elsewhere in this volume. The effect of lipid lowering on the primary or secondary prevention of lacunar stroke has not been studied specifically. In spite of its weak link as a risk factor, it is reasonable to consider possible mechanisms whereby lipids may affect lacunar stroke development. The pathogenesis of microatheroma and/or lipohyalinosis might be affected by plasma lipids, and 3-hydroxy-3-methylglutaryl coenzyme A (HMG-CoA) reductase inhibitors (statin agents) also have positive effects in arterial disease beyond lowering low-density lipoprotein cholesterol levels. For example, statins affect immune function, macrophage metabolism, inflammation, smooth muscle cell proliferation, and endothelial function, such as up-regulation of endothelial nitric oxide synthase (Koh 2000). Therefore, it is reasonable to examine the evidence for lipid-lowering treatment in the prevention of all stroke subtypes, of which lacunar stroke is a large subset.

The authors of *post hoc* analyses of four major trials with HMG-CoA reductase inhibitors have now shown that in the primary prevention of stroke in patients with coronary artery disease compared with controls, these agents are of similar efficacy to antiplatelet agents in the secondary prevention of stroke. The Scandinavian Simvastatin Survival Study (4S 1995) was associated with a 2.75 per cent stroke rate in the simvastatin group and 4.05 per cent in the placebo group. The Cholesterol and Recurrent Events Study (Sacks *et al.* 1996) was associated with a 2.11 per cent stroke rate in the pravastatin group and 3.46 per cent in the placebo group This result was statistically significant. The West of Scotland Coronary Prevention Study on healthy subjects (WOSCOPS 1992) was associated with a 1.21 per cent reduction in the pravastatin group and 1.43 per cent in the placebo group. The Long-term Intervention with Pravastatin in Ischaemic Disease (LIPID) trial (LIPID 1998) was associated with a reduced incidence of stroke at 3.7 per cent as compared with 4.5 per cent on placebo (risk reduction = 19%, $P = 0.048$). Despite this evidence, largely from studying coronary artery diseased patients, prospective randomized trials are needed in secondary stroke prevention to clarify the importance of this risk factor and its treatment.

From the LIPID study, analysis has been done on the effect of pravastatin on each of the subtypes of ischaemic stroke. There was a trend to benefit for all types, as seen in Fig. 24.5, including cardioembolic, large artery, small vessel, and 'unknown' type, but none of these small samples gave statistically significant results. However, the rate for lacunar infarction was 0.4 per cent on pravastatin compared with 0.6 per cent on placebo, and the odds ratio was better for this subtype than for any of the other subtypes (White et al. 2000).

Meta-analysis in which pooling all 16 randomized statin trials occurred, excluding LIPID (Hebert et al. 1997), also supports a risk reduction. The non-fatal stroke rate was 120/12 840 in statin-treated patients and 182/7900 in control patients, a 60 per cent reduction in risk, and the absolute difference is 1.4 per cent (95% CI 1–1.7%). A similar meta-analysis (Blauw et al. 1997) revealed 181 of 10 314 strokes in the statin group versus 261 of 10 124 strokes in the control group, which gives an odds ratio of 0.68. The absolute risk of stroke was reduced by 0.8 per cent (95% CI 0.4–1.2%). A meta-analysis of eight statin trials for coronary artery disease shows a significant reduction in atherothrombotic stroke with a risk ratio reduction of 0.76 (95% CI 0.62–0.92, $P = 0.01$) (Bucher et al. 1998). SPARCL, a currently recruiting lipid-lowering trial in TIA and ischaemic stroke with only modestly elevated serum

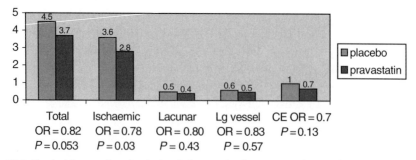

Fig. 24.5 The incidence of stroke during follow-up in the LIPID study. For the placebo arm $n = 4502$, and for the treatment arm $n = 4512$. Statistical calculations are approximate, based on data published by White et al. (2000). Lg vessel = large vessel, atherothrombotic subtype of stroke. CE = cardioembolic subtype of stroke. OR = odds of event with pravastatin/odds with placebo.

low-density lipoproteins will have a significant pool of lacunar stroke participants. This will contribute to our understanding of lipid management in this subtype of stroke (SPARCL 1998).

Conclusion Lipid-lowering therapy with pravastatin, and probably all statins, reduces the likelihood of stroke in patients with coronary artery disease. In the LIPID study, lacunar strokes were identified specifically as an outcome measure and were protected by pravastatin. More prospectively randomized trials in the secondary prevention of stroke using statins are required, but it is reasonable to treat patients with ischaemic strokes, and lipid levels in the ranges included in the CARE and LIPID trials, or higher, as a secondary prevention therapy. Lacunar strokes should not be excluded from this management approach.

Other risk factors

It was also reported recently that hyperhomocysteinaemia patients may have a high frequency of multiple lacunar strokes and ischaemic leukoencephalopoathy, although there is as yet no convincing evidence that treating hyperhomocysteinaemia will reduce the risk of subsequent stroke (Evers *et al.* 1997, Fassbender *et al.* 1999).

General conclusions

For patients with hyperacute lacunar stroke, there is a likely role for thrombolysis, similar to that seen in the large vessel stroke group. More specific research into this important issue is required.

There is reasonable evidence from the published literature that lacunar strokes should be managed with acute aspirin therapy within 48 h of stroke onset. Antiplatelet agents should be used for secondary prevention. Risk factor management should include blood pressure control, lipid lowering, and glycaemic control, and consideration should be given to the role of ramipril irrespective of blood pressure. For almost all of these concluding remarks, the evidence is obtained by extrapolation from studies that include a large proportion of lacunar stroke in a total pool of ischaemic stroke, and attempts at subgroup analyses usually reveal non-significant statistical trends in favour of the therapy in question. For each treatment option above, there is no tendency for the lacunar group to fare worse than other forms of ischaemic stroke.

In those patients with lacunar stroke and more than 60 per cent carotid stenosis, there is no clear evidence to support carotid endarterectomy as a means of stroke secondary prevention.

There are several large studies in progress in which further clarification of treatment options for lacunar stroke may become clear. In particular, these include the PROGRESS, SPARCL, and SPS3 studies. While they will contribute to many unresolved issues, further research should be encouraged.

Part VII

Subcortical haemorrhage

Chapter 25

MRI changes as a risk factor for intracerebral haemorrhage

F. Fazekas and G. Roob

Introduction

Small vessel disease is not only a frequent cause of ischaemic cerebral tissue damage with lacunar infarcts and leukoaraiosis but is also associated with a greater tendency for rupturing vessel walls and subsequent bleeding into the brain parenchyma. This aetiology of intracerebral haemorrhage (ICH) has been documented primarily for hypertensive small artery disease (Cole and Yates 1967, 1968, Fisher 1971, 1972). Vessel wall changes consistent with fibrinoid necrosis due to impaired endothelial transport of plasma proteins and vessel wall fibrosis have been found in regions of hypertensive ICH, and in some instances pathologists also observed outpouchings of the arterioles (Cole and Yates 1968, Fisher 1972). These pseudoaneurysms were felt to represent a first step towards rupture of the vessel wall. Significant fibrinoid necrosis together with microaneurysms has also been identified as the probable cause of intracerebral haemorrhage from cerebral amyloid angiopathy (CAA) (Vinters 1987, Vonsattel et al. 1991).

With the advent of neuroimaging technologies, it rapidly became apparent that computed tomography (CT) and, even more so, magnetic resonance imaging (MRI) are well suited to detect microangiopathy-related ischaemic lesions of the brain parenchyma. In the context of ICH, frequent occurrence of co-existing lacunar infarcts and white matter rarefaction, i.e. leukoaraiosis, was expected and confirmed first by studies using CT (Inzitari et al. 1990). From these findings, it was speculated that ischaemic tissue damage in itself might indicate a higher risk for ICH. In a comparison of 116 patients with ICH and 155 controls who had been selected randomly from CT examinations, lacunar infarction turned out to be a significant and independent predictor of intracerebral bleeding together with hypertension. An independent predictive effect of leukoaraiosis could not be substantiated, however (Inzitari et al. 1990).

MRI may add further to our insight into small vessel disorders associated with intracerebral bleeding. First, MRI surpasses CT in outlining the extent and location of ischaemic cerebral tissue damage. Secondly, MRI appears to have the potential to reveal even more direct evidence for the presence of bleeding-prone microangiopathy by the use of sequences that are highly sensitive for iron-containing compounds such as haemosiderin (Atlas *et al.* 1988). Conventional T_2-weighted spin-echo sequences primarily reflect differences in tissue T_2 relaxation. So-called gradient-echo acquisition also incorporates the dephasing of spins due to local magnetic field inhomogeneities. This so-called T_2^* effect occurs in lesions containing paramagnetic material which causes local susceptibility gradients that lead to a faster decay of transverse magnetization. Haemosiderin exerts such paramagnetic effects. As a consequence, areas containing haemosiderin appear markedly hypointense on T_2^*-weighted images (Fig. 25.1).

Whenever blood leaks into the brain parenchyma, haemoglobin from lysed erythrocytes is degraded to haemosiderin which is partly removed by macrophages, and partly remains stored at the site of bleeding. Such deposits, which previously have been detectable only at post-mortem, can now be visualized with MRI. Large accumulations of haemosiderin have always been shown by conventional T_2-weighted sequences. However, T_2^*-weighted images are even more sensitive (Atlas *et al.* 1988, Tanaka *et al.* 1999) and are also able to detect smaller amounts of haemosiderin deposition as illustrated in Fig. 25.1, which we have termed microbleeds (MBs).

Increasing experience with gradient-echo MRI techniques suggests that clinically silent extravasation of blood into the perivascular tissue is a relatively frequent phenomenon which occurs primarily in patients with ICH and causes small foci of signal loss throughout the brain (Roob and Fazekas 2000). We here will review

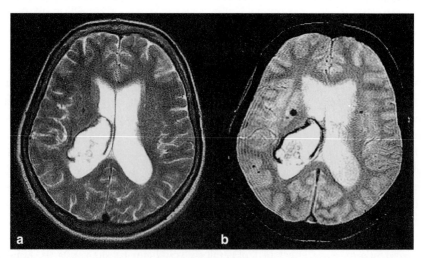

Fig. 25.1 Comparison of (a) fast spin-echo T_2-weighted (TR/TE 2900/120 ms TSE Fact 24) and (b) gradient-echo T_2^*-weighted (TR/TE 600/16 ms; flip angle 20°) images. The dark rim of haemosiderin around the thalamic haematoma is seen on both sequences but appears much more pronounced on gradient-echo T_2^*-weighted images. Similarly, a large focal hypointensity in the putamen on the same side is rarely seen on the fast spin-echo scan. A few other smaller microbleeds are seen with the gradient-echo sequence only.

available pathological support for this assumption. An overview on the frequency and distribution of MBs in various patient groups including first follow-up results will serve to address their possible clinical and therapeutic implications.

Histopathology of MBs

Focal areas of signal loss on gradient-echo T_2*-weighted images can result from various processes that affect the local susceptibility gradients. Within the brain, traces of haemosiderin were suggested as their most frequent cause, but these deposits can also have other aetiologies. Apart from spontaneous blood leakage, haemosiderin deposition may be associated with small cavernous haemangiomas or can stem from diffuse shearing injuries following head trauma. Rarely, iron particles which have been dislocated to the brain may also lead to focal signal loss. In addition, factors other than paramagnetic material can induce hypointensity on T_2*-weighted images, such as dense calcification, especially in the basal ganglia, or air bubbles following open neurosurgery. Given all these possibilities, it appeared mandatory to provide histopathological support for the assumption that foci of signal loss in ICH patients were associated primarily with haemosiderin deposits around diseased small vessels.

In an effort to achieve this, we examined the brains of 11 patients who consecutively had come to autopsy after death from an ICH (Fazekas *et al.* 1999). The ICH had been lobar in seven patients and was located in the thalamus/basal ganglia in three, and in the brainstem in one patient. Gradient-echo T_2*-weighted MRI images showed focal areas of signal loss outside the terminal ICH in seven brains. They were seen in a corticosubcortical location in six brains, in the basal ganglia/thalami in five, and infratentorially in three specimens. Correlative histopathological sections showed focal accumulation of haemosiderin-containing macrophages in 21 of 34 areas with MRI signal loss. Such deposits were most frequent in the basal ganglia adjacent to small blood vessels and were sometimes associated with minute areas of tissue necrosis. For the remaining MRI hypointensities, no specific pathological substrate was found. Haemosiderin deposits were also noted without MRI signal changes in two brains and could not be confirmed in one brain with two foci of signal loss. MRI-negative haemosiderin deposits tended to be smaller and consisted of only a few perivascular haemosiderin-laden microphages. No other abnormalities corresponding to MRI foci of signal loss were found in this study (Fazekas *et al.* 1999).

In parallel, histopathological work-up showed quite severe ischaemic damage in the majority of these 11 brains which consisted of lacunes, primarily of the basal ganglia, and extensive rarefaction of white matter. Interestingly, these ischaemic changes were not strictly correlated with either MRI hypointensities or focal haemosiderin deposits. There was evidence of moderate to severe fibrohyalinosis in all specimens, and the brains of two patients were also positive for CAA. Brains with fibrohyalinosis showed MB preferentially in the basal ganglia and thalami, but foci of blood leakage were also observed in corticosubcortical regions. Corticosubcortical MBs were detected in the

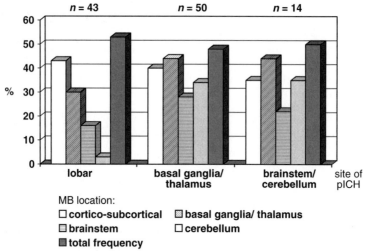

Fig. 25.2 Frequency of microbleeds in different regions of the brain in relation to the site of the symptomatic haematoma (from Roob *et al.* 2000).

brains of both patients with CAA and in the basal ganglia of one of these specimens (Fazekas *et al.* 1999).

Similar results to those in the above study were reported by Tanaka *et al.* (1999). These investigators performed post-mortem examinations of brain tissue from three patients whose MRI scans had shown small hypointense lesions. Serial histopathological sections through the sites of MRI hypointense lesions revealed foci of old haemorrhages which were characterized by perivascular haemosiderin deposits. The bleeds obviously had been caused by the rupture of ateriosclerotic microvessels measuring less than 200 μm in diameter. Gliosis and incomplete ischaemic necrosis were also seen at these sites. In one specimen, an organized pseudoaneurysm was found (Tanaka *et al.* 1999).

Together with earlier pathological observations of perivascular haemosiderin deposits in patients with microangiopathy (Fisher 1971, Vinters 1987), these studies provide strong support for the assumption that the majority of focal areas of signal loss on T_2^*-weighted MRI do represent remnants of earlier small bleeds. They also underscore the association of MBs with ischaemic tissue changes characteristic of small vessel disease.

Frequency of MBs

First observations on the frequency of foci of signal loss in ICH patients supplied quite diverse numbers (Scharf *et al.* 1994, Greenberg *et al.* 1996, Offenbacher *et al.* 1996). Small sample sizes and the pre-selection of specific patient groups are likely to have contributed to the wide range of hypointensities observed (Roob and Fazekas, 2000). It is also important to note that earlier studies have used conventional T_2-weighted sequences for all or part of their MRI examinations (Scharf et al. 1994, Offenbacher et al. 1996). As outlined above and illustrated by direct comparison, conventional T_2-weighted sequences are much less sensitive for depicting areas of haemosiderin deposition than T_2^*-weighted acquisitions (Tanaka et al. 1999). More recent studies using only T_2^*-weighted sequences suggest that MRI can document earlier MBs in about half of all patients with an ICH (Tanaka et al. 1999, Roob et al. 2000) (Table 25.1).

A finding that was not unexpected from the co-existence with lacunes and white matter damage in ICH patients was that evidence for past MBs may also be obtained in patients with ischaemic vascular disorders. This is especially true for individuals with cerebral ischaemic stroke. A careful study of 221 patients by Kwa et al. (1998) found MRI hypointensities consistent with focal haemosiderin deposits among 17 of 66 (26%) stroke patients versus three of 69 (4%) patients with myocardial infarction and 11 of 86 (13%) patients with peripheral arterial disease. Cerebral white matter lesions were an independent predictor of the presence of focal haemosiderin deposits, and the likelihood of MBs increased with the severity of white matter damage.

Rarely, MBs can also be detected in clinically asymptomatic elderly individuals. This was shown in the setting of the Austrian Stroke Prevention Study (ASPS) which is a population-based, single-centre trial on the effects of cerebrovascular risk factors on brain parenchyma and function (Schmidt et al. 1994, 1999). The ASPS prospectively follows elderly individuals who were selected randomly from the

Table 25.1 Frequency of MRI-detected old intracerebral microbleeds (MBs) in different patient populations and asymptomatic elderly individuals

Patient groups	No.	% MBs	MRI weighting	Reference
Intracerebral bleeding				
Spontaneous ICH	72	17	T_2	Scharf et al. (1994)
Primary ICH	120	23	T_2 (T_2^* in 38 patients)	Offenbacher et al. (1996)
Lobar ICH	15	80	T_2^*	Greenberg et al. (1996)
Spontaneous ICH	30	57	T_2^*	Tanaka et al. (1999)
Primary ICH	109	53	T_2^*	Roob et al. (2000)
Ischaemia				
Cerebral ischaemia	137	4	T_2	Scharf et al. (1994)
Ischaemic stroke	66	26	T_2^*	Kwa et al. (1998)
Myocardial infarction	69	4	T_2^*	Kwa et al. (1998)
Peripheral artery disease	86	13	T_2^*	Kwa et al. (1998)
Non-ICH-related neurological deficits (>50 years and/or hypertensive)	59	25	T_2^*	Tanaka et al. (1999)
Asymptomatic				
Asymptomatic elderly individuals	280	6	T_2^*	Roob et al. (1999)

official community register of the city of Graz and were free of signs or symptoms of neurological or psychiatric disorders. MRI examination of 280 individuals aged between 44 and 79 years (mean age 60 years) with a T_2^*-weighted sequence revealed one or more foci of signal loss compatible with MBs in 18 (6.4%) of these volunteers (Roob et al. 1999).

Almost all studies on MBs agree that hypertension can be regarded as the main clinically observable risk factor for these abnormalities (Roob and Fazekas 1999). This association was first highlighted by a report that attempted to define the causes of the MRI observation of multifocal hypointensities on gradient-echo sequences and found chronic hypertension as the prevailing clinical abnormality (Chan et al. 1996). The results of the ASPS with careful repeated blood pressure determinations and a wide range of values suggest a correlation of the occurrence of MBs with both elevated mean systolic and mean diastolic blood pressure (Roob et al. 1999).

Distribution of MBs

Most reports on the observation of focal hypointensities suggest that focal haemosiderin deposits can be found widely distributed throughout the brain (Offenbacher et al. 1996, Tanaka et al. 1999). In the study of multifocal hypointense lesions associated with chronic hypertension by Chan et al. (1996), however, MBs were located primarily in the basal ganglia and thalamus as well as infratentorially in the brainstem and cerebellum. Investigating patients with ischaemic vascular disease, a difference in the distribution of MBs between individuals with and without hypertension could not be confirmed (Kwa et al. 1998). In yet another setting, i.e. in patients with a lobar haematoma, Greenberg et al. (1996) observed MBs preferentially in corticosubcortical regions and felt that this pattern was strongly suggestive of CAA. It has been noted earlier that patients with CAA frequently present with repeated lobar bleeds which matches the preferred sites of vascular amyloid deposition. Evidence for MBs in specific locations could, therefore, help in differentiating various aetiologies of microangiopathy and thus might contribute to the in vivo diagnosis of CAA (Greenberg 1998).

To substantiate these assumptions, we looked specifically at the distribution of MBs in a series of 109 patients with primary ICH, i.e. spontaneous, non-traumatic intracerebral bleeding without evidence of any kind of vascular malformation or a brain tumour as the source of the haematoma (Roob et al. 2000). The overall number of MBs in these patients was quite variable and ranged from one to 90 lesions (mean 14; median 6). Most frequently, MBs were seen in corticosubcortical regions or in the basal ganglia including the thalami. MBs in the brainstem and cerebellum were observed less frequently and the white matter was spared in most instances. This is in agreement with the findings of Tanaka et al. (1999). When we compared the distribution of MBs between patients based on the site of their symptomatic haematoma, we found some correspondence between ICH location and MB

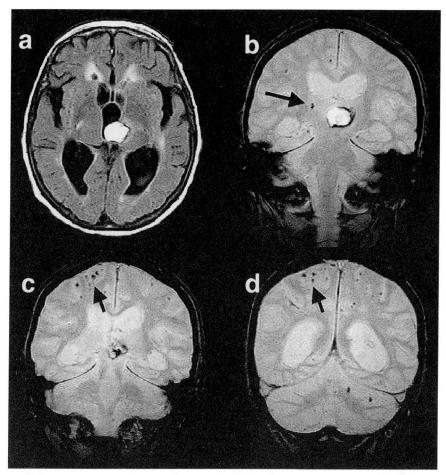

Fig. 25.3 (a) FLAIR image (TE 130 ms, TR 6000 ms, TI 1900 ms) and (b–d) gradient-echo T_2*-weighted images (TR/TE 600/16 ms; flip angle 20°) of a patient with a subacute haematoma in the left thalamus. One area of focal hypointensity is seen in the contralateral basal ganglia (arrow in b). However, many more hypointensities indicative of old MBs are seen in corticosubcortical regions (arrows in c and d) and in the cerebellum.

topography. This is illustrated in Fig. 25.2. As can be seen, the frequency of MBs in the basal ganglia/thalami and infratentorially was greater in patients with an ICH at these sites than in those with a lobar haematoma. Concerning corticosubcortical MBs, however, no clear differences emerged between ICH subgroups. Figure 25.3 illustrates such a patient with obvious discrepancy between the preferred location of MBs and the acute haematoma. Thus, we were unable to define a specific pattern of MBs that was clearly suggestive of CAA in this unselected series. Interestingly, a preferential corticosubcortical location of MBs was not even found in the normotensive patients of this study (Roob *et al.* 2000).

Longitudinal observation of MB

As haemosiderin deposits do not vanish over time, they should become more frequent with repeated episodes of blood leakage. In a first follow-up study of 24 patients, Greenberg *et al.* (1999) nicely confirmed this assumption. Seventeen individuals diagnosed with probable and seven with possible CAA were followed for a mean duration of 1.5 years. New foci of haemosiderin deposition were detected in nine (38%) patients. These new haemorrhages were seen more frequently in patients with probable amyloid angiopathy (47%) and more MBs at baseline (Greenberg *et al.* 1999).

Diagnostic impact

There is clear evidence for a strong association between the observation of focal hypointensities on gradient-echo T_2^*-weighted MRI with ischaemic cerebral tissue damage related to small vessel diseases such as lacunes and white matter rarefaction. In addition to being a further marker for microangiopathy, the detection of MBs also confirms a tendency for blood leakage through these damaged vessels. Although ischaemic and haemorrhagic events frequently appear associated, this need not always be the case, i.e. patients with marked leukoaraiosis need not always show MBs, while multiple focal hypointensities may also be seen in patients with no or minimal ischaemic tissue changes. Future research will have to clarify if and how such discrepancies relate to specific types of small vessel disorders. In addition to these pathophysiological considerations, detecting MBs in a patient with ICH clearly gives some clue as to the probable aetiology of this event and supports the assumption of a primary ICH. Together with a typical location of the presenting haematoma, such a finding frequently will reduce or abolish the need for angiography.

Whether CAA can be diagnosed on the basis of the presence and distribution of MBs is still debatable. Greenberg (1998) has suggested that a clinical diagnosis of 'probable' CAA can be made in patients aged 60 years or older with multiple haemorrhages confined to lobar brain regions and no other identifiable cause of the haemorrhage. There appears to be some association between the regional distribution of MBs and subsequent symptomatic haematomas. Great diversity in the distribution of MBs weakens this association. It could be possible, however, that certain groups of patients that certain groups of patients such as those with hereditary types of amyloid angiopathy may have a more uniform pattern of MB distribution.

Clinical aspects

Clinical expectations focus predominantly on the hope that MRI findings could improve our ability to predict an individual's risk of suffering from an ICH. This would be especially important at the start of therapies which affect the coagulation system, i.e. which may augment the risk of bleeding further. CT-documented lacunar infarcts and extensive leukoaraiosis appear to constitute such a marker. This has been shown recently in SPIRIT, a clinical study which tested the possible benefits of anticoagulation over acetyl salicylic acid in patients with transient ischaemic attack or minor ischaemic stroke [Stroke Prevention in Reversible Ischemia Trial (SPIRIT) Study Group 1997]. This trial had to be terminated prematurely because of an unacceptably high rate of intracerebral bleeds in the anticoagulated arm of the study population. This complication occurred predominantly in patients older than 75 years and in those with extensive leukoaraiosis. First, these data confirm the impact of pre-existing cerebrovascular disease on the risk of intracerebral bleeding from anticoagulation because complication rates of this unselected population of patients with cerebral ischaemic disease were much higher than in trials of anticoagulation for atrial fibrillation. Secondly, because focal hypointensities are directly indicative of previous haemorrhages, such MRI evidence might have served better to identify individuals at a higher risk of bleeding complications than leukoaraiosis, despite a similar pathogenetic background for the occurrence of both of these morphological abnormalities. Support for this hypothesis comes from a comparison of clinical and morphological findings between patients with a primary ICH and asymptomatic elderly individuals (Roob et al. 2000). In this study, we used logistic regression to identify those variables which contributed significantly and independently to the separation of both groups. These variables were the presence of MBs, the grade of periventricular hyperintensity, and the number of lacunes. No clinical or demographic variable entered this model (Roob et al. 2000).

Apart from these therapeutic considerations, MRI detection of micoangiopathy-related ischaemic damage and of MBs could also be relevant for counselling patients after their first symptomatic haematoma regarding the risk of rebleeding. Over a median interval of 22.9 ± 16.3 months, rebleeding has been observed in 53 of 989 (5.4%) patients with hypertensive ICH (Bae et al. 1999). The site of the second haemorrhage was different from the initial site in all patients. Common patterns of recurrence were ganglionic–thalamic (26.8%) and ganglionic–ganglionic (21.4%) bleeds. The lobar–lobar pattern was noted in only two patients. The risk of recurrent haemorrhage was significantly increased in those patients who had no long-term antihypertensive treatment. Similar observations were made in another study of 22 of 359 patients with recurrent primary ICH (Gonzales-Durante et al., 1999). From the preliminary experience of Greenberg et al. (1999), it can be speculated that individuals with a high number of MBs might be at greater risk of rebleeding. Also regions with the greatest number of MBs could be preferred sites of future bleeding in a given patient.

Despite all available evidence, definite conclusions on the predictive power of described MRI changes regarding future occurrence of a symptomatic ICH cannot yet be drawn. Clearly, prospective studies are needed to address these questions. At any rate, we should expect both microangiopathy-related ischaemic tissue damage and MBs to constitute markers for increased risk rather than risk factors per se. However, the magnitude of information provided by MRI with these morphological insights should definitely extend beyond that available from other clinical data.

Chapter 26

Subcortical haemorrhages

C.S. Kase

Introduction

Haemorrhage in the subcortical grey nuclei occurs in the striatum (putamen and caudate) and in the thalamus, and these locations account for the majority of cases of intracerebral haemorrhage (ICH) in clinical series. Subcortical haemorrhages are most common in the putamen (19–53% of ICHs) and thalamus (4–26% of ICHs), while those in the head of the caudate nucleus account for only 1–5 per cent of ICHs (Table 26.1). Although these various sites of ICH share a number of features, such as mechanisms and management, their clinical and imaging aspects are unique to each location, and they will be addressed separately, following the discussion of the general features that apply to all.

General features of subcortical haemorrhages

Mechanisms

The main mechanism of all forms of subcortical haemorrhage is hypertension, which accounts for a variable proportion of the cases in different series, in part reflecting biases of patient populations and referral patterns (Wolf 1994). Population studies including all anatomical sites of ICH have identified hypertension as the mechanism in as many as 89 per cent of cases (Furlan *et al.* 1979), but a decline in the prevalence and severity of hypertension in subsequent decades has resulted in figures as low as 39–49 per cent (Broderick *et al.* 1992). These differences in the impact of hypertension as the cause of ICH in general reflect, in part, factors such as the age of the population studied: the frequency of hypertension as the mechanism of ICH is higher in younger patients, in the 35–55 years range, in comparison with those older than 75 years (Drury *et al.* 1984). Other factors that account for these differences are: the inclusion in some series (Brott *et al.* 1986) but not in others (Gross *et al.* 1984) of cases of ICH with a defined, non-hypertensive mechanism, such as brain tumour or bleeding disorders; and differences in the proportion of blacks and whites in the population studied, as the former have a substantially higher prevalence of hypertension and incidence rates of ICH (Wolf 1994).

In the specific group of patients with subcortical haemorrhage, the frequency of hypertension as the cause of the ICH has been reported in the 60–65 per cent range

Table 26.1 Location of intracerebral haemorrhage

Series	n	Lobar	Caudate	Putamen	Thalamus	Pons	Cerebellum	Ventricle
Massaro et al. (1991)	209	63 (31%)	10 (5%)	51 (24.5%)	46 (22%)	11 (5%)	26 (12.5%)	–
Weisberg et al. (1991)	265	98 (37%)	10 (4%)	50 (19%)	50 (19%)	21 (8%)	28 (10%)	8 (3%)
Schütz et al. (1990)	100	27 (27%)	3 (3%)	31 (31%)	26 (26%)	3 (3%)	7 (7%)	–
Bogousslavsky et al. (1988b)	109	43 (40%)	–	46 (42%)	4 (4%)	7 (6%)	9 (8%)	–
Mohr et al. (1978)	60	14 (23%)	–	32 (53%)	7 (12%)	1 (2%)	6 (10%)	–
Brott et al. (1986)	154	73 (47%)	–	36 (23%)	15 (10%)	5 (3%)	11 (7%)	14 (10%)
Giroud et al. (1991)	87	16 (19%)	–	36 (42%)	22 (26%)	5 (4%)	8 (9%)	–
Fieschi et al. (1988)	103	31 (30%)	–	38 (37%)	18 (18%)	6 (6%)	8 (8%)	2 (2%)
Anderson et al. (1994)	60	19 (53%)	14 (23%)[a]	–	4 (7%)	4 (7%)	6 (10%)	–
Tatu et al. (2000)	343	128 (37%)	3 (1%)	112 (33%)	55 (16%)	7 (2%)	31 (9%)	7 (2%)
Bae et al. (1992)	320	33 (10%)	4 (1%)	126 (39%)	104 (33%)	23 (7%)	30 (10%)	–
Total	1810	547 (30%)	37 (2%)	565 (31%)	351 (20%)	93 (5%)	170 (10%)	31 (2%)

[a] Putamen and caudate locations together.

Table 26.2 Frequency of hypertension as the mechanism of ICH in various locations

Series	No. of ICHs	ICH location (% hypertensive)				
		Putaminal	Thalamic	Lobar	Cerebellar	Pontine
Broderick et al. (1993)	66	73%[a]		67%	73%	78%
Anderson et al. (1994)	60	61%[a]		56%	70%[b]	
Tatu et al. (2000)	350	60%	65.5%	45.3%	55%	–

[a]Putaminal and thalamic together, as 'deep'.
[b]Cerebellar and brainstem together.

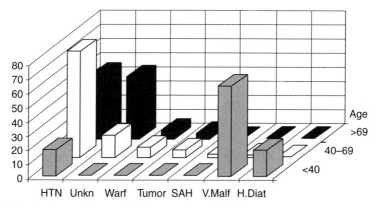

Fig. 26.1 Mechanisms of intracerebral haemorrhage in different age groups. From Schütz et al. (1990), with permission. HTN = hypertension; Unkn = unknown; Warf = warfarin; SAH = subarachnoid haemorrhage; V. Malf = vascular malformations; H. Diat = haemorrhagic diatheses.

(Anderson *et al.* 1994, Tatu *et al.* 2000), not clearly different from its frequency in other ICH locations (Table 26.2). Although there is some variation among series, these comparable figures of frequency of hypertension by ICH site have been used to argue against the concept of the predominance of deep (putaminal and thalamic) over lobar locations in patients with hypertensive ICH (Broderick *et al.* 1993). A still unresolved issue is that of an age-related predisposition for specific sites of location of ICH, which in turn has been related to its potential mechanism (Schütz *et al.* 1990) (Fig. 26.1). A commonly held notion has been that the hypertensive mechanism of ICH predominates in the young and middle-aged (Drury *et al.* 1984, Schütz *et al.* 1990), while cerebral amyloid angiopathy (with its typical lobar location of ICH) increases in prevalence with advancing age (Vinters and Gilbert 1983). This view of a diminishing importance of hypertensive ICH with advancing age has been challenged by Broderick *et al.* (1993), who have argued that the frequency of the hypertensive mechanism remains stable with advancing age, and its impact is exerted virtually equally in all the sites of ICH.

Other, non-hypertensive mechanisms of ICH tend generally to favour the lobar over the deep locations (Kase 1986). This observation applies to haemorrhages caused by cerebral amyloid angiopathy (Vinters 1987); 'cryptic' vascular malformations, especially cavernous angiomas (Simard *et al.* 1986); primary malignant and metastatic brain tumours (Kase 1994); anticoagulant and fibrinolytic agents (Hart *et al.* 1995); and sympathomimetic agents (Kase *et al.* 1987). However, in the latter group, it has been observed that ICH due to cocaine ingestion tends to be distributed more evenly between lobar and deep locations (Levine *et al.* 1990), without the lobar predominance of other 'non-hypertensive' types of ICH.

Clinical features at presentation

Headache

Headache is a commonly reported symptom at the onset of ICH. In the recent series of Tatu *et al.* (2000), headache was reported in more than one-third (36%) of the cases, and it occurred with similar frequency in the putaminal (37.5%), thalamic (34.5%), and lobar (36.7%) locations, while it was somewhat more common (58%) in the group with cerebellar haemorrhage. A higher frequency of headache at onset of cerebellar and lobar haemorrhage in comparison with the deep types (putaminal, thalamic, and caudate) has been reported in two studies (Hier *et al.* 1993, Melo *et al.* 1996). It is possible that the lower reporting of headache in cases of deep haemorrhages represents an artefact or a bias introduced by non-responders, as the highest numbers of non-responders in the study of Melo *et al.* (1996) was in the group with deep hemispheric and brainstem haematomas, which were the groups with the lowest frequency of headache. In addition to location, the study of Melo *et al.* (1996) identified female gender, meningeal signs, and signs of transtentorial herniation as features positively associated with headache at ICH presentation. In patients with putaminal ICH who reported headache (13), the majority (8/13) located the pain in the ipsilateral anterior part of the head.

Seizures

Seizures at onset of ICH are rare, generally reported with a frequency below 10 per cent in groups of ICH that include all locations (Mohr *et al.* 1978, Anderson *et al.* 1994, Tatu *et al.* 2000). However, differences in frequency of seizures by ICH location have been noted, with a higher frequency (16–36%) in lobar locations (Kase *et al.* 1982, Faught *et al.* 1989, Lipton *et al.* 1987, Massaro *et al.* 1991, Tatu *et al.* 2000), while the low frequency of seizures in the deep locations (8% for putaminal, 1.8% for thalamic) (Tatu *et al.* 2000) brings the overall frequency to the low figure of 10 per cent or less.

Progression after onset

Progression after onset is an increasingly recognized feature of ICH in all locations. The old, pre-computed tomography (CT) notion of ICH as a process completed by

1 or 2 h after onset (Herbstein and Schaumburg 1974) has been replaced by the common observation of early enlargement of ICH, facilitated by studies of repeated CT scan evaluations in the first few hours of ICH evolution (Broderick *et al.* 1990). The observed increase in ICH volume frequently is correlated with clinical deterioration, with decline in the level of consciousness and/or increase in the severity of the focal deficits (Fig. 26.2). Early neurological deterioration within the first 6–12 h is relatively common in patients with ICH (26.7% in the series of Tatu *et al.* 2000) and it can be due to a number of causes, one of which is progressive enlargement of the haematoma. This course after onset has been observed in both deep (putaminal, thalamic) and lobar ICHs, without a particular site being associated preferentially with early haematoma enlargement (Tatu *et al.* 2000). In the study of Bae *et al.* (1992), six putaminal haematomas became an average three times larger, and four of thalamic location became twice as large, generally within 24 h from onset. Recent studies (Fujii *et al.* 1994, Brott *et al.* 1997) have documented haematoma enlargement that is most prominent within the first 6 h of evolution, during which time neurological deterioration frequently is observed. Among the risk factors for such occurrence, persistent hypertension has been mentioned frequently (Kelley *et al.* 1982, Bae *et al.* 1992), but comparisons of patients with and without haematoma enlargement have not confirmed a statistically significant association between elevated blood pressure and ICH enlargement (Brott *et al.* 1997). On rare occasions, patients with putaminal ICH have a rapid, precipitous fatal clinical deterioration associated with marked enlargement of the haematoma (Wijdicks and Fulgham 1995). A process of rebleeding (rather than gradual continuous leakage) has been postulated in these instances, but no specific risk factors for it have been identified.

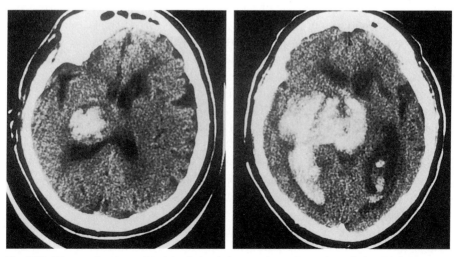

Fig. 26.2 CT scan of patient with right thalamic haemorrhage that enlarged after 3 h from onset, while the patient had progressive deterioration in the level of consciousness.

Imaging aspects of intracerebral haemorrhage

The development of CT and magnetic resonance imaging (MRI) has revolutionized the field of ICH imaging. Prior to the development of these techniques, most of the anatomical knowledge about ICH was derived from autopsy data, thus biasing the observations towards the most severe forms. The availability of CT and MRI has allowed the characterization of the whole spectrum of clinical and radiological presentations of ICH, including all sites and sizes of ICH.

CT scan is generally considered the fastest and most reliable way of documenting ICH in the acute setting, by showing the typical high-attenuation image, with its potential associated features of mass effect, intraventricular bleeding, and hydrocephalus, and accompanying subarachnoid haemorrhage (SAH). This technique also allows the documentation of a potential underlying lesion, such as a vascular malformation or tumour causing the ICH. Finally, CT also permits the evolution of the ICH to be followed to its eventual resolution, although this type of information is substantially less precise than that obtained in the acute phase: Franke *et al.* (1991) found that seven of 42 patients had no detectable CT residual lesions (despite three of them having residual neurological deficits) after a median of 9 months from ICH onset; among the 22 patients with deep ICHs, four had no residual lesions, three had only focal ventricular enlargement, one had only calcification in the area of the prior ICH, and the remaining 14 had hypodensity, six of which were slit-like. The latter was the most consistently found pattern after deep haemorrhage, while such a pattern was not observed in haemorrhages of lobar location. Similarly, Sung and Chu (1992) found in 61 patients with putaminal haemorrhage with a mean follow-up of 2.5 years that the most common residual pattern (52%) was a slit in the basal ganglia, while 29 per cent had a cavity, 8 per cent had ventricular dilatation, and only one patient (3%) had calcification at the site of the ICH; five patients (8%) had no detectable residual abnormalities from the ICH.

Advances in MRI technology have allowed a more precise diagnosis and timing of ICH, the latter based on the stages of evolution of the haemoglobin molecule within the haematoma (Dul and Drayer 1994). Although CT is still considered the diagnostic modality of choice for documenting an acute ICH, technical modifications of MRI have delineated the characteristics of ICH in the acute phase more precisely. With the use of susceptibility-weighted imaging, an echo-planar T_2^* sequence, Linfante *et al.* (1999) reported detection of ICH in the 'hyperacute' phase, within 2 h from onset. They also described the MRI anatomical features of ICH, which is composed of an isointense or hyperintense central core with a hypointense periphery on susceptibility-weighted or T_2-weighted sequences, and an external rim of vasogenic oedema, which is hypointense in T_1- and hyperintense in T_2-weighted images.

In a recent study, Dylewski *et al.* (2000) evaluated the utility of MRI in acute ICH by determining whether new diagnostic information was obtained after the use of this technique. Their results indicated that new diagnoses were uncovered by MRI in 15 of the 67 patients (22%) who underwent testing, but the diagnostic yield applied more to lobar and infratentorial ICH (30% with new diagnoses provided by MRI) than to deep haemorrhages, of which only two of 23 patients (9%) had useful new diagnostic information as a result of MRI testing. The majority of the new diagnoses after MRI were instances of amyloid angiopathy and vascular malformations (four cases each), both of which predominate in areas outside the deep grey hemispheric nuclei.

Prognosis of intracerebral haemorrhage

The mortality rates in ICH vary widely, between 20 (Bogousslavsky *et al.* 1988*b*) and 56 per cent (Silver *et al.* 1984), and are dependent on a number of features that can be determined at the time of onset. Among these, the level of consciousness and the volume of the ICH on CT scan are powerful determinants of mortality and functional outcome: a depression in the level of consciousness, measured as a Glasgow Coma Scale (GCS) score of 3–8, was correlated with a mortality of 78 per cent, in comparison with 10 per cent for those with a GCS of 9–15 (Tuhrim *et al.* 1988); and poor functional outcome and mortality were linearly correlated with increasing haematoma volume (Tatu *et al.* 2000). Other factors related to poor outcome in ICH in general have been: (i) advancing age, amount of alcohol consumed within 1 week from the ICH, and lobar and cerebellar location (Juvela 1995); the presence of hydrocephalus (Diringer *et al.* 1998, Phan *et al.* 2000); (ii) blood pressure on admission, with significantly higher mortality and worse outcome in patients with putaminal or thalamic ICH and with mean arterial pressure greater than 136 mmHg and systolic blood pressure greater than 178 mmHg (Terayama *et al.* 1997); (iii) intraventricular haemorrhage has been found to be a predictor of poor outcome in some studies (Mori *et al.* 1995), but not in others (Juvela 1995), and one study has even suggested that intraventricular bleeding is associated with improved outcome in thalamic haemorrhage (Lampl *et al.* 1995). In survivors of ICH of various locations, functional outcome [measured as being independent, with a modified Rankin scale (mRS) ≤2] is generally better in patients with lobar than with deep haemorrhages: in the study of Tatu *et al.* (2000), 43.9 per cent of patients with lobar haemorrhages reached an mRS ≤2 at 30 days, in comparison with 22.2 per cent with thalamic ICH and 16.8 per cent with putaminal ICH.

The use of evoked potentials for the prediction of outcome after ICH has gained in popularity in some centres. Kato *et al.* (1991) used median and tibial nerve somatosensory evoked potentials (SEPs) in patients with thalamic and putaminal ICH. Abnormalities were recorded in 92 per cent of arms and 81 per cent of legs tested, showing a high degree of correlation between abnormal SEPs and presence of deep haemorrhage. A common finding was an absence of SEPs in patients with haemorrhages of large size (generally associated with severe motor and sensory deficits) who were tested early after onset. On the other hand, these authors found that subsequent reappearance of SEPs was correlated with clinical improvement. In a group of 80 patients with putaminal haemorrhage, Liu *et al.* (1991) utilized SEPs and brainstem auditory evoked potentials (BAEPs) as an early guide of functional prognosis. They found that SEPs that were either normal or had prolonged central conduction time, if associated with normal BAEPs, predicted good functional outcome, while absent SEPs predicted moderate (62%) to severe (26%) disability/ death, and abnormal wave V in BAEPs was associated with severe disability (50%) or death (50%).

Recurrence of ICH is considered a rare event (Douglas and Haerer 1982, Fieschi *et al.* 1988). In a recent study, Bae *et al.* (1999) documented recurrence in 53 (5.4%) of 989 patients with ICH after a median interval of almost 2 years. The most common patterns of recurrence were an initial basal ganglionic ICH followed by either another basal ganglionic or a thalamic ICH, while two episodes of lobar ICH were distinctly uncommon. The risk of recurrent ICH was closely correlated with poor control of hypertension after the initial episode of ICH.

Putaminal haemorrhage

Clinical presentation

The early clinico-anatomical correlations in putaminal haemorrhage (Fisher 1961) were carried out in subjects who eventually died from the effects of the ICH, resulting in the description of the features associated with large, at times massive haemorrhages. These patients often presented with complete contralateral flaccid hemiplegia, conjugate eye deviation towards the side of the haematoma, contralateral hemihypaesthesia and homonymous hemianopia, and profound disturbances of consciousness, often leading to coma and death (Fisher 1961). With the advent of CT scan, it soon became apparent that a wide spectrum of severity of putaminal ICH could be correlated with the presence of haematomas of various sizes and locations within the putamen (Hier *et al.* 1977). These early clinical–CT correlations identified syndromes of small (moderate hemimotor and hemisensory deficits), moderate size ('classical' syndrome of hemiplegia, hemisensory loss, lateral gaze paresis, homo-nymous hemianopia, and either aphasia or hemi-inattention), and massive (coma, bilateral Babinski sign, fixed dilated pupils, absent extraocular movements, and death) putaminal ICH (Hier *et al.* 1977).

Clinical syndromes in relation to the location of putaminal haemorrhage

Since these early descriptions, a number of refinements in the clinico-anatomical correlations in putaminal ICH were reported by Weisberg *et al.* (1990) and Chung *et al.* (2000). The study of Weisberg *et al.* (1990) included 100 patients, and, based on observations of the pattern of haematoma extension, the authors established the following clinico-anatomical correlations.

(1) *Medial putaminal haemorrhage*: the ICH extended medially from the putamen affecting the genu and posterior limb of the internal capsule, but without extending through it; all patients had a contralateral motor deficit (hemiparesis slightly more frequently than hemiplegia) and hemisensory syndrome, but no abnormalities of ocular motility, visual fields, or level of consciousness; they were associated with no mortality and with full clinical recovery.

(2) *Lateral putaminal haemorrhage*: the haematoma originated from the lateral putamen and extended anteriorly along the external capsule, producing contralateral motor (hemiplegia more frequently than hemiparesis) and sensory deficits in all patients; more than half of these patients showed delayed neurological deterioration, and persistent deficits were more common than full recovery; both the clinical presentation and outcome in the lateral group were more severe than in the medial type, reflecting substantial differences in haematoma size (27–42 mm × 14–19 mm in the lateral type, 10 × 18 mm in the medial type).

(3) *Putaminal haemorrhage with extension to internal capsule and subcortical white matter*: these were large haematomas that extended medially through the internal capsule and superiorly into the corona radiata, causing a more severe syndrome of hemiplegia and hemianaesthesia, often but not always associated with homonymous hemianopia and conjugate ocular deviation, but generally with preserved consciousness; most patients were left with neurological sequelae, but the survival rate was 100 per cent.

(4) *Putaminal haemorrhage with subcortical and hemispheric extension*: these haematomas acquired large size as they extended into the white matter of adjacent cerebral lobes, causing mass effect on the lateral ventricle and frequently (7/19 patients) extending into the ventricular system; their clinical presentation was similar to that of the preceding group, except for having more prominence of aphasia or parietal lobe findings, and impaired consciousness (in eight of 19 patients); three of 19 patients (16%) died, and among the survivors the majority had deficits that interfered with independent living.

(5) *Putaminal–thalamic haematomas*: these were the largest haematomas, and they extended from the putamen into the thalamus (transecting the internal capsule) and into the subcortical white matter; they were associated with mass effect on the lateral and third ventricle, and all were accompanied by intraventricular haemorrhage; the clinical picture was characterized by impaired consciousness in all patients, frequently associated with hemiplegia, abnormalities of horizontal more than vertical gaze, and homonymous hemianopia; mortality for this group was 79 per cent (15/19 patients).

These clinical–CT correlations allowed the authors (Wiesberg *et al.* 1990) to delineate a number of patterns that are clinically useful: intraventricular haemorrhage was seen with large haematomas, and both features were associated with high mortality; all patients presented with combined motor and sensory deficits; the best functional outcome occurred in patients with medial or lateral putaminal haematomas that did not involve the internal capsule or the corona radiata; delayed neurological deterioration (in 8% of their cases) occurred only in patients with haematomas that extended into the cerebral hemisphere or the thalamus.

In a recent study, Chung *et al.* (2000) have analysed the clinico-anatomical correlations in putaminal haemorrhage further, based on the study of 192 patients from several institutions. These authors divided their cases into five anatomical types as middle, posteromedial, posterolateral, lateral, and massive, and related them to the presumed ruptured arterial branches leading to haematoma formation.

(1) The middle type (Fig. 26.3) resulted from rupture of medial lenticulostriate arteries, with bleeding into the medial putamen and globus pallidus, causing a benign syndrome of mild to moderate contralateral hemiparesis and hemisensory loss, with low frequency of impairment of consciousness and transient conjugate ocular deviation toward the side of the haematoma; intraventricular extension of the haemorrhage did not occur, and all patients survived. This group was equivalent to the medial putaminal haemorrhages described by Weisberg *et al.* (1990).

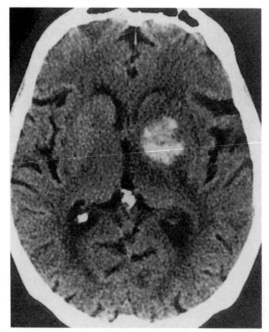

Fig. 26.3 Middle type of striatocapsular haemorrhage with minimal mass effect on the frontal horn of the left lateral ventricle, without intraventricular extension. From Chung *et al.* (2000), with permission.

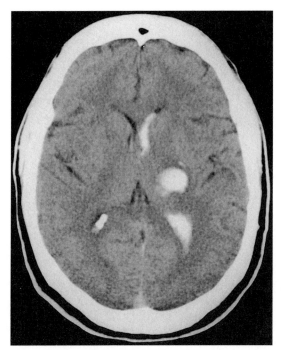

Fig. 26.4 Small posteromedial ('capsular') haemorrhage involving the posterior limb of the left internal capsule, with associated intraventricular extension.

(2) The posteromedial type (Fig. 26.4) corresponded to small haematomas confined to the posterior limb of the internal capsule ('capsular' haemorrhages), and were associated with contralateral hemiparesis, hemisensory loss, and dysarthria, resembling syndromes of lacunar infarction; the smaller haematomas did not reach the ventricular system, and were associated with no mortality and with excellent functional outcome; the bleeding vessel in this type of haemorrhage is a branch of the anterior choroidal artery, which supplies a portion of the posterior limb of the internal capsule (Chung *et al.* 2000).

(3) The posterolateral type (Fig. 26.5) was a putamino-capsular haemorrhage, and was the most common type in the series, caused by rupture of posterior branches of the lateral lenticulostriate arteries; these larger haematomas occasionally ruptured into the lateral ventricle, and produced a more severe syndrome of impaired consciousness in half of the patients, with frequent (33%) conjugate ocular deviation toward the affected hemisphere and rare (3%) contralateral eye deviation ('wrong-way' eye deviation), together with constant and generally severe contralateral hemiparesis and hemisensory loss, along with aphasia or hemineglect in dominant or non-dominant hemisphere haematomas, respectively; this group had no mortality, but 12 of 72 patients were treated surgically (stereotactic drainage of the haematoma), with excellent outcome in nine (75%).

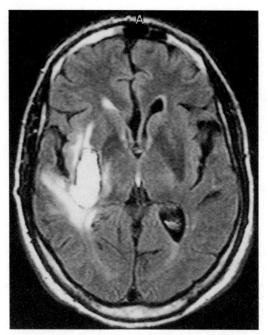

Fig. 26.5 MRI (T$_1$-weighted sequence) of a right posterolateral putaminal haemorrhage, originating from the posterior aspect of the putamen, with compression and medial displacement of the internal capsule, without intraventricular extension.

This group resembles the 'putaminal haemorrhage with subcortical and cerebral hemispheric extension' reported by Weisberg *et al.* (1990).

(4) The lateral type of haematoma (Fig. 26.6) originated for the rupture of the most lateral branches of the lenticulostriate arteries, and remained confined to an elliptical haematoma that collected itself between the putamen and the insular cortex, involving the insula > putamen > internal capsule, and producing contralateral hemiparesis, often without an associated hemisensory loss, but frequently with either aphasia or hemineglect, depending on the side of the brain involved; the outcome was generally excellent, except in cases of large haematomas, which frequently (22%) ruptured into the ventricular system, and often required surgical treatment, which was generally associated with good outcome. This 'lateral' type of putaminal ICH in the dominant hemisphere has been associated rarely with the syndrome of conduction aphasia (D'Esposito and Alexander 1995), with fluent speech and preserved comprehension but with markedly impaired repetition, thought to be due to interruption of white matter tracts (arcuate fasciculus, extreme capsule, and temporoparietal association connections) in the inferior parietal lobe.

(5) The massive type (Fig. 26.7) involved the entire striatocapsular area, and probably resulted from rupture of the same branches (posteromedial branches of

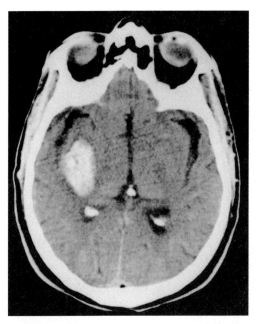

Fig. 26.6 Lateral type haemorrhage in the right putamen, as an elliptical mass located between the insula and the posterior aspect of the putamen.

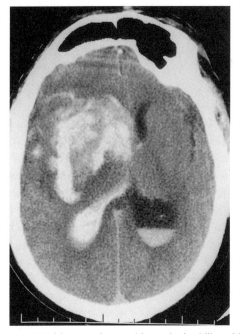

Fig. 26.7 Massive right putaminal haemorrhage with marked midline shift, ventricular extension, and hydrocephalus.

the lateral lenticulostriate arteries) that cause the posterolateral type of putaminal ICH; these patients all had a depressed level of consciousness and hemiparesis, frequently associated with ipsilateral (45%) more than contralateral (10%) conjugate eye deviation, and often progressed to coma with brainstem involvement and death (49%), despite treatment with surgical drainage of the haematoma (in 20 patients, 11 of whom died). This group corresponds to the 'putaminal–thalamic' group described by Weisberg et al. (1990).

In a separate communication, Wiesberg et al. (1992) analysed the clinical and CT features of 14 cases of massive putaminal–thalamic haemorrhage. These patients were all young African–Americans with hypertension who presented with a prodromal headache several hours before the onset of the focal deficit, all becoming hemiplegic and comatose over periods of 4–12 h. The haematomas were large, with marked mass effect and with intraventricular extension. All patients died within 72 h of onset of symptoms despite treatment of hypertension and increased intracranial pressure (ICP).

These recent clinico-anatomical studies (Weisberg et al. 1990, Chung et al. 2000) are helpful in having delineated a consistent profile of clinical presentation and prognosis, based on patterns of origin and extension of the ICH along defined anatomical structures.

Syndromes due to small putaminal haemorrhages

The availability of CT and MRI has allowed the documentation of a number of unusual presentations of small putaminal ICH, which without these imaging techniques would have been diagnosed on clinical grounds as small lacunar infarcts.

Pure motor stroke

Although rare, instances of pure motor stroke due to small putaminal–capsular haemorrhages have been documented (Tapia et al. 1983, Kim et al. 1994). The clinical presentation in such cases has been with a mild and rapidly regressive pure motor syndrome affecting the face and limbs contralaterally to a small haematoma with origin in the posterior angle of the putamen, with impingement of—but without extension into—the posterior limb of the internal capsule (Fig. 26.8). On occasions, a pure capsular haemorrhage has been described presenting with pure motor stroke and dysarthria (Chung et al. 2000), but its frequently associated compression of the lateral thalamus has resulted in a 'pure sensorimotor' stroke syndrome, rather than the less common pure motor stroke. These observations of occasional presentation of putaminal ICH with an otherwise 'typical' syndrome of lacunar infarction stress the importance of imaging in the diagnosis of acute stroke, especially in instances when anticoagulant or thrombolytic treatment is being contemplated.

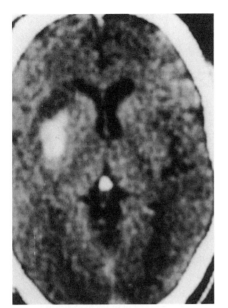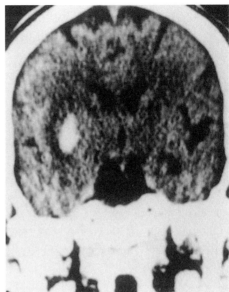

Fig. 26.8 Right small putaminal haemorrhage with clinical presentation as left 'pure motor stroke'. From Tapia *et al.* (1983) with permission.

Pure sensory stroke

The syndrome of pure sensory stroke, which is highly correlated with thalamic lacunar infarction (Fisher 1982*b*), has rarely been observed in instances of small putaminal ICH. Kim (1999) reported three (2%) such cases among a group of 152 patients with putaminal ICH, that were the result of a posteriorly located putaminal haemorrhage that was adjacent to the most posterior portion of the posterior limb of the internal capsule and the adjacent thalamus. This resulted in a contralateral hemisensory syndrome affecting superficial and deep sensory modalities, with more severe involvement of the leg than the arm and face. The imaging studies suggested a compromise of the dorsolateral aspect of the thalamus or the ascending thalamo-cortical projections located in the most posterior ('retro-lenticular') portion of the posterior limb of the internal capsule.

Hemichorea–hemiballism

This unilateral syndrome that has been associated with a lacunar infarction in either the basal ganglia, thalamus, or subthalamic nucleus (Kase *et al.* 1981) is rarely the result of a small putaminal haemorrhage (Jones *et al.* 1985, Altafullah *et al.* 1990). In both of these reports, a right putaminal haemorrhage of 'lateral' (Chung *et al.* 2000) location resulted in transient contralateral chorea and ballism, in the absence of hemiparesis, hemisensory loss, gaze paresis, or hemineglect. The prognosis was excellence in both instances, despite a moderate size haematoma in the patient reported by Jones *et al.* (1985).

Management of putaminal haemorrhage

Besides the treatment of increased ICP, the main therapeutic issues in putaminal haemorrhage centre on the choice of surgical versus non-surgical treatment. Since there have been no conclusive randomized trials comparing these two therapeutic options, most decisions are based on the results of anecdotal observations or non-randomized clinical series (Kase and Crowell 1994). The data generated from non-randomized series of patients with putaminal and lobar ICH have been inconclusive (Table 26.3), as the studies varied widely in their non-random pattern of selection of therapy, age of the populations, timing of surgery, and surgical techniques. A trend towards a benefit with surgical treatment was observed in patients with haematomas of moderate size (26–85 ml) in some studies (Volpin *et al.* 1984), and in patients operated on early (within 7 h) after ICH onset (Kaneko *et al.* 1983). The six randomized studies that have been performed are listed in Table 26.4. Although generally of small size and with some methodological flaws, these studies suggested a potential for benefit from surgery in patients who are operated on early (within 12 h) after ICH onset. This important therapeutic issue in ICH needs to be investigated further by a large-scale, randomized trial of patients with putaminal (and lobar) ICH

Table 26.3 Surgical management of ICH—non-randomized, CT scan series[a]

Study	No. of patients		Mortality	
	Surgical group	Medical group	Surgical group	Medical group
Kanaya *et al.* (1980)	410	204	18%[b]	58%[b]
Kaneko *et al.* (1983)	100	0	7%	–
Waga and Yamamoto (1983)	18	56	28%	14%
Bolander *et al.* (1983)	39	35	13%	20%
Volpin *et al.* (1984)	32[c]	34[c]	19%	44%
Kanno *et al.* (1984)		265[d]	4%[e,f]	8%[e,f]
			17%[b,e]	25%[b,e]
			86%[e,g]	96%[e,g]
Piotrowski and Rochowanski (1996)	300	0	31%	–
Schwarz *et al.* (1997)[h]	24	24	42%[e]	54%[e]

[a] From Kase (2001).
[b] Patients with moderate putaminal haemorrhage (defined as haematoma in the external capsule, but encroaching on the internal capsule).
[c] Patients with haematoma volumes of 26–85 ml.
[d] A total of 265 patients with putaminal ICH of mild, moderate, or severe character.
[e] Dead or vegetative.
[f] Patients with mild putaminal haemorrhage (defined as haematoma restricted to the external capsule).
[g] Patients with severe putaminal haemorrhage (defined as haematoma extending downward into the internal capsule, with or without extension into the midbrain).
[h] Retrospective, case–control series.

Table 26.4 Randomized clinical trials of surgical management of ICH[a]

Study	No. of patients		Mortality	
	Surgical Group	Medical group	Surgical group	Medical group
McKissock et al. (1961)	89	91	65%	51%
Juvela et al. (1989)	26	26	46%	38%
Batjer et al. (1990)	8	13	50%[b]	85%[b]
Morgenstern et al. (1998)	17	17	19%[c]	24%[c]
Zuccarello et al. (1999)	9	11	22%[d]	27%[d]
Auer et al. (1989)[e]	50	50	42%[c]	70%[c]

[a]From Kase (2001).
[b]Dead or vegetative.
[c]Mortality at 6 months.
[d]Mortality at 3 months.
[e]Surgical arm was endoscopic surgery.

subjected to surgical or non-surgical treatment. The surgical arm of the study needs to include both conventional clot evacuation by craniotomy, and the promising technique of CT-guided stereotactic haematoma drainage (Montes *et al.* 2000).

The lack of reliable information from randomized trials precludes the use of evidence-based criteria for selection of patients for surgery. However, the outcome in recent large series of patients with putaminal ICH may serve as a guide to treatment decisions. Using the new classification of putaminal ICH in defined anatomical types, Chung *et al.* (2000) observed a satisfactory outcome with non-surgical treatment of most patients with the middle, lateral, and posteromedial types, as well as in those with localized posterolateral haematomas without internal capsular extension. Surgical therapy was considered in patients with progressive compromise of the level of consciousness and focal deficits, and it included stereotactic aspiration of large posterolateral haematomas with extension into the anterior putamen and/or the posterior limb of the internal capsule. The best results were obtained in patients who were operated on within 24 h of ICH onset, and in those without evidence of haematoma extension into the lateral thalamus. In instances of massive ICH, the open surgical evacuation of the haematoma was followed by poor results, with less than 50 per cent survival, and with severe disability in the survivors, confirming the old observation that patients with large ICHs do poorly, regardless of the type of treatment used (Kase and Crowell 1994).

A special circumstance in which surgery is indicated in patients with putaminal ICH is when the bleeding has been caused by a defined lesion with potential for rebleeding, such as a vascular malformation or tumour (Broderick *et al.* 1999). In instances of the discovery of small, angiography 'occult' vascular malformations, which are generally identified by MRI, the use of microsurgical techniques allows resection with low (5%) long-term neurological morbidity (Steinberg *et al.* 2000).

Caudate haemorrhage

Haemorrhage in the head of the caudate nucleus is the least common of the 'deep' hemispheric haemorrhages, with reported frequencies of between 1 and 7 per cent of ICHs (Table 26.1; Stein *et al.* 1984). Since its mechanisms are similar to those of putaminal and thalamic haemorrhages (with predominance of hypertension), it is surprising that its frequency is so low, perhaps suggesting that the arteries whose rupture leads to this type of ICH (Heubner's artery and medial lenticulostriate arteries; Chung *et al.* 2000) are less prone to developing the hypertension-related changes that cause intraparenchymal bleeding.

Mechanisms of caudate haemorrhage

Most of the published series on caudate ICH have identified hypertension as its leading cause (Stein *et al.* 1984, Fuh and Wang 1995, Kumral *et al.* 1999). However, other causes not generally associated with deep spontaneous ICH are frequently identified, including cerebral aneurysms (Weisberg 1984), arteriovenous malformations (Waga *et al.* 1986), and the basal vascular abnormalities associated with moyamoya disease (Steinke *et al.* 1992*b*, Fuh and Wang 1995). The latter mechanism is thought to lead to ICH as a result of rupture of the anastomotic channels that develop in the area of the basal ganglia, including the head of the caudate, as a result of the progressive occlusion of trunks of the circle of Willis (Suzuki and Kodama 1983).

Clinical presentation of caudate haemorrhage

Caudate haemorrhage typically presents with sudden onset of headache, vomiting, and altered level of consciousness, resembling SAH from ruptured cerebral aneurysm (Stein *et al.* 1984, Weisberg *et al.* 1984). This clinical presentation correlates with imaging evidence of a small haematoma limited to the head of the caudate nucleus, along with intraventricular extension (Fig. 26.9). Although the clinical presentation of caudate ICH can be identical to that of aneurysmal SAH, the CT features help to distinguish them by showing absence of subarachnoid blood in the basal cisterns and interhemispheric fissure in the former (Fuh and Wang 1995), while such findings would be expected to occur regularly in SAH due to rupture of an anterior communicating artery aneurysm (Stein *et al.* 1984). Less frequently, the haematoma of the caudate head extends, in addition, into the internal capsule, and becomes associated with transient contralateral hemiparesis and ipsilateral Horner's syndrome (Stein *et al.* 1984).

In instances of either localized or more extensive caudate haemorrhages, behavioural and neuropsychological abnormalities are a prominent part of the clinical picture, producing most commonly abulia, impairment of memory (both short and long term), and abnormalities of speech, especially of verbal fluency (Stein *et al.* 1984, Fuh and Wang 1995). These deficits are thought to occur as a result of

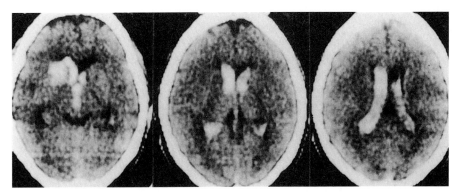

Fig. 26.9 Haemorrhage in the head of the right caudate nucleus, associated with extension into the third and lateral ventricles.

interruption of cortical–subcortical tracts between the caudate nucleus and the frontal cortex (Fuh and Wang 1995). The neuropsychological abnormalities of caudate haemorrhage have been described in detail by Fuh and Wang (1995) and by Kumral *et al.* (1999). A common pattern is that of presentation with abulia, confusion and disorientation at onset, followed by the development of a prominent amnestic syndrome, at times accompanied by language disturbances. The latter have included most often a non-fluent aphasia (Kumral *et al.* 1999), and occasional examples of transcortical motor aphasia have also been recorded (Chung *et al.* 2000). Haematomas in the non-dominant hemisphere generally do not produce unilateral disturbances of attention (Stein *et al.* 1984, Chung *et al.* 2000), although one case reported by Kumral *et al.* (1999) developed visuospatial neglect.

The generally small size and localized character of caudate haemorrhage is the reason why focal neurological deficits such as transient hemiparesis are relatively infrequent (in 30% of the 23 cases studied by Chung *et al.* 2000), while the virtually constant extension into the ventricular system accounts for the high frequency of headache and meningeal signs, resembling the onset of SAH. Rare instances of bilateral caudate ICH (Bertol *et al.* 1991) or haemorrhage associated with intra-ventricular extension with acute hydrocephalus (Stein *et al.* 1984) can have a more dramatic presentation with coma and ophthalmoplegia, the latter presumably due to oculomotor nuclei involvement as a result of aqueductal dilatation (Caplan 1994).

Prognosis and management of caudate haemorrhage

The prognosis of caudate haemorrhage is generally good, with a mortality (12%; Caplan 1994) that is substantially lower than that of all other forms of intraparenchymal haemorrhage. In addition, despite a sometimes dramatic acute presentation, patients with caudate haemorrhage tend to do well functionally, presumably due to the relatively small area of parenchymal damage that characterizes this type of ICH. This good prognosis is illustrated by an 87 per cent (20 of 23 patients) rate of normal function (mRS = 0) and 13 per cent (the remaining three patients) with minor disability (mRS = 1) due to mild residual hemiparesis in the series of Chung *et al.* (2000). Although Kumral *et al.* (1999) reported one death among six patients with caudate ICH, three of the survivors were independent 1 year after stroke onset. The good prognosis of caudate ICH not only applies to the recovery from hemiparesis but also to the eventual resolution of early neuropsycho-logical deficits: all the patients of Fuh and Wang (1995) made 'substantial recovery', with ability to return to their previous activities, and Stein *et al.* (1984) reported normalization of neurological function in seven of eight patients with prominent behavioural disturbances on presentation, including abulia, memory defects, and aphasia.

The treatment of caudate ICH is limited to supportive measures and the prevention of complications in the acute stage of the illness. In instances of severe intraventricular extension of the haemorrhage, especially if associated with hydrocephalus, ventriculostomy and ventricular drainage are recommended (Broderick *et al.* 1999), although the value of such treatment has never been assessed in a randomized prospective clinical trial.

Thalamic haemorrhage

Thalamic haemorrhage was included in the early descriptions of ICH as part of the broad group of 'deep' or 'ganglionic' haemorrhages, until the descriptions by Fisher (1959) clarified its distinct clinical presentation, with particular emphasis on its characteristic oculomotor abnormalities. Since then, a number of clinico-radiological studies have provided a great deal of detail about its clinical features, imaging aspects, prognosis, and management.

Mechanisms of thalamic haemorrhage

The main cause of thalamic haemorrhage is hypertension, this mechanism accounting for 74–83 per cent of cases in recent clinical series (Steinke *et al.* 1992a, Kumral *et al.* 1995, Chung *et al.* 1996). Other mechanisms of thalamic haemorrhage account for a few cases each in most series, including use of anticoagulant and thrombolytic agents (Dromerick *et al.* 1997), cocaine (Chung *et al.* 1996), ruptured posterior cerebral artery aneurysm (Crum and Wijdicks 2000), and cavernous malformations (Pozzatti 2000). The haemorrhages due to these mechanisms do not have clinical features that distinguish them from those caused by hypertension, except for: (i) the tendency towards recurrent bleeding in those due to cavernous angiomas; rebleeding occurred in four of the eight patients who presented with thalamic haemorrhage in the series reported by Pozzatti (2000), and the recurrence occurred at a mean interval of 18 months from the first episode of bleeding; (ii) the potential for multiple ICHs after use of cocaine (Green *et al.* 1990) and after thrombolysis, the latter illustrated by the unusual patient described by Dromerick *et al.* (1997), with bilateral simultaneous, symmetrical postero-lateral thalamic ICHs after thrombolysis with recombinant tissue plasminogen activator (rt-PA) for myocardial infarction.

Clinical presentation of thalamic haemorrhage

Thalamic ICH of moderate to large size has been associated with the 'classical' presentation, which includes various combinations of the following features:

(1) *Contralateral hemiparesis*: due to the proximity to the posterior limb of the internal capsule, thalamic-origin ICH is associated with prominent hemiparesis in about 95 per cent of cases, that is in all but a few exceptional cases of lesions that are too small and medial or dorsal to compromise the internal capsule (Steinke *et al.* 1992, Chung *et al.* 1996). In all other locations in the thalamus, ICH consistently is accompanied by hemiparesis or hemiplegia involving the face, arm, and leg to a comparable extent, to a level of complete hemiplegia in 70 per cent of the patients reported by Kumral *et al.* (1995).

(2) *Hemisensory syndrome*: as a result of the damage of thalamic tissue, patients develop prominent sensory loss, either anaesthesia or hypaesthesia affecting face, limbs, and trunk, generally for all sensory modalities, affecting as many as 85 per cent of patients with thalamic ICHs of all sizes and locations within the thalamus (Steinke *et al.* 1992*a*).

(3) *Ophthalmological signs*: in the 'classical' presentation of thalamic ICH these include paresis of upward gaze that often results in a position of downward deviation and convergence of the eyes at rest, and miotic and unreactive pupils, both due to pressure effects of the thalamic ICH over the dorsal midbrain (Fisher 1959); this is often associated with loss of vertical parallelism of the eyes that remains constant in all positions of gaze (skew deviation), and horizontal gaze disturbances; the latter most commonly correspond to the expected conjugate horizontal deviation towards the affected hemisphere, but examples of contralateral deviation ('wrong-way eyes') occasionally occur. This phenomenon has only been described in the setting of intracranial haemorrhage, never in infarction, and is related most commonly to thalamic haemorrhage, although it has rarely been seen with subdural haematoma, frontoparietal subcortical haematoma (Tijssen 1994), or SAH with dense insular clot (Pessin *et al.* 1981). The pathogenesis of this phenomenon is still controversial, but involvement of descending oculomotor tracts from the contralateral hemisphere at midbrain level is favoured, a view that has been supported by autopsy data (Tijssen 1994). Other oculomotor phenomena observed in thalamic ICH include 'acute esotropia' (markedly adducted eye contralateral to the thalamic haematoma or bilateral convergence spasm, also referred to as 'pseudo-sixth' nerve palsy) from presumed involvement at the midbrain level of supranuclear fibres with

an inhibitory effect on convergence (Gomez *et al.* 1988, Hertle and Bienfang 1990, Scoditti *et al.* 1993), as well as an instance of contralateral paralysis of convergence (Lindner *et al.* 1992). In both instances, these phenomena occurred in association with upward gaze palsy; the mechanism of the abnormalities of convergence in these cases remains speculative, the most accepted explanation being the involvement at midbrain level of supranuclear fibres concerned with convergence, supported in one case by MRI detection of a small lesion in the midbrain, ventral to the superior colliculus (Lindner *et al.* 1992).

In recent years there has been an attempt at describing the clinical syndromes associated with specific areas of involvement of the thalamus by haemorrhage (Kumral *et al.* 1995, Chung *et al.* 1996). These authors have divided the thalamic haematomas into various types depending on the topography of the haemorrhage into anterior, posteromedial, posterolateral, dorsal, and global, and have related these locations to the presumed arterial rupture within the thalamus (Chung *et al.* 1996). The clinical features in these various locations have been described as follows:

(1) Anterior type (Fig. 26.10), located in the most anterior portion of the thalamus, which is supplied by the polar or tuberothalamic artery; these haematomas are

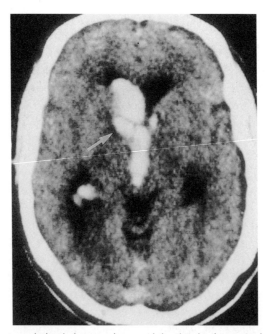

Fig. 26.10 Anterior type thalamic haemorrhage, originating in the most dorsal portion of the right thalamus (arrow), with extension into the third ventricle and frontal horn of the right lateral ventricle.

often associated with ventricular extension and are clinically characterized by behavioural abnormalities, especially memory impairment and apathy, with preserved alertness, rare and transient sensorimotor deficits, and absent ophthalmological findings.

(2) Posteromedial type (Fig. 26.11), from presumed rupture of thalamo-perforating arteries, with haematomas located in the most medial aspect of the thalamus, with frequent rupture into the third ventricle and hydrocephalus, along with extension into the midbrain, resulting in memory disturbances and behavioural abnormalities in small, localized haematomas, while the larger ones with downward extension into the midbrain are associated with early stupor or coma, along with severe motor deficits and oculomotor disturbances.

(3) Posterolateral type (Fig. 26.12) haematomas result from rupture of thalamo-geniculate arteries, producing generally large haemorrhages with frequent extension to the internal capsule and intraventricular space, associated with severe sensorimotor deficits, as well as aphasia or hemineglect in dominant or non-dominant haemorrhages, respectively; additional features of large haematomas are ipsilateral Horner's syndrome, depressed level of consciousness, and ophthalmological abnormalities (Kumral *et al.* 1995); approximately one-third of these patients developed the delayed onset of a 'thalamic pain syndrome' in the series of Chung *et al.* (1996). The aphasia of dominant posterolateral thalamic

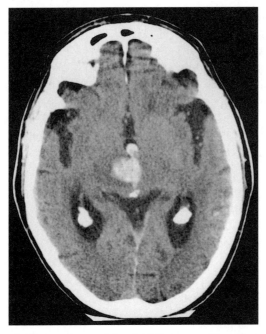

Fig. 26.11 Posteromedial haemorrhage of the right thalamus with extension into the third ventricle.

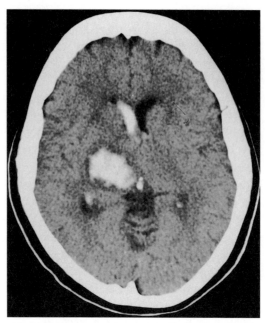

Fig. 26.12 Posterolateral thalamic haemorrhage with extension into the right lateral ventricle.

haematomas most often has been of the 'transcortical motor' type (Kumral *et al.* 1995, Karussis *et al.* 2000), except that in haematomas in the pulvinar nucleus the aphasia has been described as speech that becomes more paraphasic as the person continues to talk, eventually becoming so markedly paraphasic that it becomes jargon (Mohr *et al.* 1975); the syndromes of hemi-inattention in non-dominant thalamic haemorrhage have included a variety of features, including marked anosognosia (Karussis *et al.* 2000), in one instance with prominent associated mania (Liebson 2000), as well as examples of motor neglect or 'inertia', manifested as lack of use of limbs with normal strength (Manabe *et al.* 1999).

(4) Dorsal type (Fig. 26.13), due to rupture of branches of the posterior choroidal artery, resulting in haematomas located high in the thalamus, with frequent extension into the paraventricular white matter and the intraventricular space, with presentation characterized by mild and transient sensorimotor deficits, generally without oculomotor abnormalities, with rare confusion and memory disturbance in those located most posteriorly (in the area of the pulvinar nucleus).

(5) Global type (Fig. 26.14), with involvement of the whole extent of the thalamus by large haematomas that frequently enter the ventricular system (with associated hydrocephalus) and extend into the suprathalamic hemispheric white matter, with resulting stupor or coma, severe sensorimotor deficits, and the 'classical'

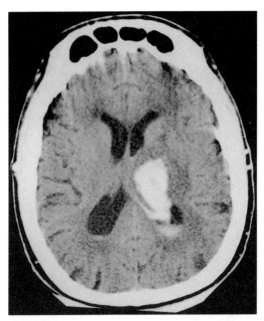

Fig. 26.13 Dorsal thalamic haemorrhage of paraventricular location, with extension into the atrium of the left lateral ventricle.

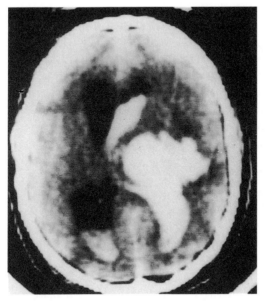

Fig. 26.14 Global thalamic haemorrhage with involvement of the whole extent of the left thalamus, and extension into the internal capsule, putamen, and ventricular space, with associated hydrocephalus and midline shift.

ophthalmological features of paralysis of upward > downward gaze, skew deviation, and small and unreactive pupils.

Syndromes of small thalamic haemorrhages

The above characterization of the specific clinical syndromes that relate to defined areas of thalamic ICH have allowed the delineation of the clinical features of moderate size and large thalamic haemorrhages. In instances of small haemorrhages, a number of different syndromes have been described, corresponding to dysfunction of one or a few isolated systems within the thalamus.

Pure sensory stroke

This syndrome, caused most often by a lacunar thalamic infarction (Fisher 1965b), has rarely been due to a small thalamic ICH (Abe *et al.* 1992, Paciaroni and Bogousslavsky 1998, Shintani *et al.* 2000). Thalamic haematomas of dorsal location have presented with a pure hemisensory syndrome in which the loss of sensation to pin-prick predominated over that of vibration and joint position sense, while motor strength was preserved, but coordination in the affected arm was abnormal with eyes closed, reflecting the 'sensory' rather than cerebellar character of the ataxia (Abe *et al.* 1992). The two patients described by Paciaroni and Bogousslavsky (1998) had involvement of all sensory modalities affecting the face, arm, and leg contralaterally to a small haemorrhage in the centre of the thalamus that involved all the ventral nuclei, the parvocellular and dorsocaudal nuclei, with sparing of the pulvinar. The haematomas were thought to have originated from rupture of thalamogeniculate branches of the posterior cerebral artery. In the study of Shintani *et al.* (2000), two patients with predominant sensory loss in the arm and leg more than the face had contralateral lesions in either the ventral–posterior–lateral (VPL) nucleus, or the ventral–posterior–medial (VPM) nucleus, while another patient with a restricted 'cheiro-oral' distribution of dysaesthesias with 'burning' quality, in the absence of sensory loss to superficial or deep modalities, had a small haematoma in the border between the VPL and VPM.

Sensory ataxic hemiparesis

A syndrome similar to the ataxic hemiparesis of lacunar infarction in the basis pontis or supracapsular hemispheric white matter (Fisher 1978b) has been reported in the setting of small thalamic haemorrhages (Dobato *et al.* 1990). However, the clinical presentation differed from that of lacunar ataxic hemiparesis in that the ataxia of the cases reported by Dobato *et al.* (1990) was due to proprioceptive sensory loss (with improvement under visual guidance, worse with eyes closed), as opposed to the cerebellar character of the ataxia in lacunar ataxic hemiparesis. The haematomas were small (mean volume, 7.2 ml), all located in the dorsolateral thalamus, associated with markedly impaired proprioception but with preserved superficial sensory modalities, and the associated hemiparesis was transient and of crural predominance.

Abnormal involuntary movements

A variety of abnormal involuntary movements have been reported in patients with generally small thalamic haemorrhages. These have included a combination of contralateral upper extremity choreiform–dystonic movements along with a pattern of rhythmic alternating movements of low frequency ('myorhythmia') in the setting of vascular lesions in the posterolateral corner of the thalamus, described in seven patients, one of whom had a focal haemorrhage (the rest being infarcts) (Lera *et al.* 2000). In most of these patients, the movement disorder occurred with a latency from the vascular event, the longest of which was 2 years in the single patient with a haemorrhage as the initial event. The reasons for the delayed onset of the unilateral dyskinesia remain uncertain. A single case of delayed onset (1 month) of a contralateral 'rubral' tremor in the arm in a patient with a small posterolateral thalamic haemorrhage with subthalamic extension was reported by Mossuto-Agatiello *et al.* (1993). Despite the 'rubral' character of the tremor (present at rest, in maintenance of postures, and in action, with maximal increase in amplitude in the latter situation), no midbrain lesions were detected with MRI. Occasionally, small thalamic haemorrhages are accompanied by contralateral ataxia, hemihypaesthesia, hemiparesis (common features of the posterolateral lesions leading to the syndrome of Dejérine–Roussy [1906]), and a motor disturbance consistent with unilateral asterixis (Donat 1980). This combination has been described in small haematomas that involve the posterolateral thalamus and the adjacent posterior limb of the internal capsule (Fig. 26.15).

Amnestic syndromes

In addition to the well-recognized syndromes of acute and persistent anterograde amnesia in the setting of anterior and posteromedial haematomas (Chung *et al.* 1995) and small paramedian haemorrhages (Saez de Ocariz *et al.* 1996) a remarkable case of transient global amnesia (TGA) has been described in a patient with a dominant hemisphere haematoma that involved the rostral–medial thalamus, with extension into the ventricular system (Chen *et al.* 1996). The episode of amnesia lasted for 10 h, during which time the patient exhibited the repetitive questioning behaviour typical of TGA, while language, praxis, visuospatial orientation, recognition of famous faces, and right–left orientation remained normal. His inability to form new memories was severe, but he exhibited no tendency to confabulate. Upon disappearance of the memory disturbance he returned to his normal baseline, and had no recurrence over a 5-year follow-up period. Based on this case and others from the literature, all of which affected the dominant thalamus, the authors interpreted the episode of TGA as secondary to involvement of the anterior and medial nuclear groups by the ICH, possibly interrupting the mamillo-thalamic tract or the ventroamygdalofugal pathway.

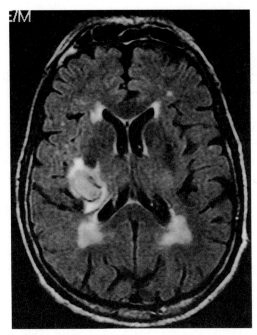

Fig. 26.15 Posterior thalamic–capsular haemorrhage associated with contralateral ataxia, hemihypaesthesia and asterixis, with mild hemiparesis.

Management of thalamic haemorrhage

The general management of thalamic haemorrhage is similar to that of other forms of ICH, in terms of treatment of hypertension, coagulopathy, and increased ICP. The issues that are more specific to thalamic haemorrhage relate to the role of surgery and other procedures intended to address the effects of intraventricular haemorrhage and hydrocephalus. The latter can at times play a major role in causing symptoms of upper brainstem dysfunction, as exemplified by a dramatic reversal of oculomotor abnormalities, including Parinaud's syndrome, after ventriculostomy (Waga *et al.* 1979). However, the use of ventriculostomy in thalamic ICH complicated by hydrocephalus and neurological deterioration in 35 patients in the series of Chung *et al.* (1996) resulted in survival of only two patients, presumably due to the fact that the majority of them had progressed to severe compromise in the level of consciousness pre-operatively. The procedure was limited to patients with large haematomas of posteromedial, posterolateral, and global type, while none of those with smaller anterior or dorsal haematomas required such treatment.

Another surgical procedure that has been used in patients with thalamic ICH is stereotactic aspiration of the haematoma, with or without the local instillation of thrombolytic agents to promote the liquefaction and easier aspiration of the clot (Niizuma *et al.* 1990, Hokama *et al.* 1993). The large experience reported by Niizuma *et al.* (1990) included 145 patients with thalamic ICH, 75 of whom were treated with stereotactic haematoma aspiration under CT guidance and with local instillation of urokinase. The procedure was used in patients with moderate size haematomas (volume > 6 ml) who had a severe motor deficit, but excluding those who were stuporous or comatose. Rebleeding occurred in two patients (3%), and two others developed meningitis that was controlled successfully with antibiotic treatment. The results in this group were good or excellent in 37 per cent, fair in 43 per cent, and poor in 13 per cent, while 7 per cent (five patients) died. Most of the good or excellent outcomes occurred in patients with haematomas of less than 15 ml, while those with hematomas in the 16–63 ml range had generally poor results, despite technically adequate haematoma aspiration. The series of Hokama *et al.* (1993) was concerned mostly with the analysis of complications following the procedure. Among 21 patients with thalamic ICH of volumes smaller than 20 ml (15 patients) or between 21 and 40 ml (six patients), two (10%) developed rebleeding, with survival but with poor neurological outcome. The authors attributed this complication to the combined effects of a coagulopathy secondary to liver disease, and poorly controlled hypertension after the procedure.

On occasions, patients with thalamic ICH and severe intraventricular haemorrhage with hydrocephalus are subjected to thrombolysis of the intraventricular haemorrhage in instances when the ventricular drainage becomes ineffective as a result of clogging of the drainage system by clot. Although this procedure needs to be evaluated prospectively as a potentially useful intervention in this setting, it has been shown recently that intraventricular fibrinolysis with rt-PA can become complicated with secondary haemorrhage, both in the parenchyma and in the ventricular space (Schwarz *et al.* 1998), suggesting that caution should be exercised in the use of this potentially hazardous procedure. The value and indications of this therapy of intraventricular haemorrhage should be defined by a prospective randomized clinical trial.

A special group that raises complex therapeutic issues is that of patients with thalamic ICH due to rupture of a cavernous angioma, which has been shown to have a high rate (50%) of recurrent bleeding (Pozzatti 2000). In those patients with multiple episodes of bleeding, the excision of the cavernoma generally has had good results, except for the occasional complication of venous haemorrhagic infarction due to excision of an associated venous angioma (Bertalanffy *et al.* 1991, Pozzatti 2000). The alternative use of radiosurgery is advocated for deep cavernous angiomas associated with recurrent small haemorrhages (Kondziolka *et al.* 1995), but the experience with this procedure in the thalamus is limited (Pozzatti 2000).

Prognosis of thalamic haemorrhage

Mortality after thalamic ICH, which has been reported in 25–52 per cent of cases (Steinke *et al.* 1992*a*, Kumral *et al.* 1995, Chung *et al.* 1996), is closely correlated with the volume of the haematoma, level of consciousness at presentation, and presence of intraventricular haemorrhage and hydrocephalus (Steinke *et al.* 1992*a*, Kumral *et al.*

Table 26.5 Early clinical and CT features indicative of poor prognosis in thalamic ICH[a]

Clinical features
Low level of consciousness at onset
Severe motor weakness, decerebrate posturing
Oculomotor abnormalities (vertical gaze paralysis, 'wrong-way eyes')
CT features
Large haematoma
Global and posteromedial types
Caudal extension of haematoma into the midbrain
Posterolateral extension of haematoma into the basal ganglia
Dense blood clot in the third ventricle
Severe hydrocephalus, mass effect, and midline shift

[a]From Chung et al. (1996).

1995, Mori et al. 1995). The size of the haematoma has long been recognized as a powerful predictor of mortality in thalamic ICH, and early writings suggested a critical diameter of approximately 3 cm, above which mortality was virtually 100 per cent (Weisberg 1979). However, subsequent series have documented survival after thalamic haemorrhage exceeding such diameters, after either conservative (Kumral et al. 1995) or surgical (stereotactic aspiration) treatment (Niizuma et al. 1990).

When comparing patients with and without intraventricular haemorrhage who were similar with regard to level of consciousness, degree of motor deficit, and presence of ophthalmoplegia, Steinke et al. (1992a) found a significantly higher mortality rate for those with intraventricular extension, leading them to the conclusion that this factor is a powerful independent predictor of mortality in thalamic haemorrhage. In addition, the different locations of haemorrhage within the thalamus generally are associated with outcomes that reflect haematoma size and type and severity of associated neurological deficits: anterior and dorsal haematomas generally had a benign course, while posterolateral, posteromedial, and global haemorrhages were associated with higher mortality rates and degree of disability in the series reported by Chung et al. (1996). The main clinical and CT features associated with poor outcome in the series of Chung et al. (1996) are listed in Table 26.5.

The functional motor outcome in survivors after thalamic haemorrhage is affected negatively by initial evidence of extension of the haematoma into the internal capsule, midbrain, or putamen, while cognitive impairment as a sequela correlates with initial disturbance of consciousness and ventricular extension of the haematoma (Mori et al. 1995). Finally, performance in activities of daily living (ADL) is influenced by advanced age and haematoma size (Mori et al. 1995), as well as by the presence of unilateral spatial neglect, aphasia, and severe degree of paresis of the lower limb (Maeshima et al. 1997).

Conclusions

Subcortical haemorrhages constitute a substantial proportion of cases of ICH. The various topographical forms correlate with well-defined syndromes that allow accurate predictions of the type and severity of their clinical manifestations and functional sequelae. Features at onset, including haematoma location and size, and associated intraventricular extension and hydrocephalus, are reliable predictors of survival in putaminal and thalamic haemorrhage. The management of subcortical haemorrhage is still for the most part non-surgical, but new surgical approaches that are emerging deserve to be tested in prospective randomized clinical trials, as they have the potential for improving the outcome of this generally severe stroke type.

References

4S (1995). Randomised trial of cholesterol lowering in 4444 patients with coronary heart disease: the Scandinavian Simvastatin Survival Study. *Lancet*, **345**, 1274–5.

Abbie, A.A. (1933). The clinical significance of the anterior choroidal artery. *Brain*, **56**, 233–46.

Abbie, A.A. (1934). The morphology of the forebrain arteriae with special reference to the evolution of the basal ganglia. *Journal of Anatomy*, **66**, 433–70.

Abboud, F.M. (1989). Ventricular syncope: is the heart a sensory organ? *New England Journal of Medicine*, **320**, 390–2.

Abbruzzese, G., Bino, G., Dall'Agata, D., Morena, M., Primavera, A., and Favale E. (1989). Somatosensory evoked potentials in the diagnosis of lacunar syndromes: comparison with EEG findings. *European Neurology*, **29** (Suppl. 2), 42–3.

Abbruzzese, G., Bino, G., Dall'Agata, D., Morena, M., Primavera, A., and Favale E. (1989). Somatosensory evoked potentials in the diagnosis of lacunar syndromes: comparison with EEG findings. European Neurology, **29** (Suppl 2), 42–3.

Abe, K., Yokoyama, R., and Yorifuji, S. (1993). Repetitive speech disorder resulting from infarcts in the paramedian thalami and midbrain. *Journal of Neurology, Neurosurgery, and Psychiatry*, **56**, 1024–6.

Abe, K., Yorifuji, S., and Nishikawa, Y. (1992). Pure sensory stroke resulting from thalamic haemorrhage. *Neuroradiology*, **34**, 205–6.

Abrahams, J.M., Hurst, R.W., Bagley, L.J., and Zager, E.L. (1999). Anterior choroidal artery supply to the posterior cerebral artery distribution: embryological basis and clinical implications. *Neurosurgery*, **44**, 1308–14.

ACAS (1995). Atherosclerosis Study. Endarterectomy for asymptomatic carotid artery stenosis. *Journal of the American Medical Association*, **273**, 1421–8.

ACCSG (1985). Persantin Aspirin Trial in cerebral ischemia. Part II: endpoint results. The American–Canadian Co-operative Study group. *Stroke*, **16**, 406–15.

Ackermann, H., Ziegler, W., and Petersen, D. (1993). Dysarthria in bilateral thalamic infarction. A case study. *Journal of Neurology*, **240**, 357–62.

Adachi, T. and Wang, X.L. (1998). Association of extracellular-superoxide dismutase phenotype with the endothelial constitutive nitric oxide synthase polymorphism. *FEBS Letters*, **433**, 166–8.

Adachi, T., Kobayashi, S., Yamaguchi, S., and Okada, K. (2000). MRI findings of small subcortical 'lacunar-like' infarction resulting from large vessel disease. *Journal of Neurology*, **247**, 280–5.

Adair, J.C. and Millikan, C. (1991). Size and distribtuion of lacunes defined by computed tomography: correlation with blood pressure and possible stroke mechanisms. *Journal of Stroke and Cerebrovascular Disease*, **1**, 158–62.

Adams, H.P., Bendixen, B.H., Kappelle, L.J., Biller, J., Love, B.B., Gordon, D.L., *et al.* (1993*b*) Classification of subtype of acute ischemic stroke. Definitions for use in a multicenter clinical trial. TOAST. Trial of Org 10172 in Acute Stroke Treatment. *Stroke*, **24** 35–41.

Adams, H.P., Damasio, H.C., Putman, S.F., and Damasio, A.R. (1983). Middle cerebral artery occlusion as a cause of isolated subcortical infarction. *Stroke*, **14**, 948–52.

Adams, H.P., Davis, P.H., Leira, E.C., Chang, K.C., Bendixen, B.H., Clarke, W.R., *et al.* (1999). Baseline NIH Stroke Scale score strongly predicts outcome after stroke: a report of the Trial of Org 10172 in Acute Stroke Treatment (TOAST). *Neurology*, 53, 126–31.

Adams, H.P., Kappelle, L.J., and Bendixen B.H. (1993*a*). The management of asymptomatic carotid stenosis. In *The handbook of cerebrovascular diseases* (ed. H.P. Adams Jr), pp 13–34. Marcel Dekker, New York.

Adams, J.H., Brierly, J.B., Connor, R.C.R., and Treip, C.S. (1966). The effects of systemic hypotension upon the human brain. Clinical and neuropathological observations in 11 cases. *Brain*, 89, 235–68.

Aggleton, J.P. (1986). Memory impairment caused by experimental thalamic lesions in monkeys. *Revue Neurologique, Paris*, 142, 418–24.

Agresti, A. (1990). *Categorical data analysis.* John Wiley & Sons, New York.

Ahmed, I. (1988). Predictive value of the electroencephalogram in acute hemispheric lesions. *Clinical Electroencephalography*, 19, 205–9.

Akiguchi, I., Ino, T., and Nabatame, H. (1987). Acute-onset amnestic syndrome with localized infarct on the dominant side. Comparison between anteriomedial thalamic lesion and PCA territory lesion. *Japanese Journal of Medicine*, 26, 15–20.

Akiguchi, I., Ito, T., Yamao, M., and Azuma, I. (1983). Acute-onset amnestic syndrome due to unilateral paramedian thalamic infarct on the dominant side. *Clinical Neurology, Tokyo*, 23, 948–55.

Alajouanine, Th. (1966). Ivan Bertrand. *Presse Medicalé*, 74, 1093–5.

Alberts, M.J. (1991). Genetic aspects of cerebrovascular disease. *Stroke*, 22, 276–80.

Alderman, M.H. (2000). Measures and meaning of blood pressure. *Lancet*, 355, 159.

Alexander, G.E. and Crutcher, D. (1990). Functional architecture of basal ganglia circuits: neural substrates of parallel processing. *Trends in Neurosciences*, 13, 266–71.

Alexander, G.E. and DeLong, M.R. (1985). Microstimulation of the primate neostriatum. l. Physiological properties of striatal microexcitable zones. *Journal of Neurophysiology*, 53, 1417–32.

Alexander, G.E., DeLong, M.R., and Strick, P.L. (1986). Parallel organization of functionally segregated circuits linking basal ganglia and cortex. *Annual Review of Neuroscience*, 9, 357–81.

Alexander, M.P., Naeser, M.A., and Palumbo, C.L. (1987). Correlations of subcortical CT lesion sites and aphasia profiles. *Brain*, 110, 961–91.

Allen, C.M.C. (1983). Clinical diagnosis of the acute stroke syndrome. *Quarterly Journal of Medicine*, 208, 515–23.

Allen, C.M.C., Hoare, R.D., Fowler, C.J., and Harrison, M.J.G. (1984). Clinico-anatomical correlations of uncomplicated stroke. *Journal of Neurology, Neurosurgery, and Psychiatry*, 47, 1251–4.

Almquist, A., Goldenberg, I.F., Milstein, S., Chen, M.Y., Chen, X.C., Hansen, R., *et al.* (1989). Provocation of bradycardia and hypotension by isoproterenol and upright posture in patients with unexplained syncope. *New England Journal of Medicine*, 320, 346–51.

Altafullah, I., Pascual-Leone, A., Duvall, K., Anderson, D.D., and Taylor, S. (1990). Putaminal hemorrhage accompanied by hemichorea–hemiballism. *Stroke*, 27, 1093–4.

Alvarez, W.C. (1946). Small infarcts of the brain. *Geriatrics*, 1, 189–216.

Alvarez, W.C. (1948). Small commonly unrecognised apoplexies. *Postgraduate Medical Journal*, 4, 96–101.

Alvarez, W.C. (1955*a*). More about little strokes. *Geriatrics*, 10, 555–62.

Alvarez, W.C. (1955*b*). The little strokes. *Journal of the American Medical Association*, 157, 1199–204.

Alvarez, W.C. (1966). *Little strokes*. pp. 157–77.

Amarenco, P., Duyckaerts, C., Tzourio, C., Hénin, D., Bousser, M., and Hauw, J.-J. (1992). The prevalence of ulcerated plaques in the aortic arch in patients with stroke. *New England Journal of Medicine*, 326, 221–5.

American Psychiatric Association (1987). Diagnostic and statistical manual of mental disorders. DSMIII, (3rd edn. American Ps;ychiatric Association, Washington, D.C.

Anastosopoulos, D. and Bronstein, A.M. (1999). A case of thalamic syndrome: somatosensory influences on visual orientation. *Journal of Neurology, Neurosurgery, and Psychiatry*, 67, 390–4.

Anderson, C.S., Chakera, T.M.H., Stewart-Wynne, E.G., and Jamrozik, K.D. (1994). Spectrum of primary intracerebral haemorrhage in Perth, Western Australia, 1989–90: incidence and outcome. *Journal of Neurology, Neurosurgery, and Psychiatry*, 57, 936–40.

Anderson, C.S., Jamrozik, K.D., Broadhurst, R.J., and Stewart.Wynne, E.G. (1994*a*). Predicting survival for 1 year among different subtypes of stroke. Results from the Perth Community Stroke Study. *Stroke*, 25, 1935–44.

Anderson, C.S., Taylor, B.V., Hankey, G.J., Stewart-Wynne, E.G., and Jamrozik, K.D. (1994*b*). Validation of a clinical classification for subtypes of acute cerebral infarction. *Journal of Neurology, Neurosurgery, and Psychiatry*, 57, 1173–9.

Andine, P., Rudolphi, K., Fredholm, B., and Hagber, H. (1990). Effect of propentofylline (HWA 285) on extracellular purines and excitatory amino acids in CA1 of rat hippocampus durring transient ischemia. *British Journal of Pharmacology*, 100, 814–8.

Angelergues, R., De Ajuriaguerra, J., and Hécaen, H. (1957). Paralysie de la verticalité du regard d'origine vasculaire. Étude anatomoclinique. *Revue Neurologique, Paris*, 96, 301–19.

Angeloni, U., Bozzao, L., Fantozzi, L., Bastianello, S., Kushner, M., and Fieschi, C. (1990). Internal borderzone infarction following acute middle cerebral artery occlusion. *Neurology*, 40, 1196–8.

Anzalone, N. and Landi, G. (1989). Non-ischaemic causes of lacunar syndromes: prevalence and clinical findings. *Journal of Neurology, Neurosurgery, and Psychiatry*, 52, 1188–90.

APT (1994). Collaborative overview of randomised trials of antiplatelet therapy. Prevention of death, myocardial infarction, and stroke by prolonged antiplatelet therapy in various categories of patients. *British Medical Journal*, 308, 81–106.

Araki, G., Mihara, H., Shizuka, M., Yunoki, K., Nagata, K., Yamaguchi, K., *et al.* (1983). CT and arteriographic comparison of patients with transient ischemic attacks—correlation with small infarction of basal ganglia. *Stroke*, 14, 276–80.

Arboix, A. and Marti-Vilalta, J.L. (1992). Lacunar syndromes not due to lacunar infarcts. *Cerebrovascular Diseases*, 2, 287–92.

Arboix, A., Marti-Vilalta, J. Pujol, J., and Garcia, J.H. (1990*b*). Lacunar cerebral infarct and nuclear magnetic resonance. A review of sixty cases. *European Neurology*, 30, 47–51.

Arboix, A., Marti-Vilalta, J.L., and Garcia, J.H. (1990*a*). Clinical study of 227 patients with lacunar infarcts. *Stroke*, 21, 842–7.

Archer, C.R., Ilinsky, I.A., Goldfader, P.R., and Smith, K.R., Jr (1981). Aphasia in thalamic stroke: CT stereotactic localization. *Journal of Computer Assisted Tomography*, 5, 27–32.

Atlas, S., Mark, A., Grossmann, R., and Gomori, J. (1988). Intracranial hemorrhage: gradient echo MR imaging at 1.5 T. Comparison with spin-echo imaging and clinical implications. *Radiology*, 168, 803–7.

Auer, L.M., Deinsberger, W., Niederkorn, K., Gell, G., Kleinert, R., Schneider, G., et al. (1989). Endoscopic surgery versus medical treatment for spontaneous intracerebral hematoma: a randomized study. *Journal of Neurosurgery*, 70, 530–5.

Awad, I.A., Johnson, P.C., Spetzler, R.F., and Hodak, J.A. (1986b). Incidental subcortical lesions identified on magnetic resonance imaging in the elderly. II. Postmortem pathological correlations. *Stroke*, 17, 1090–7.

Awad, I.A., Spetzler, R.F., Hodak, J.A., Awad, C.A., and Carey, R. (1986a). Incidental subcortical lesions identified on magnetic resonance imaging in the elderly. I. Correlation with age and cerebrovascular risk factors. *Stroke*, 17, 1084–9.

Awad, I.A., Spetzler, R.F., Hodak, J.A., Awad, C.A., Williams, F., Jr, and Carey, R. (1987). Incidental lesions noted on magnetic resonance imaging of the brain: prevalence and clinical significance in various age groups. *Neurosurgery*, 20, 222–7.

Awada, A. (1997). Blépharospasme par infarctus thalamique paramédan bilatéral. *Revue Neurologique, Paris*, 153, 62–4.

Ay, H., Buonanno, F.S., Rordorf, G., Schaefer, P.W. Schwamm, L.H., Wu, O., et al. (1999b). Normal diffusion-weighted MRI during stroke-like deficits. *Neurology*, 52, 1784–92.

Ay, H., Oliveira-Filho, J., Buonanno, F.S., Ezzeddine, M., Schaefer, P.W., Rordorf, G., et al. (1999a). Diffusion-weighted imaging identifies a subset of lacunar infarction associated with embolic source. *Stroke*, 30, 2644–50.

Aylward, E.D., Roberts-Willie, J.V., Barta, P.E. et al. (1994). Basal ganglia volume and white matter hyperintensities in patients with bipolar disorder. *American Journal of Psychiatry*, 5, 687–93.

Babikian, V. and Ropper, A.H. (1987). Binswanger's disease: a review. *Stroke*, 18, 2–12.

Backus, K.H., Pflimlin, P., and Trube, G. (1991). Actions of diazepam on the voltage-dependent Na^+ current. Comparison with the effect of phenytoin, carbamazipine, lidocaine and flumazenil. *Brain Research*, 548, 41–9.

Bae, H., Jeong, D., Doh, J., Lee, K., Yun, I., and Byun, B. (1999). Recurrence of bleeding in patients with hypertensive intracerebral hemorrhage. *Cerebrovascular Diseases*, 9, 102–8.

Bae, H.G., Lee, K.S., Yun, I.G., Bae, W.K., Choin, S.W., Byun, B.J., et al. (1992). Rapid expansion of hypertensive intracerebral hemorrhage. *Neurosurgery*, 31, 35–41.

Baird, A.E., Donnan, G.A., and Saling, M. (1991). Mechanisms and clinical features of internal watershed infarction. *Clinical and Experimental Neurology*, 28, 50–9.

Baker, P.F., Blaustein, M.P., Hodgkin, A.L., and Steinhardt, R.A. (1969). The influence of calcium on sodium efflux in squid axons. *Journal of Physiology (London)*, 200, 431–58.

Ballarin, M., Fredholm, B.B., Ambrosio, S., and Mahy, N. (1991). Extracellular levels of adenosine and its metabolites in the striatum of awake rats: inhibition of uptake and metabolism. *Acta Physiologica Scandinavica*, 142, 97–103.

Balthasar, K. and Hopf, A. (1966). Die Freund-Vogtsche Herdbildung bei supranuclearer Heberlähmung der Augen mit Lidretraktion. Zur Würdigung eines Falles von C. Freund und C.u.O. Vogt. *Deutsche Zeitschrift für Nervenheilkrankungen*, 189, 275–96.

Bamford, J. and Warlow, C. (1988). Evolution and testing of the lacunar hypothesis. *Stroke*, 19, 1074–82.

Bamford, J., Sandercock, P., Dennis, M., Burn, J., and Warlow, C. (1990). A prospective study of acute cerebrovascular disease in the community: the Oxfordshire Community Stroke Project. *Journal of Neurology, Neurosurgery, and Psychiatry*, 53, 16–22.

Bamford, J., Sandercock, P., Jones, L., and Warlow, C. (1987). The natural history of lacunar infarction: the Oxfordshire Community Stroke Project. *Stroke*, 18, 545–51.

Bamford, J., Sandercock, P., Dennis, M., Burn, J., and Warlow, C. (1991). Classification and natural history of clinically identifiable subtypes of cerebral infarction. *Lancet*, 337, 1521–6.

Baquis, G.D., Pessin, M.S., and Scott, R.M. (1985). Limb shaking—a carotid TIA. *Stroke*, 16, 444–8.

Barber, P.A., Darby, D.G., Desmond, P.M., Gerraty, R.P., Yang, Q., Li, T., *et al.* (1999*a*). Identification of major ischemic change. Diffusion-weighted imaging versus computed tomography. *Stroke*, 30, 2059–65.

Barber, P.A., Darby, D.G., Desmond, P.M., Yang, Q., Gerraty, R.P., Jolley, D., *et al.* (1998*a*). Prediction of stroke outcome with echoplanar perfusion- and diffusion-weighted MRI. *Neurology*, 51, 418–26.

Barber, P.A., Davis, S., Darby, D.G., *et al.* (1999*b*). Absent middle cerebral artery flow predicts the presence and evoluton of the ischemic penumbra. *Neurology*, 52, 1125–1132.

Barber, P.A., Davis, S.M., Infeld, B., Baird, A.E., Donnan, G.A., Jolley, D., *et al.* (1998*b*). Spontaneous reperfusion after ischemic stroke is associated with improved outcome. *Stroke*, 29, 2522–8.

Barbizet, J., Degos, J.D., Louarn, F., Nguyen, J.P., and Mas, J.L. (1981). Amnésie par lésion ischémique bi-thalamique. *Revue Neurologique, Paris*, 137, 415–24.

Barinagarrementeria, F., Vega, F., and Del Brutto, O.H. (1989). Acute hemichorea due to infarction in the corona radiata. *Journal of Neurology*, 236, 371–2.

Barkhof, F. and Valk, J. (1988). 'Top of the basilar' syndrome. A comparison of clinical and MRI findings. *Neuroradiology*, 30, 193–8.

Barnett, H.J.M., Taylor, D.W., Eliasziw, M., Fox, A.J., Ferguson, G.G., Haynes, R.B., *et al.* (1998). Benefit of carotid endarterectomy in patients with symptomatic moderate or severe stenosis for the North American Symptomatic Carotid Endarterectomy Trial Collaborators. *New England Journal of Medicine*, 339, 1415–25.

Baron, J.C., D'Antona, R., Pontano, P., Serdaru, M., Samson, Y., and Bousser, M.G. (1986). Effects of thalamic stroke on energy metabolism of the cerebral cortex. *Brain*, 109, 1243–59.

Baron, J.C., Levasseur, M., Mazoyer, B., Legault-Demare, F., Mauguière, F., Pappata, S., *et al.* (1992). Thalamocortical diaschisis: positron emission tomography in humans. *Journal of Neurology, Neurosurgery, and Psychiatry*, 55, 935–42.

Barres, B.A., Chun, L.L.Y., and Corey D.P. (1989). Glial and neuronal forms of the voltage-dependent sodium channels: Characteristics and cell-type distribution, *Neuron*, 2, 1375–88.

Barres, B.A., Chun, L.L.Y., and Corey, D.P. (1990). Ion channels in vertebrate glia. *Annual Review of Neuroscience*, 13, 441–74.

Bassetti, C., Mathis, J., Gugger, M., Lövblad, K.O., and Hess, C.W. (1996). Hypersomnia following paramedian thalamic stroke: a report of 12 patients. *Annals of Neurology*, 39, 471–80.

Basso, A., Della Sala, S., and Farabola, M. (1987). Aphasia arising from purely deep lesions. *Cortex*, 23, 29–44.

Bastian, A.J. and Thach, W.T. (1995). Cerebellar outflow lesions: a comparison of movement deficit resulting from lesions at the levels of the cerebelum and thalamus. *Annals of Neurology*, 38, 881–92.

Batjer, H.H., Reisch, J.S., Allen, B.C., Plaitier, L.J., and Su, C.J. (1990). Failure of surgery to improve outcome in hypertensive putaminal hemorrhage: a prospective randomized trial. *Archives of Neurology*, 47, 1103–6.

Baudrimont, M., Dubas, F., Joutel, A., *et al.* (1993). Autosomal dominant leukoencephalopathy and subcortical ischemic strokes: a clinicopathological study. *Stroke*, 24i, 122–5.

Baumbach, G.L. and Heistad, D.D. (1989). Remodeling of cerebral arterioles in chronic hypertension. *Hypertension*, 13, 968–72.

Baumgartner, R.W. and Regard, M. (1993). Bilateral neuropsychological deficits in unilateral paramedian thalamic infarction. *European Neurology*, 33, 195–8.

Baumgartner, R.W., Sturzenegger, M., and Mattle, H.P. (1994). Thalamic infarct with homonymous upper sectoranopia and Déjérine–Roussy syndrome. *Cerebrovascular Diseases*, 4, 55–6.

Beasley, B.A., Davenport, R.W., and Nakagawa, H. (1980). CT localisation of the thalamic syndrome. A case report. *Computerized Tomography*, 4, 243–5.

Béhague, P. (1952). Pierre Marie intime. *Revue Neurologique, Paris*, 86, 733–40.

Benhaiem-Sigaux, N., Gray, F., Gherardi, R., Roucayrol, A.M., and Poirier, J. (1987). Expanding cerebellar lacunes due to dilation of the perivascular space associated with Binswanger's subcortical arteriosclerotic encephalopathy. *Stroke*, 18, 1087–92.

Benveniste, H., Drejer, J., Schousboe, A., and Diemer, N. (1984). Elevation of the extracellular concentrations of glutamate and aspartate in rat hippocampus during transient cerebral ischaemia monitored by intracerebral microdialysis. *Journal of Neurochemistry*, 43, 1369–74.

Berger, K., Ajani, U.A., Kase, C.S., Gaziano, J.M., Buring, J.E., Glynn, R.J. (1999). Light-to-moderate alcohol consumption and the risk of stroke among U.S. male physicians. *New England Journal of Medicine*, 341, 1557–64.

Bertalanffy, H., Gilsbach, J.M., Eggert, H.R., and Seeger, W. (1991). Microsurgery of deep-seated cavernous angiomas: report of 26 cases. *Acta Neurochirurgica*, 108, 91–9.

Bertol, V., Gracia-Naya, M., Oliveros, A., and Gros, B. (1991). Bilateral symmetric caudate hemorrhage. *Neurology*, 41, 1157–8.

Bertrand, I. (1923). *Les Processus de Désintégration Nerveuse*. Paris, Masson.

Besson, G., Bogousslavsky, J., and Regli, F. (1991). Posterior choroidal-artery infarct with homonymous horizontal sectoranopia. *Cerebrovascular Diseases*, 1, 117–20.

Besson, G., Hommel, M., and Perret J. (1992). Historical aspects of the lacunar concept. *Cerebrovascular Diseases*, 1, 306–10.

Bewermeyer, H., Dreesbach, H.A., Rackl, A., Neveling, M., and Heiss, W.D. (1985). Presentation of bilateral thalamic infarction on CT, MRI and PET. *Neuroradiology*, 27, 414–9.

Bhatia, K. and Marsden, C. (1994). The behavioural and motor consequences of focal lesions of the basal ganglia in man. *Brain*, 117, 859–76.

Biller, J., Merchut, M., and Emanuele, M.A. (1984). Nonhemorrhagic infarction of the thalamus. *Neurology*, 34, 1269–70.

Biller, J., Sand, J.J., Corbett, J.J., Adams, H.P., Jr, and Dunn, V. (1985). Syndrome of the paramedian thalamic arteries: clinical and neuro-imaging correlation. *Journal of Clinical Neuro-ophthalmology*, 5, 217–23.

Black, J.A., Dib-Hajj, S., McNabola, K., Jeste, S., Rizzo, M.A., Kocsis, J.D., *et al.* (1996). Spinal sensory neurons express multiple sodium channel -subunit mRNAs. *Molecular Brain Research*, 43,117–32.

Blackwood, W., Hallpike, J.F, Kocen, R.S., and Mair, W.G.P. (1969). Atheromatous disease of the carotid arterial system and embolism from the heart in cerebral infarction: a morbid anatomical study. *Brain*, 92, 897–910.

Bladin, C.F. and Chambers, B.R. (1993). Clinical features, pathogenesis, and computed tomographic characteristics of internal watershed infarction. *Stroke*, 24, 1925–32.

Bladin, C.F. and Chambers, B.R. (1994). Frequency and pathogenesis of hemodynamic stroke. *Stroke*, 25, 2179–82.

Bladin, P.F. and Berkovic, S.F. (1984). Striatocapsular infarction. Large infarcts in the lenticulostriate arterial territory. *Neurology*, 34, 1423–30.

Blass, J.P., Hoyer, S., and Nitsch, R. (1991). A translation of Otto Binswanger's article, 'The delineation of the generalized progressive paralyses'. *Archives of Neurology*, 48, 961–72.

Blaustein, M.P. and Santiago, E.M. (1977). Effects of internal and external cations and of ATP on sodium–calcium and calcium–calcium exchange in squid axons. *Biophysics Journal*, 20, 79–111.

Blauw, G., Lagaay, A., Smelt, A. and Westendorp, R. (1997). Stroke, statins, and cholesterol: a meta-analysis of randomized, placebo-controlled, double-blind trials with HMG-CoA reductase inhibitors. *Stroke*, 28, 946–50.

Blecic, S.A., Bogousslavsky, J., van Melle, G., and Regli, F. (1993). Isolated sensorimotor stroke: a reevaluation of clinical, topographic and ethiological patterns. *Cerebrovascular Diseases*, 3, 357–63.

Boerwinkle, E., Doris, P.A., and Fornage, M. (1999). Field of needs. The genetics of stroke. *Circulation*, 99, 331–3.

Bogousslavsky, J. (1989). Syndromes oculomoteurs résultant de lésions mésencéphaliques chez l'homme. *Revue Neurologique, Paris*, 145, 546–59.

Bogousslavsky, J. (1991a). Brain or nosology lacunes? *Cerebrovascular Diseases*, 1, 305.

Bogousslavsky, J. (1991b). Topographic patterns of cerebral infarcts. Correlation with etiology. *Cerebrovascular Diseases*, 1, 61–8.

Bogousslavsky, J. (1992). The plurality of subcortical infarction. *Stroke*, 23, 629–631.

Bogousslavsky, J. and Regli, F. (1984a). Cerebral infarction with transient signs (CITS): do TIA's correspond to small deep infarcts in internal carotid artery occlusion? *Stroke*, 15, 536–9.

Bogousslavsky, J. and Regli, F. (1984b). Upgaze palsy and monocular paresis of downward gaze from ipsilateral thalamo-mesencephalic infarction: a vertical 'one-and-a-half' syndrome. *Journal of Neurology*, 231, 43–5.

Bogousslavsky, J. and Regli, F. (1986a). Unilateral watershed cerebral infarcts. *Neurology*, 36, 373–7.

Bogousslavsky, J. and Regli, F. (1986b). Borderzone infarctions distal to internal carotid artery occlusion: prognostic implications. *Annals of Neurology*, 20, 346–50.

Bogousslavsky, J. and Regli, F. (1992). Centrum ovale infarcts. Subcortical infarction in the superficial territory of the MCA. *Neurology*, 42, 1992–8.

Bogousslavsky, J., Ferrazzini, M., Regli, F., Assal, G., Tanabe, H., and Delaloye-Bischof, A. (1988e). Manic delirium and frontal-like syndrome with para-median infarction of the right thalamus. *Journal of Neurology, Neurosurgery, and Psychiatry*, 51, 116–9.

Bogousslavsky, J., Martin, R., and Moulin, T. (1992). Homolateral ataxia and crural paresis: a syndrome of anterior cerebral artery territory infarction. *Journal of Neurology, Neurosurgery, and Psychiatry*, 55, 1146–9.

Bogousslavsky, J., Miklossy, J., Deruaz, J. P., Regli, F., and Assal, G. (1986a). Unilateral left paramedian infarction of thalamus and midbrain: a clinico-pathological study. *Journal of Neurology, Neurosurgery, and Psychiatry*, 49, 686–94.

Bogousslavsky, J., Miklossy, J., Regli, F., Deruaz, J.-P., Assal, G., and Delaloye, B. (1988c). Subcortical neglect: neuropsychological, SPECT, and neuropathological correlations with anterior choroidal artery territory infarction. *Annals of Neurology*, 23, 448–52.

Bogousslavsky, J., Regli, F., and Assal, C.J. (1988d). Acute transcortical mixed aphasia: a carotid occlusion syndrome with pial and watershed infarcts. *Brain*, 111, 631–41.

Bogousslavsky, J., Regli, F., and Assal, G. (1986b). The syndrome of tubero-thalamic artery territory infarction. *Stroke*, 17, 434–41.

Bogousslavsky, J., Regli, F., and Maeder, P. (1991*a*). Intracranial large-artery disease and 'lacunar' infarction. *Cerebrovascular Diseases*, 1, 154–9.

Bogousslavsky, J., Regli, F., and Schneider, C. (1981). Les ramollissements dans le territoire de l'artère cérébrale posterieure. Syndromes cliniques, manifestations initiales, facteurs de risque. Etude de 50 cas. *Médecine et Hygiène*, 39, 3469–78.

Bogousslavsky, J., Regli, F., and Uske, A. (1988*a*). Thalamic infarcts: clinical syndromes, etiology and prognosis. *Neurology*, 38, 837–48.

Bogousslavsky, J., Regli, F., Delaloye, B., Delaloye-Bischof, A., Assal,G., and Uské, A. (1991*b*). Loss of psychic selfactivation with bithalamic infarction. Neurobehavioural, CT, MRI and SPECT correlates. *Acta Neurologica Scandinavica*, 83, 309–16.

Bogousslavsky, J., Regli, F., Ghika, J., and Feldmeyer, J.J. (1984). Painful ataxic hemiparesis. *Archives of Neurology*, 41, 892–3.

Bogousslavsky, J., van Melle, G., and Regli, F. (1988*b*). The Lausanne Stroke Registry: analysis of 1000 consecutive patients with first stroke. *Stroke*, 19, 1083–92.

Boiten, J. (1991). Lacunar stroke. A prospective clinical and radiological study. Thesis. Maastricht.

Boiten, J. and Lodder, J. (1991*a*). Lacunar infarcts. Pathogenesis and validity of the clinical syndromes. *Stroke*, 22, 1374–78.

Boiten, J., and Lodder, J. (1991*b*). Isolated monoparesis is usually caused by superficial infarction. *Cerebrovascular Diseases*, 1, 337–40.

Boiten, J. and Lodder, J. (1992). Large striatocapsular infarcts: clinical presentation and pathogenesis in comparison with lacunar and cortical infarcts. *Acta Neurologica Scandinavica*, 86, 298–303.

Boiten, J. and Lodder, J. (1993). Prognosis for survival, handicap and recurrence of stroke in lacunar and superficial infarction. *Cerebrovascular Diseases*, 3, 221–6.

Boiten, J., Lodder, J., and Kessels, F. (1993). Two clinically distinct lacunar infarct entities? A hypothesis. *Stroke*, 24, 652–6.

Boiten, J., Luyckx, G.J., Kessels, F., and Lodder, J. (1996). Risk factors for lacunes. *Neurology*, 47, 1109.

Boiten, J., Rothwell, P.M., Slattery, J., and Warlow, C.P. for the European Carotid Surgery Trialists' Collaborative Group (1997). Frequency and degree of carotid stenosis in small centrum ovale infarcts as compared to lacunar infarcts. *Cerebrovascular Diseases*, 7, 138–43.

Boiten, J., Rothwell, P.M., Slattery, J., Warlow, C.P., for the European Carotid Surgery Trialists' Collaborative Group. (1996). Ischaemic lacunar stroke in the European Carotid Surgery Trial. Risk factors, distribution of carotid stenosis, effect of surgery and type of recurrent stroke. *Cerebrovascular Diseases*, 6, 281–7.

Bokura, H. and Robinson, R.G. (1997). Long-term cognitive impairment associated with caudate stroke. *Stroke*, 28, 970–5.

Bolander, H.G., Kourtopoulos, H., Liliequist, B., and Wittboldt, S (1983). Treatment of spontaneous intracerebral haemorrhage: a retrospective analysis of 74 consecutive cases with special reference to computer tomographic data. *Acta Neurochirgica*, 67, 19–28.

Bonhoeffer, K. (1928). Klinisch-anatomische Beitäge zur Pathologie des Sehhügels und der Regio subthalamica. I. Ein Sehhügelherd. *Monatsschrift für Psychiatrie und Neurologie*, 67, 253–71.

Borruat, F.X. and Maeder, P. (1995). Sectoranopia after head trauma: evidence of lateral geniculate body lesion on MRI. *Neurology*, 45, 590–2.

Boucher, M. (1982). Charles Foix, sa vie—son oeuvre. In *Conférences Lyonnaises d'histoire de la Neurologie et de la Psychiatrie* (ed. M. Boucher), pp. 201–18, Documentation médicale Oberval, Lyon.

Bousser, M. And Tournier Lasserve, E. (1994*a*). Summary of the first International workshop on CADASIL. *Stroke*, 25, 704–7.

Bousser, M., Eschwege, E., Haguenau, M., *et al.* (1983). 'AICLA' controlled trial of aspirin and dipyridamole in secondary prevention of atherothrombotic cerebral ischemia. *Stroke*, 14, 5–14.

Bousser, M., Tournier-Lasserve, E., Aylward, R., Tourbah, A., Dormart, D., Romero, N., *et al.* (1988). Recurrent strokes in a family with diffuse white-matter abnormalities—a new mitochondrial cytopathy? *Journal of Neurology*, 235 (suppl. 1), S4–5.

Bousser, M.G. Tournier-Lasserve, E. (1994*b*). Summary of the proce4edings of the First International Workshop on CADASIL. Paris, May 19–21, 1993. *Stroke*, 25, 704–7.

Bozzao, L., Fantozzi, L.M., Bastianello, S., Bozzao, A., and Fieschi, C. (1989). Early collateral blood supply and late parenchymal brain damage in patients with middle cerebral artery occlusion. *Stroke*, 20, 735–40.

Braffman, B.H., Zimmerman, R.A., Trojanowski, J.Q., Gonatas, N.K., Hickey, W.F., and Schlaepfer, W.W. (1988). Brain MR: pathologic correlation with gross and histopathology. 2. Hyperintense white-matter foci in the elderly. *American Journal of Neuroradiology*, 9, 629–36.

Brage, D., Morea, R., and Copello, A. (1961). Syndrome nécrotique tegmento-thalamique avec mutisme akinétique (étude clinique et anatomo-pathologique). *Revue Neurologique, Paris*, 104, 126–37.

Brainin, M., Seiser, A., Czvitkovits, B., and Pauly, E. (1992). Stroke subtype is and age-independent predictor of first-year survival. *Neuroepidemiology*, 11, 190–5.

Brant-Zawadski, M., Fein, G., Van Dyke, C., Kiernan, R., Davenport, L., and de Groot, J. (1985). MR imaging of the aging brain: patchy white-matter lesions and dementia. *American Journal of Neuroradiology*, 6, 675–82.

Brass, L.M., Isaacsohn J.L., Merikangas K.R., and Robinette C.D. (1992). A study of twins and stroke. *Stroke*, 23, 221–3.

Brigell, M., Babikian, V., and Goodwin, J.A. (1984). Hypometric saccades and low-gain pursuit resulting from a thalamic hemorrhage. *Annals of Neurology*, 15, 374–8.

Brissaud, E. (1894). Maladies de l'encéphale. In *Traité de Médecine*, tome VI (ed. J.-M., Charcot, C. Bouchard, and E. Brissaud.), pp. 144–168. Masson, Paris.

Brissaud, E. (1899). *Leçons sur les Maladies Nerveuses*. Deuxième série. (Hôpital Saint-Antoine), Masson, Paris.

Britton, M., Helmers, C., and Samuelsson, K. (1987). High-dose acetylsalicylic acid after cerebral infarction. A Swedish Cooperative Study. *Stroke*, 18, 325–34.

Brodal A. (1973). Self-observations and neuro-anatomical considerations after a stroke. *Brain*, 96, 675–94.

Broderick, J.P., Adams, H.P., Barsan, W., Feinberg, W., Feldmann, E., Grotta, J., *et al.* (1999). Guidelines for the management of spontaneous intracerebral hemorrhage: a statement for healthcare professionals from a special writing group of the Stroke Council, American Heart Association. *Stroke*, 30, 905–15.

Broderick, J.P., Brott, T., Tomsick, T., and Leach A. (1993). Lobar hemorrhage in the elderly: the undiminishing importance of hypertension. *Stroke*, 24, 49–51.

Broderick, J.P., Brott, T., Tomsick, T., Huster, G., and Miller, R. (1992). The risk of subarachnoid and intracerebral hemorrhages in blacks as compared with whites. *New England Journal of Medicine*, 326, 733–6.

Broderick, J.P., Brott, T.G., Tomsick, T., Barsan, W., and Spilker, J. (1990). Ultra-early evaluation of intracerebral hemorrhage. *Journal of Neurosurgery*, 72, 195–9.

Broderick, J.P., Hagen, T., Brott, T., and Tomsick, T. (1995). Hyperglycemia and hemorrhagic transformation of cerebral infarcts. *Stroke*, 26, 484–7.

Brott, T., Broderick, J., Kothari, R., Barsan, W., Tomsick, T., Sauerbeck, L., *et al.* (1997). Early hemorrhage growth in patients with intracerebral hemorrhage. *Stroke*, 28, 1–5.

Brott, T., Thalinger, K., and Hertzberg, V. (1986). Hypertension as a risk factor for spontaneous intracerebral hemorrhage. *Stroke*, 17, 1078–83.

Brower, M.C., Rollins, N., and Roach E.S. (1996). Basal ganglia and thalamic infarction in children. Cause and clinical features. *Archives of Neurology*, 53, 1252–6.

Brown, B., Cukingnan, R., DeRoven, T., *et al.* (1985). Improved graft patency in patients treated with platelet-inhibiting therapy after coronary bypass surgery. *Circulation*, 72, 138–46.

Brown, D.A. and Marsh, S. (1978). Axonal GABA-receptors in mammalian peripheral nerve trunks. *Brain Research*, 156, 187–91.

Brown, G.G., Kieran, S., and Patel, S. (1987). Memory functioning following a left medial thalamic hemorraghe. *Neurology*, 37, 171.

Brown, J.J., Hesselink, J.R., and Rothrock, J.F. (1988). MR and CT of lacunar infarcts. *American Journal of Roentgenology*, 151, 367–72.

Brown, M.M., Pelz, D.M., and Hachinski, V.C. (1990). White matter vasodilatory reserve is impaired in patients with cerebrovascular disease and diffuse periventricular lacunes. *Journal of Neurology*, 237, 157.

Brown, R.D., Whisnant, J.P., Sicks, J.D., O'Fallon, W.M., and Wiebers, D.O. (1996). Stroke incidence, prevalence, and survival. Secular trends in Rochester, Minnesota, through 1989. *Stroke*, 27, 373–80.

Brun, A. and Englund, E. (1986). A white matter disorder in dementia of the Alzheimer type: a pathoanatomical study. *Annals of Neurology*, 91, 253–62.

Brun, A., Fredriksson, K., and Gustafson, L. (1992). Pure subcortical arteriosclerotic encephalopathy (Binswanger's disease): a clinicopathologic study. Part 2: pathologic features. *Cerebrovascular Diseases*, 2, 87–92.

Bruno, A., Adams, H.P., Biller, J., Rezai, K., Cornell, S., and Aschenbrener, C.A. (1988). Cerebral infarction due to moyamoya disease in young adults. *Stroke*, 19, 826–33.

Bruno, A., Graff-Radford, N.R., Biller, J., and Adams, H.P. (1989). Anterior choroidal artery territory infarction: a small vessel disease. *Stroke*, 20, 616–9.

Bruyn, R.P.M. (1989). Thalamic aphasia. A conceptional critique. *Journal of Neurology*, 236, 21–5.

Bryan, R.N., Cai, J., Burke, G., Hutchinson, R.G., Liao, D., Toole, J.F., *et al.* (1999). Prevalence and anatomic characteristics of infarct-like lesions on MR images of middle-aged adults: the atherosclerosis risk in communities study. *American Journal of Neuroradiology*, 20, 1273–80.

Brückmann, H., Kottlarek, F., Biniek, R., and Roßberg, C. (1989). Stammganglieninfarkte in Kindesalter—neuroradiologische Befunde und Differntialdignostik. *Klinische Pädiatrie*, 201, 78–85.

Bucher, H., Griffith, L., and Guyatt, G. (1998). Effect of HMGcoA reductase inhibitors on stroke: a meta-analysis of randomized, controlled trials. *Annals of Internal Medicine*, 128, 89–95.

Buge, A., Escourolle, R., Hauw, J.J., Rancurel, G., Gray, F., and Tempier, P. (1979). Syndrome pseudobulbaire aigu par infarctus bilateral limité du territoire des artères choroidiennes anterieures. *Revue Neurologique, Paris*, 135, 313–8.

Byrom, F.B. (1954). The pathogenesis of hypertensive encephalopathy and its relation to the malignant phase of hypertension; experimental evidence from the hypertensive rat. *Lancet*, 2, 201–11.

Büttner, J. (1960). Die Blutgefässe im menschlichen Thalamus. *Acta Anatomica*, **41**, 279–99.

Büttner-Ennever, J.A., Büttner, U., Cohen, B., and Baumgartner, G. (1982). Vertical gaze paralysis and rostral interstitial nucleus of the medial longitudinal fasciculus. *Brain*, **105**, 125–49.

Cabin, H.S., Clubb, K.S., Hall, C., Perlmutter, R.A., and Feinstein, A.R. (1990). Risk of systemic embolization of atrial fibrillation without mitral stenosis. *American Journal of Cardiology*, **65**, 1112–6.

Cacciatore, A. and Russo, L.S. (1991). Lacunar infarction as an embolic complication of cardiac and arch angiography. *Stroke*, **22**, 1603–5.

Caffery, J.M., Eng, D.L., Black, J.A., Waxman, S.G., and Kocsis, J.D. (1992). Three types of sodium channels in adult rat dorsal root ganglion neurons. *Brain Research*, **592**, 283–97.

Cahalan, M. (1978). Local anesthetic block of sodium channels in normal and pronase-treated squid giant axon. *Biophysics Journal*, **23**, 285–311.

Camargo, C.A. (1989). Moderate alcohol consumption and stroke. The epidemiologic evidence. *Stroke*, **20**, 1611–26.

Cambier, J., Elghozi, D., and Graveleau, P. (1982). *Neuropsychologie des lésions du thalamus*. Masson, Paris.

Cambier, J., Elghozi, D., and Strube, E. (1980). Lésions du thalamus droit avec syndrome de l'hémisphère mineur. Discussion du concept de négligence thalamique. *Revue Neurologique, Paris*, **136**, 105–16.

Cambier, J., Graveleau, Ph., Decroix, J.P., Elghozi, D., and Masson, M. (1983). Le syndrome de l'artère choroidienne anterieure, étude neuropsychologique de 4 cas. *Revue Neurologique, Paris*, **139**, 553–9.

Canadian Cooperative. (1978). A randomized trial of aspirin and sulfinpyrazone in threatened stroke. The Canadian Cooperative Study Group (CCSG). *New England Journal of Medicine*, **299**, 53–9.

Cantu, C., Villarreal, J., Soto, J.L., and Barinagarrementeria, F. (1998). Cerebral cysticercotic arteritis: detection and follow-up by transcranial Doppler. *Cerebrovascular Diseases*, **8**, 2–7.

Caplan, L.R. (1976). Lacunar infarction: a neglected concept. *Geriatrics*, **31**, 71–5.

Caplan, L.R. (1980). 'Top of the basilar' syndrome. *Neurology*, **30**, 72–9

Caplan, L.R. (1989). Intracranial branch atheromatous disease: a neglected, understudied, and underused concept. *Neurology*, **39**, 1246–50.

Caplan, L.R. (1991). Diagnosis and treatment of ischaemic stroke. *Journal of the American Medical Association*, **266**, 2413–8.

Caplan, L.R. (1994). Caudate hemorrhage. In *Intracerebral hemorrhage* (ed. C.S. Kase and L.R. Caplan), pp. 329–40. Butterworth-Heinemann, Boston.

Caplan, L.R. (1996). Penetrating branch artery and lacunar disease. In *Posterior circulation disease*. pp. 381–443. Blackwell Science, Oxford.

Caplan, L.R. and Helgason, C.M. (1995), Caudate infarcts. In *Lacunar and other subcortical infarctions* (ed. G. Donnan, B. Norrving, J. Bamford, and J. Bogousslavsky), pp. 117–30. Oxford University Press.

Caplan, L.R. and Schoene, W.C. (1978). Clinical features of subcortical arteriosclerotic encephalopathy (Binswanger disease). *Neurology*, **28**, 1206–15.

Caplan, L.R. and Stein, R.W. (1986). Small vessel disease. In *Stroke: a clinical approach*, pp. 167–77. Butterworths, London Wellington.

Caplan, L.R. and Young, R.R. (1972). EEG findings in certain lacunar stroke syndromes. *Neurology*, 22, 403.

Caplan, L.R., Babikian, V., Helgason, C., Hier, D.B., De Witt, D., Patel D., *et al.* (1985). Occlusive disease of the middle cerebral artery. *Neurology*, 35, 975–82.

Caplan, L.R., Dewitt, D., Pessin, M.S., Gorelick, P.B., and Adelman, L.S. (1988). Lateral thalamic infarcts. *Archives of Neurology*, 45, 959–64.

Caplan, L.R., Schmahmann, J.D., Kase, C.S., Feldman, E., Baquis, G., Greenberg, J.P., *et al.* (1990). Caudate infarcts. *Archives of Neurology*, 47, 133–43.

CAPRIE (1996). A randomised, blinded, trial of clopidogrel versus aspirin in patients at risk of ischaemic events (CAPRIE). *Lancet*, 348, 1329–39.

Carmelli, D., DeCarli, C., Swan, G.E., Jack, L.M., Reed, T., Wolf, P.A., and Miller, B.L. (1998). Evidence for genetic variance in white matter hyperintensity volume in normal elderly male twins. *Stroke*, 29, 1177–81.

Carter, A.M., Catto, A.J., Bamford, J.M., and Grant, P.J. (1999). Association of the platelet glycoprotein IIb HPA-3 polymorphism with survival after acute ischemic stroke. *Stroke*, 30, 2606–11.

Caruso, G., Vincentelli, F., Giudicelli, G., Grisoli, F., Xu, T., and Gouaz, A. (1990). Perforating branches of the basilar bifurcation. *Journal of Neurology*, 73, 259–65.

CAST (1997). CAST: randomised placebo-controlled trial of early aspirin use in 20,000 patients with acute ischaemic stroke. *Lancet*, 349, 1641–9.

Castaigne, P., Buge, A., Cambier, J., Escourolle, R., Brunet, P., and Degos, J.D. (1966). Démence thalamique d'origine vasculaire par ramollissement bilatéral, limité au territoire du pédicule rétromamillaire. A propos de deux observations anatomo-cliniques. *Revue Neurologique, Paris*, 114, 89–107.

Castaigne, P., Buge, A., Escourolle, R., and Masson, M. (1962). Ramollissement pédonculaire médian tegmento-thalamique avec ophtalmoplégie et hypersomnie (étude anatomo-clinique). *Revue Neurologique, Paris*, 106, 357–67.

Castaigne, P., Lhermitte, F., Buge, A., Escourolle, R., Hauw, J.J., and Lyon-Caen, O. (1981). Paramedian thalamic and midbrain infarcts: clinical and neuropathological study. *Annals of Neurology*, 10, 127–48.

Catsman-Berrevoets, C.E. and Van Harskamp, F. (1988). Compulsive pre-sleep behavior and apathy due to the bilateral thalamic stroke: response to bromocriptine. *Neurology*, 38, 647–9.

Catterall, W.A. (1981). Inhibition of voltage-sensitive sodium channels in neuroblastoma cells by antiarrythmic drugs. *Molecular Pharmacology*, 20, 356–62.

Catto, A., Carter, A., Barrett, J.H., Stickland, M., Bamford, J., Davies, A., *et al.* (1996). Angiotensinogen-converting enzyme insertion/deletion polymorphism and cerebrovascular disease. *Stroke*, 27, 435–40.

Catto, A.J., Kohler, H. P., Bannan, S., Stickland, M., Carter, A., and Grant, P.J. (1998). Factor XIII Val 34 Leu: a novel association with primary intracerebral hemorrhage. *Stroke*, 29, 813–6.

Catto, A.J., Kohler, H.P., Coore, J., Mansfield, M.W., Stickland, M.H., and Grant, P.J. (1999). Association of a common polymorphism in the factor XIII gene with venous thrombosis. *Blood*, 93, 906–8.

Cayatte, A.J., Palacino, J.J., Horten, K., and Cohen, R.A. (1994). Chronic inhibition of nitric oxide production accelerates neointima formation and impairs endothelial function in hypercholesterolemic rabbits. *Arteriosclerosis and Thrombosis*, 14, 753–9.

Ceballos-Baumann, A., Passingham, R., Marsden, C., and Brooks, D. (1995). Motor reorganization in acquired dystonia. *Archives of Neurology*, 37, 746–57.

Ceccaldi, M. and Milandre, L. (1994). A transient fit of laugher as the inaugural symptom of capsular–thalamic infarction. *Neurology*, 44, 1762.

Ceccaldi, M., Poncet, M., Milandre, L., and Rouyer, C. (1994). Temporary forced laughter after unilateral strokes. *European Neurology*, 34, 36–9.

Cerveto, L., Lagnado, L., Perry, R., Robinson, D., and McNaughton, P. (1989). Extrusion of calcium from rod outer segments is driven by both sodium and potassium gradients. *Nature*, 337, 740–3.

Chabriat, H., Bousser, M.G., and Pappata, S. (1995*a*). Cerebral autosomal dominant arteriopathy with subcortical infarcts and leukoencephalopathy: a positron emission tomography study in two affected family members. *Stroke*, 26, 1729–30.

Chabriat, H., Joutel, A., Vahedi, K., Iba-Zizen, M.T., Tournier-Lasserve, E., Bousser, M.G. (1996). CADASIL (cerebral autosomal dominant arteriopathy with subcortical infarcts and leukoencephalopathy). *Journal Maladies Vasculaires*, 21, 277–82.

Chabriat, H., Joutel, A., Vahedi, K., Iba-Zizen, M.T., Tournier-Lasserve, E., Bousser, M.G. (1997). CADASIL. Cerebral autosomal dominant arteriopathy with subcortical infarcts and leukoencephalophathy. *Rev Neurologique, Paris*, 153, 376–85.

Chabriat, H., Mrissa, R., Levy, C., Vahedi, K., Taillia, H., Iba-Zizen, M.T., *et al.* (1999*a*). Brain stem MRI signal abnormalities in CADASIL. *Stroke*, 30, 457–9.

Chabriat, H., Pappata, S., Ostergaard, L., Clarck, C.A., Poupon, C., Vahedi, K., *et al.* (2000). Cerebral hemodynamics in CADASIL before and after acetazolamide challenge assessed with MRI bolus tracking. *Stroke*, 31, in press.

Chabriat, H., Pappata, S., Poupon, C., Clarck, C.A., Vahedi, K., Poupon, F., *et al.* (1999*b*). Clinical severity in CADASIL related to ultrastructural damage in white matter. *In-vivo* study with diffusion tensor MRI. *Stroke*, in press.

Chabriat, H., Tournier-Lasserve, E., Vahedi, K., Leys, D., Joutel, A., Nibbio, A., *et al.* (1995*b*). Autosomal dominant migraine with MRI white-matter abnormalities mapping to the CADASIL locus. *Neurology*, 45, 1086–91.

Chabriat, H., Vahedi, K., Iba-Zizen, M.T., Joutel, A., Nibbio, A., Nagg, T., *et al.* (1995*c*). Clinical spectrum of CADASIL: a study of 7 families. Cerebral autosomal dominant arteriopathy with subcortical infarcts and leukoencephalopathy. *Lancet*, 346, 934–9.

Challa, V.R., Bell, M.A., and Moody, D.M. (1990). A combined haematoxylin–eosin, alkaline phosphatase and high resolution microradiographic study of lacunes. *Clinical Neuropathology*, 9, 196–204.

Chalmers, J., Neal, B., and MacMahon, S. (2000). PROGRESS (Perindopril Protection Against Recurrent Stroke Study): regional characteristics of the study population at baseline. PROGRESS Management Committee. *Journal of Hypertension*, 18 (Suppl. 1), S13–9.

Chambers, B.R., Brooder, R.J., and Donnan, G.A. (1991). Proximal PCA occlusion simulating MCA occlusion. *Neurology*, 41, 385–90.

Chamorro, A., Sacco, R.L., Mohr, J.P, Foulkes M.A., Kase C.S., Tatemichi T.K., *et al.* (1991). Clinical–computed tomographic correlations of lacunar infarction in the stroke data bank. *Stroke*, 22, 175–81.

Chan, S., Kartha, K., Yoon, S., Desmond, D., and Hilal, S. (1996). Multifocal hypointense cerebral lesions on gradient-echo MRI are associated with chronic hypertension. *American Journal of Neuroradiology*, 17, 1821–7.

Chassagnon, C., Boucher, M., Tommasi, M., Bianchi, G.S., and Moene, Y. (1969). Démence thalamique d'origine vasculaire (observation anatomoclinique). *Journal Médical de Lyon*, 50, 1153–66.

Chaves, C.J., Silver, B., Schlaug, G., Dashe, J., Caplan, L.R., and Warach, S. (2000). Diffusion- and perfusion-weighted MRI patterns in borderzone infarcts. *Stroke*, 31, 1090–6.

Chen, C.-J. and Barkovich, (1998). A hyperplastic anterior choroidal artery with double persistent anastamotic channels. *American Journal of Neuroradiology*, 19, 1758–60.

Chen, W.H., Liu, J.S., Wu, S.C., and Chang, Y.Y. (1996). Transient global amnesia and thalamic hemorrhage. *Clinical Neurology and Neurosurgery*, 98, 309–11.

Chen, Z., Sandercock, P., Pau, H., *et al.* (2000). Indications for early aspirin use in acute ischemic stroke. A combined analysis of 40 000 randomized patients from the Chinese Acute Stroke Trial and the International Stroke Trial. *Stroke*, 31, 1240.

Chimowitz, M.I., Furlan, A.J., Sial, C.A., Paranandi, L., and Beck, G.J. (1991). Etiology of motor and sensory stroke: a prospective study of the predictive value of clinical and radiological features. *Annals of Neurology*, 30, 519–25.

Chinny, T.A. (1904). Sur un cas de syndrome thalamique. *Revue Neurologique, Paris*, 12, 505–11.

Chiray, M., Foix, C., and Nicolesco, J. (1923). Hémitremblement du type de la sclérose en plaques par lésion rubro-thalamo-sousthalamique. Syndrome de la région supéro-externe du noyau rouge avec atteinte silencieuse ou non du thalamus. *Annales de Médecine, Paris*, 14, 173–91.

Choi, D., Sudarsky, L., Schachter, S., Biber, M., and Burke, P. (1983). Medial thalamic hemorrhage with amnesia. *Archives of Neurology*, 40, 611–3.

Chung, C.M., Caplan, L.R., Yamamoto, Y., Chang, H.M., Lee, S., Song, H., *et al.* (2000). Striatocapsular haemorrhage. *Brain*, 123, 1850–62.

Chung, C.S., Caplan, L.R., Han, W., Pessin, M.S., Lee, K.H., and Kim, S.M. (1996). Thalamic hemorrhage. *Brain*, 119, 1873–86.

Clark, J.M. and Albers G.W. (1995). Vertical gaze palsies from medial thalamic infarctions without midbrain involvement. *Stroke*, 26, 1467–70.

Clarke, R., Shipley, M., Lewington, S., *et al.* (1999). Underestimation of risk associations due to regression dilution in long-term follow-up of prospective studies. *American Journal of Epidemiology*, 150, 341–53.

Clarke, S., Assal, G., Bogousslavsky, J., Regli, F., Townsend, D.W., Leenders, K.L., and Blecic, S. (1994). Pure amnesia after unilateral left polar thalamic infarct: topographic and sequential neuropsychological and metabolic (PET) correlates. *Journal of Neurology, Neurosurgery, and Psychiatry*, 57, 27–34.

Clavier, I., Hommel, M., Besson, G., Noëlle, B., and Ferjus Perret, J.E. (1994). Long-term prognosis of symptomatic lacunar infarcts. A hospital-based study. *Stroke*, 25, 2005–9.

Cohen, J.A., Gelfer, C.E., and Sweet, R.D. (1980). Thalamic infarction producing aphasia. *Mount Sinai Journal of Medicine*, 47, 398–404.

Cohen, L., Bolgert, F., Timsit, S., and Chermann, J.F. (1994). Anomia for proper names after left thalamic infarctions. *Journal of Neurology, Neurosurgery, and Psychiatry*, 57, 1283–4.

Cole, F. and Yates, P. (1967). Intracerebral microaneurysms and small cerebrovascular lesions. Brain, 90, 759–70.

Cole, F. and Yates, P. (1968). Comparative incidence of cerebrovascular lesions in normotensive and hypertensive patients. *Neurology*, 18, 255–9.

Cole, M., Winkelman, M.D., Morris, J.C., Simon, J.E., and Boyd, T.A. (1992). Thalamic amnesia: Korsakoff syndrome due to left thalamic infarction. *Journal of the Neurological Sciences*, 110, 62–7.

Collins, R., Peto, R., MacMahon, S., Hebert, P., Fiebach, N.H., Eberlein, K.A. (1990). Blood pressure, stroke, and coronary heart disease. *Lancet*, **335**, 827–38.

Combarros, O., Polo, J.M., Pascual, J., and Berciano, J. (1991). Evidence of somatotopic organization of the sensory thalamus based on infarction in the nucleus ventralis posterior. *Stroke*, **22**, 1445–7.

Come P.C., Riley M.F., Bivas N.K., (1983) Roles of echocardiography and arrythmia monitoring in the evaluation of patients with suspected systemic embolism. Ann Neurol 13,527–531.

Confort-Gouny, S., Vion-Dury, J., Nicoli, F., Dano, P., Donnet, A., Grazziani, N., *et al.* (1993). A multiparametric data analysis showing the potential of localized proton MR spectroscopy of the brain in the metabolic characterization of neurological diseases. *Journal of the Neurological Sciences*, **118**, 123–33.

Cooper, I. (1955). Surgical occlusion of the anterior choroidal artery in parkinsonism. *Surgery, Gynecology and Obstetrics*, **99**, 207–19.

Cordery, R.J. and Rossor, M.N. (1999). Bilateral thalamic pain secondary to bilateral thalamic infarcts relieved by a further unilateral ischaemic episode. *European Journal of Neurology*, **6**, 717–9.

Croisille, P., Turjman, F., Croisile, B., Tournut, P., Laharotte, J.C., Aimard, G., *et al.* (1994). Striatocapsular infarction: MRI and MR angiography. *Neuroradiology*, **36**, 430–1.

Crosson, B., Parker, J.C., Kim, K.K., Wanen, R.L., Kepes., J.J., and Tully, R. (1986). A case of thalamic aphasia with postmortem verification. *Brain and Language*, **29**, 301–14.

Crum, B.A. and Wijdicks, E.F. (2000). Thalamic hematoma from a ruptured posterior cerebral artery aneurysm. *Cerebrovascular Diseases*, **10**, 475–7.

Csornai, M. (1974). Über Störungen der vertikalen Blickbewegeungen und des Bewusstseins bei Heiden des mesodiencephalen Übergangsgebietes. *Archiv für Psychiatrie und Nervenkrankheiten*, **219**, 79–88.

Cummins, T.R. and Waxman, S.G. (1997). Down-regulation of tetrodotoxin-resistant sodium currents and up-regulation of a rapidly repriming tetrodotoxin-sensitive sodium current in small spinal sensory neurons following nerve injury. *Journal of Neuroscience*, **17**, 3503–14.

Cummins, T.R., Dib-Hajj, S.D., Black, J.A., Akopian, A.N., Wood J.N., and Waxman, S.G. (1999). A novel persistent tetrodotoxin-resistant sodium current in SNS-null wild-type small primary sensory neurons. *Journal of Neuroscience*, **19**, RC43 (1–6).

D'Esposito, M. and Alexander, M.P. (1995). Subcortical aphasia: distinct profiles following left putaminal hemorrhage. *Neurology*, **45**, 38–41.

Damasio, A.R., Damasio, H., Rizzo, M., Varney, N., and Gersh, F. (1982). Aphasia with non-hemorrhagic lesions in the basal ganglia and internal capsule. *Archives of Neurology*, **39**, 15–20.

Damasio, H. (1983). A computed tomographic guide to the identification of cerebral vascular territories. *Archives of Neurology*, **40**, 138–42.

Danziger, N., Meary, E., Mercier, B., Samson, Y., and Rancurel, G. (1997). Hallucinose visuelle et hyperhédonisme au cours d'un infarctus pontique et thalamique. *Revue Neurologique, Paris*, **153**, 679–83.

Davies, M.J. (2000). The pathophysiology of acute coronary syndromes. *Heart*, **83**, 361–6.

Davis P. and Ransom, B.R. (1987). Anoxia and CNS white matter: *in vitro* studies using the rat optic nerve. *Society for Neuroscience Abstracts*, **13**, 1634.

Davis, S.M., Tress, B., Barber, P.A., Darby, D., Parsons, M., Gerraty, R., *et al.* (2000). Echoplanar magnetic resonance imaging in acute stroke. *Journal of Clinical Neuroscience*, **7**, 3–8.

Davis, S.M., Tress, B.M., Dowling, R., Donnan, G.A., Kiers, L., and Rossiter, S.C. (1989) Magnetic resonance imaging in posterior circulation infarction: impact on diagnosis and management. *Australian and New Zealand Journal of Medicine*, 19, 219–25.

Davous, P. and Bequet, D. (1995). CADASIL. Un nouveau modèle de démence souscorticale. *Revue Neurologique, Paris*, 151, 634–9.

Davous, P. and Fallet-Bianco, C. (1991). Démence sous-corticale familiale avec leucoencèphalopathie artériopathique. Observation clinicopathologique. *Revue Neurologique, Paris*, 5, 376–84.

Davous, P., Bianco, C., Duval-Lota, A.M., de Recondo, J., Vedrenne, C., and Roudot, P. (1984). Aphasie par infarctus thalamique paramédian gauche. Observation anatomo-clinique. *Revue Neurologique, Paris*, 140, 711–9.

Dawson, T.M. and Starkebaum, G. (1999). Isolated central nervous system vasculitis associated with hepatitis C infection. *Journal of Rheumatology*, 26, 2273–6.

DCCT (1993). The effect of intensive treatment of diabetes on the development and progression of long-term complications in insulin-dependent diabetes mellitus. *New England Journal of Medicine*, 329, 977–86.

De Boucaud, P., Vital, C., and De Boucaud, D. (1968). Démence thalamique d'origine vasculaire. *Revue Neurologique, Paris*, 119, 461–8.

de Haan, R.J., Limburg, M., Van der Meulen, J.H.P., Jacobs, H.M., and Aaronson, N.K. (1995). Quality of life after stroke. Impact of stroke type and lesion location. *Stroke*, 26. 402–8.

De Reuck, J.L. (1971). The human periventricular blood supply and the anatomy of cerebral infarctions. European Neurology, 5, 321–34.

De Smet, Y. (1986). Le syndrome thalamique de Dejérine–Roussy. Prolégomènes. *Revue Neurologique, Paris*, 142, 259–66.

De Weerd, A.W., Veldhuizen, R.J., Veering, M.M., Poortvliet, D.C.J., and Jonkman, E.J. (1988). Recovery from cerebral ischaemia. EEG, cerebral blood flow and clinical symptomatology in the first three years after a stroke. *Electroencephalography and Clinical Neurophysiology*, 70, 197–204.

Dechambre, A. (1838). Mémoire sur la curabilité du ramollissement cérébral. *Gazette Médical de Paris*, 6, 305–14

Decroix, J.P., Graveleau, Ph., Masson, M., and Cambier, J. (1986). Infarction in the terrirtory of the anterior choroidal artery. A clinical and computerized study of 16 cases. *Brain*, 109, 1071–85.

Dehaene, I. (1982). Bilateral thalamo-subthalamic infarction. *Acta Neurologica Belgica*, 82, 253–61.

Dejérine, J. and Egger, M. (1903). Contribution à l'étude de la physio-pathologique de l'incoordination motrice. *Revue Neurologique, Paris*, 11, 397–405.

Dejérine, J. and Long, E. (1898). Sur quelques dégénérescences du tronc encéphalique de l'homme étudiées par la méthodde de Marchi. Sur les connections de la couche optique avec la corticalité cerebrale. Sur la localisation de l'hémianesthésie dite capsulaire. *Comptes Rendus de la Société de Biologie, Paris*, 50, 864–7, 1131–4.

Dejérine, J. and Roussy, G. (1906). Le syndrome thalamique. *Revue Neurologique, Paris*, 14, 521.

Del Brutto, O.H. (1992). Neurocysticercosis and cerebrovascular disease: a review. *Journal of Neurology, Neurosurgery, and Psychiatry*, 55, 252–4.

del Mar Sáez de Ocariz, M., Nader, J.A., Santos, J.A., and Bautista, M. (1996). Thalamic vascular lesions: risk factors and clinical course for infarcts and hemorrhages. *Stroke*, 27, 1530–6.

Del Ser, T., Bermejo, F., Portera, A., Arredondo, J.M., Bouras, C., and Constantinidis, J. (1990). Vascular dementia: a clinicopathological study. *Journal of the Neurological Sciences*, 96, 1–17.

Del Sette, M., Eliasziw, M., Streifler, J.Y., Hachinski, V.C., Fox, A.J., Barnett, H.J.M., for the North American Symptomatic Carotid Endarterectomy (NASCET) Group (2000). Internal borderzone infarction: a marker for severe stenosis in patients with symptomatic internal carotid artery disease. *Stroke*, 31, 631–6.

Delay, J. and Brion, S. (1962). *Les démences tardives*. Masson, Paris.

DeLeo, J., Schubert, P., and Kreutzberg, G.W. (1988). Propentofylline (HWA285) protects hippocampal neurones of mongolian gerbils against ischemic damage in the presence of an adenosine antagonist. *Neuroscience Letters*, 84, 307–11.

DeLeo, J.P.S. and Kreutzberg, G.W. (1988). Protection against ischemic brain damage using propentofylline in gerbils. *Stroke*, 19, 1535–9.

Demeurisse, G. Derouck, M. Coekaerts M.J., Deltenre, P., Van Nechel, C., Demol, O., and Capon, A. (1979). Study of two cases of aphasia by infarction of the left thalamus, without cortical lesion. *Acta Neurologica Belgica*, 79, 450–9

Derdeyn, C.P., Powers, W.J., Moran, C.J., Cross, D.T., 3rd, and Allen, B.T. (1995). Role of Doppler US in screening or carotid atherosclerotic disease. *Radiology*, 197, 635–43.

Derex, L., Ostrowsky, K., Nighoghossian, N., and Trouillas, P. (1997). Severe pathological crying after left anterior choroidal artery infarct. Reversibility with paroxetine treatment. *Stroke*, 28, 1464–6.

Derouesne, C., Gray, F., Escourelle, R., and Castaigne, P. (1987). 'Expanding cerebral lacunae' in a hypertensive patient with normal pressure hydrocephalus. *Neuropathology and Applied Neurobiology*, 13, 309–20.

Derouesne, C., Yelnik, A., and Castaigne, P. (1985). Deficit sensitif isolé par infarctus dans la territoire de l'artère choroidienne antérieure. *Revue Neurologique, Paris*, 141, 311–4.

Desmond, D.W., Moroney, J.T., Lynch, T., Chan, S., Chin, S.S., Mohr, J.P. (1999). The natural history of CADASIL: a pooled analysis of previously published cases. *Stroke*. 30, 1230–3.

Desmond, D.W., Tatemichi, T.K., Rosen, W.G., Stern, Y., Friedman, D.P., Mohr, J.P., *et al.* (1992). Serial neuropsychological findings five years after left anterior thalamic infarction. *International Journal of Neuroscience*, 63, 235–6.

Destee, A., Muller, J.P., Vermersch, P., Pruvo, J.P., and Warot, P. (1990). Hémiballisme hémichorée. Infarctus striatal. *Revue Neurologique, Paris*, 146, 150–2.

Devic, M., Michel, F., and Lenglet, J.P. (1964). Nystagmus retractorius, paralysie de la verticalité, aréflexie pupillaire et anomalie de la posture du regard par ramollissement dans le territoire de la choroïdienne postérieure. *Revue Neurologique, Paris*, 110, 399–404.

Dib-Hajj, S.D., Tyrrell, L., Black, J.A., and Waxman, S.G. (1998). NaN, a novel voltage-gated Na channel preferentially expressed in peripheral sensory neurons and down-regulated following axotomy. *Proceedings of the National Academy of Sciences of the USA*, 95, 8963–8.

Dichgans, M. and Petersen, D. (1997). Angiographic complications in CADASIL [letter]. *Lancet*, 349, 776–7.

Dichgans, M., Filipi, M., Brüning, R., Iannucci, G., Berrchten-breiter, C., Minicucci, L., *et al.* (1999). Quantitative MRI in CADASIL. *Neurology*, 52, 1361–7.

Dichgans, M., Ludwig, H., Muller-Hocker, J., Messerschmidt, A., Gasser, T. (2000). Small in-frame deletions and missense mutations in CADASIL: clinical findings in 102 cases. *Annals of Neurology*, 44, 731–9.

Dichgans, M., Mayer, M., Uttner, I., Bruning, R., Muller-Hocker, J., Rungger, L., *et al.* (1998). The phenotypic spectrum of CADASIL: clinical findings in 102 cases. *Annals of Neurology*. 44, 731–9.

Dickmann, E. and Müller, E. (1985). Lakunäre Hirninfarkte. *Zeitschrift für Gerontologie*, 18, 222–5.

Dide, M. and Durocher, A. (1904). Un cas de syndrome thalamique avec autopsie. *Revue Neurologique, Paris*, 12, 808–14.

Diener, H., Cunha, L., Forbes, H., Sivenius, J., Smets, P., and Lowenthal, J. (1996). European Stroke Prevention Studies 2: dipyridamole and acetyl salicylic acid in the secondary prevention of stroke. *Journal of the Neurological Sciences*, 143, 1–13.

Dieterich, M. and Brandt, T. (1993). Thalamic infarctions: differential effects on vestibular function in the roll plane (35 patients). *Neurology*, 43, 1732–40.

Diringer, M.N., Edwards, D.F., and Zazulia, A.R. (1998). Hydrocephalus: a previously unrecognized predictor of poor outcome from supratentorial intracerebral hemorrhage. *Stroke*, 29, 1352–7.

Dixon, S., Pais, S., *et al.* (1982). Natural history of nonstenotic, asymptomatic ulcerative lesions of the carotid artery. A further analysis. *Archives of Surgery*, 117, 1493–8.

Dobato, J.L., Villanueva, J.A., and Gimenez-Roldan, S. (1990). Sensory ataxic hemiparesis in thalamic hemorrhage. *Stroke*, 21, 1749–53.

Dobkin, B.H. (1983). Heparin for lacunar stroke in progression. *Stroke*, 14, 421–3.

Doi, Y., Yoshinari, M., Yoshizumi, H., Ibayashi, S., Wakisaka, M., and Fujishima, M. (1997). Polymorphism of the angiotensin-converting enzyme (ACE) gene in patients with thrombotic brain infarction. *Atherosclerosis*, 132, 145–50.

Domasio, H. (1983). A computed tomographic guide to the identification of cerebral vascular territories. *Archives of Neurology*, 40, 138–42.

Donat, J.R. (1980). Unilateral asterixis due to thalamic hemorrhage. *Neurology*, 30, 83–4.

Donnan, G. A., Tress, B., Bladin, P. F. (1982). A prospective study of lacunar infarction using computerized tomography. Neurology, 32, 49–56.

Donnan, G.A. (1992). Investigation of patients with stroke and transient ischaemic attacks. *Lancet*, 339, 473–7.

Donnan, G.A., Bladin, P.F., Berkovic, S.F., Longley, W.A., and Saling, M.M. (1991). The stroke syndrome of striatocapsular infarction. *Brain*, 114,51–70.

Donnan, G.A., McNeil, J.J., Adena, M.A., Doyle, A.E., O'Malley, H.M., and Neill, G.C. (1989). Smoking as a risk factor for cerebral ischaemia. *Lancet*, 2, 643–7.

Donnan, G.A., Norrving, B., Bamford, J., and Bogousslavsky, J. (1993). Subcortical infarction: classification and terminology. *Cerebrovascular Diseases*, 3, 248–251.

Donnan, G.A., Tress B., and Bladin, P.F. (1982). A prospective study of lacunar infarction using computerized tomography. Neurology, 32, 49–56.

Douglas, M.A. and Hearer, A.F. (1982). Long-term prognosis of hypertensive intracerebral hemorrhage. *Stroke*, 13, 488–91.

Dozono, K., Ishii, N., Nishihara, Y., and Horie A. (1991). An autopsy study of the incidence of lacunes in relation to age, hypertension, and arteriosclerosis. *Stroke*, 22, 993–6.

Dromerick, A.X., Meschia, J.F., Kumar, A., and Hanton, R.E. (1997). Simultaneous bilateral thalamic hemorrhages following the administration of intravenous tissue plasminogen activator. *Archives of Physical Medicine and Rehabilitation*, 78, 92–4.

Drury, I., Whisnant, J.P., and Garraway, W.M. (1984). Primary intracerebral hemorrhage: impact of CT on incidence. *Neurology*, 34, 653–7.

Dubois, B., Pillon, B., De Saxcé, H., Lhermitte, F., and Agid, Y. (1986). Disappearance of Parkinsonian signs after spontaneous vascular 'thalamotomy'. *Archives of Neurology*, 43, 815–7.

DuBois-Poulsen, A., Guillaume, J., and Magis, C. (1956). La ligature de l'artère choroidienne antérieure. *Bulletin et Mémoires Societé Française Opthalmologie*, 69, 450–65.

Dul, K. and Drayer, B.P. (1994). CT and MRI imaging of intracerebral hemorrhage. In *Intracerebral hemorrhage* (ed. C.S. Kase and L.R. Caplan), pp. 73–93. Butterworth-Heinemann, Boston.

Dunker, R.O. and Harris, A.B. (1976). Surgical anatomy of the proximal anterior cerebral artery. *Journal of Neurosurgery*, **44**, 359–67.

Dupré, E. and Devaux, A. (1901). Foyers lacunaires de désintégration cérébrale (note sur le processus histogénique). *Revue Neurologique, Paris*, **9**, 653–7.

Durand-Fardel, M. (1842). Mémoire sur une altération particulière de la substance blanche. *Gazette Médicale de Paris*, **10**, 23–6, 33–8.

Durand-Fardel, M. (1843). *Traité du Ramollissement du Cerveau*. Baillière. Paris.

Durand-Fardel, M. (1854). *Traité Clinique et Pratique des Maladies des Vieillards*. Baillière, Paris.

Duret, H. (1874). Recherches anatomiques sur la circulation de l'encéphale. *Archives de Physiologie Normale et Pathologigue, Paris*, **6**, 60–91, 316–58.

Dutch (1993). Trial of secondary prevention with atenolol after transient ischemic attack or non-disabling ishemic stroke. *Stroke*, **24**, 543–8.

Dyken, M.L. (1991). Stroke risk factors. In *Prevention of stroke* (ed. J.W. Norris and V.C. Hachinski), pp. 83–101. Springer-Verlag, New York.

Dylewski, D.A., Morgenstern, L.B., and Demchuck, A.M. (2000). Utility of magnetic resonance imaging in acute intracerebral hemorrhage. *Journal of Neuroimaging*, **10**, 78–83.

EAFT. (1993). Secondary prevention in non-rheumatic atrial fibrillation after transient ischaemic attack or minor stroke. EAFT (European Atrial Fibrillation Trial) Study Group. *Lancet*, **342**, 1255–62.

Earnest, M.P., Fahn, S., and Karp, J.H. (1974). Normal pressure hydrocephalus and hypertensive cerebrovascular disease. *Archives of Neurology*, **31**, 262–6.

ECST Collaborative Group (1995). Risk of stroke in the distribution of an asymptomatic carotid artery. *Lancet*, **345**, 209–12.

ECST Collaborative Group (1998). Randomised trial of endarterectomy for recently symptomatic carotid stenosis: final results of the MRC European Carotid Surgery Trial. *Lancet*, **351**, 1379–87.

Elbaz, A. and Amarenco, P. (1999). Genetic susceptibility and ischaemic stroke. *Current Opinion in Neurology*, **12**, 47–55.

Elbaz, A., Poirier, O., Canaple, S., Chédru, F., Cambien, F., and Amarenco, P. on behalf of the GÉNIC investigators (2000a). The association between the Va134Leu polymorphism in the factor XIII gene and brain infarction. *Blood*, **95**, 586–91.

Elbaz, A., Poirier, O., Moulin, T., Chédru, F., Cambien, F., and Amarenco, P. on behalf of the GÉNIC investigators. (2000b). The association between the Glu298Asp polymoprhism in the endothelial constitutive nitric oxide synthase gene and brain infarction. *Stroke*, **31**, 1634–1639.

Elghozi, D., Strube, E., Signoret, J.L., Cambier, J., and Lhermitte, F. (1978). Quasi-aphasie lors de lésion du thalamus. Relation du trouble du langage et de l'activation élective de l'hémisphére gauche dans 4 observations de lésions thalamiques gauches et droites. *Revue Neurologique, Paris*, **134**, 557–74.

Erkinjuntti, T. (1987a). Differential diagnosis between Alzheimer's disease and vascular dementia: evaluation of common clinical methods. *Acta Neurologica Scandinavica*, **76**, 433–42.

Erkinjuntti, T. (1987b). Types of multi-infarct dementia. *Acta Neurologica Scandinavica*, **75**, 391–9.

Escourolle, R. and Poirier, J. (1977). *Manuel Élémentaire de Neuropathologie*. Masson, Paris.

Eslinger, P.J., Warner, G.C., Gratton, L.M., and Easton, J.D. (1991). 'Frontal lobe' utilization behavior associated with paramedian thalamic infarction. *Neurology*, **41**, 450–2.

ESPRIT (2000). ESPRIT protocol version 7 date 10/03/2000.

ESPS (1990). European Stroke Prevention Study. ESPS Group. *Stroke*, **21**, 1122–30.

Estes, M., Chimowitz, M., Awad, I., *et al.* (1991). Sclerosing vasculopathy of the central nervous system in non-elderly demented patients. *Archives of Neurology*, **48**, 631–6.

Evers, S., Koch, H., Grotemeyer, K.H., Lange, B., Deufel, T., and Ringelstein, E.B. (1997). Features, symptoms, and neurophysiological findings in stroke associated with hyperhomocysteinemia. *Archives of Neurology*, **54**, 1276–82.

Façon, E., Stériade, M., and Wertheim, N. (1958). Hypersomnie prolongée engendrée par des lésions bilatérales du système activateur médial. Le syndrome thrombotique de la bifurcation du tronc basilaire. *Revue Neurologique, Paris*, **98**, 117–33.

Falcone, N., Fensore, C., Lanzetti, A., Lazzarino, L.G., Nappo, A., Nicolai, A., *et al.* (1986). Considerazioni cliniche e correlazioni EEG–TC negli infarti lacunari. *Rivista di Neurologia*, **56**, 396–410.

Faris, A.A., Poser, C.M., Wilmore, D.W., and Agnew, C.H. (1963). Radiologic visualization of neck vessels in healthy men. *Neurology*, **13**, 386–91.

Farrell, B., Godwin, J., and Richards, S.C.W. (1991). The United Kingdom transient ischaemic attack (UK-TIA) aspirin trial: final result. *Journal of Neurology, Neurosurgery, and Psychiatry*, **54**, 1044–54.

Fassbender, K., Mielke, O., Bertsch, T., Nafe, B., Froschen, S., and Hennerici, M. (1999). Homocysteine in cerebral macroangiography and microangiopathy. *Lancet*, **353**, 1586–7.

Faught, E., Peters, D., Bartolucci, A., Moore, L., and Miller, P.C. (1989). Seizures after primary intracerebral hemorrhage. *Neurology*, **39**, 1089–93.

Fazekas, F., Kleinert, R., Roob, G., Kleinert, G., Kapeller, P., Schmidt, R., *et al.* (1999). Histopathologic analysis of foci of signal loss in gradient-echo T2*-weighted MR images in patients with spontaneous intracerebral hemorrhage: evidence of microangiopathy-related microbleeds. *American Journal of Neuroradiology*, **20**, 637–42.

Feigin, I. and Prose, P. (1959). Hypertensive fibrinoid arteritis of the brain and gross cerebral hemorrhage. A form of hyalinosis. *Archives of Neurology*, **1**, 98–110.

Feinberg, W.M. and Rapcsak, S.Z. (1989). 'Peduncular hallucinosis' following paramedian thalamic infarction. *Neurology*, **39**, 1535–6.

Feinberg, W.M., Seeger, J.F., Carmody, R.F., Anderson, D.C., Hart, R.G., and Pearce, L.S. (1990). Epidemiologic features of asymptomatic cerebral infarction in patients with nonvalvular atrial fibrillation. *Archives of Internal Medicine*, **150**, 2340–4.

Feldmeyer, J.J., Bogousslavsky, J., and Regli, F. (1984). Astérixis uni-ou bilatéral en cas de lésion thalamique ou pariétale: un trouble moteur afférentiel? *Schweizeriche Medizinische Wochenschrift*, **114**, 167–71.

Fensore, C., Lazzarino, L.G., Nappo, A., and Nicolai, A. (1988). Language and memory disturbances from mesencephalo-thalamic infarcts. A clinical CT study. *European Neurology*, **28**, 51–6.

Fern, R., Ransom, B., and Waxman, S.G. (1996). Autoprotective mechanisms in the CNS. *Molecular and Chemical Neuropathology*, **27**, 107–29.

Fern, R., Ransom, B.R., and Waxman, S.G. (1995b). Voltage-gated calcium channels in CNS white matter: role in anoxic injury. *Journal of Neurophysiology*, **74**, 369–77.

Fern, R., Ransom, B.R., Stys, P.K., and Waxman, S.G. (1993). Pharmacological protection of CNS white matter during anoxia: actions of phenytoin, carbamazepine and diazepam. *Journal of Pharmacology and Experimental Therapeutics*, **266**, 1549–55.

Fern, R., Waxman, S.G., and Ransom, B.R. (1994). Modulation of anoxic injury in CNS white matter by adenosine and interaction between adenosine and GABA. *Journal of Neurophysiology*, **72**, 2609–16.

Fern, R., Waxman, S.G., and Ransom, B.R. (1995a). Endogenous GABA attenuates CNS white matter dysfunction following anoxia. *Journal of Neuroscience*, 15, 699–708.

Ferrand, J. (1902). *Essai sur l'hémiplégie des Vieillards. Les Lacunes de Desintégration Cérébrale.* Jules Rousset, Paris.

Ferro, J.M. and Kertesz, A. (1984). Posterior internal capsule infarction associated with neglect. *Archives of Neurology*, 41, 422–24.

Fields, W., Lemak, N., Frankowski, R., and Hardy, R. (1979). Controlled trial of aspirin in cerebral ischemia (AITIA Study). *Thromb Haemost*, 41, 135–41.

Fieschi, C., Carolei, A., Fiorelli, M., Argentino, C., Bozzao, L., Fazio, C., *et al.* (1988). Changing prognosis of primary intracerebral hemorrhage: results of a clinical and computed tomographic follow-up study of 104 patients. *Stroke*, 19, 192–5.

Fiorelli, M., Toni, D., Bastianello, S., Sacchetti, M.L., Sette, G., Falcou, A., *et al.* (2000). Computed tomography findings in the first few hours of presumed ischemic stroke: implications for the clinician. *Journal of Neurological Sciences*, 173, 10–17.

Fisher, C.M. (1951). Occlusion of the internal carotid artery. *Archives of Neurology*, 65, 346–77.

Fisher, C.M. (1959). The pathologic and clinical aspects of thalamic hemorrhage. *Transactions of the American Neurological Association*, 84, 56–9.

Fisher, C.M. (1961). Clinical syndromes in cerebral hemorrhage. In *Pathogenesis and treatment of cerebrovascular disease* (ed. W.S. Fields), pp. 318–42. Charles C. Thomas, Springfield.

Fisher, C.M. (1965a). Lacunes: small, deep cerebral infarcts. *Neurology*, 15, 774–84.

Fisher, C.M. (1965b). Pure sensory stroke involving face, arm, and leg. *Neurology*, 15, 76–80.

Fisher, C.M. (1965c). Homolateral ataxia and crural paresis. A vascular syndrome. *Journal of Neurology, Neurosurgery, and Psychiatry*, 28, 48–55.

Fisher, C.M. (1965d). Pure motor hemiplegia of vascular origin. *Archives of Neurology*, 13, 130–40.

Fisher, C.M. (1967). A lacunar stroke: the dysarthria–clumsy hand syndrome. *Neurology*, 17, 614–7.

Fisher, C.M. (1969). The arterial lesion underlying lacunes. *Acta Neuropathologica (Berlin)*, 12, 1–15.

Fisher, C.M. (1971). Pathological observations in hypertensive cerebral hemorrhage. *Journal of Neuropathology and Experimental Neurology*, 30, 536–50.

Fisher, C.M. (1972). Cerebral miliary aneurysms in hypertension. *American Journal of Pathology*, 66, 313–30.

Fisher, C.M. (1976). In Scheinberg P (ed): *Cerebrovascular diseases. 10th Princeton Conference* (ed. P. Scheinberg), pp. 50–3. Raven Press, New York.

Fisher, C.M. (1977). Bilateral occlusion of the basilar artery branches. *Journal of Neurology, Neurosurgery, and Psychiatry*, 40, 1182–9.

Fisher, C.M. (1978a). Thalamic pure sensory stroke: a pathologic study. *Neurology*, 28, 1141–4.

Fisher, C.M. (1978b). Ataxic hemiparesis: a pathologic study. *Archives of Neurology*, 35, 126–8.

Fisher, C.M. (1979). Capsular infarcts. The underlying vascular lesions. *Archives of Neurology*, 36, 65–73.

Fisher, C.M. (1982a). Lacunar strokes and infarcts: a review. *Neurology*, 32, 871–6.

Fisher, C.M. (1982b). Pure sensory stroke and allied conditions. *Stroke*, 13, 434–47.

Fisher, C.M. (1985). The ascendancy of the diastolic blood pressure. *Lancet*, 2, 1349–50.

Fisher, C.M. (1986). Unusual vascular events in the territory of the posterior cerebral artery. *Canadian Journal of Neurological Sciences*, 13, 1–7.

Fisher, C.M. (1991). Lacunar infarcts: a review. *Cerebrovascular Diseases*, 1, 311–20.

Fisher, C.M. and Caplan, L.R. (1971). Basilar artery branch occlusion: a cause of pontine infarction. *Neurology*, 21, 900–5.

Fisher, C.M. and Cole, H. (1965). Homolateral ataxia and crural paresis: a vascular syndrome. *Journal of Neurology, Neurosurgery, and Psychiatry*, 28, 48–65.

Fisher, C.M. and Curry, H.B. (1965). Pure motor hemiplegia of vascular origin. *Archives of Neurology*, 13, 30–44.

Fisher, C.M. and Ojemann, R.G. (1986). A clinico-pathologic study of carotid endarterectomy plaques. *Revue Neurologique, Paris*, 142, 573–89.

Fisher, C.M. and Tapia, J. (1987). Lateral medullary infarction extending to the lower pons. *Journal of Neurology, Neurosurgery, and Psychiatry*, 50, 620–624.

Fisher, C.M., Karnes, W., and Kubik, C. (1961). Lateral medullary infarction: the pattern of vascular occlusion. *Journal of Neuropathology and Experimental Neurology*, 20, 323–79.

Fisher, M., Lingley, J.F., Blumenfeld, A., and Felice, K. (1989). Anterior choroidal artery territory infarction and small vessel disease. *Stroke*, 20, 1591–2.

Fisher, M., Smith, T.W., and Jacobs, R. (1988). Pure motor hemiplegia secondary to a saccular basilar artery aneurysm. *Stroke*, 19, 104–7.

FISS (1998). Fraxiparine in Ischemic Stroke Study (FISS bis) (abstract). *Cerebrovascular Diseases*, 8 (Suppl, 4), 19.

Fitzimons, R.B. and Wolfenden, W.H. (1991). Migraine coma. Meningitic migraine with cerebral oedema associated with a new form of autosomal dominant cerebellar ataxi. *Brain*, 108, 555–77.

Foix, C. (1923). *Titres et travaux scientifiques*. Masson, Paris.

Foix, C. and Hillemand, P. (1925). Les syndromes de la région thalamique. *Presse Médicale*, 1, 113–7.

Foix, C. and Levy, M. (1927). Les ramollissements sylviens: syndromes des lésions en foyer du territoire de l'artère sylvienne et de ses branches. *Revue Neurologique, Paris*, 43, 1–51.

Foix, C. and Schiff-Wertheimer, S. (1926). Semiologie des hémianopsies au cours du ramollissement cérébral. *Revue d'Oto-neuro-oculistique*, 4, 561–84.

Foix, C., Chavany, H., Hillemand, P., and Schiff Wertheimer, S. (1925). Oblitération de l'artère choroidienne antérieure. Ramollissement de son territoire cérébral, hémiplégie, hémianesthésie, hémianopsie. *Bulletin de la Societé d'Ophtalmologie de Paris*, 27, 221–3.

Foix, C. and Nicolesco, I. (1923). Contribution à l'étude des grands syndromes de désintégration sénile cérébro-mésencéphalique. *Presse Médicale*, 92, 957–63.

Foulkes, M.A., Wolf, P.A., Price, T.R., Mohr, J.P., and Hier, D.B. (1988). The stroke data bank: design, methods, and baseline characteristics. *Stroke*, 19, 547–54.

Franck, G., Salmon, E., Sadzot, B., and Van der Linden, M. (1986). Etude hémodynamique et métabolique par tomographie à émission de positons d'un cas d'atteinte ischémique thalamo-capsulaire droite. *Revue Neurologigue, Paris*, 142, 475–9.

Franco, R.F., Reitsma, P.H., Lourenco, D., Maffei, F.H., Morelli, V., Tavella, M.H., *et al.* (1999). Factor XIII Va134Leu is a genetic factor involved in the aetiology of venous thrombosis. *Thrombosis and Haemostasis*, 81, 676–9.

Franke, C.L., van Swieten, J.C., and van Gijn, J. (1991). Residual lesions on computed tomography after intracerebral hemorrhage. *Stroke*, 22, 1530–3.

Fredriksson, K., Aver, R.N., Kalimo, H. Nordborg, C., Olsson, Y., and Johansson, B.B. (1985). Cerebrovascular lesions in stroke prone spontaneously hypertensive rats. *Acta Neuropathologica*, 68, 284–94.

Fredriksson, K., Brun, A., and Gustafson, L. (1992). Pure subcortical arteriosclerotic encephalopathy (Binswanger's disease): a clinicopathologic study. Part 1: clinical features. *Cerebrovascular Diseases*, 2, 82–6.

Fredriksson, K., Nordborg, C., Kalimo, H., Olsson, Y., and Johansson, B.B. (1988). Cerebral microangiopathy in stroke-prone spontaneously hypertensive rats. An immunohistochemical and ultrastructural study. *Acta Neuropathologica*, 54, 183–8.

Frequin, S.T.F.M., Linssen, W.H.J.P., Pasman, J.W., Hommes, O.R., Merx, H.L. (1991). Recurrent prolonged coma due to basilar artery migraine. A case report. *Headache*, 31, 75–81.

Friedman, J.H. (1985). Syndrome of diffuse encephalopathy due to nondominant thalamic infarction. *Neurology*, 35, 1524–6.

Frisen L. (1979). Quadruple sectoranopia and sectorial optic atrophy: a syndrome of the distal anterior choroidal artery. *Journal of Neurology, Neurosurgery, and Psychiatry*, 42, 590–4.

Frisén, L., Holmegaard, L., and Rosencrantz, M. (1978). Sectorial optic atrophy and homonymous, horizontal sectoranopia: a lateral choroidal artery syndrome? *Journal of Neurology, Neurosurgery, and Psychiatry*, 41, 374–80.

Fuh, J.-L. and Wang, S.-J. (1995). Caudate hemorrhage: clinical features, neuropsychological assessments and radiological findings. *Clinical Neurology and Neurosurgery*, 97, 296–9.

Fujii, Y., Tanaka, R., Takeuchi, S., Koike, T., Minakawa, T., and Sasaki, O. (1994). Hematoma enlargement in spontaneous intracerebral hemorrhage. *Journal of Neurosurgery*, 80, 51–7.

Fukatsu, R., Fujii, T., Yamadori, A., Nagasawa, H., and Sakurai, Y. (1997). Persisting childish behavior after bilateral thalamic infarcts. *European Neurology*, 37, 230–5.

Fung, V.S.C., Morris, J.G.L., Leicester, J., Soo, Y.S., and Davies, L. (1997). Clonic perseveration following thalamofrontal disconnection: a distinctive movement disorder. *Movement Disorders*, 12, 378–85.

Furby, A., Vahedi, K., Force, M., *et al.* (1998). Differential diagnosis of a vascular leukoencephalopathy within a CADASIL family: use of skin biopsy electron microscopy study and direct genotypic screening. *Journal of Neurology*, 245, 734–40.

Furlan, A.J., Whisnant, J.P., and Elveback, L.R. (1979). The decreasing incidence of primary intracerebral hemorrhage: a population study. *Annals of Neurology*, 5, 367–73.

Furuta, A., Nobuyoshi, N., Nishihara, Y., and Honie, A. (1991). Medullary arteries in aging and dementia. *Stroke*, 22, 442–6.

Futrell, N., Millikan, C., Watson, B.D., Dietrich, W.D., and Ginsberg, M. (1989). Embolic stroke from a carotid arterial source in the rat: pathology and clinical implications. *Neurology*, 39, 1050–6.

Galizzi, J., Borsotto, M., Barhanin, J., Fossett, M., and Lazdunski, M. (1986). Characterization and photoaffinity labeling of receptor sites for the Ca^{2+} channel inhibitors d-*cis*-diltiazem, (+)-depridil, desmethoxyverapamil, and (+)-PN 200–110 in skeletal muscle transverse tubule membranes. *Journal of Biological Chemistry*, 261, 1393–1397.

Gallassi, R., Morreale, A., Montagna, P., Sacquegna, T., Di Sarro, R., and Lugaresi, E. (1991). Binswanger's disease and normal-pressure hydrocephalus: clinical and neuropsychological comparison. *Archives of Neurology*, 48, 1156–9.

Gan, R., Sacco, R.L., Kargman, D.E., Roberts, J.K., Boden-Albala, B., and Gu, Q. (1997). Testing the validity of the lacunar hypothesis: the Northern Manhattan Stroke Study experience. *Neurology*, 48, 1204–11.

Gandolfo, C., Caponnetto, C., Del Sette, M., Santoloci, D., and Loeb, C. (1988). Risk factors in lacunar syndromes: a case–control study. *Acta Neurologica Scandinavica*, 77, 22–6.

Gandolfo, C., Del Sette, M., Finocchi, C., Calautti, C., and Loeb, C. (1998). Internal borderzone infarction in patients with ischemic stroke. *Cerebrovascular Diseases*, **8**, 255–8.

Gandolfo, C., Moretti, C., Dall'Agata, D., Primavera, A., Brusa, G., and Loeb, C. (1986). Long-term prognosis of patients with lacunar syndromes. *Acta Neurologica Scandinavica*, **74**, 234–9.

Garcia, J.H., Lassen, N.A., Weiller C., Sperling B., and Nakagawa, J. (1995). Ischemic stroke and incomplete infarction. *Stroke*, **27**, 761–5.

Garcia, M., King, V., Shevell, J., Slaughter, R., Saurex, K., Winquist, R., and Kaczorowski, G. (1990). Amiloride analogs inhibit L-type calcium channels and display calcium entry blocker activity. *Journal of Biological Chemistry*, **265**, 3673–771.

Garcia-Albea, E., Cabello, A., and Franch, O. (1987). Subcortical arteriosclerotic encephalopathy (Binswanger's disease): a report of five patients. *Acta Neurologica Scandinavica*, **75**, 295–303.

Garcin, R. and Lapresle, J. (1954). Syndrome sensitif de type thalamique et à topographie cheiro-orale par lésion localisée du thalamus. *Revue Neurologique, Paris*, **90**, 124–9.

Garcin, R. and Lapresle, J. (1960). Deuxième observation personnelle du syndrome de type thalamique à topographie cheiro-orale par lésion localisée du thalamus. *Revue Neurologique, Paris*, **103**, 474–81.

Garcin, R. and Lapresle, J. (1969). Incoordination cérébelleuse du membre inférieur par lésion localisée dans la région interne du thalamus contralatéral. *Revue Neurologique, Paris*, **120**, 5–13.

Gastaut, H., Naquet, R., and Vigouroux, R.A. (1971). The vascular syndrome of the parieto-temporal-occipital triangle based on 18 cases. In *Cerebral circulation and stroke* (ed. K.-J. Zülch), pp. 82–91. Springer-Verlag, Berlin.

Gatto, E.M., Zurrú, M.C., Rugilo, C., Mitre, S., Pardal, A.M., Martinez, M., and Pardal, M.M.F. (1998). Focal myoclonus associated with posterior thalamic hematoma. *Movement Disorders*, **13**, 182–4.

Gautier, J.C. (1976). Cerebral ischemia in hypertension. In *Vascular disease of the central nervous system* (ed. R.W. Ross Russel) pp. 181–209. Churchill Livingstone, Edinburgh.

Gent, M., Barnett, H., Sackett, D., Taylor, D. (1980). A randomized trial of aspirin and sulfinpyrazone in patients with threatened stroke. Results and methodologic issues. *Circulation*, **62**, V97–105.

Gent, M., Blakely, J.A., Easton, J.D., *et al.* (1989). The Canadian–American ticlopidine study (CATS) in thromboembolic stroke. *Lancet*, **1**, 1215–20.

Gentilini, M., De Renzi, E., and Crisi, G. (1987). Bilateral paramedian thalamic artery infarcts: report of 8 cases. *Journal of Neurology, Neurosurgery, and Psychiatry*, **50**, 900–9.

Geny, C., Yulis, J., Azoulay, A., Brugières, P., Saint-Val, C., and Degos, J.D. (1991). Thalamic infarction following lingual herpes zester. *Neurology*, **41**, 1846.

George, A.E., de Leon, M.J., and Gentes, C.I. (1986). Leukoencephalopathy in normal and pathologic aging: CT of brain lucencies. *American Journal of Neuroradiology*, **7**, 561–6.

Georgiadis, A.L., Yamamoto, Y., Kwan, E.S., Pessin, M.S., and Caplan L.R. (1999). Anatomy of sensory findings in patients with posterior cerebral artery territory infarction. *Archives of Neurology*, **56**, 835–8.

Gérald, J.M., Bouton, R., Van Nechel, Ch., and Cordonnier, M. (1998). Diploplie verticale révélatrice d'un infarctus de l'artère horoïdienne postérieure. *Revue Neurologique, Paris*, **154**, 401–7.

Gerber, O. and Gudesblatt, M. (1986). Bilateral paramedian thalamic infarctions: a CT study. *Neuroradiology*, **28**, 128–31.

Gerraty, R.P., Parsons, M., Barber, P.A., Darby, D.G., Yang, Q., Desmond, P.M., *et al.* (2001). Examining the lacunar hypothesis with diffusion and perfusion MRI (abstract). *Stroke*, in press.

Ghidoni, E., Pattacini, F., Galimberti, D., and Aguzzoli, L. (1989). Lacunar thalamic infarcts and amnesia. *European Neurology*, **29** (Suppl. 2), 13–15.

Ghika, J., Bogousslavsky, J., and Regli, F. (1989). Infarcts in the territory of the deep perforators from the carotid system. Neurology, **39**, 507–12.

Ghika, J., Bogousslavsky, J., and Regli, F. (1995). Delayed unilateral akathisia with posterior thalamic infarct. *Cerebrovascular Diseases*, **5**, 55–8.

Ghika, J., Bogousslavsky, J., Henderson, J., Maeder, P., and Regli, F. (1994). The 'jerky dystonic unsteady hand': a delayed motor syndrome in posterior thalamic infarctions. *Journal of Neurology*, **241**, 537–42.

Ghika, J.A., Bogousslavsky, J., and Regli, F. (1990). Deep perforators from the carotid system: template of the vascular territories. *Archives of Neurology*, **47**, 1097–100.

Gibbs, J.M., Leenders, K.L., Wise, R.J.S., and Jones, T. (1984). Evaluation of cerebral perfusion reserve in patients with carotid-artery occlusion. *Lancet*, **1**, 310–4.

Gillilan, L. (1968). The arterial and venous blood supplies to the forebrain (including the internal capsule) of primates. *Neurology*, **18**, 653–70.

Giroud, M., Gras, P. Chadan, N., Beuriat, P., Milan, C., Arveun, P., et al. (1991). Cerebral hemorrhage in a French prospective population study. *Journal of Neurology, Neurosurgery, and Psychiatry*, **54**, 595–8.

Giroud, M., Gras, P., Milan, C., Arveux, P., Beuriat, P., Vion, P., and Dumas, R. (1991). Natural history of lacunar syndromes. Contribution of the Dijon registry of cerebrovascular complications. *Revue Neurologique, Paris*, **147**, 566–72.

Glass, J.D., Levey, A.I., and Rothstein, J.D. (1990). The dysarthria–clumsy hand syndrome: a distinct clinical entity related to pontine infarction. *Annals of Neurology*, **27**, 487–94.

Goldblatt, D., Markesbery, W., and Reeves, A.G. (1974). Recurrent hemichorea following striatal lesions. *Archives of Neurology*, **31**, 51–4.

Goldenberg, G., Podreka, I., Pfaffelmeyer, N., Wessely, P., and Deecke, L. (1991). Thalamic ischemia in transient global amnesia: a SPECT study. *Neurology*, **41**, 1748–52.

Goldenberg, G., Wimmer, A., and Maly, J. (1983). Amnesic syndrome with a unilateral thalamic lesion: a case report. *Journal of Neurology*, **229**, 79–86.

Goldman, S., Copeland, J., Moritz, T., et al. (1988). Improvement in early saphenous vein graft patency after coronary artery bypass surgery with antiplatelet therapy: results of a Veterans Administration cooperative study. *Circulation*, **77**, 1324–32.

Goldman, S., Copeland, J., Moritz, T., et al. (1989). Saphenous vein graft patency 1 year after coronary artery bypass msurgery and effects of antiplatelet therapy: results of a Veterans Administration cooperative study. *Circulation*, **80**, 1190–207.

Gomez, C.R., Gomez, S.M., and Selhorst, J.B. (1988). Acute thalamic esotropia. *Neurology*, **38**, 1759–62.

Gonzales-Duarte, A., Cantu, C., Ruizsandoval, J., and Barinagarrementeria, F. (1998). Recurrent primary cerebral hemorrhage: frequency, mechanisms, and prognosis. *Stroke*, **29**, 1802–5.

Gonzalez, R., Schaefer, P., Buonanno, F.S., et al. (1999). Diffusion weighted MR imaging: diagnostic accuracy within 6 hours of stroke onset. *Radiology*, **210**, 155–62.

Goodman, L.S. and Gilman, A.G. (1987). *The pharmacological basis of therapeutics.* Macmillan Publishing Company, New York.

Gorczyca, W. and Mohr, G. (1987), Microvascular anatomy of Heubner's recurrent artery. *Neurological Research*, **9**, 254–64.

Gordon, D., Bendixen, B., *et al.* Interphysician agreement in the diagnosis of subtypes of acute ischemic stroke: implications for clinical trials. *Neurology*, **43**, 1021–7.

Gorelick, P.B., Amico, L.L., Ganellen, R., and Benevento L.A. (1988). Transient global amnesia and thalamic infarction. *Neurology*, **38**, 496–9.

Gorelick, P.B., Budzenski, C., Hier, D.B., Hermann, B.P., and Benevento, L. (1985). Thalamic infarction: neuropsychometric, language and CT correlates. *Neurology*, **35** (Suppl. 1), 180.

Gorelick, P.B., Hier, D.B., Benevento, L., Levitt, S., and Tan, W. (1984). Aphasia after left-thalamic infarction. *Archives of Neurology*, **41**, 1296–8.

Gorman, M.J., Dafer, R., and Levine, S.R. (1998). Ataxic hemiparesis: critical appraisal of a lacunar syndrome. *Stroke*, **29**, 2549–55.

Gorsselink, E.L. and Lodder, J. (1985). Pure sensory stroke, with lacunar infarction in the posterior ventral thalamus on CT. *Clinical Neurology and Neurosurgery*, **87**, 45–6.

Gorsselink, E.L., Peeters, H.P.M., and Lodder, J. (1984). Causes of small deep infarcts detected by CT. *Clinical Neurology and Neurosurgery*, **86**, 271–3.

Gorter, J.W., Algra, A., van Gijn, J., Kappelle, L.J., Koudstaal, P.J., Tjeerdsma, H.C., on behalf of the SPIRIT Study Group. (1997). SPIRIT: predictors of anticoagulant-related bleeding complications in patients after cerebral ischemia. *Cerebrovascular Diseases*, **7** (Suppl. 4), 3.

Goto, K., Ishii, N., and Fukasawa, H. (1981). Diffuse white-matter disease in the geriatric population. *Radiology*, **141**, 687–95.

Goto, K., Tagawa, K., Uemura, K., Ishii, K., and Takahashi, S. (1979). Posterior cerebral artery occlusion: clinical, CT, and angiographic correlation. *Radiology*, **132**, 357–68.

Graffagnino, C., Gasecki, A.P., Doig, G.S., and Hachinski, V.C. (1994). The importance of family history in cerebrovascular disease. *Stroke*, **25**, 1599–604.

Graff-Radford, N.R., Damasio, H., Yamada, T., Eslinger, P.J., and Damasio, A.R. (1985*a*). Non-hemorrhagic thalamic infarction. Clinical, neuropsychological and electrophysiological findings in four anatomic groups defined by computerized tomography. *Brain*, **108**, 485–516.

Graff-Radford, N.R., Eslinger, P.J., Damasio, A.R., and Yamada, T. (1984). Nonhemorrhagic infarction of the thalamus: behavioral, anatomic and physiologic correlates. *Neurology*, **34**, 14–23.

Graff-Radford, N.R., Schelper, R.L., Ilinsky, I.A., and Damasio, H. (1985*b*). CT and postmortem study of a nonhemorrhagic thalamic infarction. *Archives of Neurology*, **42**, 761–3.

Graff-Radford, N.R., Tranel, D., Van Hoesen, G., and Brandt, J.P. (1990). Diencephalic amnesia. *Brain*, **113**, 1–25.

Graham, G.D., Kalvach, P., Blamire, A.M., Brass, L.M., Fayad, P.B., and Prichard, J.W. (1995). Clinical correlates of proton magnetic resonance spectroscopy findings after acute cerebral infarction. *Stroke*, **26**, 225–9.

Gratton, J.A., Sauter, A., Rudin, M., Lees, K.R., McColl, J., Reid, J.L., *et al.* (1998). Susceptibility to cerebral infarction in the stroke-prone spontaneously hypertensive rat is inherited as a dominant trait. *Stroke*, **29**, 690–4.

Graveleau, P., Vider, F., Masson, M., and Cambier, J. (1986). Négligence thalamique. *Revue Neurologique, Paris*, **142**, 425–30.

Gray, F., Dubas, F., Roullet, E., and Escourolle, R. (1985). Leukoencephalopathy in diffuse haemorrhagic cerebral amyloid angiopathy. *Annals of Neurology*, **18**, 54–9.

Gray, F., Robert, F., Labrecque, R., *et al.* (1994*a*). Autosomal dominant arteriopathic leuko-encephalopathy and alzheimer's disease. *Neuropathology and Applied Neurobiology*, **20**, 22–30.

Green, R.M., Kelly, K.M., Gabrielsen, T., Levine, S.R., and Vanderzant, C. (1990). Multiple intracerebral hemorrhages after smoking 'crack' cocaine. *Stroke*, **21**, 957–62.

Greenberg, S. (1998). Cerebral amyloid angiopathy: prospects for clinical diagnosis and treatment. *Neurology*, 51, 690–4.

Greenberg, S., Finkelstein, S., and Schaefer, P. (1996). Petechial hemorrhages accompanying lobar hemorrhage: detection by gradient echo MRI. *Neurology*, 46, 1751–4.

Greenberg, S., O'Donnell, H., Schaefer, P., and Kraft, E. (1999). MRI detection of new hemorrhages: potential marker of progression in cerebral amyloid angiopathy. *Neurology*, 22, 1135–8.

Grond, M., Stenzel, C., Schmulling, S., Rudolf, J., Neveling, M., Lechleuthner, A., Schneweis, S., Heiss, W.D. (1998). Early intravenous thrombolysis for acute ischemic stroke in a community-based approach. *Stroke*, 29, 1544–9.

Groothuis, D.R., Duncan, G.W., and Fisher, C.M. (1977). The human thalamocortical sensory path in the internal capsule: evidence from a small capsular haemorrhage causing a pure sensory stroke. *Annals of Neurology*, 2, 328–31.

Gross, C.R., Kase, C.S., Mohr, J.P., Cunningham, S.C., and Baker, W.E. (1984). Stroke in South Alabama: incidence and diagnostic features. A population-based study. *Stroke*, 15, 249–55.

Gruner, J.E. and Feuerstein, J. (1966). Troubles de la conscience et tronc cérébral. Corrélations anatomo-cliniques. In *Clinical experiences in brain stem disorders* (Acta 25 Conventus Neuropsychiatricus et EEG Hungarici) (ed.I. L. Juhàsz), pp. 293–6. Vàllalat, Budapest.

Grünthal, E. (1942). Uber thalamische Demenz. *Monatsschrift für Psychiatrie und Neurologie*, 106, 114–28.

Grzyska, U., Freitag, J., and Zeumer, H. (1990). Selective cerebral intrarterial DSA. Complication rate and control of risk factors. *Neuroradiology*, 32, 296–9.

Guberman, A. and Stuss, D. (1983). The syndrome of bilateral paramedian thalamic infarction. *Neurology*, 33, 540–6.

Gubner, R.S. (1962). Systolic hypertension: a pathogenetic entity. Significance and therapeutic considerations. *American Journal of Cardiology*, 9, 773–6.

Gueyffier, F., Boissel, J., Boutitie, F., *et al.* (1997). Effect of antihypertensive treatment in patients having already suffered from stroke. *Stroke*, 28, 2557.

Gueyffier, F., Froment, A., and Gouton, M. (1996). New meta-analysis of treatment trials of hypertension. *Journal of Human Hypertension*, 10, 1–8.

Guillain, G. (1952). Pierre Marie. Sa vie et son oeuvre scientifique. *Revue Neurologique, Paris*, 86, 726–33.

Guiraud-Chaumeil, B., Rascol, A., David, J., Boneu, B., Clanet, M., and Bierme. (1982). Prévention des récidives des accidents vasculaires cérébraux ischémiques par les anti-agrégants plaquettaires. *Revue Neurologique, Paris*,

Gupta, S.R., Naheedy, M.H., Young, J.C., Ghobrial, M., Rubino, F.A., and Hindo, W. (1988). Periventricular white matter changes and dementia: clinical, neuropsychological, radiological, and pathological correlation. *Archives of Neurology*, 45, 637–41.

Gustafsson, F. (1997). Hypertensive arteriolar necrosis revisited. *Blood Pressure*, 6, 71–7.

Gutierrez-Molina, M., Caminero-Rodriguez, A., Martinez Garcia, C., *et al.* (1994). Small arterial granular degeneration in familial Binswanger's syndrome. *Acta Neuropathologica*, 87, 98–105.

Gutmann, D.H. and Scherer, S. (1989). Magnetic resonance imaging of ataxic hemiparesis localized to the corona radiata. *Stroke*, 20, 1571–3.

Gutrecht, J.A., Zamani, A.A., and Pandya, D.N. (1992). Lacunar thalamic stroke with pure cerebellar and proprioceptive deficits. *Journal of Neurology, Neurosurgery, and Psychiatry*, 55, 854–6.

Haber, S.N., Groenewegen, H.J., Grove, E.O., and Nauta, W.J.H. (1985). Efferent connections of the ventral pallidum in the rat. Evidence of a dual striato-pallidofugal pathway. *Journal of Comparative Neurology*, **235**, 322–35.

Hachinski, V.C., Potter, P., and Merskey, H. (1987). Leuko-araiosis. *Archives of Neurology*, **44**, 21–3.

Hacke, W., Brott, T., Caplau, L., *et al.* (1999). Thrombolysis in acute ischemic stroke: controled trials and clinical experience. *Neurology*, **53** (7 Suppl. 4), S3–14.

Hacke, W., Kaste, M., Fieschi, C., Toni, D., Lesaffre, E., von Kummer, R., *et al.* for the European Cooperative Acute Stroke Study Group (1995). Safety and efficacy of intravenous thrombolysis with a recombinant tissue plasminogen activator in the treatment of acute hemispheric stroke.. *Journal of the American Medical Association*, **274**, 1017–25.

Hacke, W., Kaste, M., Fieschi, C., von Kummer, R., Davalos, A., Meier, D., *et al.* (1998). Randomised double-blind placebo-controlled trial of thrombolytic therapy with intravenous alteplase in acute ischaemic stroke (ECASS II). Second European–Australasian Acute Stroke Study Investigators. *Lancet*, **352**, 1245–51.

Haferkamp, G. (1977). Das Krankheitsbild des lakunären Hirninfarktes. *Aktuelle Neurologie*, **4**, 115–20.

Hagberg, H., Andersson, P., Lacarewicz, J., Jacobson, I., Butcher, S., and Sanberg, M., (1987). Extracellular adenosine, inosine, hypoxanthine, and xanthine in relation to tissue nucleotides and purines in rat striatum during transient ischemia. *Journal of Neurochemistry*, **49**, 227–31.

Haguenau, M.D. (1965). Contribution à l'étude des syndromes sensitifs cheiro-oraux. Thèse. R. Foulon et Cie, Paris.

Hamilton, S.A. on behalf of the Standard Treatment with activase to Reverse Stroke (STARS) Investigators. (1999). Post approval experience with intravenous t-PA for treatment of acute stroke: a phase IV multicenter, prospective, monitored study.*Cerebrovascular Diseases*, **9** (Suppl. 1), 125.

Hankey, G.J. and Eikelboom, J.W. (1999). Homocysteine and vascular disease. *Lancet*, **354**, 407–13.

Hankey, G.J. and Stewart-Wynne, E.G. (1988). Amnesia following thalamic hemorrhage. Another stroke syndrome. *Stroke*, **19**, 776–8.

Hankey, G.J., Sudlow, C., and Dunbabiu, D. (2000). Thienopyridines or aspirin to prevent stroke and other serious vascular events in patients at high risk of vascular disease? A systematic review of the evidence from randomized trials. *Stroke*, **31**, 1779–84.

Hankey, G.J., Warlow, C.P., and Sellar, R.J. (1990). Cerebral angiographic risk in mild cerebrovascular disease. *Stroke*, **21**, 209–22.

Hansen, A. (1985). Effect of anoxia on ion distribution in the brain. *Physiological Reviews*, **65**, 101–48.

Hansson, L., Zanchetti, A., Carruthers, S., *et al.* (1998). Effects of intensive blood-pressure lowering and low-dose aspirin in patients with hypertension: principal results of the Hypertension Optimal Treatment (HOT) randomised trial. HOT Study Group. *Lancet*, **351**, 1755–62.

Hart, R.G., Boop, B.S., and Anderson, D.C. (1995). Oral anticoagulants and intracranial hemorrhage: facts and hypotheses. *Stroke*, **26**, 1471–7.

Hashimoto, R., Yoshida, M., and Tanaka, Y. (1995). Utilization behavior after right thalamic infarction. *European Neurology*, **35**, 58–62.

Hauw, J.J. (1988). Leuko-araiosis: the brain interstitial atrophy (atrophie interstitielle du cerveau) of Durand-Fardel. *Archives of Neurology*, **45**, 140.

Haymaker, W. (1951). Cécile and Oskar Vogt. On the occasion of her 75th and his 80th birthday. *Neurology*, **1**, 179–204.

Haymaker W. (1969). In: *Bing's Local Siagnosis in Neurological Diseases*. Mosby, Saint Louis.

Hebert, P.R., Gaziano, J.M, Chan, K.S., and Hennekens, C.H. (1997). Cholesterol lowering with statin drugs, risk of stroke, and total mortality. *Journal of the American Medical Association*, 228, 313–21.

Heiserman, J.E., Dean, B.L., Hodak, J.A., Flom, R.A., Bird, C.R., Drayer, B.P., *et al.* (1994). Neurologic complications of cerebral angiography. *American Journal of Neuroradiology*,15, 1401–7.

Helgason, C., Caplan, L.R., Goodwin, J., and Hedges, T., III (1986). Anterior choroidal artery territory infarction. Report of cases and review. *Archives of Neurology*, 43, 681–6.

Helgason, C., Wilbur, A., Weiss, A., Redmond, J., and Kingsbury, N.A. (1988). Acute pseudobulbar mutism due to discrete bilateral capsular infarction in the territory of the anterior choroidal artery. *Brain*, 11, 507–24.

Helgason, C.M. (1995). Anterior choroidal artery territory infarction. In *Lacunar and other subcortical infarctions* (ed. G.A. Donnan, B. Norrving, J. Bamford, and J. Bogousslavsky), pp. 131–8. Oxford University Press, Oxford.

Helweg, S., Larsson, H., Henricksen, O., and Sorensen, P.S. (1988). Ataxic hemiparesis: three different locations of lesions studied by MRI. *Neurology*, 38, 1322–4.

Henderson, V.W., Alexander, M.P., and Naeser, M.A. (1982). Right thalamic injury, impaired visuospatial perception and alexia. *Neurology*, 32, 235–40.

Hennerici, M., Daffertshofer, M., and Jakobs, L. (1998). Failure to identify cerebral infarct mechanisms from topography of vascular territory lesions. *American Journal of Neuroradiology*, 19, 1067–74.

Hennerici, M., Hulsbomer, H., *et al.* (1987). Natural history of asymptomatic extracranial arterial disease: results of a long-term prospective study. *Brain*, 110, 777–91.

Heo, J.H. and Choi, B.O. (1996). Hemiataxia–hypesthesia in thalamic hemorrhage. Significance of the sensory deficit patterns and presence or absence of weakness. *European Neurology*, 36, 243–4.

Herbstein, D.J. and Schaumburg, H.H. (1974). Hypertensive intracerebral hematoma: an investigation of the initial hemorrhage and rebleeding using chromium Cr^{51}-labeled erythrocytes. *Archives of Neurology*, 30, 412–4.

Herman, L.H., Ostrowski, A.Z., and Gurdjian, E.S. (1963). Perforating branches of the middle cerebral artery. *Archives of Neurology*, 8, 32–4.

Hertle, R.W. and Bienfang, D.C. (1990). Oculographic analysis of acute esotropia secondary to a thalamic hemorrhage. *Journal of Clinical Neuro-ophthalmology*, 10, 21–6.

Hier, D.B., Babcock, D.J., Foulkes, M.A., Mohr, J.P., Price, T.R., and Wolf, P.A. (1993). Influence of site on course of intracerebral hemorrhage. *Journal of Stroke and Cerebrovascular Diseases*, 3, 65–74.

Hier, D.B., Davis, K.R., Richardson, E.R., and Mohr, J.P. (1977). Hypertensive putaminal hemorrhage. *Annals of Neurology*, 1, 152–9.

Hier, D.B., Foulkes, M.A., Swiontoniowski, M., Sacco, R.L., Gorelick, P.B., Mohr, J.P., *et al.* (1991). Stroke recurrence within 2 years after ischemic infarction. *Stroke*, 22, 155–61.

Hijdra, A., Verbeeten, B., and Verhulst, J.A.P.M. (1990). Relation of leukoaraiosis to lesion type in stroke patients. *Stroke*, 21, 890–4.

Hill, G.S. (1970). Studies on the pathogenesis of hypertensive vascular disease. Effects of high-pressure intra-arterial injections in rats. *Circulation Research*, 27, 657–68.

Hojer-Pedersen, E. and Petersen, O.F. (1989). Changes of blood flow in the cerebral cortex after subcortical ischaemic infarction. *Stroke*, 20, 211–6.

Hokama, M., Tanizaki, Y., Mastuo, K., Hongo, K., and Kobayashi, S. (1993). Indications and limitations for CT-guided stereotaxic surgery of hypertensive intracerebral haemorrhage, based on the analysis of postoperative complications and poor ability of daily living in 158 cases. *Acta Neurochirurgica*, **125**, 27–33.

Hollenhorst, R.W. (1958). Ocular manifestations of insufficiency or thrombosis of the internal carotid artery. *Transactions of the American Ophthalmology Society*, **58**, 474–506.

Holmgreen, H., Leijon, G., Boivie, J., Johanson, I., and Ilievska, L. (1990). Central post-stroke pain. Somatosensory evoked potentials in relation to location of the lesion and sensory signs. *Pain*, **40**, 43–52.

Hommel, M. and Bogousslavsky, J. (1991). The spectrum of vertical gaze disturbances in unilateral upper midbrain stroke. *Neurology*, **41**, 1229–34.

Hommel, M., Besson, G., Le Bas, J.F., Gaio, J.M., Pollak, P., Borgel, F., *et al.* (1990*a*). Prospective study of lacunar infarction using magnetic resonance imaging. *Stroke*, **21**, 546–54.

Hommel, M., Besson, G., Pollak, P., Kahane, P., Le Bas, J.F., and Perret, J. (1990*b*). Hemiplegia in posterior cerebral artery occlusion. *Neurology*, **40**,1496–9.

Hommel, M., DuBois, F., Pollak, P., Francois, A., Borgel, F., Gaio, J.M., *et al.* (1985). Syndrome de l'artère choroidienne antérieure gauche avec troubles du language et apraxie constructive. *Revue Neurologique, Paris*, **141**, 137–42.

Hommel, M., Gaio, J. M., Pollak, P., Borgel, F., and Perret, J. (1987). Hémiparésie ataxique par lacune thalamique. *Revue Neurologique, Paris*, **143**, 602–4.

HOPE (2000). Effects of ramipril on cardiovascular and microvascular outcomes in people with diabetes mellitus: results of the HOPE study and MICRO-HOPE substudy. *Lancet*, **355**, 253–9.

Horowitz, D.H., Tuhrim, S., Weinberger, J., and Rudolph, S.H. (1992). Mechanisms in lacunar infarction. *Stroke*, **23**, 325–7.

Horowitz, S.H., Zito, J.L., Donnarumma, R., Patel, M., and Alvir, J. (1991). Computed tomographic–angiographic findings within the first five hours of cerebral infarction. *Stroke*, **22**, 1245–53.

Hougaku, H., Matsumoto, M., *et al.* (1994). Asymptomatic carotid lesions and silent cerebral infarction. *Stroke*, **25**, 566–70.

Howard, G., Evans, G.W., Crouse, J.R., Toole, J.F., Ryu, J.E., Tegeler, C. (1994). A prospective reevaluation of transient ischemic attacks as a risk factor for death and fatal or nonfatal cardiovascular events. *Stroke*, **25**, 342–5.

Hoyt, W.F. (1975). Geniculate hemianopias: incongruous visual defects from partial involvement of the lateral geniculate body. *Proceedings of the Australian Association of Neurologists*, **12**, 7–16.

Huang, C.Y., Woo, E., Yu, Y.L., and Chan, F.L. (1987). When is sensorimotor stroke a lacunar syndrome? *Journal of Neurology, Neurosurgery, and Psychiatry*, **50**, 720–6.

Hughes, W. (1965). Hypothesis—origin of lacunes. *Lancet*, **2**, 19–21.

Hupperts, R.M., Lodder, J., Heuts-van Raak, E.P., and Kessels, F. (1994). Infarcts in the anterior choroidal artery territory. Anatomical distribution, clinical syndromes, presumed pathogenesis and early outcome. *Brain*, **117**, 825–34.

Hupperts, R.M., Warlow, C.P., Slattery, J., and Rothwell, P.M. (1997*a*). Severe stenosis of the internal carotid artery is not associated with borderzone infarcts in patients randomised in the European Carotid Surgery Trial. *Journal of Neurology*, **244**, 45–50.

Hupperts, R.M.M., Lodder, J., Heuts-van Raak, L., and Kessels, F. (1997*b*). Borderzone small deep infarcts: vascular risk-factors and relationship with signs of small- and large-vessel disease. *Cerebrovascular Diseases*, **7**, 280–3.

Hutchinson, M., O'Riordan, J., Javed, M., *et al.* (1995). Familial hemiplegic migraine and autosomal dominant arteriopathy with leukoencephalopathy (CADASIL). *Annals of Neurology*, 38, 817–24.

Imaizumi, T., Kocsis, J.D., and Waxman, S.G. (1999). The role of voltage-gated Ca^{2+} channels in anoxic injury of spinal cord white matter, *Brain Research*, 817, 84–92.

Ince, B., Petty, G.W., Brown, R.D., Jr, Chu, C.P., Sicks, J.D., and Whisnant, J.P. (1998). Dolichoectasia of the intracranial arteries in patients with first ischemic stroke: a population-based study. *Neurology*, 50,1694–8.

International Headache Society (1988). Classification and diagnostic criteria for headache disorders, cranial neuralgias and facial pain. *Cephalalgia*, Suppl. 7, 8.

Inzitari, D., Cadelo, M., Marranci, M.L., Pracucci, G., and Pantoni, L. (1997). Vascular deaths in elderly neurological patients with leukoaraiosis. *Journal of Neurology, Neurosurgery, and Psychiatry*, 62, 177–81

Inzitari, D., Di Carlo, A.S., Mascalchi, M., Pracucci, G., and Amaducci, L. (1995). The cardiovascular outcome of patient with motor impairment and extensive leukoaraiosis. *Archives of Neurology*, 52, 687–91.

Inzitari, D., Diaz, F., Fox, A., Hachinski, V.C., Steingart, A., Lau, C., *et al.* (1987). Vascular risk factors and leukoaraiosis. *Archives of Neurology*, 44, 42–7.

Inzitari, D., Eliasziw, M., Sharpe, B.L., Fox, A.J., Barnett, H.J.M., for the North American Symptomatic Carotid Endarterectomy Trial Group (2000). Risk factors and outcome of patients with carotid artery stenosis presenting with lacunar stroke. *Neurology*, 54, 660–6.

Inzitari, D., Giordano, G., Ancona, A., Pracucci, G., Mascalchi, M., and Amaducci, L. (1990). Leukoaraiosis, intracerebral hemorrhage, and arterial hypertension. *Stroke*, 21, 1419–23.

Iragui, V.J. and McCutchen, C.B. (1982). Capsular ataxic hemiparesis. *Archives of Neurology*, 39, 528–9.

Isaka, Y., Okamoto, M., Ashida, K., and Imaizumi, M. (1994). Decreased cerebrovascular dilatory capacity in subjects with asymptomatic periventricular hyperintensities. *Stroke*, 25, 375–81.

IST (1997). The international stroke trial (IST): a randomised trial of aspirin, subcutaneous heparin, both or neither among 19435 patients with acute ischemic stroke. *Lancet*, 349, 1569–81.

Jack, J.J.B., Noble, D., and Tsien, R.W. (1983). *Electric current flow in excitable cells.* Oxford University Press, London.

Jackel, R.J. and Harner, R.N. (1989). Computed EEG topography in acute stroke. *Neurophysiologie Clinique*, 19, 185–97.

Jackel, R.J., Dhaduk, V., Hooker, M., Mawhinney-Hee, M., and Harner, R.N. (1987). Computed EEG topography in acute stroke. *Neurology*, 37 (Suppl. 1), 364.

Jacobs, L., Anderson, P.J., and Bender, M.B. (1973). The lesions producing paralysis of downward but not upward gaze. *Archives of Neurology*, 28, 319–23.

Jacobson, K.A., van Galen, P.J.M., and Williams, M. (1992). Adenosine receptors: pharmacology, structure–activity relationships, and therapeutic potential. *Journal of Medical Chemistry*, 35, 407–22.

Jain, K.K. (1964). Some observations on the anatomy of the middle cerebral artery. *Canadian Journal of Surgery*, 7, 134–9.

Jakimowicz, W., Stefanko, S., and Pajak, B. (1968). Ramollissements du thalamus dans le territoire des pédicules artériels venant de la cérébrale postérieure. *Acta Medica Polonia*, 9, 447–54.

Janati, A., Kidwai, S., Balachdran, S., Dang, M.T., and Harrington, D. (1987). A comparative study of electroencephalography and computed axial tomography in recent cerebral infarction. *Clinical Electroencephalography*, 18, 20–5.

Jankovic, J. and Patel, S.C. (1983). Blepharospasm associated with brainstem lesions. *Neurology*, 33, 1237–40.

Jeffs, B., Clark, J.S., Anderson, N.H., Gratton, J., Brosnan, M.J., Gauguier, D., *et al.* (1997). Sensitivity to cerebral ischaemic insult in a rat model of stroke is determined by a single genetic locus. *Nature Genetics*, 16, 364–7.

Johnson, E., Lanes, S., Wentworth, Cr., Safferfield, M., Abebe, B., and Dicker, L. (1999). A metaregression analysis of the dose–response effect of aspirin on stroke. *Archives of Internal Medicine*, 159, 1248–53.

Jones, H.R., Baker, R.A., and Kott, H. S. (1985). Hypertensive putaminal hemorrhage presenting with hemichorea. *Stroke*, 16, 130–1.

Jonkman, E.J., Van Huffelen, A.C., and Pfurtscheller, G. (1986). Quantitative EEG in cerebral ischemia. In *Clinical applications of computer analysis of EEG and other neurophysiological signs* (ed. F.H. Lopes da Silva, W. Storm van Leeuwen, and A. Rémond), pp. 205–37. Elsevier, Amsterdam.

Jørgensen, L. and Torvik, A. (1969). Ischaemic cerebrovascular diseases in an autopsy series. Part 2. Prevalence, location, pathogenesis and clinical course of cerebral infarcts. *Journal of the Neurological Sciences*, 9, 285–320.

Jousilahti, P., Rastenyte, D., Tuomilehto, J., Sarti, C., and Vartiainen, E. (1997). Parental history of cardiovascular disease and risk of stroke: a prospective follow-up of 14 371 middle-aged men and women in Finland. *Stroke*, 28, 1361–6.

Joutel, A. and Tournier-Lasserve, E. (1998). Notch signalling pathway and human diseases. *Seminars in Cell and Developmental Biology*, 9, 619–25.

Joutel, A., Andreux, F., Gaulis, S., *et al.* (2000a). The ectodomain of the Notch3 receptor accumulates within the cerebrovasculature of CADASIL patients. *Journal of Clinical Investigation*, 105, 597–605.

Joutel, A., Corpechot, C., Ducros, A., *et al.* (1996). Notch3 mutations in CADASIL, a hereditary adult-onset condition causing stroke and dementia. *Nature*, 383, 707–10.

Joutel, A., Dodick, D.D., Parisi, J.E., *et al.* (2000b). *De novo* mutation in the *Notch3* gene causing CADASIL. *Annals of Neurology*, 47, 388–91.

Jungquist, G., Hanson, B.S., Isacsson, S.-O., Janzon, K., Steen, B., and Lindell, S.-E. (1991). Risk factors for carotid artery stenosis: an epidemiological study of men aged 69 years. *Journal of Clinical Epidemiology*, 44, 347–53.

Junque, C., Pujol, J., Vendrell, P., Bruna, O., Jodar, M., Ribas, J.C., *et al.* (1990). Leukoaraiosis on magnetic resonance imaging and speed of mental processing. *Archives of Neurology*, 47, 151–6.

Juvela, S. (1995). Risk factors for impaired outcome after spontaneous intracerebral hemorrhage. *Archives of Neurology*, 52, 1193–200.

Juvela, S., Heiskanen, O., Poranen, A., Valtonen, S., Kuurne, T., Kabre, M., *et al.* (1989). The treatment of spontaneous intracerebral hemorrhage: a prospective randomized trial of surgical and conservative treatment. *Journal of Neurosurgery*, 70, 755–8.

Kaczorowski, G.H., Slaughter, R.S., King, V.F., and Garcia, M.L. (1989). Inhibitors of sodium–calcium exchange: identification and development of probes of transport activity, *Biochimica et Biophysica Acta*, 998, 287–302.

Kanaya, H., Yukawa, H., Itoh, Z., Kutsuzawa, H., Kagawa, M., Kanno, T., *et al.* (1980). Grading and the indications for treatment in ICH of the basal ganglia (cooperative study in Japan). In *Spontaneous intracerebral haematomas: advances in diagnosis and therapy* (ed. H.W. Pia, C. Langmaid, and J. Zierski), pp. 268–74. Springer-Verlag, Heidelberg.

Kaneko, M., Tanaka, K., Shimada, T., Sato, K., and Uemura, K. (1983). Long-term evaluation of ultra-early operation for hypertensive intracerebral hemorrhage in 100 cases. Journal of Neurosurgery, **58**, 838–42.

Kang, D.W., Roh, J.K., Lee, Y.S., Song, I.C., Yoon, B.W., and Chang, K.H. (2000). Neuronal metabolic changes in the cortical region after subcortical infarction: a proton MR spectroscopy study. *Journal of Neurology, Neurosurgery, and Psychiatry*, **69**, 222–7.

Kanno, T., Sano, H., Shinomiya, Y., Katada, K., Nagata, J., Hoshino, M., *et al.* (1984). Role of surgery in hypertensive intracerebral hematoma: a comparative study of 305 nonsurgical and 154 surgical cases. *Journal of Neurosurgery*, **61**, 1091–9.

Kaplan, H.A. (1965). The lateral perforating branches of the anterior and middle cerebral arteries. *Journal of Neurosurgery*, **23**, 305–10.

Kaplan, H.A. and Ford, D.H. (1966). *The brain vascular system*, pp. 46–69. Elsevier, Amsterdam.

Kaplan, R.F., Estol, C.J., Damasio, H., Tettenborn, B., and Caplan, L.R. (1991). Bilateral polar artery thalamic infarcts. *Neurology*, **41** (Suppl. 1), 329.

Kappelle, L.J. and Van Gijn, J. (1986). Lacunar infarcts. *Clinical Neurology and Neurosurgery*, **88**, 3–17.

Kappelle, L.J., Koudstaal, P.J., Van Gijn, J., Ramos, L.M.P., and Keunen, J.E.E. (1988). Carotid angiography in patients with lacunar infarcts—a prospective study. *Stroke*, **19**, 1093–6.

Kappelle, L.J., Ramos, L.M.P., and Van Gijn, J. (1989). The role of computed tomography in patients with lacunar stroke in the carotid territory. *Neuroradiology*, **31**, 316–9.

Kappelle, L.J., Van Huffelen, A.C., and Van Gijn, J. (1990). Is the EEG really normal in lacunar stroke? *Journal of Neurology, Neurosurgery, and Psychiatry*, **53**, 63–6.

Kappelle, L.J., van Latrum, J.C., van Swieten, J.C., Algra, A., Koudstaal, P.J., van Gijn, J, for the Dutch TIA Trial Study Group (1995). Recurrent stroke and transient ischaemic attack or minor ischaemic stroke: does the distinction between small and large vessel disease remain true to type? *Journal of Neurology, Neurosurgery, and Psychiatry*, **59**, 127–31.

Karabelas, G., Kalfakis, N., Kasvikis, I., and Vassilopoulos, D. (1985). Unusual features in a case of bilateral paramedian thalamic infarction. *Journal of Neurology, Neurosurgery, and Psychiatry*, **48**, 186.

Karalis, D.G., Chandrasekaran, K., Victor, M.F., Ross, J.J., and Mintz, G.S. (1991). Recognition and embolic potential of intraaortic atherosclerotic debris. *Journal of the American College of Cardiology*, **17**, 73–8.

Karni, A., Sadeh, M., Blatt, I., and Goldhammer, Y. (1991). Cogan's syndrome complicated by lacunar brain infarcts. *Journal of Neurology, Neurosurgery, and Psychiatry*, **54**, 169–71.

Karussis, D., Leker, R.R., and Abramsky, O. (2000). Cognitive dysfunction following thalamic stroke: a study of 16 cases and review of the literature. *Journal of the Neurological Sciences*, **172**, 25–9.

Kase, C.S. (1986). Intracerebral hemorrhage: non-hypertensive causes. *Stroke*, **17**, 590–5.

Kase, C.S. (1994). Intracranial tumors. In *Intracerebral hemorrhage* (eds. C.S. Kase and L.R. Caplan), pp. 243–61. Butterworth-Heinemann, Boston.

Kase, C.S. (2001). Intracerebral hemorrhage. In *Clinical trials in neurology* (ed. J. Bogousslavsky and J. Biller), pp. 49–62. Butterworth-Heinemann, Boston.

Kase, C.S. and Crowell, R.M. (1994). Prognosis and treatment of patients with intracerebral hemorrhage. In *Intracerebral hemorrhage* (eds. C.S. Kase and L.R. Caplan), pp. 467–89. Butterworth-Heinemann, Boston.

Kase, C.S., Foster, T.E., Reed, J.E., Spatz, E.L., and Girgis, G.N. (1987). Intracerebral hemorrhage and phenylpropanolamine use. *Neurology*, **37**, 399–404.

Kase, C.S., Maulsby, G.O., Mohr, J.P., and DeJuan, E. (1981). Hemichorea–hemiballism and lacunar infarction in the basal ganglia. *Neurology*, 31, 452–5.

Kase, C.S., Williams, J.P., Wyatt, D.A., and Mohr, J.P. (1982). Lobar intracerebral hematomas: clinical and CT analysis of 22 cases. *Neurology*, 32, 1146–50.

Kashihara, M. and Matsumoto, K. (1985). Acute capsular infarction. *Neuroradiology*, 27, 248–53.

Kastrup, O., Schwarz, M., Ringelstein, E.B., and Weiller, C. (1992). Morphometric differentiation of large embolic and haemodynamic subcortical infarcts. *Cerebrovascular Diseases*. 2, 233.

Kato, H., Sugawara, Y., Ito, H., Onodera, K., Sato, C., and Kogure, K. (1991). Somatosensory evoked potentials following stimulation of median and tibial nerves in patients with localized intracerebral hemorrhage: correlations with clinical and CT findings. *Journal of the Neurological Sciences*, 103, 172–8.

Kato, M., Miyashita, N., Hikosaka, O., Matsumura, M., Usui, S., and Kori, A. (1995). Eye movements in monkeys with local dopamine depletion in the caudate nucleus. I. Deficits in spontaneous saccades. *Journal of Neuroscience*, 15, 912–27.

Katz, D.I, Alexander, M.P., and Mandell, A.M. (1987). Dementia following strokes in the mesencephalon and diencephalon. *Archives of Neurology*, 44, 1127–33.

Kawakami, Y., Chikama, M., Tanimoto, T., and Shimamura, Y. (1989). Radiological studies of the cheiro-oral syndrome. *Journal of Neurology*, 236, 177–81.

Kawamura, M., Takahashi, N., and Hirayama, K. (1988). Hemichorea and its denial in a case of caudate infarction diagnosed by magnetic resonance imaging. *Journal of Neurology, Neurosurgery, and Psychiatry*, 51, 590–1.

Kayser-Gatchalian, N.C. and Neundorfer, B. (1980). The prognostic value of the EEG in ischemic cerebral insults. *Electroencephalography and Clinical Neurophysiology*, 57, 343–6.

Kazui, S., Levi, C.R., Jones, E.F., Quang, L., Calafiore, P., and Donnan, G.A. (2001). Lacunar stroke: transesophageal echocardiographic factors influencing long-term prognosis. *Cerebrovascular Diseases*, in press.

Kelley, R.E., Berger, J.R., Scheinberg, P., and Stokes, N. (1982). Active bleeding in hypertensive intracerebral hemorrhage: computed tomography. *Neurology*, 32, 852–6.

Kertesz, A., Black, S.E., Tokar, G., Benke, T., Carr, T., and Nicholson, L. (1988). Periventricular and subcortical hyperintensities on magnetic resonance imaging: 'rims, caps and unidentified bright objects'. *Archives of Neurology*, 45, 404–8.

Kertesz, A., Polk, M., and Carr, T. (1990). Cognition and white matter changes on magnetic resonance imaging in dementia. *Archives of Neurology*, 47, 387–91.

Kessler, C., Kummer, R., and Von Herold, S. (1982). Zur etiologie der doppel-seitigen, symmetrischen Thalamusläsion. *Nervenarzt*, 53, 406–10.

Kessler, C., Spitzer, C., Stauske, D., Mende, S., Stadlmuller, J., Walther, R., et al. (1997). The apolipoprotein E and beta-fibrinogen G/A-455 gene polymorphisms are associated with ischemic stroke involving large-vessel disease. *Arteriosclerosis, Thrombosis, and Vascular Biology*, 17, 2880–4.

Khodorov, B.I. (1991). Role of inactivation in local anesthetic action. *Annals of the New York Academy of Sciences*, 625, 224–8.

Khoury, M.J. and Yang, Q.H. (1998). The future of genetic studies of complex human diseases: an epidemiologic perspective. *Epidemiology*, 9, 350–4.

Kidwell, C.S., Saver, J.L., Mattiello, J., Starkman, S., Vinuela, F., Duckwiler, G., et al. (2000). Thrombolytic reversal of acute human cerebral ischemic injury shown by diffusion/perfusion magnetic resonance imaging. *Annals of Neurology*, 47, 462–9.

Kiely, D.K., Wolf P.A., Cupples L.A., Beiser A.S., and Myers R.H. (1993). Familial aggregation of stroke. The Framingham Study. *Stroke*, 24, 1366–71.

Kim, J.S. (1992). Delayed onset hand tremor caused by cerebral infarction. *Stroke*, 23, 292–4.

Kim, J.S. (1994). Restricted acral sensory syndrome following minor stroke. Further observation with special reference to differential severity among individual digits. *Stroke*, 25, 2497–502.

Kim, J.S. (1996). Restricted nonacral sensory syndrome. *Stroke*, 27, 988–90.

Kim, J.S. (1997). Cheiro-oral syndrome with vivid recollection of past in thalamic infarction. *European Neurology*, 37, 253–4.

Kim, J.S. (1999). Lenticulocapsular hemorrhages presenting as pure sensory stroke. *European Neurology*, 42, 128–31.

Kim, J.S., Im, J.H., Kwon, S.U., Kang, J.H., and Lee, M.C. (1998). Micrographia after thalamo-mesencephalic infarction: evidence of striatal dopaminergic hypofunction. *Neurology*, 51, 625–7.

Kim, J.S., Lee, J.H., and Lee, M.C. (1994). Small primary intracerebral hemorrhage: clinical presentation of 28 cases. *Stroke*, 25, 1500–6.

Kim, J.W., Kim, S.H., and Cha, J.K. (1999). Pseudochoreoathethosis in four patients with hypesthesic ataxic hemiparesis in a thalamic lesion. *Journal of Neurology*, 246, 1075–1079.

Kimura, M., Tanaka, A., and Yoshinaga, S. (1992). Significance of periventricular hemodynamics in normal pressure hydrocephalus. *Neurosurgery*, 30, 701–4.

Kinkel, W.R., Jacobs, L., Polachini, I., Bates, V., and Heffner, R.R., Jr (1985). Subcortical arteriosclerotic encephalopathy (Binswanger's disease): computed tomographic, nuclear magnetic resonance, and clinical correlations. *Archives of Neurology*, 42, 951–9.

Kinney, H.C., Korein, J., Panigrahy, A., Dikkes, P., and Goode, R. (1994). Neuropathological findings in the brain of Karen Ann Quinlan. The role of thalamus in the persistent vegetative state. *New England Journal of Medicine*, 330, 1469–75.

Kirkpatrick, J.B. and Hayman, L.A. (1987). White-matter lesions in MR imaging of clinically healthy brains of elderly subjects: possible pathologic basis. *Radiology*, 162, 509–11.

Kleist, K. (1950). Oskar Vogt 80 Jahre, Cécile Vogt 75 Jahre. *Archives of Psychiatry Zeitsch Neurology*, 185, 619–23.

Kleist, K., and Gonzalo, J. (1938). Über Thalamus- und Subthalamus Syndrome und die Störungen einzelner Thalamuskerne. *Monatsschrift für Psychiatrie und Neurologie*, 99, 87–130.

Kleyman, T. R. and Cragoe, E.J.J. (1988). Amiloride and its analogs as tools in the study of ion transport. *Journal of Membrane Biology*, 105, 1–21.

Kloster, F.E. (1975). Diagnosis and management of complications of prosthetic heart valves. *American Journal of Cardiology*, 35, 872–85.

Knibestöl, M., Hägg, E., and Liliequist, B. (1988). Discrepancies between CT and EEG findings after acute cerebrovascular disease. *Uppsala Journal of Medical Sciences*, 93, 63–9.

Kobari, M., Ishihara, N., and Yunoki, K. (1987). Bilateral thalamic infarction associated with selective downward gaze paralysis. *European Neurology*, 26, 246–51.

Kobari, M., Meyer, J.S., and Ichijo, M. (1990a). Leukoaraiosis, cerebral atrophy, and cerebral perfusion in normal aging. *Archives of Neurology*, 47, 161–5.

Kobari, M., Meyer, J.S., Ichijo, M., and Oravez, W.T. (1990b). Leukoaraiosis: correlation of MR and CT findings with blood flow, atrophy, and cognition. *American Journal of Neuroradiology*, 11, 273–81.

Koh, K. (2000). Effects of statins on vascular wall: vasomotor function, inflammation, and plaque stability. *Cardiovascular Research*, 47, 648–57.

Kohler, H.P., Ariens, R.A., Whitaker, P., and Grant, P.J. (1998a). A common coding polymorphism in the FXIII A-subunit gene (FXIIIVal34Leu) affects cross-linking activity. *Thrombosis and Haemostasis*, **80**, 704.

Kohler, H.P., Futers, T.S., and Grant, P.J. (1999). Prevalence of three common polymorphisms in the A-subunit gene of factor XIII in patients with coronary artery disease—association with FXIII activity and antigen levels. *Thrombosis and Haemostasis*, **81**, 511–5.

Kohler, H.P., Stickland, M.H., OsseiGerning, N., Carter, A., Mikkola, H., and Grant, P.J. (1998b). Association of a common polymorphism in the factor XIII gene with myocardial infarction. *Thrombosis and Haemostasis*, **79**, 8–13.

Kolisko, A. (1891). *Uber die Beziehung der arteria choroidea anterior zum hinteren Schenkel der inneren Kapsel des Gehirnres*. A. Holder, Vienna.

Kölmel, H.W. (1991). Peduncular hallucinations. *Journal of Neurology*, **238**, 457–9.

Kömpf, D., Oppermann, J., Künig, F., Talmon-Gros, S., and Babaian, E. (1984). Vertikale Blickpause und thalamische Demenz. Syndrom der posterioren thalamo-subthalamischen paramedianen Arterie. *Nervenarzt*, **55**, 625–36.

Kondziolka, D., Lunsford, D., Flickinger, J.C., and Kestle, J.R.W. (1995). Reduction of hemorrhage risk after stereotactic radiosurgery of cavernous malformations. *Journal of Neurosurgery*, **83**, 825–31.

Kooistra, C.A. and Heilman, K.M. (1988). Memory loss from a subcortical white matter infarct. *Journal of Neurology, Neurosurgery, and Psychiatry*, **51**, 866–9.

Kori, A., Miyashita, N., Kato, M., Hikosaka, O., Usui, S., and Matsumura, M. (1995), Eye movements in monkeys with local dopamine depletion in the caudate nucleus. II. Deficits in voluntary saccades. *Journal of Neuroscience*, **15**, 928–41.

Kosner, S. and Sparr, S.A. (1992). Inverse cheiro-oral syndrome. *Annals of Neurology*, **32**, 266–7.

Kotila, M., Hokkanen, L., Laaksonen, R., and Valanne, L. (1994). Long-term prognosis after left tuberothalamic infarction: a study of 7 cases. *Cerebrovascular Diseases*, **4**, 44–50.

Koto, A., Rosenberg, G., Zingesser, L.H., Horoupian, D., and Katzman, R. (1977). Syndrome of normal pressure hydrocephalus: possible relation to hypertensive and arteriosclerotic vasculopathy. *Journal of Neurology, Neurosurgery, and Psychiatry*, **40**, 73–9.

Krapf, H., Widder, B., and Skalej, M. (1998). Small rosarylike infarctions in the centrum ovale suggest haemodynamic failure. *American Journal of Neuroradiology*, **19**, 1479–84.

Kritchevsky, M., Graff-Radford, N.R., and Damasio, A.R. (1987). Normal memory after damage to medial thalamus. *Archives of Neurology*, **44**, 959–62.

Krul, J.M.J., Van Gijn, J., Ackerstaff, R.G.A., Eikelboom, B.C., Theodorides, T., and Vermeulen, F.E.E. (1989). Site and pathogenesis of infarcts associated with carotid endarterectomy. *Stroke*, **20**, 324–8.

Krystkowiak, P., Martinat, P., Defebvre, L., Pruvo, J.P., Leys, D., and Destée, A. (1998). Dystonia after stratopallidal and thalamic stroke: clinicoradiological correlations and pathophysiological mechanisms. *Journal of Neurology, Neurosurgery, and Psychiatry*, **65**, 703–8.

Kubota, M., Yamaura, A., Ono, J., Itani, T., Tachi, N., Ueda, K., *et al.* (1997). Is family history an independent risk factor for stroke? *Journal of Neurology, Neurosurgery, and Psychiatry*, **62**, 66–70.

Kucharczyk, J., Vexler, Z.S., Roberts, T.P., Asgari, H.S., Mintorovitch, J., Derugin, N., *et al.* (1993). Echo-planar perfusion-sensitive MR imaging of acute cerebral ischemia. *Radiology*, **188**, 711–7.

Kulisevsky, J., Avila, A., Roig, C., and Escartín, A. (1993a). Unilateral blepharospam stemming from a thalamomesencephalic lesion. *Movement Disorders*, **8**, 239–40.

Kulisevsky, J., Berthier, M.L., and Pujol, J. (1993*b*). Hemiballismus and secondary mania following a right thalamic infarction. *Neurology*, 43, 1422–4.

Kuller, L.H., Shemanski, L., Manolio, T., Haan, M., Fried, L., Bryan, N., *et al.* (1998). Relationship between ApoE, MRI findings, and cognitive function in the Cardiovascular Health Study. *Stroke*, 29, 388–98.

Kumral, E., Evyapan, D., and Balkir, K. (1999). Acute caudate vascular lesions. *Stroke*, 30, 100–8.

Kumral, E., Kocaer, T., Ertubey, N.O., and Kumral, K. (1995). Thalamic hemorrhage: a prospective study of 100 patients. *Stroke*, 26, 964–70.

Kuwert, T., Hennerici, M., Langen, K.J., Aulich, A., Herzog, H., Sitzer, M., *et al.* (1991). Regional cerebral glucose consumption measured by PET in patients with unilateral thalamic infarction. *Cerebrovascular Diseases*, 1, 327–36.

Kwa, V., Franke, C., Verbeeten, B., and Stam, J. (1998). Silent intracerebral microhemorrhages in patients with ischemic stroke. *Annals of Neurology*, 44, 372–7.

Labauge, R., Pages, M., Marty-Double, C., Blard, J.M., Boukobza, M., and Salvaing, P. (1981). Occlusion du tronc basilaire. *Revue Neurologique, Paris*, 137, 545–71.

Lai, M.L., Hsu, Y.I., Ma, S., and Yu, C.Y. (1995). Magnetic resonance spectroscopic findings in patients with subcortical ischemic stroke. *Chung Hua I Hsueh Tsa Chih (Taipei)*, 56, 31–5.

Laloux, P. and Brucher, J.M. (1991). Lacunar infarctions due to cholesterol emboli. *Stroke*, 22, 1440–4.

Lammie, G.A. (1998). The role of oedema in lacune formation. *Cerebrovascular Diseases*, 8, 246.

Lammie, G.A. and Wardlaw, J.M. (1999). Small centrum ovale infarcts—a pathological study. *Cerebrovascular Diseases*, 9, 82–90.

Lammie, G.A., Brannan, F., and Wardlaw, J.M. (1998). Incomplete lacunar infarction (type 1b lacunes). *Acta Neuropathologica*, 96, 163–71.

Lammie, G.A., Brannan, F., Slattery, J., and Warlow, C.P. (1997). Nonhypertensive cerebral small-vessel disease—an autopsy study. *Stroke*, 28, 2222–9.

Lammie, G.A., Rakshi, J., Rossor, M.N., *et al.* (1995). Cerebral autosomal dominant arteriopathy with subcortical infarcts and leukoencephalopathy (CADASIL)—confirmation by cerebral biopsy in 2 cases. *Clinical Neuropathology*, 14, 201–6.

Lammie, G.A., Sandercock, P.A.G., and Dennis, M.S. (1999). Recently occluded intracranial and extracranial carotid arteries. Relevance of the unstable atherosclerotic plaque. *Stroke*, 30, 1319–25.

Lampl, Y., Gilad, R., Eshel, Y., and Sarova-Pinhas, I. (1995). Neurological and functional outcome in patients with supratentorial hemorrhages. *Stroke*, 26, 2249–53.

Landau, W.M. (1989). Clinical neuromythology VI. Au clair de lacune: holy, wholly, holey logic. *Neurology*, 39, 725–30.

Landi, G., Anzalone, N., and Vaccari, U. (1984). CT evidence of posterolateral thalamic infarction in pure sensory stroke. *Journal of Neurology, Neurosurgery, and Psychiatry*, 47, 570–1.

Landi, G., Anzalone, N., Cella, E., Boccardi, E., and Musicco, M. (1991). Are sensorimotor strokes lacunar strokes? A case–control study of lacunar and non-lacunar strokes. *Journal of Neurology, Neurosurgery, and Psychiatry*, 54, 1063–8.

Landi, G., Cella, E., Boccardi, E., and Musicco, M. (1992). Lacunar versus non-lacunar infarcts: pathogenetic and prognostic differences. *Journal of Neurology, Neurosurgery, and Psychiatry*, 55, 441–45.

Lanoe, Y., Pedetti, L., Lanoe, A., Mayer, J.M., and Evrard, S. (1994). Aphasie par lésion isolée du centre semi-ovale: apport de la mesure du débit sanguin cérébral. *Revue Neurologique, Paris*, 150, 430–4.

Laplane, D., Baulac, M., and Carydakis, C. (1986). Négligence motrice d'origine thalamique. *Revue Neurologique, Paris*, 142, 375–9.

Laplane, D., Escourolle, R., Degos, J.D., Sauron, B., and Massiou, H. (1982). La négligence motrice d'origine thalamique. A propos de deux cas. *Revue Neurologique, Paris*, 138, 201–11.

Lapresle, J. and Hagueneau, M. (1973). Anatomo-clinical correlation in focal thalamic lesions. *Zeitschrift für Neurologie*, 205, 29–46.

Lassen, N.A. (1982). Incomplete cerebral infarction: focal incomplete ischemic tissue necrosis not leading to emollision. *Stroke*, 13, 522–3.

Lassen, N.A., Olsen, T.S., Hougaard, K., and Skriver, E. (1983). Incomplete infarction: a CT negative irreversible ischaemic brain lesion. *Journal of Cerebral Blood Flow and Metabolism*, 3 (Suppl. 1), S602–3.

Lauterbach, E.C. (1994). Fluoxetine withdrawal and thalamic pain. *Neurology*, 44, 983–4.

Lazzarino, C.G., Nicolai, A., Valassi, F., and Biasizzo, E. (1991). Language disturbances from mesencephalon–thalamic infarcts: identification of thalamic nuclei by CT-reconstruction. *Neuroradiology*, 33, 300–304.

Lazzarino, L.G. and Nicolai, A. (1988). Aphonia as the only speech disturbance from bilateral thalamic infarction. *Clinical Neurology and Neurosurgery*, 90, 265–7.

Lechi, A. and Macchi, G. (1974). Le syndrome du pédicule artériel rétro-mamillaire. *Acta Neurologica Belgica*, 74, 13–24.

Lechner, H., Schmidt, R., Bertha, G., Justich, E., Offenbacher, H., and Schneider, G. (1988). Nuclear magnetic resonance image white matter lesions and risk factors for stroke in normal individuals. *Stroke*, 19, 263–5.

Lee, L.J., Kidwell, C.S., Alger, J., Starkman, S., and Saver, J.L. (2000). Impact on stroke subtype diagnosis of early diffusion-weighted magnetic resonance imaging and magnetic resonance angiography. *Stroke*, 31, 1081–9.

Lee, M.S., Kim, Y.D., Kim, J.T., and Lyoo, C.H. (1998). Abrupt onset of transient pseudo-choreoathetosis associated with proprioceptive sensory loss as a result of a thalamic infarction. *Movement Disorders*, 13, 184–6.

Lee, M.S., Lee S.A., Heo, J.H., and Choi, I.S. (1993). A patient with a resting tremor and a lacunar infarction at the border between the thalamus and the internal capsule. *Movement Disorders*, 8, 244–6.

Lee, N., Roh, J.K., and Nyung, H. (1989). Hypesthetic ataxic hemiparesis in a thalamic lacune. *Stroke*, 20, 819–21.

Leenders, K.L., Frackowiak R.S.J., Quinn, N., Brooks, D., Sumner, D., and Marsden C.D. (1986). Ipsilateral blepharospasm and contralateral hemidystonia and parkinsonism in a patient with a unilateral rostral brainstem–thalamic lesion: structural and functional abnormalities studied with CT, MRI, and PET scanning. *Movement Disorders*, 1, 51–58.

Lehéricy, S., Vidailhet, M., Dormont, D., Piérot, L., Chiras, J., Mazetti, P., et al. (1996). Striatopallidal and thalamic dystonia: a magnetic resonance imaging anatomoclinical study. *Archives of Neurology*, 53, 241–50.

Leifer, D., Buonanno, F.S., and Richardson, E.P., Jr (1990). Clinicopathologic correlations of cranial magnetic resonance imaging of periventricular white matter. *Neurology*, 40, 911–8.

Lellouch, A. (1986). Histoire de la vieillesse et de ses maladies (del'antiquité au XIXe siècle). La contribution de Jean-Martin Charcot (1825–1893) et des médecins des hospices Parisiens. Thèse (Philosophie), Panthéon-Sorbonne, Paris.

Lemak, N., Fields, W., and Gary, H.J. (1986). Controlled trial of aspirin in cerebral ischemia: an addendum. *Neurology*, 36, 705–10.

Lera, G., Scipione, O., Garcia, S., Cammarota, A., Fischbein, G., and Gershanik, O. (2000). A combined pattern of movement disorders resulting from posterolateral thalamic lesions of a vascular nature: a syndrome with clinico-radiologic correlation. *Movement Disorders*, 15, 120–6.

Levasseur, M., Baron, J.C., Sette, G., Legault-Demare, F., Pappata, S., Mauguière, F., *et al.* (1992). Brain energy metabolism in bilateral paramedian infarcts: a positron emission tomography study. *Brain*, 115, 795–807.

Levine, R.L, Lagreze, H.L., Dobkin, J.A., and Turski, P.A. (1988). Large subcortical hemispheric infarctions. Presentation and prognosis. *Archives of Neurology*, 45, 1074–7.

Levine, S.R., Brust, J.C.M., Futrell, N., Ho, K.L., Blake, D., Millikan, C.H., *et al.* (1990). Cerebrovascular complications of the use of the 'crack' form of alkaloidal cocaine. *New England Journal of Medicine*, 323, 699–704.

Lev-Ram, V. and Grinvald, A. (1987). Activity-dependent calcium transients in central nervous system myelinated axons revealed by the calcium indicator FURA-2. *Biophysics Journal*, 52, 571–6.

Levy, R.H., Dreifuss, F.E., Mattson, R.H., Meldrum, B.S., and Penry, J.K. (1989). *Antiepileptic drugs*. Raven Press, New York.

Levy, R.H., Duyckaerts, C., and Hauw, J.-J. (1995). Massive infarcts involving the territory of the anterior choroidal artery and cardioembolism. *Stroke*, 26, 609–13.

Ley, J. (1932). Contribution à l'étude du ramollissement cérébral, envisagée au point de vue de la pathogénie de l'ictus apoplectique. *Journal de Neurologie et de Psychiatrie*, 32, 785 and 895.

Leys, D., Mounier-Vehier, F., Lavenu, I., Rondepierre, P., and Pruvo, J.P. (1994*a*). Anterior choroidal artery territory infarcts. Study of presumed mechanisms. *Stroke*, 25, 837–42.

Leys, D., Mounier-Vehier, F., Rondepierre, P., Leclerc, X., Godefroy, O., Marchau, M., Jr, *et al.* (1994*b*). Small infarcts in the centrum ovale: study of predisposing factors. *Cerebrovascular Diseases*, 4, 83–7.

Lhermitte, F., Gautier, J.C., Marteau, R., and Chain, F. (1963). Troubles de la conscience et mutisme akinétique: étude anatomoclinique d'un ramollissement paramédian bilatéral du pédoncule cérébral et du thalamus. *Revue Neurologique, Paris*, 109, 115–31.

Li, M., West, J.W., Numann, R., Murphy, B.J., Scheuer, T., and Catterall, W.A. (1993). Convergent regulation of sodium channels by protein kinase C and cAMP-dependent protein kinase. *Science*, 261, 1039–42.

Li, S., Mealing, G.A.R., Morley, P., and Stys, P.K. (1999). Novel injury mechanism in anoxia and trauma of spinal cord white matter: glutamate release via reverse Na^+-dependent glutamate transport. *Journal of Neuroscience*, 19, 1–9.

Liao, D.P., Myers, R., Hunt, S., Shahar, E., Paton, C., Burke, G., *et al.* (1997). Familial history of stroke and stroke risk: the Family Heart Study. *Stroke*, 28, 1908–12.

Liebson, E. (2000). Anosognosia and mania associated with right thalamic haemorrhage. *Journal of Neurology, Neurosurgery, and Psychiatry*, 68, 107–8.

Lindgren, A., Staaf, G., Geiger, B., Brockstedt, S., Stahlberg, F., Holtas, S., *et al.* (2000). Clinical lacunar syndromes as predictors of lacunar infarcts. A comparison of acute clinical lacunar syndromes and findings on diffusion-weighted MRI. *Acta Neurologica Scandinavica*, 101, 128–34.

Lindner, K., Hitzengerger, P., Drlicek, M., and Grisold, W. (1992). Dissociated unilateral convergence paralysis in a patient with thalamotectal haemorrhage. *Journal of Neurology, Neurosugery and Psychiatry*, 55, 731–3.

Linfante, I., Llinas, R.H., Caplan, L.R., and Warach, S. (1999). MRI features of intracerebral hemorrhage within 2 hours from symptom onset. *Stroke*, **30**, 2263–7.

LIPID Study Group (1998). Prevention of cardiovascular events and death with pravastatin in patients with coronary heart disease and a broad range of initial cholesterol levels. The Long-Term Intervention with Pravastatin in Ischaemic Disease (LIPID) Study Group. *New England Journal of Medicine*, **339**, 1349–57.

Lipton, R.B., Berger, A.R., Lesser, M.L., Lantos, G., and Portenoy, R.K. (1987). Lobar vs thalamic and basal ganglion hemorrhage: clinical and radiographic features. *Journal of Neurology*, **234**, 86–90.

Lisovoski, F., Koskas, P., Dubard, T., Dessarts, I., Dehen, H., and Cambier, J. (1993). Left tuberothalamic artery territory infarction: neuropsychological and MRI features. *European Neurology*, **33**, 181–4.

Liu, C.-W., Chu, N.-S., and Ryu, S.-J. (1991). CT, somatosensory and brainstem auditory evoked potentials in the early prediction of functional outcome in putaminal hemorrhage. *Acta Neurologica Scandinavica*, **84**, 28–32.

Lodder, J. and Baard, W.C. (1981). Paraballism caused by bilateral hemorrhagic infarction in the basal ganglia. *Neurology*, **31**, 484–6.

Lodder, J., Bamford, J., Kappelle, J., and Boiten, J. (1994). What causes false clinical prediction of small, deep infarcts. *Stroke*, **25**, 86–91.

Lodder, J., Bamford, J.M., Sandercock, P.A.G., Jones, L.N., and Warlow, C.P. (1990). Are hypertension or cardiac embolism likely causes of lacunar infarction? *Stroke*, **21**, 375–81.

Lodder, J., Boiten, J., Raak, L., and Heuts van Raak, L. (1991). Sensorimotor syndrome relates to lacunar rather than to non-lacunar cerebral infarction. *Journal of Neurology, Neurosurgery, and Psychiatry*, **54**, 1097.

Loeb, C., Gandolfo, C., Mancardi, G.L., Primavera, A., and Tassinari, T. (1986). The lacunar syndromes: a review with personal contribution. In *Cerebrovascular disease: research and clinical management*, Vol. 1 (ed. H. Lechner, J.S. Meyer, and E. Ott), pp. 107–56. Elsevier, Amsterdam.

Loizou, L.A., Kendall, B.E., and Marshall, J. (1981). Subcortical arteriosclerotic encephalopathy: a clinical and radiological investigation. *Journal of Neurology, Neurosurgery, and Psychiatry*, **44**, 294–304.

Longstreth, W.T., Bernick, C., Manolio, T.A., Bryan, N., Jungreis, C.A., and Price, T.R. (1998). Lacunar infarcts defined by magnetic resonance imaging of 3660 elderly people: the cardiovascular health study. *Archives of Neurology*, **55**, 1217–25.

LoPachin, R.M., Jr and Stys, P.K. (1995). Elemental composition and water content of rat optic nerve myelinated axons and glial cells: effects of *in vitro* anoxia and reoxygenation. *Journal of Neuroscience*, **15**, 6735–46.

Lotz, P.R., Ballinger, W.E., and Quisling, R.G. (1986). Subcortical arteriosclerotic encephalopathy: CT spectrum and pathologic correlation. *American Journal of Neuroradiology*, **7**, 817–22.

Louarn, F., Gray, F., Degos, J.D., Meyrignac, C., and Poirier, J. (1986). Syndrome de l'hémisphère mineur par infarctus thalamique droit: un cas anatomoclinique. *Revue Neurologique, Paris*, **142**, 777–82.

Louis, E.D., Lynch, T., Ford, B., Greene, P., Bressman, S.B., and Fahn S. (1996). Delayed-onset cerebellar syndrome. *Archives of Neurology*, **53**, 450–4.

Lovblad, K.O., Laubach, H.J., Baird, A.E., Curtin, F., Schlaug, G., Edelman, R.R., *et al.* (1998). Clinical experience with diffusion-weighted MR in patients with acute stroke. *American Journal of Neuroradiology*, **19**, 1061–6.

Lownie, S.P. and Gilbert, J.J. (1990). Hemichorea and hemiballismus: recent concepts. *Clinical Neuropathology*, 9, 46–50.

Luco, C., Hoppe, A., Schweitzer, M., Vicuna, X., and Fantin, A. (1992). Visual field defects in vascular lesions of the lateral geniculate body. *Journal of Neurology, Neurosurgery, and Psychiatry*, 55, 12–15.

Ludbrook, J. (1998). Multiple comparison procedures updated. *Clinical and Experimental Pharmacology and Physiology*, 25, 1032–7.

Lyrer, P.A., Engelter, S., Radu, E.W., and Steck, A.J. (1997). Cerebral infarcts related to isolated middle cerebral artery stenosis. *Stroke*, 28, 1022–7.

Ma, K.C. and Olsson, Y. (1993). Structural and vascular permeability abnormalities associated with lacunes of the human brain. *Acta Neurologica Scandinavica*, 88, 100–7.

Ma, K.C. and Olsson, Y. (1997). The role of chronic brain edema in the formation of lacunes in Binswanger's encephalopathy. Histopathology and immunohistochemical observations. *Cerebrovascular Diseases*, 7, 324–31.

Macdonald, R.L., Kowalczuk, A., and Johns, L. (1995). Emboli enter penetrating arteries of monkey brain in relation to their size. *Stroke*, 26, 1247–50.

Macdonell, R.A.L., Donnan, G.A., Bladin, P.F., Berkovic, S.F., and Wriedt, C.H.R. (1988). The electroencephalogram and acute ischemic stroke. Distinguishing cortical from lacunar infarction. *Archives of Neurology*, 45, 520–4.

Mackenzie, E.T., Strandgaard, T.S., Graham, D.I., Jones, J.V., Harper, A.M., and Farrar, J.K. (1976). Effects of acutely induced hypertension in cats on pial arteriolar caliber, local cerebral flow, and the blood–brain barrier. *Circulation Research*, 39, 33–41.

MacLeod, M.J., Dahiyat, M.T., Cumming, A., Meiklejohn, D., Shaw, D., and St Clair, D. (1999). No association between Glu/Asp polymorphism of NOS3 gene and ischemic stroke. *Neurology*, 53, 418–20.

MacMahon, S., Peto, R., Cutler, J., Collins, R., Sarlie, P., Neaton, J. (1990). Blood pressure, stroke, and coronary heart disease. *Lancet*, 335, 765–74.

Madden, K.P., Karanjia, P.N., Adams, H.P., Jr, Clarke, W.R. and the TOAST investigators. (1995). Accuracy of initial stroke subtype diagnosis in the TOAST study. *Neurology*, 45, 1975–79.

Maeshima, S., Truman, G., Smith, D.S., Nobuyuki, D., Itakura, T., and Komai, N. (1997). Functional outcome following thalamic haemorrhage: relationship between motor and cognitive functions and ADL. *Disability and Rehabilitation*, 11, 459–64.

Magarelli, N., Scarabino, T., Simeone, A.L., Florio, F., Carriero, A., Salvolini, U., *et al.* (1998). Carotid stenosis: a comparison between MR and spiral CT angiography. *Neuroradiology*, 40, 367–73.

Malamut, B.L., Graff-Radford, N., Chawluk, J., Grossman, R.I., and Gur, R.C. (1992). Memory in a case of bilateral thalamic infarction. *Neurology*, 42, 163–9.

Malandrini, A., Carrera, P., Ciacci, G., *et al.* (1997). Unusual clinical features and early brain MRI lesions in a family with cerebral autosomal dominant arteriopaty. *Neurology*, 48, 1200–3.

Manabe, Y., Kashibara, K., Ota, T., Shohmori, T., and Abe, K. (1999). Motor neglect following left thalamic hemorrhage: a case report. *Journal of the Neurological Sciences*, 171, 69–71.

Mano, Y., Nakamuro, T., Takayanagi, T., and Mayer R.F. (1993). Ceruletide therapy in action tremor following thalamic hemorrhage. *Journal of Neurology*, 240, 144–8.

Maraist, T.A., Soloman, D.H., Rarohn R.J., and Bazan, C. (1991). Thalamic ataxia. *Neurology*, 41 (Suppl. 1), 125.

Marie, P. (1901a). Des foyers lacunaires de désintégration et de différents autres états cavitaires du cerveau. *Revue de Medicine, Paris*, 21, 281–98.

Marie, P. (1901b). Foyers lacunaires de désintégration différents autres états cavitaires du cerveau. In *Pierre Marie. Travaux et mémoires. Tome deuxieme.* pp. 71–89. Masson et Cie, Paris, 1928.

Marie, P. (1906). Le syndrome thalamique. Discussion. *Revue Neuroloqique, Paris,* 12, 555–6.

Marinkovic, S.V., Gibo, H., Nikodijevic, I., and Petrovic, P. (1999). The surgical anatomy of the perforating branches of the anterior choroidal artery. *Surgical Neurology,* 52, 30–36.

Marinkovic, S.V., Milisavlejevic, M.M., and Kovacevic, M.S. (1986). Anastomoses among the thalamo-perforating branches of the posterior cerebral artery. *Archives of Neurology,* 43, 811–4.

Marinković, S.V., Milisavljević, M.M., Kovaćević, M.S., and Stevic, Z.D. (1985). Perforating branches of the middle cerebral artery. *Stroke,* 16, 1022–9.

Markowitsch, H.J. (1982). Thalamic mediodorsal nucleus and memory: a critical evaluation of studies in animals and man. *Neuroscience and Biobehavioral Reviews,* 6, 351–80.

Markowitsch, H.J. (1988). Diencephalic amnesia: a reorientation towards tracts? *Brain Research Reviews,* 13, 351–70.

Markowitsch, H.J., von Cramon, D.Y., Hofman, E., Sick, C.-D., and Kinzler, P. (1990). Verbal memory deterioration after unilateral infarct of the internal capsule in an adolescent. *Cortex,* 26, 597–609.

Marks, M.P. (1996). Computed tomography angiography. *Neuroimaging Clinics of North America,* 6, 899–909.

Markus, H.S., Ali, N., Swaminathan, R., Sankaralingam, A., Molloy, J., and Powell, J. (1997). A common polymorphism in the methylenetetrahydrofolate reductase gene, homocysteine, and ischemic cerebrovascular disease. *Stroke,* 28, 1739–43.

Markus, H.S., Barley J., Lunt R., Bland J.M., Jeffery S., Carter N.D., et al. (1995). Angiotensin-converting enzyme gene deletion polymorphism. A new risk factor for lacunar stoke but not carotid atheroma. Stroke, 26, 1329–33.

Markus, H.S., Ruigrok, Y., Ali, N., and Powell, J.F. (1998). Endothelial nitric oxide synthase exon 7 polymorphism, ischemic cerebrovascular disease, and carotid atheroma. *Stroke,* 29, 1908–11.

Marshall, V.G., Bradlay, W.G., Marshall. C.E., Bhoopat, T., and Rhodes, R.H. (1988). Deep white matter infarction: correlation of MR imaging and histopathologic findings. *Radiology,* 167, 517–22.

Marti-Vilalta, J.L. and Arboix, A. (1999). The Barcelona Stroke Registry. *European Neurology,* 41, 135–42.

Martin, J.J. (1970). Sémiologie et neuropathologie thalamiques humaines. *Acta Neurologica Belgica,* 70, 771–94.

Martin, N., Hadley, M., et al. (1986). Management of asymptomatic carotid atherosclerosis. *Neurosurgery,* 18, 505–13.

Masdeu, J.C. and Gorelick, P.B. (1988). Thalamic astasia: inability to stand after unilateral thalamic lesions. *Annals of Neurology,* 23, 596–603.

Masdeu, J.C. and Rosenberg, M. (1987). Midbrain diencephalic horizontal gaze paresis. *Journal of Clinical Neuro-ophthalmology,* 7, 227–34.

Massaro, A.R., Sacco, R.L., Mohr, J.P., Foulkes, M.A., Tatrmichi, T.K., Price, T.R., et al. (1991). Clinical discriminators of lobar and deep hemorrhages: the Stroke Data Bank. *Neurology,* 41, 1881–8.

Massey, E.W., Goodman, J.C., Stewart, C., and Brannon, W.L. (1979). Unilateral asterixis: motor integrative dysfunction in focal vascular disease. *Neurology,* 29, 1180–2.

Masson, C., Krespi, Y., Denninger, M.H., Vertichel, P.,Cambier, J., and Masson, M. (1994). Infarctus hippocampo-thalamique: une forme limitée d'infarctus du territoire de l'artère cérébrale postérieure. *Revue Neurologique, Paris*, **150**, 385–7.

Masson, M., Decroix, J.P., Hénin, D., Dairou, R., Graveleau, Ph., and Cambier, J. (1983). Syndrome de l'artère chorodienne antérieure. Etude clinique et tomodensitométrique de 4 cas. *Revue Neurologique, Paris*, **139**, 547–52.

Mast, H., Thompson, J.L.P., Lee, S.H., Mohr, J.P., and Sacco, R.L. (1995). Hypertension and diabetes mellitus as determinants of multiple lacunar infarcts. *Stroke*, **26**, 30–3.

Masuda, J., Tanaka, K., Omae, T., Ueda, K., and Sadoshima, S. (1983). Cerebrovascular diseases and their underlying vascular lesions in Hisayama, Japan—a pathological study of autopsy cases. Stroke, **14**, 934–40.

Matsui, T. and Hirano, A. (1978). *An atlas of the human brain for computerised tomography*. Igaku-shoin Ltd, Tokyo.

Matsuki, N., Quandt, F.N., Ten Eick, R.E., and Yeh, J.Z. (1984). Characterization of the block of sodium channels by phenytoin in mouse neuroblastoma cells. *Journal of Pharmacology and Experimental Therapeutics*, **228**, 523–30.

Mattle, H.P., Kent, C., Edelman, R., Atkinson, D.J., and Skillman, J. (1989). Evaluation of the extracranial carotid arteries: correlation of magnetic resonance angiography, duplex ultrasonography, and conventional angiography. *Journal of Vascular Surgery*, **13**, 838–45.

Matute, C., Sanchez-Gomez, M.V., Martinez-Millian, L., and Miledi, R. (1997). Glutamate receptor-mediated toxicity in optic nerve oligodendrocytes. *Proceedings of the National Academy of Sciences of the USA*, **94**, 8830–5.

Mauguière, F. and Desmedt, J.E. (1988). Thalamic pain syndrome of Dejérine–Roussy. Differentiation of 4 subtypes assisted by SEP data. *Annals of Neurology*, **45**, 1312–20.

Mauguière, F., Gonnaud, P.M., Ibanez, V., and Schott, B. (1987). Potentiels évoqués somesthésiques précoces et déficits sensitifs dans les lésions thalamiques et juxta-thalamiques. Etude clinique, électrophysiologique, et scanner X chez 70 patients. *Revue Neurologique, Paris*, **143**, 643–56.

Mayer, J.M., Lanoe, Y., Pedetti, L., and Fabry, B. (1992). Anterior choroidal-artery territory infarction and carotid occlusion. *Cerebrovascular Diseases*, **2**, 315–6.

Mayes, A.R., Mendell, P.R., Mann, D., and Pickering, A. (1988). Location of lesions in Korsakoff's syndrome: neuropsychological and neuropathological data on two patients. *Cortex*, **24**, 367–88.

Mazaux, J.M., Orgogozo, J.M., Henry, P., and Loiseau, P. (1979). Troubles du langage au cours des lésions thalamiques. Etude par le test de Goodglass et Kaplan. *Revue Neurologique, Paris*, **135**, 59–64.

McDonald, J.W., Althomsons, S.P., Hyrc, K.L., Choi, D.W., and Goldberg, M.P. (1998). Oligodendrocytes from forebrain are highly vulnerable to AMPA/kainate receptor-mediated excitotoxicity. *Nature Medicine*, **4**, 291–7.

McFarling, D., Rothi, L.J., and Heilman, K.M. (1982). Transcortical aphasia from ischemic infarcts of the thalamus: a report of two cases. *Journal of Neurology, Neurosurgery, and Psychiatry*, **45**, 107–12.

McGilchrist, I., Goldstein, L.H., Jadresic, D., and Fenwick, P. (1993). Thalamo-frontal psychosis. *British Journal of Psychiatry*, **163**, 113–5.

McKissock, W., Richardson, A., and Taylor, J. (1961). Primary intracerebral haemorrhage: a controlled trial of surgical and conservative treatment in 180 unselected cases. *Lancet*, **2**, 221–6.

McQuinn, B.A. and O'Leary, D.H. (1987). White matter lucencies on computed tomography, subacute arteriosclerotic encephalopathy (Binswanger's disease) and blood pressure. *Stroke*, **18**, 900–5.

Mead, G. and O'Neill, P.A. (1999). Carotid disease in acute stroke: a review. *Journal of Stroke and Cerebrovascular Diseases*, **8**, 197–206.

Mead, G.E., Lewis, S.C., Wardlaw, J.M., Dennis, M.S., and Warlow, C.P. (1999). Should computed tomography appearance of lacunar stroke influence patient management? *Journal of Neurology, Neurosurgery, and Psychiatry*, **67**, 682–4.

Mead, G.E., Shingler, H., Farrell, A., O'Neill, P.A., and McCollum, C.N. (1998). Carotid disease in acute stroke. *Age and Ageing*, **27**, 677–82.

Meghji, P., Tuttle, J.B., and Rubio, R. (1989). Adenosine formation and release by embryonic chick neurones and glia in cell culture. *Neurochemistry*, **53**, 1852–69.

Mehler, M.F. (1989). The rostral basilar artery syndrome: diagnosis, etiology, prognosis. *Neurology*, **39**, 9–16.

Meissner, I., Sapir, S., Kokmen, E., and Stein, S.D. (1987). The paramedian diencephalic syndrome: a dynamic phenomenon. *Stroke*, **18**, 380–5.

Melo, T.P. and Bogousslavsky, J. (1992). Hemiataxia–hypesthesia: a thalamic stroke syndrome. *Journal of Neurology, Neurosurgery, and Psychiatry*, **55**, 581–4.

Melo, T.P., Bogousslavsky, J., Moulin, T., Nader, J., and Regli, F. (1992*b*). Thalamic ataxia. *Journal of Neurology*, **239**, 331–7.

Melo, T.P., Bogousslavsky, J., Van Melle, G., and Regli, F. (1992*a*). Pure motor stroke: a reappraisal. *Neurology*, **42**, 789–98.

Melo, T.P., Pinto, A.N., and Ferro, J.M. (1996). Headache in intracerebral hematomas. *Neurology*, **47**, 494–500.

Mendez, A. and Estanol, B. (1993). Small, deep, penetrating cerebral artery embolic cerebral infarct or embolic lacune? *Stroke*, **24**, 328.

Mendez, M., Adams, N., and Lewandowski, K. (1989), Neurobehavioral changes associated with caudate lesions. *Neurology*, **39**, 349–54.

Mene, P., Pugliese, F., and Cinotti, G.A. (1991). Regulation of Na^+/Ca^{++} exchange in cultured human mesanglial cells. *American Journal of Physiology*, **261**, F466–73.

Mennemeier, M., Fennell, E., Valenstein, E., and Heilman, K.M. (1992). Contributions of the left intralaminar and medial thalamic nuclei to memory: comparisons and report of a case. *Archives of Neurology*, **49**, 1050–8.

Metter, E.J., Riege, W.H., Hanson, W.R., Kuhl, D.E., Phelps, M.E., and Squire, L.R. (1983). Comparison of metabolic rates, language and memory in subcortical aphasias. *Brain and Language*, **19**, 33–47.

Metz, R.J., Dupuis, M.J.M., and Jean, D. (1993). Troubles oculomoteurs dus à un infarctus thalamo-pédonculaire par dissection de l'artère vertébrale. *Revue Neurologique, Paris*, **149**, 799–801.

Michel, D., Laurent, B., Foyatier, N., Blanc, A., and Portafaix, M. (1982). Infarctus thalamique paramédian gauche. Etude de la mémoire et du langage. *Revue Neurologique, Paris*, **138**, 533–50.

Midgard, R., Aarli, J.A., Julsrud, O.J., and Odegaard, H. (1989). Symptomatic hemidystonia of delayed onset. Magnetic resonance demonstration of pathology in the putamen and caudate nucleus. *Acta Neurologica Scandinavia*, **79**, 27–31.

Mikkola, H., Syrjala, M., Rasi, V., Vahtera, E., Hamalainen, E., Peltonen, L., *et al.* (1994). Deficiency in the A-subunit of coagulation factor XIII: two novel point mutations demonstrate different effects on transcript levels. *Blood*, **84**, 517–25.

Miklossy, J., Van der Loos, H., Deruaz, J.P., Bogousslavsky, J., and Regli, F. (1987). Thalamic aphasia and neglect: cortical involvement as shown by anterograde axonal degeneration in the human brain. In *Cellular thalamic mechanisms*, Proceedings of the International Brain Research Organization, Verona.

Milandre, L., Brosset, C., Gabriel, B., and Khalil, R. (1993). Mouvements involontaires transitoires et infarctus thalamiques. *Revue Neurologique, Paris*, **149**, 402–6.

Milisavljevic, M., Marinkovic, S.V., Gibo, H., and Puskas, L.F. (1991). The thalamogeniculate perforators of the PCA: the microsurgical anatomy. *Neurosurgery*, **28**, 523–30.

Miller, V.T. (1983). Lacunar stroke. A reassessment. *Archives of Neurology*, **40**, 129–34.

Millikan, C. and Futrell, N. (1990). The fallacy of the lacune hypothesis. *Stroke*, **21**, 1251–7.

Millikan, C.H., Siekert, R.G., and Shick, R.M. (1955). Studies in cerebrovascular disease. V. The use of anticoagulant drugs in the treatment of intermittent insufficiency of the internal carotid arterial system. *Mayo Clinic Proceedings*, **30**, 578–86.

Mills, R.P. and Swanson, P.D. (1978). Vertical oculomotor apraxia and memory loss. *Annals of Neurology*, **4**, 149–53.

Minematsu, K., Li, L., Sotak, C.H., Davis, M.A., and Fisher, M. (1992). Reversible focal ischemic injury demonstrated by diffusion-weighted magnetic resonance imaging in rats. *Stroke*, **23**, 1304–11.

Miwa, H., Hatori, K., Kondo, T., Imai, H., and Mizuno, Y. (1996). Thalamic tremor: case reports and implications of the tremor-generating mechanism. *Neurology*, **46**, 75–9.

Miyao, S., Takano, A., Teramoto, J., and Takahashi, A. (1992). Leukoaraiosis in relation to prognosis for patients with lacunar infarction. *Stroke*, **23**, 1434–8.

Mochizuki, Y., Oishi, M., and Takasu, T. (1997). Cerebral blood flow in single and multiple lacunar infarctions. *Stroke*, **28**, 1458–60.

Mohr, J. (1982). Lacunes. *Stroke*, **13**, 3–11.

Mohr, J.P. (1986). Lacunes. In *Stroke: pathophysiology, diagnosis and management* (ed. H.J.M. Barnett, J.P. Mohr, B.M.Stein, and F.M. Yatsu,), pp. 475–96. Churchill Livingstone, New York.

Mohr, J.P. and Martí-Vilalta, J.M. (1998). Lacunes. In *Stroke: pathophysiology, diagnosis and management.* (ed. H.J.M. Barnett, J.P. Mohr, B.M. Stein, and F. Yatsu), pp. 599–622. 3rd edn. Churchill Livingstone, New York.

Mohr, J.P., Caplan, L.R., Melski, J.W., Goldstein, R.J., Duncan, G.W., Kistler, J.P., *et al.* (1978). The Harvard Cooperative Stroke Registry: a prospective registry. *Neurology*, **28**, 754–62.

Mohr, J.P., Kase, C.S., Meckler, R.J., and Fisher, C.M. (1977). Sensorimotor stroke due to thalamocapsular ischemia. *Archives of Neurology*, **34**, 734–41.

Mohr, J.P., Steinke, W., Timsit, S.G., Sacco, R.L., and Tatemichi, T.K. (1991). The anterior choroidal artery does not supply the corona radiata and lateral ventricular wall. *Stroke*, **22**, 1502–.

Mohr, J.P., Watters, W.C., and Duncan, G.W. (1975). Thalamic hemorrhage and aphasia. *Brain and Language*, **2**, 3–17.

Molina, C., Sabin, J.A., Montaner, J., Rovira, A., Abilleira, S., and Codina, A. (1999). Impaired cerebrovascular reactivity as a risk marker for first-ever lacunar infarction. A case control study. *Stroke*, **30**, 2296–301.

Molnár, L. (1958–1959). Die lokal diagnostische Bedeutung der vertikalen Blicklähmung. Beitrage zur Symptomatologie und Faseranatomie des mesodiencephalen Übergangsgebietes. *Archiv für Psychiatrie und Nervenkrankheiten vereinigt mit Zeitschrift für die Gesamte Neurologie und Psychiatrie*, **198**, 523–34.

Moniz, E. (1940). *Die cerebrale arteriographie und phlebographie.* Springer, Berlin.

Montes, J.M., Wong, J.H., Fayad, P.B., and Awad, I.A. (2000). Stereotactic computed tomographic-guided aspiration and thrombolysis of intracerebral hematoma: protocol and preliminary experience. *Stroke*, **31**, 834–40.

Moody, D.M., Bell, M.A., and Challa, V.R. (1990). Features of the cerebral vascular pattern that predict vulnerability to perfusion or oxygenation deficiency: an anatomic study. *American Journal of Neuroradiology*, **11**, 431–9.

Moonis, M., Jain, S., Prasad, K., Mishra, N.K., Goulatia, R.K., and Maheshwari, M.C. (1988). Left thalamic hypertensive haemorrhage presenting as transient global amnesia. *Acta Neurologica Scandinavica*, **77**, 331–4.

Moore, M.T. (1954). Perivascular encephalolysis. *Archives of Neurology and Psychiatry*, **71**, 344–57.

Moore, W., Boren, C., *et al.* (1978). Natural history of nonstenotic, asymptomatic ulcerative lesions of the carotid artery. *Archives of Surgery*, **113**, 1352–9.

Moreaud, O., Charnallet, A., David, D., Cinotti, L., and Pellat, J. (1996). Frontal lobe syndrome after a left genu capsular infarction. *European Neurology*, **36**, 322–4.

Moreaud, O., Pellat, J., Charnallet, A., Carbonnel, S., and Brennen, T. (1995). Déficit de la production et de l'apprentissage de noms propres après lésion ischémique tubéro-thalamique gauche. *Revue Neurologique, Paris*, **151**, 93–9.

Morgenstern, L.B., Frankowski, R.F., Shedden, P., Pasteur, W., and Grotta, J.C. (1998). Surgical treament for intracerebral hemorrhage (STICH): a single-center, randomized clinical trial. *Neurology*, **51**, 1359–63.

Mori, E., Yamadori, A., and Mitani, Y. (1986). Left thalamic infarction and disturbance of verbal memory: a clinico-anatomical study with a new method of CT stereotaxic lesion localization. *Annals of Neurology*, **20**, 671–6.

Mori, S., Sadoshina, S., Ibayashi, S., Fujishima, M., and Iino, K. (1995). Impact of thalamic hematoma on six-month mortality and motor and cognitive functional outcome. *Stroke*, **26**, 620–6.

Morillo, A. and Cooper, I. (1955). Occlusion of the anterior choroidal artery. *American Journal of Ophthalmology*, **40**, 796–801.

Moriwaki, H., Matsumoto, M., Hashikawa, K., *et al.* (1997). Hemodynamic aspect of cerebral watershed infarction: assessment of perfusion reserve using iodine-123-iodoamphetamine SPECT. *Journal of Nuclear Medicine*, **38**, 1556–62.

Mossuto-Agatiello, L., Puccetti, G., and Castellano, A.E. (1993). 'Rubral' tremor after thalamic haemorrhage. *Journal of Neurology*, **241**, 27–30.

Moulton, A.W., Singer, D.E., and Haas, J.S. (1991). Risk factors for stroke in patients with nonrheumatic atrial fibrillation: a case study. *American Journal of Medicine*, **91**, 156–61.

Mounier-Vehier, F., Leys, D., Godefroy, O., Rondepierre, Ph., Marchau, M., Jr, and Pruvo, J.P. (1994). Borderzone infarct subtypes: preliminary study of the presumed mechanism. *European Neurology*, **34**, 11–15.

Mull, M., Schwarz, M., and Thron, A. (1997). Cerebral hemispheric low-flow infarcts in arterial occlusive disease. Lesion patterns and angiomorphological conditions. *Stroke*, **28**, 118–23.

Muller, J.P., Destée, A., Steinling, M., Pruno, J.P., and Warot, P. (1989). Infarctus bithalamique paramédian: 1 cas avec IRM et tomographie d'émission gamma. *Revue Neurologique, Paris*, **141**, 732–4.

Muroi, A., Hirayama, K., Tanno, Y., Shimizu, S., Watanabe, T., and Yamamoto T. (1999). Cessation of stuttering after bilateral thalamic infarction. *Neurology*, **53**, 890–1.

Müller, A., Baumgartner, R.W., Röhrenbach, C., and Regard, M. (1999). Persistent Klüver–Bucy syndrome after bilateral thalamic infarction. *Neuropsychiatry, Neuropsychology, and Behavioral Neurology*, 12, 136–9.

Nadeau, S.E., Jordan, J.E., Mishra, S.K., and Haerer, A.F. (1993). Stroke rates in patients with lacunar and large vessel cerebral infarctions. *Journal of the Neurological Sciences*, 114, 128–37.

Nadeau, S.E., Roeltgen, D.P., Sevush, S., Ballinger, W.E., and Watson, R.T. (1994). Apraxia due to a pathogically documented thalamic infarction. *Neurology*, 44, 2133–7.

Naeser, M.A., Alexander, M.P., Helm-Estabrooks, N., Levine, H.L., Laughlin, S.A., and Geschwind, N. (1982). Aphasia with predominantly subcortical lesion sites. *Archives of Neurology*, 39, 2–14.

Nagaratnam, N., Wong, V., and Jeyaratnam, D. (1998). Left anterior choroidal artery infarction and uncontrollable crying. *Journal of Stroke and Cerebrovascular Disease*, 7, 263–4.

Nagata, K., Araki, G., Mizukami, M., Hyodo, A. (1984). Topographic electroencephalographic study of ischemic vascular disease. In Brain ischemia: Quantitative EEG and imaging techniques. Progress in brain research (ed G. Pfurtscheller, E.J.Jonkman, F.H. Lopes da Silva), pp. 271–286. Elsevier, Amsterdam.

Nakano, S., Yokogami, K., Ohta, H., Goya, T., and Wakisaka, S. (1995). CT-defined large subcortical infarcts: correlation of location with site of cerebrovascular occlusive disease. *AmericanJournal of Neuroradiology*, 16, 1581–5.

Narahashi, T., Anderson, N., and Moore, J. (1967). Comparison of tetrodotoxin and procaine in internally perfused squid giant axons. *Journal of General Physiology*, 50, 1413–28.

Nasreddine, Z.S. and Saver, J.L. (1997). Pain after thalamic stroke: right diencephalic predominance and clinical features in 180 patients. *Neurology*, 48, 1196–9.

National Institute of Neurological Disorders and Stroke (1990). Classification of cerebrovascular diseases III. *Stroke*, 21, 637–676.

National Institute of Neurological Disorders and Stroke rt-PA Stroke Study Group (1995). Tissue plasminogen activator for acute ischemic stroke. *New England Journal of Medicine*, 333, 1581–7.

Neau, J.P. and Bogousslavsky, J. (1996). The syndrome of posterior choroidal artery territory infarction. *Annals of Neurology*, 39, 779–88.

Nelson, R.F., Pullicino, P., Kendall, B.E., and Marshall, J. (1980). Computed tomography in patients presenting with lacunar syndromes. *Stroke*, 11, 256–61.

Neumann-Haefelin, T., Moseley, M.E., and Albers, G.W. (2000). New magnetic resonance imaging methods for cerebrovascular disease: emerging clinical applications. *Annals of Neurology*, 47, 559–70.

Nichelli, P., Bahmanian-Bebahani, G., Gentilini, M., and Vecchi, A. (1988). Preserved memory abilities in thalamic amnesia. *Brain*, 111, 1337–53.

Nicolai, A., Lazzarino, L.G., and Biasutti, E. (1996). Large striatocapsular infarcts: clinical features and risk factors. *Journal of Neurology*, 243, 44–50.

Nicolaou, M., DeStefano, A.L., Gavras, I., Cupples, L.A., Manolis, A.J., Baldwin, C.T., *et al.* (2000). Genetic predisposition to stroke in relatives of hypertensives. *Stroke*, 31, 487–92.

Nicolesco, J. (1959). Travaux scientifiques, Bucarest, Paris. *Editions de l'Académie de la République Populaire Roumaine*, Masson, Paris.

Niculescu, S.I. (1992). *Ion T Niculescu maestri, prieteni, contemporani Eminescu*. Bucarest.

Niizuma, H., Yonemitsu, T., Jokura, H., Nakasato, N., Suzuki, J., and Yoshimoto, T. (1990). Stereotactic aspiration of thalamic hematoma. *Stereotactic and Functional Neurosurgery*, 54/55, 438–44.

NINDS (1995). Tissue plasminogen activator for acute ischemic stroke. *New England Journal of Medicine*, 333, 1581–7.

Nishida, N., Ogata, J., Yutani, C., Minematsu, K., and Yamaguchi, T. (2000). Cerebral artery thrombosis as a cause of striatocapsular infarction. A histopathological case study. *Cerebrovascular Diseases*, 10, 151–4.

Nishiuma, S., Kario, K., Nakanishi, K., Yakushijin, K., Kageyama, G., Matsunaka, T., et al. (1997). Factor VII R353Q polymorphism and lacunar stroke in Japanese hypertensive patients and normotensive controls. *Blood, Coagulation, and Fibrinolysis*, 8, 525–30.

Nishiuma, S., Kario, K., Yakushijin, K., Maeda, M., Murai, R., Matsuo, T., et al. (1998). Genetic variation in the promoter region of the beta-fibrinogen gene is associated with ischemic stroke in a Japanese population. *Blood, Coagulation, and Fibrinolysis*, 9, 373–9.

Nishizaki, T., Yamauchi, R., Tanimoto, M., and Okada, Y. (1988). Effects of temperature on the oxygen consumption in thin slices from different brain regions. *Neuroscience Letters*, 86, 301–5.

Noda, S., Mizoguchi, M., and Yamamoto A. (1993). Thalamic experimental hallucinosis. *Journal of Neurology, Neurosurgery, and Psychiatry*, 56, 1224–6.

Noguchi, K., Nagayoshi, T., Watanabe, N., Kanazawa, T., Toyoshima, S., Morijiri, M., et al. (1998). Diffusion-weighted echo-planar MRI of lacunar infarcts. *Neuroradiology*, 40, 448–51.

Norris, J.W. and Hachinski, V.C. (1991). Stroke prevention: past, present, and future. In *Prevention of stroke* (ed. J.W. Norris and V.C. Hachinski), pp. 1–15. Springer, New York.

Norris, J.W. and Zhu, C.Z. (1992). Silent stroke in carotid stenosis. *Stroke*, 23, 483–5.

Norris, J.W., Zhu, C.Z., et al. (1992). Vascular risks of asymptomatic carotid stenosis. *Stroke*, 22, 1485–90.

Norrving, B. (1999). Diffusion-weighted MRI findings in patients with the capsular warning syndrome. *Stroke*, 30, 259.

Norrving, B. and Cronqvist, S. (1989). Clinical and radiological features of lacunar versus nonlacunar minor stroke. *Stroke*, 20, 59–64.

Norrving, B. and Staaf, G. (1991). Pure motor stroke from presumed lacunar infarct. Incidence, risk factors and initial course. *Cerebrovascular Diseases*, 1, 203–9.

Notsu, Y., Nabika, T., Park, H.Y., Masuda, J., and Kobayashi, S. (1999). Evaluation of genetic risk factors for silent brain infarction. *Stroke*, 30, 1881–6.

Numann, R., Hauschka, S.D., Catterall, W.A., and Scheuer, T. (1994). Modulation of skeletal muscle sodium channels in a satellite cell line by protein kinase C. *Journal of Neuroscience*, 14, 4226–36.

Nuwer, M.N., Jordan, S., and Ahn, S. (1987a). Quantitative EEG is abnormal more often than routine EEG in mild stroke. *Neurology*, 37 (Suppl 1), 369.

Nuwer, M.N., Jordan, S., and Ahn, S. (1987b). Evaluation of stroke using EEG frequency analysis and topographic mapping. *Neurology*, 37, 1153–9.

O'Brien, A., Rajkumar, C., and Bulpitt, C. (1999). Blood pressure lowering for the primary and secondary prevention of stroke: treatment of hypertension reduces the risk of stroke. *Cardiovascular Risk*, 6, 203–5.

O'Regan, M.H., Kocsis, J.D., and Waxman S.G. (1991). Nimodipine and nifedipine enhance synaptic transmission in CA1 pyramidal neurons. *Experimental Brain Research*, 84, 224–8.

O'Regan, M.H., Kocsis, J.D., and Waxman, S.G. (1990). Depolarization-dependent actions of dihydropyridines on synaptic transmission in the *in vitro* rat hippocampus. *Brain Research*, 527, 181–91.

O'Regan, M.H., Simpson, R.E., Perkins, L.M., and Phillis, J.W. (1992). Adenosine receptor agonists inhibit the release of γ-aminobutyric acid (GABA) from the ischemic rat cerebral cortex. *Brain Research*, 582, 22–6.

Offenbacher, H., Fazekas, F., Schmidt, R., Koch, M., Fazekas, G., and Kapeller, P. (1996). MR of cerebral abnormalities concomitant with primary intracerebral hematomas. *American Journal of Neuroradiology*, 17, 573–8.

Oglen, M.P., Mateer, C.A., and Wyler, A.R. (1984). Alterations in visually related eye movements following left pulvinar damage in man. *Neuropsychologia*, 22, 187–96.

Ohkubo, Y., Kishikawa, H., Araki, E., *et al.* (1995). Intensive insulin therapy prevents the progression of diabetic microvascular complications in Japanese patients with non-insulin-dependent diabetes mellitus: a randomized prospective 6-year study. *Diabetes Research and Clinical Practice*, 28, 103–17.

Okuno, T., Takao, T., Ito, M., Konishi, Y., Mikawa, H., and Nakano, Y. (1980). Infarction of the internal capsule in children. *Journal of Computer Assisted Tomography*, 4, 770–4.

Oliveira-Filho, J., Ay, H., Schaefer, P.W., Buonanno, F.S., Chang, Y., Gonzalez, R.G., *et al.* (2000). Diffusion-weighted magnetic resonance imaging identifes the 'clinically relevant' small-penetrator infarcts. *Archives of Neurology*, 57, 1009–14.

Olsen, T.S., Bruhn, P., and Oberg, R.G.E. (1986). Cortical hypoperfusion as a possible cause of 'aubcortical aphasia'. *Brain*, 109, 393–410.

Olsen, T.S., Skriver, E.B., and Herning, M. (1985). Cause of cerebral infarction in the carotid territory. Its relation to the size and location of the infarct and to the underlying vascular lesion. *Stroke*, 16, 459–66.

Olsson, G.-B., Söderfelt, B., and Samuelsson, M. (1996). Life satisfaction in persons with lacunar infarction—a comparative analysis of two measures of life satisfaction. *International Journal of Rehabilitation Research*, 19, 321–5.

Olszewski, J. (1950). Cécile and Oskar Vogt. *Archives of Neurology and Psychiatry*, 64, 813–22.

Ono, S., Matsuzaki, M., Toma, Y., Michishigee, H., Okuda, F., and Kusukawa, R. (1989). Assessment of atherosclerotic lesions in thoracic aorta by transesophageal echocardiography. *Circulation*, 80 (Suppl. II), 11–12.

Orgogozo, J.M. and Bogousslavsky, J. (1989). Lacunar syndromes. In *Vascular diseases Part II. Handbook of clinical neurology* (ed. J.F. Toole), pp. 235–69. Elsevier, Amsterdam.

Otonello, G. A., Regesta, G., and Tanganelli, T. (1980). Correlation and discrepancies between clinical aspects, EEG and CT brainscan data in ischaemic cerebral disease. In *EEG and clinical neurophysiology* (ed H. Lechner and A. Aranibar), pp. 148–62. Exerpta Medica, Amsterdam.

Ott, B.R. and Saver, J.L. (1993). Unilateral amnestic stroke. Six new cases and review of the literature. *Stroke*, 24, 1033–42.

Otto, S., Büttner, T., Schöls, L., Windmeier, D.T., and Przuntek, H. (1995). Head tremor due to bilateral thalamic and midbrain infarct. *Journal of Neurology*, 242, 608–9.

Paciaroni, M. and Bogousslavsky, J. (1998). Pure sensory syndromes in thalamic stroke. *European Neurology*, 39, 211–7.

Padovan, C.S., Bise, K., Hahn, J., Sostak, P., Holler, E., Kolb, H.J., *et al.* (1999). Angiitis of the central nervous system after allogeneic bone marrow. *Stroke*, 30, 1651–6.

Pantoni, L. and Garcia, J.H. (1995). The significance of cerebral white matter abnormalities 100 years after Binswanger's report: a review. *Stroke*, 26, 1293–301.

Pantoni, L. and Garcia, J.H. (1997). Pathogenesis of leukoaraiosis: a review. *Stroke*, 28, 652–9.

Pappata, S., Mazoyer, B., Tran Dim, S., Cambon, H., Levasseur, M., and Baron, J.C. (1990). Effects of capsular or thalamic stroke on metabolism in the cortex and cerebellum: a PET study. *Stroke*, 21, 519–24.

PARIS (1980). Persantine and aspirin in coronary heart disease. *Circulation*, 62, 449–61.

Paroni Sterbini, G.L., Massuto Agatiello, L., Stocchi, A., and Solivetti, F.M. (1987). CT of ischemic infarctions in the territory of the anterior choroidal artery: a review of 28 cases. *American Journal of Neuroradiology*, 8, 229–32.

Parsons, M.W., Li, T., Barber, P.A., Yang, Q., Darby, D.G., Desmond, P.M., *et al.* (2000). Combined ¹H MR spectroscopy and diffusion-weighted MRI improves the prediction of stroke outcome. *Neurology*, 55, 498–506.

Pedroza, A., Dujovny, M., Artero, J.C., Umansky, F., Berman, S.K., Diaz, F.G., *et al.* (1987*a*). Microanatomy of the posterior communicating artery. *Neurosurgery*, 20, 228–35.

Pedroza, A., Dujovny, M., Cabeduzo-Artero, J., Umansky, F., Kim Berman, S., Diaz, F.G., *et al.* (1987*b*). Microanatomy of the pre-mammilary artery. *Acta Neurochirurgica*, 86, 50–5.

Pelletier, J., Cabanot, C., Lévrier, O., Thuillier, J.N., and Chérif, A.A. (1997). Angiodysplasie de type Moya-Moya révélée par des des mouvements anormaux involuntaires choréiformes au cours d'une contraception orale. A propos de 2 cas. *Revue Neurologique, Paris*, 153, 393–7.

Peltonen, M., Stegmayr, B., and Asplund, K. (1998). Time trends in long-term survival after stroke: the Northern Sweden Multinational Monitoring of Trends and Determinants in Cardiovascular Disease (MONICA) study, 1985–1994. *Stroke*, 29, 1358–65.

Pepin, E.P. and Auray-Pepin L. (1993). Selective dorsolateral frontal lobe dysfunction associated with diecephalic amnesia. *Neurology*, 43, 733–41.

Perani, D., Vallar, G., Cappa, S., Messa, C., and Fazio, F. (1987). Aphasia and neglect after subcortical stroke. A clinical/cerebral perfusion correlation study. *Brain*, 110, 1211–29.

Percheron, G. (1973). The anatomy of the arterial supply of the human thalamus and its use for the interpretation of the thalamic vascular pathology. *Zeitschrift für Neurologie*, 205, 1–13.

Percheron, G. (1976). Les artères du thalamus humain. II. Artères et territoires thalamiques paramédians de l'artère basilaire communicante. *Revue Neurologique, Paris*, 132, 309–24.

Percheron, G. (1977). Les artères du thalamus humain. Territoire des artères choroòdiennes (III–V). *Revue Neurologique, Paris*, 133, 547–59.

Pereira, A.C., Saunders, D.E., Doyle, V.L., Bland, J.M., Howe, F.A., Griffiths, J.R., *et al.* (1999). Measurement of initial *N*-acetyl aspartate concentration by magnetic resonance spectroscopy and initial infarct volume by MRI predicts outcome in patients with middle cerebral artery territory infarction. *Stroke*, 30, 1577–82.

Perry, I.J., Refsum, H., Morris, R.W., Ebrahim, S.B., Ueland, P.M., and Shaper, A.G. (1995). Prospective study of serum total homocysteine concentration and risk of stroke in middle-aged British men. *Lancet*, 346, 1395–8.

Pertuiset, B., Aron, D., Dilenge, D., *et al.* (1962). Les syndromes de l'artere choroidienne anterieure: étude clinique et radiologique. *Revue Neurologique, Paris*, 106, 286–94.

Pessin, M.S., Adelman, L.S., Prager, R.J., Lathi, E.S., and Lange, D.J. (1981). 'Wrong way eyes' in supratentorial hemorrhage. *Annals of Neurology*, 9, 79–81.

Petersen, P., Madsen, E.B., Brun, B., Pedersen, F., Gylvensted, C., and Boysen, G. (1987). Silent cerebral infarction in chronic atrial fibrillation. *Stroke*, 18, 1098–100.

Petiot, P., Croisile, B., Confavreux, C., Aimard, G., Trillet, M., French, P., *et al.* (1991). Thalamic stroke and congenital factor V deficiency. *Stroke*, 22, 1606.

Petit, H., Rousseaux, M., Clarisse, J., and Delafosse, A. (1981). Troubles oculocéphalomoteurs et infarctus thalamo-sousthalamique bilatéral. *Revue Neurologique, Paris*, 137, 709–22.

Petrescu, A. (1978). Doua Commemorari: Charles Foix (1882–1927) si prof. Ion T. Niculescu (1895–1957) si 20 de ani de la moartealor. *Neurol. Psihiatr., Neurochir*, 23, 151–6.

Petty, G.W., Brown, R.D., Whisnant, J.P., Sicks, J.D., O'Fallon, W.M., and Wiebers, D.O. (1999). Ischemic stroke subtypes—a population-based study of incidence and risk factors. *Stroke*, 30, 2513–16.

Petty, G.W., Brown, R.D.J., Whisnant, J.P., Sicks, J.D., O'Fallon, W.M., and Wiebers, D.O. (2000). Ischemic stroke subtypes: a population-based study of functional outcome, survival, and recurrence. *Stroke*, 31, 1062–8.

Pfurtscheller, G., Aranibar, A. (1977). Event-related cortical desynchronization detected by power measurements of scalp EEG. *Electroencephalography and Clinical Neurophysiology*, 42, 817–26.

Pfurtscheller, G., Sager, W., and Wege, W. (1981). Correlations between CT-scan and sensorimotor EEG rhythms in patients with cerebrovascular disorders. *Electroencephalography and Clinical Neurophysiology*, 52, 473–85.

Phan, T.G., Koh, M., Vierkant, R.A., and Wijdicks, E.F.M. (2000). Hydrocephalus is a determinant of early mortality in putaminal hemorrhage. *Stroke*, 31, 2157–62.

Philip, I., Plantefeve, G., Vuillaumier-Barrot, S., Vicaut, E., LeMarie, C., Henrion, D., *et al.* (1999). G894T polymorphism in the endothelial nitric oxide synthase gene is associated with an enhanced vascular responsiveness to phenylephrine. *Circulation*, 99, 3096–8.

Physician's Health Study Group (1988). Preliminary report: findings from the aspirin component of the ongoing Physicians Health Study. *New England Journal of Medicine*, 318, 262–4.

Pierrot-Deseilligny, C., Chain, F., Gray, F., Serdaru, M., Escourolle, R., and Lhermitte, F. (1982). Parinaud's syndrome. Electro-oculographic and anatomical analyses of 6 vascular cases with deductions about vertical gaze organization in the premotor structures. *Brain*, 105, 667–96.

Piotrowski, W.P. and Rochowanski, E. (1996). Operative results in hypertensive intracerebral hematomas in patients over 60. *Gerontology*, 42, 339–47.

Plets, C., De Reuck, J., Van der Eecken, H., and Vanderbergh, R. (1970). The vascularization of the human thalamus. *Acta Neurologica Belgica*, 70, 685–767.

Poirier, J. (1983). Giant cerebral lacunae due to dilatation of the perivascular space: a case report. *Clinical Neuropathology*, 2, 138–40.

Poirier, J. and Derouesné, C. (1984). Cerebral lacunae. A proposed new classification. *Clinical Neuropathology*, 3, 266.

Poirier, J. and Derouesné, C. (1985). Le concept de lacune cérébrale de 1838 à nos jours. *Revue Neurologique, Paris*, 141, 3–17.

Poirier, J., Barbizet, J., Gaston, A., and Meyrignac, C. (1983). Démence thalamique. Lacunes expansives du territoire thalamo-mésencéphalique paramédian. Hydrocéphalie par sténose de l'aqueduc de Sylvius. *Revue Neurologique, Paris*, 139, 349–58.

Pollanen, M.S. and Deck, J.H. (1990). The mechanism of embolic watershed infarction, experimental studies. *Canadian Journal of Neurological Science*, 17, 395–8.

Pollock, H., Hutchings, M., Weller, R.O., and Zhang, E.-T. (1997). Perivascular spaces in the basal ganglia of the human brain: their relationship to lacunes. *Journal of Anatomy*, 191, 337–46.

Pop, G., Sutherland, G.R., Koudstaal, P.J., Sit, T.W., de Jong, G., and Roelandt, J.R.T.C. (1990). Transesophageal echocardiography in the detection of intracardiac embolic sources in patients with transient ischemic attacks. *Stroke*, 21, 560–5.

Poppi, U. (1928a). La sindrome anatomo-clinica conseguente a lesione dell'arteria coroidea anteriore. *Rivista di Neurologia*, 1, 466–75.

Poppi, U. (1928b). Sindrome talamo-capsulare per rammollimento nel territorio dell'arteria coroidea anteriore. *Rivista di Patologia Nervosa e Mentale*, 33, 505–42.

Powers, J.M. (1985). Blepharospasm due to unilateral diencephalon infarction. *Neurology*, 35, 283–4.

Pozzati, E. (2000). Thalamic cavernous malformations. *Surgical Neurology*, 53, 30–40.

Primavera, A., Folis, E., Romangnoli, P., Ruffinengo, U., and Barolini, A. (1984). The EEG in lacunar strokes. *Stroke*, 15, 579–80.

PROGRESS (1996). Blood pressure lowering for the secondary prevention of stroke: rationale and design for PROGRESS. *Journal of Hypertension*, 14, 541–6.

Prospective Studies Collaboration (1995). Cholesterol, diastolic blood pressure, and stroke: 13.000 strokes in 450.000 people in 45 prospective cohorts. *Lancet*, 346, 1647–53.

Puel, M., Cardebat, D., Demonet, J.F., Elghozi, D., Cambier, J., Guiraud-Chaumeil, B., *et al.* (1986). Le rôle du thalamus dans les aphasies sous-corticales. *Revue Neurologique, Paris*, 142, 431–40.

Pujol, J., Junque, C., Vendrell, P., Capdevila, A., and Marti-Vilalta, J.L. (1991). Cognitive correlates of ventricular enlargement in vascular patients with leuko-araiosis. *Acta Neurologica Scandinavica*, 84, 237–42.

Pullicino, P, Lichter, D., and Benedict, R. (1994). Micrographia with cognitive dysfunction: minimal sequela of a putaminal infarct [case report]. *Movement Disorders*, 3, 371–73.

Pullicino, P., Nelson, R.F., Kendall, B.E., and Marshall J. (1980). Small deep infarcts diagnosed on computed tomography. *Neurology*, 30, 1090–6.

Pullicino, P., Ostow, P., Miller, L., *et al.* (1995). Pontine ischemic rarefaction. *Ann Neurol*, 37, 460–466.

Pullicino, P.M. (1993). Pathogenesis of lacunar infarcts and small deep infarcts. *Advances in Neurology*, 62, 125–40.

Radue, E.W. and Moseley, I.F. (1978). Carotid artery occlusion and computed tomography. *Neuroradiology*, 17, 7–12.

Ragno, M., Tournier-Lasserve, E., Fiori, M., *et al.* (1995). An italian kindred with cerebral autosomal dominant arteriopathy with subcortical infarcts and leukoencephlopathy (CADASIL). *Annals of Neurology*, 38, 231–6.

Ragsdale, D.S., Scheuer, T., and Catterall, W.A. (1991). Frequency and voltage-dependent inhibition of type IIA Na^+ channels, expressed in a mammalian cell line, by local anesthetic, antiarrhythmic, and anticonvulsant drugs. *Molecular Pharmacology*, 40, 756–65.

Raiha, I., Tarvonen, S., Kurki, T., Rajala, T., and Sourander, L. (1993). Relationship between vascular factors and white matter low attenuation of the brain. *Acta Neurologica Scandinavia*, 87, 286–9.

Ranalli, P.J., Sharpe, J.A., and Fletcher, W.A. (1988). Palsy of upward and downward saccadic, pursuit, and vestibular movements with a unilateral midbrain lesion. Pathophysiologic correlations. *Neurology*, 38, 14–22.

Rand, R., Brown, W., and Stern, E. (1956). Surgical occlusion of anterior choroidal arteries in parkinsonism: clinical and neuropathological findings. *Neurology*, 6, 390–401.

Ransom, B.R. and Philbin, D.M. (1992). Anoxia-induced extracellular ionic changes in CNS white matter: the role of glial cells. *Canadian Journal of Physiology and Pharmacology*, 70, 181–9.

Ransom, B.R., Walz, W., Davis, P.K., and Carlina, W.G. (1992). Anoxia-induced changes in extracellular K^+ and pH in mammalian central white matter. *Journal of Cerebral Blood Flow and Metabolism*, 12, 593–602.

Ransom, B.R., Waxman, S.G., and Davis, P.K. (1990). Anoxic injury of CNS white matter: protective effect of ketamine. *Neurology*, **40**, 1399–404.

Rascol, A., Clanet, M., Manelfe, C., Guiraud, B., and Bonafe, A. (1982). Pure motor hemiplegia: CT study of 30 cases. *Stroke*, **13**, 11–7.

Rasgado-Flores, H. and Blaustein, M.P. (1987). Na/Ca exchange in barnacle muscle cells has a stoichiometry of 3 $Na^+/1$ Ca^{2+}. *American. Journal of Physiology*, **252**, C499–504.

Rastenyte, D., Tuomilehto J., and Sarti C. (1998). Genetics of stroke—a review. *Journal of the Neurological Sciences*, **153**, 132–45.

Read, S.J., Pettigrew, L., Schimmel, L., Levi, C.R., Bladin, C.F., Chambers, B.R., *et al*. (1998a). White matter medullary infarcts: acute subcortical infarction in the centrum ovale. *Cerebrovascular Diseases*, **8**, 289–95.

Regli, L., Regli, F., Maeder, P., and Bogousslavsky, J. (1993). Magnetic resonance imaging with gadolinium contrast agent in small deep (lacunar) cerebral infarcts. *Archives of Neurology*, **50**, 175–80.

Reilly, M., Connoly, S., Stack, J., Martin, E.A., and Hutchinson, M. (1992). Bilateral paramedian infarction: a distinct but poorly recognized stroke syndrome. *Quarterly Journal of Medicine*, **297**, 63–70.

Reuther, R., and Dorndorf, W. (1978). Aspirin in patients with cerebral ischaemia and normal angiograms or non-surgical lesions. Acetylsalicylic Acid in Cerebral Ischaemia and Coronary heart Disease. Stuttgart, Germany *Schattauer*, 97–106.

Rezek, D.L., Morris, J.C., Fulling, K.H., and Gado, M.H. (1987). Periventricular white matter lucencies in senile dementia of the Alzheimer type and in normal aging. *Neurology*, **37**, 1365–8.

Rhoton, A., Kiyotaka, F., and Fradd, B. (1979). Microsurgical anatomy of the anterior choroidal artery. *Surgical Neurology*, **12**, 171–87.

Ricci, S., Flaminio, F.O., Celani, M.G., Marini, M., Antonini, D., Bartolini, S., *et al*. (1991). Prevalence of internal carotid-artery stenosis in subjects older than 49 years: a population study. *Cerebrovascular Diseases*, **1**, 16–9.

Richfield, E.K., Twyman, R., and Berent, S. (1987). Neurologic syndrome following bilateral damage to the head of the caudate nucleus. *Annals of Neurology*, **22**, 768–71.

Ring, B.A. (1971). Occlusio supra occlusionem: intracranial occlusions following carotid thrombosis as diagnosed by cerebral angiography. *Stroke*, **2**, 487–93.

Ringelstein, E.B., Koschorke, S., Holling, A., Thron, A., Lambertz, H., and Minale, C. (1989). Computed tomographic patterns of proven embolic brain infarctions. *Annals of Neurology*, **26**, 759–65.

Ringelstein, E.B., Sievers, C., Ecker, S., Schneider, P.A., and Otis, S.M. (1988). Noninvasive assessment of CO_2 induced cerebral vasomotor reactivity in normal individuals and patients with internal carotid artery occlusions. *Stroke*, **19**, 963–9.

Ringelstein, E.B., Zeumer, H., and Angelou, D. (1983). The pathogenesis of strokes from internal carotid artery occlusion. Diagnostic and therapeutical implications. *Stroke*, **14**, 867–75.

Ringelstein, E.B., Zeumer, H., and Schneider, R. (1985). Der Beitrag der zerebralen Computertomogtaphie zur Differentialtypologie und Differentialtherapie des ischänischen Grosshirninfarktes. *Fortschriftte der Neurologie und Psychiatrie*, **53**, 315–36.

Ringelstein, E.B.,Biniek, R., Weiller, C., Ammeling, B., Nolte, P.N., and Thron, A. (1992). Type and extent of hemispheric brain infarctions and clinical outcome in early and delayed middle cerebral artery recanalization. *Neurology*, **42**, 289–98.

Robbins, J.A., Sagar, K.B., French, M., and Smith, P.J. (1983). Influence of echocardiography on management of patients with systemic emboli. *Stroke*, 14, 546–9.

Roland, E.H., Poskitt, K., Rodriguez, E., Lupton, B.A., and Hill, A. (1998). Perinatal hypoxic–ischemic thalamic injury: clinical features and neuroimaging. *Annals of Neurology*, 44, 161–6.

Roman, G.C. (1987). Senile dementia of the Binswanger type: a vascular form of dementia in the elderly. *Journal of the American Medical Association*, 258, 1782–8.

Roman, G.C. (1996). From UBOs to Binswanger's disease. Impact of magnetic resonance imaging on vascular dementia research. *Stroke*, 27, 1269–73.

Romanul, F.C.A. and Abramowicz, A. (1964). Changes in brain and pial vessels in arterial border zones. *Archives of Neurology*, 11, 40–65.

Rondot, P., De Recondo, J., Davous, P., Bathien, N., and Coignet, A. (1986). Infarctus thalamique bilatéral avec mouvements anormaux et amnésie durable. *Revue Neurologique, Paris*, 142, 398–405.

Roob, G., Schmidt, R., Kapeller, P., Lechner, A., Hartung, H., and Fazekas, F. (1999). MRI evidence of past cerebral microbleeds in a healthy elderly population: the Austrian Stroke Prevention Study. *Neurology*, 52, 991–4.

Roob, G. and Fazekas, F. (2000). Magnetic resonance imaging of cerebral microbleeds. *Current Opinion in Neurology*, 13, 69–73.

Roob, G., Lechner, A., Schmidt, R., Flooh, E., Hartung, H., and Fazekas, F. (2000). Frequency and location of microbleeds in patients with primary intracerebral hemorrhage. *Stroke*, 31, 2665–9.

Rosenblum, W.I. (1993). The importance of fibrinoid necrosis as the cause of cerebral hemorrhage in hypertension. Commentary. *Journal of Neuropathology and Experimental Neurology*, 52, 11–3.

Ross, E.D. (1985). Modulation of the affect and nonverbal communication by the right hemisphere. In *Principles of Behavioral Neurology* (ed. M.-M. Mesulam). p. 239. Davis, Philadelphia.

Roßerg, C. and Mennel, H.D. (1986). Über ein-und doppelseitige Infarkte im Versorgungsgebiet der A. thalamoperforata posterior: neuropathologische Befunden. *Nervenarzt*, 57, 29–34.

Roßerg, C., Boccalini, P., and Wagner, H.J. (1992). Über Infarkte im Versorgungsgebiet arteriae lenticulostriatae. Eine neuropathologische und postmortal-neuroradiologische Analyse. *Klinische Neuroradiologie*, in press.

Rothrock, J.F., Lyden, P.D., Hesselink, J.R., Brown, J.J., and Healy, M.E. (1987). Brain magnetic resonance imaging in the evaluation of lacunar stroke. *Stroke*, 18, 781–6.

Röther, J., Schleper, B., Fiehler, J., Kucinski, T., Knab, R., Bohuslavizki, K.H., *et al.* (2001). The fate of saved tissue at risk of infarction. In *Proceedings of the 9th Annual Meeting of the International Society of Magnetic Resonance in Medicine*, Glasgow.

Rousseaux, M., Cabaret, M., Bernati, T., Pruvo, J.P., and Steinling, M. (1998). Déficit résiduel du rappel verbal après un infarctus de la veine cérébrale interne gauche. *Revue Neurologique, Paris*, 154, 401–7.

Rousseaux, M., Cabaret, M., Lesoin, F., Devos P., Dubois, F., and Petit, H. (1986). Bilan de l'amnésie des infarctus thalamiques restreints—6 cas. *Cortex*, 22, 213–28.

Rousseaux, M., Kassiotis, P., Signoret, J.L., Cabaret, M., and Petit, H. (1991). Syndrome amnésique par infarctus restreint du thalamus antérieur droit. *Revue Neurologique, Paris*, 147, 809–18.

Rousseaux, M., Muller, P., Gahide, I., Mottin, Y., and Romon, M. (1996). Disorders of smell, taste and food intake in a patient with a dorsomedial thalamic infarct. *Stroke*, 27, 2328–30.

Rousseaux, M., Petit, H., Hache, J.C., Devos, P., Dubois, F., and Warot, P. (1985). La motricité oculaire et céphalique dans les infarctus de la région thalamique. *Revue Neurologigue, Paris*, 141, 391–403.

Rousseaux, M., Steinling, M., Griffié, G., Quint, S., Cabaret, M., Lesoin, F., *et al.* (1990). Corrélations de l'aphasie thalamique avec le débit sanguin cérébral. *Revue Neurologique, Paris*, 146, 345–53.

Rousseaux, M., Steinling, M., Kassiotis, P., and Lesoin, F. (1989). Débit sanguin cérébral et infarctus thalamiques. Confrontations topographiques et neuropsychologiques. *Revue Neurologique, Paris*, 145, 140–7.

Roussy, G. (1927). Charles Foix. *Revue Neurologique, Paris*, 43, 441–6.

Roussy, G. and Foix, C. (1910). Etude anatomique sur coupes sériées d'un cas d'hémianesthésie par lésion corticale. *Revue Neurologique, Paris*, xx, 660–2.

Rowley, H.A., Lowenstein, D.H., Rowbotham, M.C., and Simon R.P. (1989). Thalamomesencephalic strokes after cocaine abuse. *Neurology*, 39, 428–30.

Rubattu, S., Ridker, P., Stampfer, M.J., Volpe, M., Hennekens, C.H., and Lindpaintner, K. (1999). The gene encoding atrial natriuretic peptide and the risk of human stroke. *Circulation*, 100, 1722–6.

Rubattu, S., Volpe, M., Kreutz, R., Ganten, U., Ganten, D., and Lindpaintner, K. (1996). Chromosomal mapping of quantitative trait loci contributing to stroke in a rat model of complex human disease. *Nature Genetics*, 13, 429–34.

Ruchoux, M.M. and Maurage, C.A. (1997). CADASIL: cerebral autosomal dominant arteriopathy with subcortical infarcts and leukoencephalopathy. *Journal of Neuropathology and Experimental Neurology*, 56, 947–64.

Ruchoux, M.M., Chabriat, H., Bousser, M.G., *et al.* (1994). Presence of ultrastructural arterial lesions in muscle and skin vessels of patients with CADASIL.*Stroke*, 25, 2291–2.

Ruchoux, M.M., Guerrouaou, D., Vandenhaute, B., *et al.* (1995). Systemic vascular smooth muscle cell impairment in cerebral autosomal dominant arteriopathy with subcortical infarcts and leukoencephlopathy. *Acta Neuropathologica*, 89, 500–12.

Rudolphi, K.A., Schubert, P., Parkinson, F.E., and Fredholm, B.B. (1992). Neuroprotective role of adenosine in cerebral ischemia. *Trends in Pharmacological Science*, 13, 439–45.

Sabbadini, G., Francia, A., Calandriello, L., *et al.* (1995). Cerebral autosomal dominant arteriopathy with subcortical infarcts and leukoencephalopathy (CADASIL). Clinical, neuroimaging, pathological and genetic study of a large Italian family. *Brain*, 118, 207–15.

Sacco, R.L., Bello, J.A., Traub, R., and Brust, J.C.M. (1987). Selective proprioceptive loss from a thalamic lacunar stroke. *Stroke*, 18, 1160–3.

Sacco, R.L., Benjamin, E.J., Broderick, J.P., Dyken, M., Easton, J.D., Feinberg, W.M. (1997). Risk factors. Stroke, 28, 1507–17.

Sacco, R.L., Shi, T., Zamanillo, M.C., and Kargman, D.E. (1994). Predictors of mortality and recurrence after hospitalized cerebral infarction in an urban community: the Northern Manhattan Stroke Study. *Neurology*, 44, 626–34.

Sacco, S.E., Whisnant, J.P., Broderick, J.P., Phillips, S.J., and O'Fallon, W.M. (1991). Epidemiological characteristics of lacunar infarcts in a population. *Stroke*, 22, 1236–41.

Sachdeva, K. and Woodward, K.G. (1989). Caudal thalamic infarction following intranasal methamphetamine use. *Neurology*, 39, 305–6.

Sacks, F., Pfeffer, M., Moye, L.A., *et al.* (1996). The effect of pravastatin on coronary events after myocardial infarction in patients with average cholesterol levels. *New England Journal of Medicine*, **335**, 1001–9.

Saez de Ocariz, M.D.M., Nader, J.A., Santos, J.A., and Bautista, M. (1996). Thalamic vascular lesions: risk factors and clinical course for infarcts and hemorrhages. *Stroke*, **27**, 1530–6.

Sage, J.I. and Lepore, F.E. (1983). Ataxic hemiparesis from lesions of the corona radiata. *Archives of Neurology*, **40**, 449–50.

Sainio, K., Stenberg, D., Keskimèki, I., Muuronen, A., and Kaste, M. (1983). Visual and spectral EEG analysis in the evaluation of the outcome in patients with ischemic brain infarction. *Electroencephalography and Clinical Neurophysiology*, **56**, 117–24.

Saito, I., Segawa, H., Shiokawa, Y., Taniguchi, M., and Tsutsumi, K. (1987). Middle cerebral artery occlusion: correlation of computed tomography and angiography with clinical outcome. *Stroke*, **18**, 863–8.

Sakatani, K., Black, J.A., and Kocsis, J.D. (1992). Transient presence and functional interaction of endogenous $GABA_A$ receptors in developing optic nerve. *Proceedings of the Royal Society of London, Series B*, **247**, 155–61.

Salamon, G. (1973). *Atlas de la vascularisation artérielle du cerveau chez l'homme*, 2nd edn. Sandoz, Paris.

Salamon, G., Boudouresques, J., Combalbert, A., Khalil, R., Faure, J., and Guidecelli G. (1966). Les artères lenticulo-striées. Etude artériographique. Leur intérêt dans le diagnostic des hématomes intracérébraux. *Revue Neurologique, Paris*, **114**, 361–73.

Salgado, A.V., Ferro, J.M., and Gouveia-Oliveira, A. (1996). Long-term prognosis of first-ever lacunar strokes. A hospital-based study. *Stroke*, **27**, 661–6.

Salgado, E.D, Weinstein, M., Furlan, A.F., Modic, M.T., Beck, G.J., Estes, M., *et al.* (1986). Proton magnetic resonance imaging in ischemic cerebrovascular disease. *Annals of Neurology*, **20**, 502–7.

SALT TSCG (1991). Swedish Aspirin Low-Dose Trial (SALT) of 75 mg aspirin as secondary prophylaxis after cerebrovascular ischaemic events. The SALT Collaborative Group. *Lancet*, **338**, 1345–9.

Salvi, F., Michelucci, R., Plasmati, R., *et al.* (1992). Slowly progressive familial dementia with recurrent strokes and white matter hypodensities on CT scan. *Italian Journal of Neurological Sciences*, **13**, 135–40.

Samuelsson, M., Lindell, D., and Norrving, B. (1996*a*). Presumed pathogenic mechanisms of recurrent stroke after lacunar infarction. *Cerebrovascular Diseases*, **6**, 128–36.

Samuelsson, M., Lindell, D., and Olsson, G.-B. (1994). Lacunar infarcts: a 1-year clinical and MRI follow-up study. *Cerebrovascular Diseases*, **3**, 221–6.

Samuelsson, M., Soderfeldt, B., and Olsson, G.B. (1996*b*). Functional outcome in patients with lacunar infarction. *Stroke*, **27**, 842–6.

Sandercock, P., Molyneux, A., and Warlow, C. (1985). Value of computed tomography in patients with stroke: Oxfordshire Community Stroke Project. *British Medical Journal*, **290**, 193–7.

Santamaria, J., Graus, F., Rubio, F., Arbizu, T., and Peres, J. (1983). Cerebral infarction of the basal ganglia due to embolism from the heart. *Stroke*, **14**, 911–14.

Sarangi, S., San Pedro, E.C., and Mountz, J.M. (2000). Anterior choroidal artery infarction presenting as a progressive cognitive deficit. *Clinical Nuclear Medicine*, **25**, 187–90.

Saris, S. (1983). Chorea caused by caudate infarction. *Archives of Neurology*, **40**, 590–1.

Sato, M., Tanaka, S., and Kohama, A. (1987). 'Top of the basilar' syndrome. Clinico-radiological evaluation. *Neuroradiology*, **29**, 354–9.

Schaid, D.J. and Rowland, C. (1998). Use of parents, sibs and unrelated controls for detection of associations between genetic markers and disease. *American Journal of Human Genetics*, **63**, 1492–506.

Scharf, J., Brauherr, E., Forsting, M., and Sartor, K. (1994). Significance of haemorrhagic lacunes on MRI in patients with hyperintense cerebrovascular diseases and intracerebral haemorrhage. *Neuroradiology*, **37**, 504–8.

Schauf, C.L., Davis, F.A., and Marber, J. (1974). Effects of carbamazepine on the ionic conductances of myxicola giant axons. *Journal of Pharmacology and Experimental Therapeutics*, **189**, 538–43.

Schaul, N., Green, L., Peyster, R., and Gotman, J. (1986). Structural determinants of electroencephalographic findings in acute hemispheric lesions. *Annals of Neurology*, **20**, 703–11.

Scheltens, P., Barkhof, F., Leys, D., Wolters, E.C., Ravid, R., and Kamphorst, W. (1995). Histopathologic correlates of white matter changes on MRI in Alzheimer's disease and normal aging. *Neurology*, **45**, 883–8.

Scheltens, P., Erkinjuntti, T., Leys, D., Wahlund, L.O., Inzitari, D., del Ser, T., *et al.* (1998). White matter changes on CT and MRI: an overview of visual rating scales. European Task Force on Age-Related White Matter Changes. *European Neurology*, **39**, 80–9.

Schlaepfer, W.W. (1977). Structural alterations of peripheral nerve induced by the calcium ionophore A23187. *Brain Research*, **136**, 1–9.

Schlaepfer, W.W. and Bunge, R.P. (1973). Effects of calcium ion concentration on the degeneration of amputated axons in tissue culture. *Journal of Cell Biology*, **59**, 456–70..

Schlangers, J. (1991). Novation et histoire. In *Les concepts scientifiques, invention et pouvoir* (ed. I. Stengers and J. Schlangers) pp. 101–131. Gallimard, Paris.

Schlesinger, B. (1976). *The upper brainstem in the human: its nuclear configuration and vascular supply*. Springer, New York.

Schmidt, R., Lechner, H., Fazekas, F., Niederkorn, K., Reinhart, B., Grieshofer, P., *et al.* (1994). Assessment of cerebrovascular risk profiles in healthy persons: definition of research goals and the Austrian Stroke Prevention Study. *Neuroepidemiology*, **13**, 308–13.

Schmidt, R., Schmidt, H., Fazekas, F., Schumacher, M., Niederkorn, K., Kapeller, P., *et al.* (1997). Apolipoprotein E polymorphism and silent microangiopathy-related cerebral damage. Results of the Austrian Stroke Prevention Study. *Stroke*, **28**, 951–6.

Schmidt, R., Fazekas, F., Kapeller, P., Schmidt, H., and Hartung, H. (1999). MRI white matter hyperintensities: three-year follow-up of the Austrian Stroke Prevention Study. *Neurology*, **53**, 132–9.

Schneider, A., Gutbrod, K, Hess, W., and Schroth, G. (1996). Memory without context: amnesia with confabulations after infarction of the right capsular genu. *Journal of Neurology, Neurosurgery, and Psychiatry*, **61**, 186–93.

Schonewille, W.J, Tuhrim, S., Singer, M.B., and Atlas, S.W. (1999). Diffusion-weighted MRI in acute lacunar syndromes: a clinical–radiological correlation study. *Stroke*, **30**, 2066–2069.

Schoop, W. and Levy, H. (1983). Prevention of peripheral arterial occlusive disease with antiaggregants. *Thrombosis and Haemostasis*, **50**, 137.

Schott, B., Laurent, B., and Mauguière, F. (1986). Les douleurs thalamiques. Étude critique de 43 cas. *Revue Neurologique, Paris*, **142**, 308–15.

Schott, B., Mauguière, F., Laurent, B., Serclerat, O., and Fisher, C. (1980). L'amnésie thalamique. *Revue Neurologigue, Paris*, **136**, 117–30.

Schroder, J.M., Sellhaus, B., and Jorg, J. (1995). Identification of the characterisitc vascular changes in a sural nerve biopsy of a case with cerebral autosomal dominant arteriopathy with subcortical infarcts and leukoencephalopathy (CADASIL). *Acta Neuropathologica*, **89**, 116–21.

Schuster, P. (1936). Beitrège zur Pathologie des Thalamus opticus. I. Mitteilung: Kasuistik. Gefèssgebiet der A. thalamo-geniculata, der A. thalamo-perforata, der A. tubero-thalamica und der A.lenticulo-optica. *Archiv für Psychiatrie und Nervenkrankheiten*, **105**, 358–432.

Schütz, H., Bödeker, R.H., Damian, M., Krack, P., and Dorndorf, W. (1990). Age-related spontaneous intracerebral hematoma in a German community. *Stroke*, **21**, 1412–8.

Schwartz, J.R. and Grigat, G. (1989). Phenytoin and carbamazepine: potential-and-frequency-dependent block of Na currents in mammalian myelinated nerve fibers. *Epilepsia*, **30**, 286–94.

Schwartz, P. (1930). Die Arten der Schlaganfälle des Gehirns und ihre Entstehung. Zweiter Teil. Morphologie der apoplektischen Insulte. *Monographien aus dem Gesamtgebeit der Neurologie und Psychiatrie.* pp. 61–70. Springer, Berlin.

Schwarz, G.A. and Barrows, L.J. (1960). Hemiballism without involvement of Luys body. *Archives of Neurology*, **21**, 420–34.

Schwarz, S., Jauss, M., Krieger, D., Dörfe,r A., Albert, F., and Hacke, W. (1997). Haematoma evacuation does not improve outcome in spontaneous supratentorial intracerebral haemorrhage: a case–control study. *Acta Neurochirurgica*, **139**, 897–904.

Schwarz, S., Schwab. S., Steiner, H.-H., and Hacke, W. (1998). Secondary hemorrhage after intraventricular fibrinolysis: a cautionary note: a report of two cases. *Neurosurgery*, **42**, 659–63.

Scoditti, U., Colonna, F., Bettoni, L., and Lechi, A. (1993). Acute esotropia from small thalamic hemorrhage. *Acta Neurologica Belgica*, **93**, 290–4.

Segarra, J.M. (1970). Cerebral vascular disease and behavior. I. The syndrome of the mesencephalic artery (basilar artery bifurcation). *Archives of Neurology*, **22**, 408–18.

Serra Catafan, J., Rubio, F., and Peres Serra, J. (1992). Peduncular hallucinosis associated with posterior thalamic infarction. *Journal of Neurology*, **239**, 89–90.

Sgouropoulos, P., Baron, J.C., Samson, Y., Bousser, M.G., Comar, D., and Castaigne, P. (1985). Sténoses serrés et occlusions persistantes de l'artère cérébrale moyenne. *Revue Neurologique, Paris*, **141**, 698–705.

Shacklett, D., O'Connor, P., Dormant, C.N., Linn, D., and Carter, J. (1984). Congruous and incongruous sectorial visual defects with lesions of the lateral geniculate nucleus. *American Journal of Ophthalmology*, **98**, 283–90.

Sharma, P. (1998). Meta-analysis of the ACE gene in ischaemic stroke. *Journal of Neurology, Neurosurgery, and Psychiatry*, **64**, 227–30.

Sharp, F.R., Rando, T.A., Greenberg, A.S., Brown, L., and Sagar S.M. (1994). Pseudochoreoathetosis: movements associated with loss of proprioception. *Archives of Neurology*, **51**, 1103–9.

SHEP Study. (1991). Prevention of stroke by anti-hypertensive drug treatment in older persons with isolated systolic hypertension: final results of the Systolic Hypertension in the Elderly Program. *Journal of the American Medical Association*, **265**, 3255–64.

Shimada, N., Graf, R., Rosner, G., and Heiss, W.D. (1993). Ischemia-induced accumulation of extracellular amino acids in cerebral cortex, white matter, and cerebrospinal fluid. *Journal of Neurochemistry*, **60**, 66–71.

Shimasaki, Y., Yasue, H., Yoshimura, M., Nakayama, M., Kugiyama, K., Ogawa, H., *et al.* (1998). Association of the missense Glu298Asp variant of the endothelial nitric oxide synthase gene with myocardial infarction. *Journal of the American College of Cardiology*, **31**, 1506–10.

Shintani, S., Tsuruoka, S., and Shiigai, T. (2000). Pure sensory stroke caused by a cerebral hemorrhage: clinical–radiologic correlations in seven patients. *American Journal of Neuroradiology*, **21**, 515–20.

Shinton, R. and Beevers, G. (1989). Meta-analysis of relation between cigarette smoking and stroke. *British Medical Journal*, **298**, 789–94.

Shuaib, A. and Hachinski, V.C. (1991). Mechanisms and management of stroke in the elderly. *Canadian Medical Association Journal*, **145**, 433–43.

Shuren, J.E., Jacobs, D.H., and Heilman K.M. (1997). Diencephalic temporal order amnesia. *Journal of Neurology, Neurosurgery, and Psychiatry*, **62**, 163–8.

Shuren, J.E., Maher, L.M., Heilman, K.M. (1994). Role of the pulvinar ideomotor praxis. *Journal of Neurology, Neurosurgery, and Psychiatry*, **57**, 1282–3.

Sieben, G., De Reuck, J., and Van der Eecken, H. (1977). Thrombosis of the mesencephalic artery. A clinicopathological study of 2 cases and its correlation with the arterial vascularization. *Acta Neurologica Belgica*, **77**, 151–62.

Siesjo, B. and Bengston, F. (1989). Calcium fluxes, calcium antagonists, and calcium related pathology in brain ischaemia, hypoglycemia, and spreading depression: a unifying hypothesis. *Journal of Cerebral Blood Flow and Metabolism*, **9**, 127–40.

Signoret, J.L. and Goldenberg, G. (1986). Troubles de la mémoire lors des lésions du thalamus chez l'homme. *Revue Neurologique, Paris*, **142**, 445–8.

Sigwald, J. and Monnier, M. (1936). Syndrome thalamo-hypothalamique avec hémitremblement (ramollissement du territoire artériel thalamo-perforé). *Revue Neurologique, Paris*, **66**, 616–31.

Silver, F.L., Norris, J.W., Lewis, A.J., and Hachinski, V.C. (1984). Early mortality following stroke: a prospective review. *Stroke*, **15**, 492–6.

Simard, J.M., Garcia-Bengochea, F., Ballinger, W.E., *et al.* (1986). Cavernous angioma: a review of 126 collected and 12 new clinical cases. *Neurosurgery*, **18**, 162–72.

Singer, M.B., Chong, J., Lu, D., Schonewille, W.J., Tuhrim, S., and Atlas, S.W. (1998). Diffusion-weighted MRI in acute subcortical infarction [published erratum appears in *Stroke* 1998 Mar;29(3):731]. *Stroke*, **29**, 133–6.

Sittig, O. (1914). Klinische Beiträge zur Lehre von den sensiblen Kinden-zentren. *Prager Medizinische Wochenschrift*, **39**, 548–50.

Skehan, S.J., Hutchinson, M., and MacErlaine, D.P. (1995). Cerebral autosomal dominant arteriopathy with subcortical infarcts and leukoencephalopathy: MR findings. *American Journal of Neuroradiology*, **16**, 2115–9.

Skoog, B., Lernfelt, S., Landahl, B., Palmertz, L.-A., Andreasson, L., Nilsson, G., *et al.* (1996). 15-year longitudinal study of blood pressure and dementia. *Lancet*, **347**, 1141–5

Skyhof Olsen, T., Bruhn, P., and Oberg, R.G.E. (1986). Cortical hypoperfusion as a possible cause of 'subcortical aphasia'. *Brain*, **109**, 393–410.

Smith, M.S. and Laguna, J.F. (1981). Upward gaze paralysis following unilateral pretectal infarction. CT correlation. *Archives of Neurology*, **38**, 127–9.

Sodeyama, N., Tamaki, M., and Sugishita, M. (1995). Persistent pure verbal amnesia and transient aphasia after left thalamic infarction. *Journal of Neurology*, **242**, 289–94.

Soisson, T., Cabanis, E.A., Iba-Zizen, M.T., Bousser, M.G.,Laplane, D., and Castaigne, P. (1982). Pure motor hemiplegia and computed tomography, 19 cases. *Journal of Neuroradiology*, **9**, 304–22.

Soler, R., Vivancos, F., Muñoz-Torrero, J.J., Arpa, J., and Barreiro, P. (1999). Postural tremor after thalamic infarction. *European Neurology*, **42**, 180–1.

Solomon D.H., Barohn, R.J., Bazan, C., and Grissom J. (1994). The thalamic ataxia syndrome. *Neurology*, 44, 810–4.

Soloway, H.B. and Aronson, S.M. (1964). Atheromatous emboli to central nervous system. *Archives of Neurology*, 11, 657–67.

Sontheimer, H. and Waxman, S.G. (1992). Ion channels in spinal cord astrocytes *in vitro*: II Biophysical and pharmacological analysis of two Na$^+$ current types. *Journal of Neurophysiology*, 68, 1000–11.

Sorensen, A., Buonanno, F., Gonzalez, R.G., Schwamm, L.H., Lev, M.H., Huang-Hellinger, F.R., *et al.* (1996). Hyperacute stroke: evaluation with combined multisection, diffusion weighted, and hemodynamically weighted echoplanar MR imaging. *Radiology*, 199, 391–401.

Sorensen, P., Pedersen, H., Marquardsen, J., *et al.* (1983). Acetylsalicylic acid in the prevention of stroke in patients with reversible cerebral ischemic attacks. A Danish cooperative study. *Stroke* 14, 15–22.

Sorteberg, A., Sorteberg, W., Lindegaard, K.F., Bakke, J.S., and Nornes, H. (1996). Haemodynamic classification of symptomatic obstructive carotid artery disease. *Acta Neurochirurgica*, 138, 1079–86.

Sourander, P. And Walinder, J. (1977). Hereditary mutli-infarct dementia Morphological and clinical studies of a new disease. *Acta Neuropathologica*, 39, 247–254.

Speedie, L.J. and Heilman, K.M. (1982). Amnestic disturbance following infarction of the left dorsomedial nucleus of the thalamus. *Neuropsychologia*, 20, 597–604.

Speedie, L.J. and Heilman, K.M. (1983). Anterograde memory deficit for visuospatial material after infarction of the right thalamus. *Archives of Neurology*, 40, 183–6.

Spence, J.D., Sibbald, W.J., and Cape, R.D. (1978). Pseudohypertension in the elderly. *Clinical Science and Molecular Medicine*, 55 Suppl, 399–402.

Spiegel, E.A., Wycis, H.T., Orchinik, C., and Freed, H. (1956). Thalamic chronotaxis. *The American Journal of Psychiatry*, 113, 97–105.

Spielman, R.S. and Ewens, W.J. (1996). The TDT and other family-based tests for linkage disequilibrium and association. *American Journal of Human Genetics*, 59, 983–9.

Spielman, R.S. and Ewens, W.J. (1998). A sibship test for linkage in the presence of association: the sib transmission/disequilibrium test. *American Journal of Human Genetics*, 62, 450–8.

Spolveri, S., Baruffi, M.C., Cappelletti, C., Semerano, F., Rossin, S., Pracucci, G. (1998). Vascular risk factors linked to multiple lacunar infarcts. *Cerebrovascular Diseases*, 8, 152–7.

Staaf, G., Lindgren, A., and Norrving, B. (2000). Lacunar infarcts: a 10-year follow-up study. *Stroke*, 31, 2827.

Staaf, G., Samuelsson, M., Lindgren, A., and Norrving, B. (1998). Sensorimotor stroke; clinical features, MRI findings, and cardiac and vascular concomitants in 32 patients. *Acta Neurologica Scandinavica*, 97, 93–8.

Stafstrom, C.E., Schwindt, P.C., Chubb, M.C., and Crill, W.E. (1985). Properties of persistent sodium conductance and calcium conductance of layer V neurons from cat sensorimotor cortex *in vitro.Journal of Neurophysiology*, 53, 153–70.

Stapf, C., Hofmeister, C., Hartmann, A., Marx, P., and Mast, H. (2000). Predictive value of clinical lacunar syndromes for lacunar infarcts on magnetic resonance brain imaging. *Acta Neurologica Scandinavica*, 101,13–8.

Starkstein, S.E., Robinson, R.G., Berthier, M.C., Parikh, R.M., and Price, T.R. (1988). Differential mood changes following basal ganglia vs thalamic lesions. *Archives of Neurology*, 45, 725–30.

Steegman, A.T. and Roberts, D.J. (1935). The syndrome of the anterior choroidal artery: report of a case. *Journal of the American Medical Association*, **104**, 1695–7.

Stein, B.M., McCormick, W.F., Rodriguez, J.N., and Taveras, J.M. (1962). Postmortem angiography of cerebral vascular system. *Archives of Neurology*, **7**, 545–59.

Stein, R.W., Kase, C.S., Hier, D.B., Caplan, L.R., Mohr, J.P., Hemmati, M., *et al.* (1984). Caudate hemorrhage. *Neurology*, **34**, 1549–54.

Steinberg, G.K., Chang, S.D., Gewirtz, R.J., and Lopez, J.R. (2000). Microsurgical resection of brainstem, thalamic, and basal ganglia angiographically occult vascular malformations. *Neurosurgery*, **46**, 260–70.

Steingart, A., Hachinski, V.C., Lau, C., Fox, A.J., Diaz, F., Cape, R., *et al.* (1987). Cognitive and neurologic findings in subjects with diffuse white matter lucencies on computed tomographic scan (leukoaraiosis). *Archives of Neurology*, **44**, 32–5.

Steinke, W., Sacco, R., Mohr, J.P., Foulkes, M.A., Tatemichi, T.K., and Wolf, P.A. (1992a). Thalamic stroke: presentation and prognosis of infarcts and hemorrhages. *Archives of Neurology*, **49**, 703–10.

Steinke, W., Schwartz, A., and Hennerici, M. (1996). Topography of cerebral infarction associated with carotid artery dissection. *Journal of Neurology*, **243**, 323–8.

Steinke, W., Tatemichi, T.K., Mohr, J.P., Massaro, A., Prohovnik, I., and Solomon, R.A. (1992b). Caudate hemorrhage with moyamoya-like vasculopathy from atherosclerotic disease. *Stroke*, **23**, 1360–3.

Stell, R., Davis, S., and Carroll, W.M. (1994). Unilateral asterixis due to a lesion of the ventrolateral thalamus. *Journal of Neurology, Neurosurgery, and Psychiatry*, **57**, 878–80.

Stephens, R. and Stilwell, D. (1969). *Arteries and veins of the human brain*. Charles C. Thomas, Springfield.

Sterbini, G.L.P., Agatiello, L.M., Stocchi, A., and Solivetti, F.M. (1987). CT of ischemic infarctions in the territory of the anterior choroidal artery: a review of 28 cases. *American Journal of Neuroradiology*, **8**, 229–232.

Stern, K. (1939). Severe dementia associated with bilateral symmetrical degeneration of the thalamus. *Brain*, **62**, 157–71.

Stole, S. (1988). Comparison of effects of selected local anesthetics on sodium and potassium channels in mammalian neurons. *General Physiology and Biophysics*, **7**, 177–89.

Strandgaard, S. and Paulson, O.B. (1984). Cerebral autoregulation. *Stroke*, **15**, 413–6.

Streifler, J.Y., Eliasziw, M., Benavente, O.R., Hachinski, V.C., Fox, A.J., and Barnett, H.J. (1995). Lack of relationship between leukoaraiosis and carotid artery disease. The North American Symptomatic Carotid Endarterectomy Trial. *Archives of Neurology*, **52**, 21–4.

Streifler, J.Y., Fox, A.J., Wong, C.J., Hachinski, V.C., and Barnett, H.J.M. (1992). Importance of 'silent' brain infarctions in TIA patients with high-grade carotid stenosis: results from NASCET. *Archives of Neurology*, **49**, 657–67.

Strichartz, G. (1976). Molecular mechanisms of nerve block by local anesthetics. *Anesthesiology*, **45**, 421–41.

Strichartz, G.R. (1973). The inhibition of sodium currents in myelinated nerve by quaternary derivatives of lidocaine. *Journal of General Physiology*, **62**, 37–57.

Stroke Prevention by Aggressive Reduction of Cholesterol Levels (SPARCL) Protocol 981-124. study protocol 1998; August 6.

Stroke Prevention in Reversible Ischemia Trial (SPIRIT) Study Group (1997). A randomised trial of anticoagulants versus aspirin after cerebral ischemia of presumed arterial origin. *Annals of Neurology*, 42, 857–65.

Stuss, D.T., Guberman, A., Nelson, R., and Larochelle, S. (1988). The neuropsychology of paramedian thalamic infarction. *Brain and Cognition*, 8, 348–78.

Stys, P. (1995). Protective effects of antiarrhythmic agents against anoxic injury in CNS white matter. Journal of Cerebral Blood Flow and Metabolism, 15, 425–32.

Stys, P.K. and Lesiuk, H. (1996). Correlation between electrophysiological effects of mexiletine and ischemic protection in CNS white matter. *Journal of Neuroscience*, 71, 27–36.

Stys, P.K. and LoPachin, R.M. (1998). Mechanisms of calcium and sodium fluxes in anoxic myelinated central nervous system axons. *Neuroscience*, 82, 21–32.

Stys, P.K., Ransom, B.R., and Waxman, S.G. (1991). Compound action potential of nerve recorded by suction electrode: a theoretical and experimental analysis. *Brain Research.* 546, 18–32.

Stys, P.K., Ransom, B.R., and Waxman, S.G. (1992b). Tertiary and quaternary local anesthetics protect CNS white matter from anoxic injury at concentrations that do not produce excitability. *Journal of Neurophysiology*, 67, 236–40.

Stys, P.K., Ransom, B.R., Waxman, S.G., and Davis, P.K. (1990). Role of extracellular calcium in anoxic injury of mammalian central white matter. *Proceedings of the National Academy of Sciences of the USA*, 87, 4212–6.

Stys, P.K., Sontheimer, H., Ransom, B.R., and Waxman, S.G. (1993). Non-inactivating, tetrodotoxin-sensitive Na^+ conductance in rat optic nerve axons. *Proceedings of the National Academy of Sciences of the USA*, 90, 6976–80.

Stys, P.K., Waxman, S.G., and Ransom, B.R. (1992a). Ionic mechanisms of anoxic injury in mammalian CNS white matter: role of Na^+ channels and Na^+–Ca^{2+} exchanger. *Journal of Neuroscience*, 12, 430–9.

Stys, P.K., Waxman, S.G., and Ransom, B.R. (1992c). Effects of temperature on evoked electrical activity and anoxic injury in CNS white matter. *Journal of Cerebral Blood Flow and Metabolism*, 12, 977–86

Sulkava, R. and Erkinjuntti, T. (1987). Vascular dementia due to cardiac arrhythmias and systemic hypotension. *Acta Neurologica Scandinavica*, 76, 123–8.

Summergrad, P. and Peterson, B. (1988). Binswanger's disease (Part I): the clinical recognition of subcortical arteriosclerotic encephalopathy in elderly neuropsychiatric patients. *Journal of Geriatric Psychiatry and Neurology*, 2, 123–33.

Sung, C.Y. and Chu, N.S. (1992). Late CT manifestations in spontaneous putaminal haemorrhage. *Neuroradiology*, 3/4, 200–4.

Sunohara, N., Mukoyama, M., Mano, Y., and Satoyoshi, E. (1984). Action induced rhythmic dystonia: an autopsy case. *Neurology*, 34, 321–7.

Suzuki, J. and Kodama, N. (1983). Moyamoya disease: a review. *Stroke*, 14, 104–9.

Swanson, R.A. and Schmidley, J.W. (1985). Amnestic syndrome and vertical gaze palsy: early detection of bilateral thalamic infarction by CT and NMR. *Stroke*, 16, 823–7.

Szelies, B., Herholz, K., Pawlik, G., Karbe, H., Hebold, I., and Heiss, W.D. (1991). Widespread functional effects of discrete thalamic infarction. *Archives of Neurology*, 48, 178–82.

Szirmai, I., Guseo, A., and Molnár, M. (1977). Bilateral symmetrical softening of the thalamus. *Journal of Neurology*, 217, 57–65.

Tabaton, M., Mancardi, G., and Loeb, C. (1985). Generalized chorea due to bilateral small deep cerebral infarcts. *Neurology*, 35, 588–9.

Taillia, H., Chabriat, H., Kurtz, A., *et al.* (1998) Cognitive alterations in non-demented CADASIL patients. *Cerebrovascular Diseases*, 8, 97–101.

Takagi, S. and Shinohara, Y. (1981). Internal carotid occlusion: volume of cerebral infarction, clinical findings, and prognosis. *Stroke*, 12, 835–9.

Takahashi, S., Goto, K., Fukasawa, H., Kawata, Y., Uemura, K., and Suzuki, K. (1985). Computed tomography of cerebral infarction along the distribution of the basal perforating arteries. Part 1: striate arterial group. *Radiology*, 155, 107–18.

Takahashi, S., Ishii, K., Matsumoto, K., Higano, S., Ishibashi, T., Suzuki, M., *et al.* (1994). The anterior choroidal artery syndrome. II. CT and/or MR in angiographically verified cases. *Neuroradiology*, 36, 340–5.

Takahashi, S., Suga, T., Kawata, Y., and Sakamoto, K. (1990). Anterior choroidal artery: angiographic analysis of variations and anomalies. *American Journal of Neuroradiology*, 11, 719–29.

Takano, T., Kimura, K., Nakamura, M., Fukunaga, R., Kusunoki, M., Etani, H., *et al.* (1985). Effect of small deep hemispheric infarction on the ipsilateral cortical blood flow in man. *Stroke*, 16, 64–69.

Takayama, Y., Sugishita, M., Kido, T., Ogawa, M., Fukuyama, H., and Akiguchi, I. (1994). Impaired stereoacuity due to a lesion in the left pulvinar. *Journal of Neurology, Neurosurgery, and Psychiatry*, 57, 652–4.

Talairach, J. and Tournoux, P. (1988). *Coplanar stereotaxic atlas of the human brain*. George Thieme, New York.

Tan, M.J. and Halsey, J.H. (1990). Lacunar infarction due to middle cerebral artery stenosis. *Stroke*, 21, 1759.

Tanaka, A., Ueno, Y., Nakayama, Y., Takano, K., and Takebayashi, S. (1999). Small chronic hemorrhages and ischemic lesions in association with spontaneous intracerebral hematomas. *Stroke*, 30, 1637–42.

Tanaka, A., Yoshinaga, S., Nakayama, Y., Kimura, M., and Tomonaga, M. (1996). Cerebral blood flow and clinical outcome in patients with thalamic hemorrhages: a comparison with putaminal hemorrhages. *Journal of the Neurological Sciences*, 144, 191–7.

Tanaka, M., Kondo, S., Hirai, S., Ishiguro, K., Ishihara, T., Morimatsu, M. (1992). Crossed cerebellar diaschisis accompanied by hemiataxia: a PET study. *Journal of Neurology, Neurosurgery, and Psychiatry*, 55, 121–5.

Tanaka, Y., Tanaka, O., Mizuno, Y., and Yoshida, M. (1989). A radiologic study of dynamic processes in lacunar dementia. *Stroke*, 20, 1488–93.

Tanridag, O. and Kirshner, H.S. (1985). Aphasia and agraphia in lesions of the posterior internal capsule and putamen. *Neurology*, 35, 1797–801.

Tapia, J.F., Kase, C.S., Sawyer, R.H., and Mohr, J.P. (1983). Hypertensive putaminal hemorrhage presenting as pure motor hemiparesis. *Stroke*, 14, 505–6.

Tarvonen-Schröder, S., Roytta, M., Raiha, I., Kurki, T., Rajala, T., and Sourander, L. (1996). Clinical features of leuko-araiosis. *Journal of Neurology, Neurosurgery, and Psychiatry*, 60, 431–6.

Tashiro, K., Matsumoto, A., Hamada, T., and Moriwaka, F. (1987). The aetiology of mirror writing: a new hypothesis. *Journal of Neurology, Neurosurgery, and Psychiatry*, 50, 1572–8.

Tatemichi , T.K., Desmond, D.W., Prohovnik, I., Cross, D.T., Gropen, T.I., Mohr, J.P., *et al.* (1992*b*). Confusion and memory loss from capsular genu infarction: a thalamo-cortical disconnection syndrome? *Neurology*, 42, 1966–79.

Tatemichi, T.K., Steinke, W., Duncan, C., Bello, J.A., Odel, J.G., Behrens, M.M., *et al.* (1992*a*). Paramedian thalamopeduncular infarction: clinical syndromes and magnetic resonance imaging. *Annals of Neurology*, 32, 162–71.

Tatu, L., Moulin T., El Mohamad R., Vuillier F., Rumbach L., and Czorny A. (2000). Primary intracerebral hemorrhages in the Besançon stroke registry: initial clinical and CT findings, early course and 30-day outcome in 350 patients. *European Neurology*, 43, 209–14.

Tatu, L., Moulin, T., Bogousslavsky, J., and Duvernoy, H. (1998). Arterial territories of the human brain: cerebral hemispheres. *Neurology*, 50, 1699–1708.

Tatu, L., Moulin, T., Martin, V., Chavot, D., and Rumbach, L. (1996*b*). Hemiataxia–hypesthesia and small thalamic primary hemorrhages. *Cerebrovascular Diseases*, 6, 166–7.

Tatu, L., Moulin, Th., Chavot, T., Bergès, S., Chopard, J.L., and Rumbach, L. (1996*a*). Hallucinations et infarctus thalamique. *Revue Neurologique, Paris*, 152, 557–9.

TDTSG Tospwaatiaonis TDTTSG (1993). Trial of secondary prevention with atenolol after transient ischemic attack or non-disabling ishemic stroke. *Stroke* 24, 543–548.

Tegeler, C.H., Shi, F., and Morgan, T. (1991). Carotid stenosis in lacunar stroke. *Stroke*, 22, 1124–8.

Tei, H., Uchiyama, S., Koshimizu, K., Kobayashi, M., and Ohara, K. (1999). Correlation between symptomatic, radiological and etiological diagnosis in acute ischemic stroke. *Acta Neurologica Scandinavica*, 99, 192–5.

Ten Holter, J. and Tijssen, C. (1988). Cheiro-oral syndrome: does it have a specific localizing value? *European Neurology*, 28, 326–30.

Terayama, Y., Tanahashi, N., Fukuuchi, Y., and Gotoh, F. (1997). Prognostic value of admission blood pressure in patients with intracerebral hemorrhage. *Stroke*, 28, 1185–8.

Thajeb, P. (1993). Large vessel disease in Chinese patients with capsular infarcts and prior ipsilateral transient ischaemia. *Neuroradiology*, 35, 190–5.

Theron, J. and Newton, T.H. (1976). The anterior choroidal artery. Anatomic and radiographic study. *Journal of Neuroradiology*, 3, 5–30.

Thomas, A. and Chiray, M. (1904). Sur un cas de syndrome thalamique. *Revue Neurologique, Paris*, 12, 505–11.

Thrift, A., McNeil, J., Forbes, A., and Donnan, G. (1999). Risk of primary intracerebral haemorrhage associated with aspirin and non-steroidal anti-inflammatory drugs: case-control study. *British Medical Journal*, 318, 759–64.

Tijssen, C.C. (1994). Contralateral conjugate eye deviation in acute supratentorial lesions. *Stroke*, 25, 1516–9.

TOAST (1998). Low molecular weight heparinoid, ORG 10172 (danaparoid), and outcome after acute ischemic stroke: a randomized controlled trial. *Journal of the American Medical Association*, 279, 1265–72.

Tobler, H.G., and Edwards, J.E. (1988). Frequency and location of atherosclerotic plaques in the ascending aorta. *Journal of Thoracic and Cardiovascular Surgery*, 96, 304–6.

Tolonen, U. (1984). Parametric relationship between four different quantitative EEG methods in cerebral infarction. In *Brain ischemia: quantitative EEG and imaging techniques. Progress in brain research* (ed. G. Pfurtscheller, E.J. Jonkman, and F.H. Lopesda Silva), pp. 51–64. Elsevier, Amsterdam.

Tolonen, U., Ahnonen, A., Sulg, I.A., Knikka, J., Kallanranta, T., Koskinen, M., *et al.* (1980). Serial measurements of quantitative EEG and cerebral blood flow and circulation time after brain infarction. *Acta Neurologica Scandinavica*, 63, 145–55.

Tommasi, M. (1982). Cécile (1875–1962) et Oskar (1870–1959) Vogt. In *Conférences Lyonnaises d'histoire de la neurologie et de la psychiatrie* (ed. M. Boucher), pp. 191–9. Documentation médicale Oberval, Lyon.

Toni, D. And Falcou, A. (1999). Prevention after lacunar infarction: what changes? In *Prevention of ischemic stroke* (ed. C. Fieschi, M. Fisher), pp. 157–67. Martin-Dunitz.

Toni, D., Del Duca, R., Fiorelli, M., Sacchetti, M.L., Bastainello, S., Giubilei, F., *et al.* (1994). Pure motor hemiparesis and sensorimotor stroke. Accuracy of very early clinical diagnosis of lacunar strokes. *Stroke*, **25**, 92–6.

Toni, D., Fiorelli, M., Bastianello, S., Falcou, A., Sette, G., Ceschin, V., *et al.* (1997). Acute ischemic strokes improving during the first 48 hours of onset: predictability, outcome and possible mechanisms—a comparison with early deteriorating strokes. *Stroke*, **28**, 10–14.

Toni, D., Fiorelli, M., De Michele, M., Bastianello, S., Sacchetti, M.L., Montinaro, E., *et al.* (1995*a*). Clinical and prognostic correlates of stroke subtype misdiagnosis within 12 hours from onsetn. *Stroke*, **26**, 1837–40.

Toni, D., Fiorelli, M., Gentile, M., Bastianello, S., Sacchetti, M.L., Argentino, C., *et al.* (1995*b*). Progressing neurological deficit secondary to aute ischemic stroke—a study on predictability, pathogenesis and prognosis. *Archives of Neurology*, **52**, 670–5.

Toni, D., Iweins, F., von Kummer, R., Busse, O., Bogousslavsky, J., Falcou, A., *et al.* (2000). Identification of lacunar infarcts before thrombolysis in the ECASS I study. *Neurology*, **54**, 684–8.

Torvik, A. (1984). The pathogenesis of watershed infarcts in the brain. *Stroke*, **15**, 221–3.

Torvik, A. and Jørgensen, L. (1966). Thrombotic and embolic occlusions of the carotid arteries in an autopsy series. Part 2. Cerebral lesions and clinical course. *Journal of the Neurological Sciences*, **3**, 410–32.

Torvik, A. and Skullerud, K. (1982). Watershed infarcts in the brain caused by micro emboli. *Clinical Neuropathology*, **1**, 99–105.

Tournier-Lasserve, E., Iba-Zizen, M.T., Romero, N., *et al.* (1991). Autosomal dominant syndrome with stroke-like episodes and leukoencephalopathy. *Stroke*, **22**, 1297–302

Tournier-Lasserve, E., Joutel, A., Melki, J., *et al.* (1993) Cerebral autosomal dominant arteriopathy with subcortical infarcts and leukoencephalopathy maps to chromosome 19q12. *Nature Genetics*, **3**, 256–259.

Trelles, O. (1987). Cécile y Oskar Vogt, veintecinco años despues. *Revista Neuro-Psiquiat.*, **50**, 207–20.

Trillet, M., Croisile, B., Tourniaire, D., and Schott, B. (1990). Perturbations de l'activite motrice volontaire et lésions des noyaux caudes. *Revue Neurologique, Paris*, **146**, 338–44.

Trillet, M., Vighetto, A., Croisile, B., Charles, N., and Aimard, G. (1995). Hémiballisme avec libération thymo-affective et logorrhée par hématome du noyau sous-thalamique gauche. *Revue Neurologique, Paris*, **151**, 416–9.

Trojanowski, J.Q. and Lafontaine, M.H. (1981). Neuroanatomical correlates of selective downgaze paralysis. *Journal of the Neurological Sciences*, **52**, 91–101.

Trojanowski, J.Q. and Wray, S.H. (1980). Vertical gaze ophthalmoplegia: selective paralysis of downward gaze. *Neurology*, **30**, 605–10.

Trouillas, P., Derex, L., Nighoghossian, N., Honnorat, J., Li, W., Neuschwander, P., *et al.* (2000). rtPA intravenous thrombolysis in anterior choroidal artery territory stroke. *Neurology*, **54**, 666.

Trouillas, P., Nighoghossian, N., Derex, L., Adeleine, P., Honnorat, J., Neuschwander, P., *et al.* (1998). Thrombolysis with intravenous rtPA in a series of 100 cases of acute carotid territory stroke: determination of etiological, topographic, and radiological outcome factors. *Stroke*, 29, 2529–40.

Tuhrim, S., Dambrosia, J.M., Price, T.R., Mohr, J.P., Wolf, P.A., Heyman, A., *et al.* (1988). Prediction of intracerebral hemorrhage survival. *Annals of Neurology*, 24, 258–63.

Turner, R., Holman, R., Stratton, I., *et al.* (1998). Tight blood pressure control and risk of macrovascular and microvascular complications in type 2 diabetes: UKPDS 38. *British Medical Journal*, 317, 703–13.

Tuszynski, M.H. and Petito, C.K. (1988). Ischemic thalamic aphasia with pathologic confirmation. *Neurology*, 38, 800–2.

Tuszynski, M.H., Petito, C.K., and Levy, D.E. (1989). Risk factors and clinical manifestations of pathologically verified lacunar infarctions. *Stroke*, 20, 990–9.

Ueda, S., Weir, C.J., Inglis, G., Murray, G.D., Muir, K.W., and Lees, K.R. (1995). Lack of association between angiotensin converting enzyme insertion/deletion polymorphism and stroke. *Journal of Hypertension*, 13, 1597–601.

Uhlenbrock, D. and Sehlen, S. (1989). The value of T_1-weighted images in the differentiation between MS, white matter lesions, and subcortical arteriosclerotic encephalopathy (SAE). *Neuroradiology*, 31, 203–12.

Uldry, P.A., Regli, F., and Bogousslavsky, J. (1988). Cerebral angiography and recurrent strokes following *Borrelia burgdorferi* infection. *Journal of Neurology, Neurosurgery, and Psychiatry*, 50, 1703–4.

Unlu, M., de Lange, R.P., de Silva, R., *et al.* (2000). Detection of complement factor B in the cerebrospinal fluid of patients with cerebral autosomal dominant arteriopathy with subcortical infarcts and leukoencephalopathy disease using two-dimensional gel electrophoresis and mass spectrometry. *Neuroscience Letters*, 282, 149–152.

Vahedi, K., Chabriat, H., Ducros, A., *et al.* (1996). Analysis of CADASIL clinical natural history in a series of 134 patients belonging to 17 families linked to chromosome 19. *Neurology*, 46, A211.

Van Bogaert, L. (1952). L'amyotrophie Charcot-Marie. *Revue Neurologique, Paris*, 86, 745–53.

Van Bogaert, L. (1955). Encéphalopathie sous-corticale progressive (Binswanger) à évolution rapide chez deux soeurs. *Med Hellen*, 24, 961–72.

Van Damme, H., Demoulin, J.C., and Limet, R. (1991). Lacunar infarctions and carotid artery disease. *Lancet*, 337, 1361–2.

Van Der Werf, Y.D., Weerts, J.G.E., Jolles, J., Witter, M.P., Lindeboom, J., and Scheltens Ph. (1999). Neuropsychological correlates of a right unilateral lacunar thalamic infarction. *Journal of Neurology, Neurosurgery, and Psychiatry*, 66, 696–7.

Van Huffelen, A.C., Poortvliet, D.C.J., Van der Wulp, C.J.M., and Magnus, O. (1980). Quantitative EEG in cerebral ischemia. A. Parameters for the detection of abnormalities in 'normal' EEGs in patients with acute unilateral cerebral ischemia (AUCI). In *EEG and clinical neurophysiology* (ed. H. Lechner and A. Aranibar), pp. 163–72. Excerpta Medica, Amsterdam.

Van Huffelen, A.C., Poortvliet, D.C.J., and Van der Wulp, C.J.M. (1984). Quantitative electroencephalography in cerebral ischemia. Detecion of abnormalities in 'normal' EEGs. In *Brain ischemia: quantitative EEG and imaging techniques. Progress in brain research* (ed. G. Pfurtscheller, E.J. Jonkman, and F.H. Lopes daSilva), pp. 3–28. Elsevier, Amsterdam.

Van Swieten, J.C., Staal, S., Kappelle, L.J., Derix, M.M., and van Gijn, J. (1996). Are white matter lesions directly associated with cognitive impairment in patients with lacunar infarcts? *Journal of Neurology*, 243, 196–200.

Van Swieten, J.C., Van den Hout, J.H.W., Van Ketel, B.A., Hijdra, A., Wokke, J.H.J., and Van Gijn, J. (1991). Periventricular lesions in the white matter on magnetic resonance imaging in the elderly. A morphometric correlation with arteriolosclerosis and dilated perivascular spaces. *Brain*, 114, 761–74.

Van Wylen, D.G.L., Park, T.S., Rubio, R., and Berne, R.M. (1986). Increases in cerebral interstitial fluid adenosine concentration during hypoxia, local potassium infusion, and ischemia. *Journal of Cerebral Blood Flow and Metabolism*, 6, 522–8.

Van Zagten, M., Boiten, J., Kessels, F., and Lodder, J. (1996). Significant progression of white matter lesions and small deep (lacunar) infarcts in patients with stroke. *Archives of Neurology*, 53, 650–55.

Van Zandvoort, M.J.E., Kappelle, L.J., Algra, A., and De Haan, E.H.F. (1998). Decreased capacity for mental effort after single supratentorial lacunar infarct may affect performance in everyday life. *Journal of Neurology, Neurosurgery, and Pschiatry*, 65, 697–702.

Van den Bergh, R. and Van der Eecken, H. (1968). Anatomy and embryology of cerebral circulation. In *Progress in brain research*, Vol. 30 (ed. W. Luyendijk), pp. 1–25. Elsevier, Amsterdam.

Van den Bergh, R. (1969). The periventricular intracerebral blood supply. In *Research in the cerebral circulation, Third International Salzberg Conference* (ed. J.S. Meyer, H. Lechner, and O. Eichorn), pp. 52–650. Charles C. Thomas, Springfield.

Van der Drift, J.H.A., Visser, S.L., Jonkman, E.J., and Van derSteen, A. (1980). Clinical value of EEG in transient ischaemic attacks. In *EEG and clinical neurophysiology* (ed. H. Lechner and A. Aranibar), pp. 163–72. Exerpta Medica, Amsterdam.

Van der Eecken, H. (1969). Arterial topography and architecture of the intracerebral arterial demarcation zones of the human adult and foetus. In *Research in the cerebral circulation, Third International Salzberg Conference* (ed. J.S. Meyer, H. Lechner, and O. Eichorn), pp. 42–51. Charles C. Thomas, Springfield.

Van der Eeken, H.M. and Adams, R.D. (1953). The anatomy and functional significance of the meningeal arterial anastomoses of the human brain. *Journal of Neuropathology and Experimental Neurology*, 12, 132–57.

Van der Grond, J., van Everdingen, K.J., Eikelboom, B.C., Kenéz, J., and Mali, W.P.T.M. (1999). Assessment of borderzone ischemia with a combined MR imaging–MR angiography–MR spectroscopy protocol. *Journal of Magnetic Resonance Imaging*, 9, 1–9.

Veniant, M., Ménard, J., Bruvenal, P., Morley, S., Gonzales, M. F., and Mullins, J. (1996). Vascular damage without hypertension in transgenic rats expressing prorenin exclusively in the liver. *Journal of Clinical Investigation*, 98, 1966–70.

Verin, M., Rolland, Y., Landgraf, F., *et al.* (1995). New phenotype of the cerebral autosomal dominant arteriopathy mapped to chromosome 19: migraine as the prominent clinical feature. *Journal of Neurology, Neurosurgery, and Psychiatry*, 59, 579–85.

Vermersch, A.-I., Gaymard, B.M., Rivaud-Perchoux, S., Ploner, C.J., Agid, Y., and Pierrot-Deseilligny, C. (1999). Memory guided saccade deficit after caudate nucleus lesion. *Journal of Neurology, Neurosurgery, and Psychiatry*, 66, 524–7.

Verret, J.M. and Lapresle, J. (1986). Sémiologie motrice du thalamus. *Revue Neurologique, Paris*, 142, 368–74.

Versino, M., Simonetti, F., Egitto, M.G., Ceroni, M., Cosi, V., and Beltrami, G. (1999). Lateral gaze synkinesis on downward attempts with paramedian thalamic and midbrain infarct. *Journal of Neurology, Neurosurgery, and Psychiatry*, 67, 696–7.

Viader, F., Cambier, J., Luft, A., Pousin, J.C., Méric, P., and Mamo H. (1987). Etude du débit sanguin cérébral par injection intra-veineuse de Xénon 133 lors de lésions thalamiques et juxta-thalamiques. *Revue Neurologique, Paris*, **143**, 729–36.

Viader, F., Masson, M., Marion, M.H., and Cambier, J. (1984). Infarctus cérébral dans le territoire de l'artère choroidienne antérieure avec trouble oculomoteur. *Revue Neurologique, Paris*, **140**, 668–70.

Victor, M., Adams, R.D., and Collins, G.H. (1971). *The Wernicke–Korsakoff syndrome*. Blackwell, Oxford.

Vighetto, A., Confavreux, C., Boisson, D., Aimard, G., and Devic, M. (1986). Paralysie de l'abaissement du regard et amnésie globale durable par lésion thalamo-sous-thalamique bilatérale. *Revue Neurologique, Paris*, **142**, 449–55.

Villard, E. and Soubrier, F. (1996). Molecular biology and genetics of the angiotensin-I-converting enzyme: potential implications in cardiovascular diseases. *Cardiovascular Research*, **32**, 999–1007.

Vinters, H.V. and Gilbert, J.J. (1983). Cerebral amyloid angiopathy: incidence and complications in the aging brain. II: the distribution of amyloid vascular changes. *Stroke*, **14**, 924–8.

Vinters, H.V. (1987). Cerebral amyloid angiopathy: a critical review. *Stroke*, **18**, 311–24.

Vogt, C., Vogt, O. (1920). Zur Lehre der Erkrankungen des striäten Systems. *Journal für Psychologie und Neurologie*, **25**, 627–848.

Volpe, M., Laccarino, G., Vecchione, C., Rizzoni, D., Russo, R., Rubattu, S., *et al.* (1996). Association and cosegregation of stroke with impaired endothelium-dependent vasorelaxation in stroke-prone, spontaneously hypertensive rats. *Journal of Clinical Investigation*, **98**, 256–61.

Volpin, L., Cervellini, P., Colombo, F., Zanusso, M., and Benedetti, A. (1984). Spontaneous intracerebral hematomas: a new proposal about the usefulness and limits of surgical treatment. *Neurosurgery*, **15**, 663–6.

Von Cramon, D. and Zihl, J. (1979). Roving eye movements with bilateral symmetrical lesions of the thalamus. *Journal of Neurology*, **221**, 105–12.

Von Cramon, D.Y., Hebel, N., and Schur, U. (1985). A contribution to the anatomical basis of thalamic amnesia. *Brain*, **108**, 993–1008.

Von Kummer, R., Bozzao, L., and Manelfe, C. (1995). *Early CT diagnosis of hemispheric brain infarction*. Springer, Berlin.

Vonsattel, J., Myers, R., Hcedley-Whyte, T., Ropper, A., Bird, E., and Richardson, E. (1991). Cerebral amyloid angiopathy without and with cerebral hemorrhages: a comparative histological study. *Annals of Neurology*, **30**, 637–49.

van Domburg, P.H.M.F., ten Donkelaar, H.J., and Notermans S.L.H. (1996). Akinetic mutism with bithalamic infarction. Neurophysiological correlates. *Journal of the Neurological Sciences*, **139**, 58–65.

van Kooten, F., Maasland, L., Dippel, D.W.J., Kluft, C., Grobbee, D.E., and Koudstaal, P.J. (1997). CT-scan abnormalities in relation to dementia in patients with stroke. *Cerebrovascular Diseases*, **7** (Suppl. 14), 42.

van der Zwan, A., Hillen, B., Tulleken, C.A.F., Dujovny, M., and Dragovic, L. (1992). Variability of the territories of the major cerebral arteries. *Journal of Neurosurgery*, **77**, 927–40.

Vuilleumier, P., Ghika-Schmid, F., Bogosslavsky, J., Assal, G., and Regli, F. (1998). Persistent recurrence of hypomania and prosopoaffective agnosia in a patient with right thalamic infarct. *Neuropsychiatry, Neuropsychology, and Behavioral Neurology*, **11**, 40–4.

WHO Task Force on Stroke and Other Cerebrovascular Disorders: Stroke 1989 (1989). Recommendations on stroke prevention, diagnosis, and therapy. *Stroke*, **20**, 1407–1431.

WOSCOPS (1992). A coronary primary prevention study of Scottish men aged 45–64 years. *Journal of Clinical Epidemiology*, **45**, 849–60.

Waga, S. and Yamamoto, Y. (1983). Hypertensive putaminal hemorrhage: treatment and results: is surgical treatment superior to conservative one? *Stroke*, **14**, 480–5.

Waga, S., Okada, M., and Yamomoto, Y. (1979). Reversibility of Parinaud syndrome in thalamic hemorrhage. *Neurology*, **29**, 407–9.

Wakamori, M., Kaneda, M., Oyama, Y., and Akaike, N. (1989). Effects of chlordiazepoxide, chlorpromaxine, diazepam, diphenylhydantoin, flunitrazepam and haloperidol on the voltage-dependent sodium current of isolated mammalian brain neurons. *Brain Research*, **494**, 374–8.

Wall, M., Slamovits, T.L., Weissberg, L.A., and Trufaut, S.A. (1986). Vertical gaze ophthalmoplegia from infarction in the area of the posterior thalamo-subthalamic paramedian artery. *Stroke*, **17**, 546–55.

Wallesch, C.W., Kornhuber, H.H., Kunz, T., and Brunner, R.J. (1983). Neuropsychological deficits associated with small unilateral thalamic lesions. *Brain*, **106**, 141–52.

Walther, H. (1945–1946). Ueber einen Dèmmerzustand mit triebhafter Erregung nach Thalamusschèdigung. *Monatsschrift für Psychiatrie und Neurologie*, **111**, 1–16.

Wang, G.K., Brodwick, M.S., Eaton, D.C., and Strichartz, G.R. (1987). Inhibition of sodium currents by local anesthetics in chloramine-T-treated squid axons. The role of channel activation. *Journal of General Physiology*, **89**, 645–67.

Wang, X.L., Mahaney, M.C., Sim, A.S., Wang, J., Blangero, J., Almasy, L., et al. (1997). Genetic contribution of the endothelial constitutive nitric oxide synthase gene to plasma nitric oxide levels. *Arteriosclerosis, Thrombosis, and Vascular Biology*, **17**, 3147–53.

Wannamethee, S.G., Shaper, A.G., and Ebrahim, S. (1996). History of parental death from stroke or heart trouble and the risk of stroke in middle-aged men . *Stroke*, **27**, 1492–8.

Warach, S., Dashe, J., and Edelman, R. (1996). Clinical outcome in ischemic stroke predicted by early diffusion weighted and perfusion magnetic resonance imaging: a preliminanry analysis. *Journal of Cerebral Blood Flow and Metabolism*, **16**, 53–9.

Warach, S., Gaa, J., Siewert, B., Wielopolski, P., and Edelman, R.R. (1995). Acute human stroke studied by whole brain echo planar diffusion-weighted magnetic resonance imaging. *Annals of Neurology*, **37**, 231–41.

Wartiovaara, U., Perola, M., Mikkola, H., Totterman, K., Savolainen, V., Penttila, A., et al. (1999). Association of FXIII Val134Leu with decreased risk of myocardial infarction in Finnish males. *Atherosclerosis*, **142**, 295–300.

Waterston, J.A., Brown, M.M., Butler, P., and Swash, M. (1990). Small deep cerebral infarcts associated with occlusive internal carotid artery disease. *Archives of Neurology*, **47**, 953–7.

Watson, R.T., Valenstein, E., and Heilman, K.M. (1987). Thalamic neglect. Possible role of the medial thalamus and nucleus reticularis in behavior. *Archives of Neurology*, **38**, 501–6.

Waxman, S., Black, J., Ransom, B., and Stys, P. (1994). Anoxic injury of rat optic nerve: ultrastructural evidence for coupling between Na^+ influx and Ca^{2+}-medicated injury in myelinated CNS axons. *Brain Research*, **644**, 197–204.

Waxman, S.G., Black, J.A., Ransom, B.R., and Stys, P.K. (1993). Protection of the axonal cytoskeleton in anoxic optic nerve by decreased extracellular calcium. *Brain Research*, **614**, 137–45.

Waxman, S.G., Black, J.A., Stys, P.K., and Ransom, B.R. (1992). Ultrastructural concomitants of anoxic injury and early post-anoxic recovery in rat optic nerve. *Brain Research*, **574**, 105–19.

Waxman, S.G., Ransom, B.R., and Stys, P.K. (1991). Non-synaptic mechanisms of calcium-mediated injury in CNS white matter. *Trends in Neuroscience*, 14, 461–8.

Wechsler, L. (1988). Ulceration and carotid artery disease. *Stroke*, 19, 650–3.

Weiller, C., Chollet, F., Friston, K.J., Wise, R.J.S., and Frackowiak, R.S.J. (1992) Functional reorganization of the brain in recovery from striatocapsular infarction in man. *Annals of Neurology*, 31, 465–72.

Weiller, C., Ringelstein, E.B., Reiche, W., Thron, A., and Buell, U. (1990). The large striatocapsular infarct. A clinical and pathophysiological entity. *Archives of Neurology*, 47, 1085–91.

Weiller, C., Ringelstein, E.B., Reiche, W., and Buell, U. (1991a). Clinical and hemodynamic aspects of low-flow infarcts. *Stroke*, 22, 1117–23.

Weiller, C., Ringelstein, E.B., Reiche, W., and Buell, U. (1991b). The role of the vascular factor in aphasia and neglect after subcortical stroke. *Journal of Cerebral Blood Flow and Metabolism*, 11, S662.

Weiller, C., Willmes, K., Reiche, W., Thron, A., Isensee, Ch., Buell, U., et al. (1993) The case of aphasia or neglect after striatocapsular infarction. *Brain*, 116, 1509–25.

Weisberg, L.A., Elliott, D., and Shamsnia, M. (1992). Massive putaminal–thalamic nontraumatic hemorrhage. *Computerized Medical Imaging and Graphics*, 16, 353–7.

Weisberg, L.A., Shamsnia, M., and Elliott, D. (1991). Seizures caused by nontraumatic parenchymal brain hemorrhages. *Neurology*, 41, 1197–9.

Weisberg, L.A., Stazio, A., Elliot, D., and Shamsnia, M. (1990). Putaminal hemorrhage: clinical–computed tomographic correlations. *Neuroradiology*, 32, 200–6.

Weisberg, L.A. (1979). Computed tomography and pure motor hemiparesis. *Neurology*, 29, 490–5.

Weisberg, L.A. (1982). Lacunar infarcts. Clinical and computed tomographic correlations. *Archives of Neurology*, 39, 37–40.

Weisberg, L.A. (1984). Caudate hemorrhage. *Archives of Neurology*, 41, 971–4.

Weisberg, L.A. (1988). Diagnostic classification of stroke, especially lacunes. *Stroke*, 19, 1071–3.

Weller, M., Petersen, D., Dichgans, J., et al. (1996). Cerebral angiography complications link CADASIL to familial hemiplegic migraine. *Neurology*, 46, 844.

White, H., Simes, R., Anderson, N., et al. (2000). Pravastatin therapy and the risk of stroke. *New England Journal of Medicine*, 343, 317–26.

Wijdicks, E.F.M. and Fulgham, J.R. (1995). Acute fatal deterioration in putaminal hemorrhage. *Stroke*, 26, 1953–5.

Willow, M., Gonoi, T., and Catterall, W.A. (1985). Voltage clamp analysis of the inhibitory actions of diphenylhydantoin and carbamazepine on the voltage-sensitive sodium channels in neuroblastoma cells. *Molecular Pharmacology*, 27, 549–58.

Willow, M., Kuenzel, E.A., and Catterall, W.A. (1984). Inhibition of voltage-sensitive sodium channels in neuroblastoma cells and synaptosomes by the anticonvulsant drugs diphenylhydantoin and carbamazepine. Molecular Pharmacology, 25, 228–35.

Wilterdink, J. and Easton, D. (1999). Dipyridamole plus aspirin in cerebrovascular disease. *Archives of Neurology*, 56, 1087–92.

Winocur, G., Oxbury, S., Roberts, R., Agnetti, V., and Davis, C. (1984). Amnesia in a patient with bilateral lesions to the thalamus. *Neuropsychologia*, 22, 123–43.

Wodarz, R. (1980). Watershed infarctions and computed tomography. A topographical study in cases with stenosis or occlusion of the carotid artery. *Neuroradiology*, 19, 245–8.

Wolf, P.A., Cobb, J.L., D'Agostino, R.B. (1992*a*). Epidemiology of stroke. In *Stroke. pathophysiology, diagnosis, and management* (ed. H.J.M. Barnett, J.P. Mohr, B.M. Stein, and F.M. Yatsur), pp. 3–29. Churchill Livingstone, New York.

Wolf, P.A., D'Agostino, R.B., Kannel, W.B., Bonita, R., and Belanger, A.J. (1988). Cigarette smoking as a risk factor for stroke. The Framingham study. *Journal of the American Medical Association*, **259**, 1025–9.

Wolf, P.A., D'Agostino, R.B., O'Neal, M.A., Sytkowski, P., Kase, C.S., Belanger, A.J. (1992*b*). Secular trends in stroke incidence and mortality: the Framingham Study. Stroke, **23**, 1551–5.

Wolf, P.A. (1994). Epidemiology of intracerebral hemorrhage. In *Intracerebral Hemorrhage* (ed. C.S. Kase and L.R. Caplan), pp. 21–30. Butterworth-Heinemann, Boston.

Wolfe, N., Linn, R., Babikian, V.L., Knoefel, J.E., and Albert, M. (1990). Frontal systems impairment following multiple lacunar infarcts. *Archives of Neurology*, **47**, 129–32.

Wollner, L., McCarthy, S.T., Soper, N.D.W., and Macy, D.J. (1979). Failure of cerebral auto-regulation as a cause of brain dysfunction in the elderly. *British Medical Journal*, **1**, 1117–8.

WOSCOPS (1992). A coronary primary prevention study of Scottish men aged 45–64 years: trial design. *Journal of Clinical Epidemiology*, **45**, 849–860.

Wurtz, R.H. and Hikosaka, O. (1986). Role of the basal ganglia in the initiation of saccadic eye movements. *Progress in Brain Research*, **64**, 175–90.

Yahashi, Y., Kario, K., Shimada, K., and Matsuo, M. (1998). The 27-bp repeat polymorphism in intron 4 of the endothelial cell nitric oxide synthase gene and ischemic stroke in a Japanese population. *Blood, Coagulation, and Fibrinolysis*, **9**, 405–9.

Yamamoto, H. and Bogousslavsky, J. (1998). Mechanisms of second and further strokes. *Journal of Neurology, Neurosurgery, and Psychiatry*, **64**, 771–6.

Yamamoto, Y., Akiguchi, I., Oiwa, K., Hayashi, M., and Kimura, J. (1998). Adverse effect of nighttime blood pressure on the outcome of lacunar infarct patients. *Stroke*, **29**, 570–76.

Yamanaka, K., Fukuyama, H., and Kimura, J. (1996). Abulia from unilateral capsular genu infarction: report of two cases. *Journal of the Neurological Sciences*, **143**, 181–4.

Yamanouchi, H., Nagura, H., *et al.* (1983). Anticoagulant vs antiplatelet therapy as prophylactic effect against cerebral infarction. *Neurological Medicine (Tokyo)*, **18**, 373–82.

Yamanouchi, H., Sugiura, S., and Tomonaga, M. (1989). Decrease in nerve fibres in cerebral white matter in progressive subcortical vascular encephalopathy of Binswanger type: an electron microscopic study. *Journal of Neurology*, **236**, 382–7.

Yamauchi, H., Fukuyama, H., and Shio, H. (2000). Corpus callosum atrophy in patients with leukoaraiosis may indicate global cognitive impairment. *Stroke*, **31**, 1515–20.

Yamauchi, H., Fukuyama, H., Harada, K., *et al.* (1990*a*). White matter hyperintensities may correspond to areas of increased blood volume: correlative MR and PET observations. *Journal of Computer Assisted Tomography*, **14**, 905–8.

Yamauchi, H., Fukuyama, H., Kimura, J., Konishi, J., and Kameyama, M. (1990*b*). Hemodynamics in internal carotid artery occlusion examined by positron emission tomography. *Stroke*, **21**, 1400–6.

Yamauchi, H., Fukuyama, H., Nagahama, Y., Shiozaki, T., Nishizawa, S., Konishi, J., *et al.* (1999). Brain arteriolosclerosis and hemodynamic disturbance may induce leukoaraiosis. *Neurology*, **53**, 1833–8.

Yamauchi, H., Fukuyama, H., Nagahama, Y., *et al.* (1996). Evidence of misery perfusion and risk for recurrent stroke in major cerebral arterial occlusive diseases from PET. *Journal of Neurology, Neurosurgery, and Psychiatry*, **61**, 18–25.

Yamauchi, H., Fukuyama, H., Yamaguchi, S., Miyoshi, T., Kimura, J., and Konishi, J. (1991). High-intensity area in the deep white matter indicating hemodynamic compromise in internal carotid artery occlusive disorders. *Archives of Neurology*, 48, 1067–71.

Yamori, Y., Horie, R., Handa, H., Sato, M., and Fukose, M. (1976). Pathogenetic similarity of strokes in stroke-prone spontaneously hypertensive rats and humans. *Stroke*, 7, 46–53.

Yanagihara, T., Housser, O.W., and Klass, D.W. (1981). Computed tomography and EEG in cerebrovascular disease. *Archives of Neurology*, 38, 597–600.

Yanagihara, T., Piepgras, D.G., and Klass, D.W. (1985). Repetitive involuntary movement associated with episodic cerebral ischaemia. *Annals of Neurology*, 18, 244–50.

Yasuda, Y., Akiguchi, I., Ino, M., Nabatabe, H., and Kameyama, M. (1990). Paramedian thalamic and midbrain infarcts associated with palilalia. *Journal of Neurology, Neurosurgery, and Psychiatry*, 53, 797–9.

Yates, P.O. (1975). Epidemiology of cerebral haemorrhages. In *Maladies Vasculaires cérébrales, Cerebrovascular Diseases*. Conférences de la Salpêtriére 24–25 avril 1975, (ed. P. Castaigne, F. Lhermitte, and J.-C. Gautier) pp. 29–46. Paris, Baillière.

You, R., McNeil, J.J., O'Malley, H.M., Davis, S.M., and Donnan, G.A. (1995). Risk factors for lacunar infarction syndromes. *Neurology*, 45(8), 1483–7.

Yusuf, S., Sleight, P., Pogue, J., Bosch, J., Davies, R., and Dagenais, G. (2000). Effects of an angiotensin-converting-enzyme inhibitor, ramipril, on cardiovascular events in high-risk patients. The Heart Outcomes Prevention Evaluation Study Investigators. *New England Journal of Medicine*, 342, 145–53.

Zee, R.Y., Ridker, P.M., Stampfer, M.J., Hennekens, C.H., and Lindpaintner, K. (1999). Prospective evaluation of the angiotensin-converting enzyme insertion/deletion polymorphism and the risk of stroke. *Circulation*, 99, 340–3.

Zeumer, H., Ringelstein, E.B., and Klose, K.C. (1981). Lakunare Infarkte im Computer tomogramm. Angiographische Befunde und differentialdiagnostische Gesichts-punkte. *Fortschritte auf dem Gebiete der Röntgenstrahlen und der neuen bildgehenden Verfahren*, 134, 488–94.

Zhange, W., Chun Ma, K., Andersen, O., et al. (1994). The microvascular changes in cases of hereditary multi-infarct disease of the brain. *Acta Neuropathologica*, 87, 317–24.

Zhu, C. and Norris, J. (1991). A therapeutic window for carotid endarterectomy in patients with asymptomatic carotid stenosis. *Canadian Journal of Surgery*, 34, 437–40.

Ziegler, D.K., Kaufman, A., and Marshall, H.E. (1977). Abrupt memory loss associated with thalamic tumor. *Archives of Neurology*, 38, 545–8.

Zola-Morgan, S. and Squire, L.R. (1985). Amnesia in monkey after lesions of the mediodorsal nucleus of the thalamus. *Annals of Neurology*, 17, 558–64.

Zorzon, M., Masè, G., Iona, L.G., and Cazzato, G. (1986). Elettroencefalogramma ed infarti lacunari. *Rivista di Neurologia*, 56, 293–9.

Zuccarello, M., Brott, T., Derex, L., Kothari, R., Saverbeck, L., Tew, J., et al. (1999). Early surgical treatment for supratentorial intracerebral hemorrhage: a randomized feasibility study. *Stroke*, 30, 1833–9.

Zülch, K.-J. (1961a). Über die Entstehung und Lokalisation der Hirninfarkte. *Zentralblatt Fur Neurochirurgie (Leipzig)*, 21, 158–78.

Zülch, K.-J. (1961b). Die Pathogenese von Massenblutung und Erweichung unter besonderer Beruecksichtigung klinischer Gesichtspunkte. *Acta Neurochirurgica Supplementum (Wien)*, 7, 51–117.

Zülch, K.-J. (1985). The cerebral infarct: pathology, pathogenesis and computed tomography. Springer-Verlag, Berlin.

Index

Entries in bold refer to illustrations. Those in italic refer to tables.